RENAL PHYSIOLOGY:
Principles and Functions

An integrated analysis of
renal–body fluid regulating systems

ESMAIL KOUSHANPOUR, Ph.D.

Associate Professor of Physiology
Northwestern University Medical School
Chicago, Illinois

1976
W. B. SAUNDERS COMPANY · Philadelphia · London · Toronto

W. B. Saunders Company: West Washington Square
Philadelphia, PA 19105

1 St. Anne's Road
Eastbourne, East Sussex BN21 3UN, England

833 Oxford Street
Toronto, M8Z 5T9, Canada

Library of Congress Cataloging in Publication Data

Koushanpour, Esmail.

Renal physiology.

Includes index.

1. Kidneys.   2. Body fluids.   I. Title. [DNLM: 1. Kidney
   —Physiology.   2. Body fluids—Physiology. WJ300 K867]

QP249.K68   612'.463   75-12489

ISBN 0-7216-5493-2

Renal Physiology, Principles and Functions   ISBN 0-7216-5493-2

Last digit is the print number: 9   8   7   6   5   4   3   2   1

PREFACE

Physiologists and clinicians are keenly aware of the truth in the century-old statement by Claude Bernard that constancy of internal milieu is pre-requisite to a normal life. The mechanisms by which this constancy of internal environment or "homeostasis" is maintained involve the dynamic interplay of several organ systems, of which the kidney is the most prominent. However, few textbooks on renal function have even attempted to, much less succeeded in, explaining this dynamic interaction to medical and allied health students.

This interdependence is well demonstrated by patients with primary or secondary renal disease, who often exhibit a wide variety of clinical symptoms, seemingly unrelated to the failure of the kidney. Included in these symptoms are: hypertension, of both the arterial and the portal vein variety, fluid retention in dependent extremities, often accompanied by acute renal failure, congestive heart failure, and liver cirrhosis, as well as acid-base disturbances associated with abnormal metabolism, such as diabetes mellitus and gastrointestinal disorders. Although not readily apparent, a careful analysis of the patient's physical and laboratory findings, as well as of the physiology of renal function, would reveal that most, if not all, of these unrelated symptoms can be traced to some disturbance in normal renal regulatory functions. Therefore, to facilitate an intelligent approach to the diagnosis of the underlying cause and the management of the clinical symptoms, it is necessary to acquire a thorough understanding of the renal function in relation to its dynamic interaction with other major organ systems involved in homeostatic regulation.

This book has developed from a 20-lecture course in renal physiology given for the past 12 years by the author to medical students at Northwestern University Medical School. It is an attempt to present an integrated, quantitative analysis of renal function and its role in body fluid homeostasis. The book uses the systems analysis and synthesis approach, which represents a significant departure from the traditional and conventional presentation of the subject. The understanding that such an approach provides is not descriptive, but mechanistic; it imposes mathematical rigor on conceptual processes. It facilitates the search for key factors, alternate possibilities, and missing links that guide experimentation in fruitful directions. At each stage of progress, it summarizes in unambiguous form the current state of understanding so that deficiencies are well exposed to prod further efforts. This approach does not replace experimental ingenuity nor depth of knowledge of the subject, but facilitates and stimulates both. Therefore, application of systems analysis to the study of renal function developed in the present book represents a new and novel approach to the description of this complex physiological system.

This book consists of 13 chapters and two appendices. The first chapter presents an overview of the renal-body fluid regulating system. It not only introduces the reader to the author's approach to the subject, but also brings into focus the unique role the kidney plays in the regulation of body fluid homeostasis. Chapters 2 through 11 are devoted to a rigorous and mechanistic description of body fluids and renal function. Where appropriate, sufficient background materials are included in each chapter so as to minimize the need for review. For example, Chapter 7 gives a detailed analysis of the biochemical and quantitative concepts necessary to understand the mechanisms of renal transport and the concentration and dilution of urine discussed in Chapters 8, 9, and 11. To better understand the role of the kidney in the regulation of acid-base balance, an extensive discussion of buffers and associated concepts as well as respiratory regulation of acid-base are included in Chapter 10. In this way, the materials in each chapter not only introduce and develop systematically some aspects of renal function, but they also provide the necessary background for the materials presented in the succeeding chapters. Furthermore, unlike other books on the subject, in which the anatomy of the kidney is treated separately, we have integrated the anatomical information with the discussion of kidney function. Also, at the end of each chapter, numerous problems are included, which are designed to further the students' understanding of the materials covered in the text.

Chapters 12 and 13 are devoted to a detailed and integrated analysis and synthesis of the renal-body fluid regulating system, in the light of what has been presented before, and from the standpoints of both normal and pathophysiological disturbances. Included are a mechanistic description of renal function in disease and the extent of its involvement in conditions such as acute glomerulonephritis, pyelonephritis, nephrotic syndrome, hypertension, liver cirrhosis and congestive heart failure. It is hoped that these clinical examples will provide a clear demonstration to the reader of the utility and relevance of the materials presented earlier and contribute to his understanding of the diverse processes which underlie a disease state.

Appendix A is an attempt to introduce the student to the principles of systems analysis and synthesis and its potential application to physiological systems. Appendix B presents a mathematical background for the principle of dilution used in this book. Finally, at the end of the book we have provided answers to some of the problems given at the end of each chapter, designed to increase the understanding of the student of the principles presented in the text.

As written, this book should fulfill the needs of all types of students, including those with little or no mathematical background. At first glance, the quantitative and rigorous approach to the subject may be considered somewhat beyond the need of the medical students. Our experience at Northwestern University Medical School has proved otherwise. The materials presented and the systems analysis approach were received enthusiastically not only by the medical students, but also by the physical therapy and medical technology students. Of course, for the latter group we minimized the extent of mathematical notations, but we made no compromise in the flow and functional diagram approach.

Finally, although the author's primary goal has been to write a book which satisfies the needs of several groups of students, it could be of special interest to researchers in renal physiology as well as medical practitioners. For the latter audience, it should provide a fresh approach to a complex field hitherto not within easy grasp.

It would be impossible to acknowledge and adequately thank everyone who has helped make this book possible. The author is indebted to Professor John S. Gray, who not only introduced him to systems analysis and its application to physiological systems, but also helped with the development of some aspects of the book, especially the acid-base chapter. I wish to express my sincere appreciation to many former medical students, who made invaluable contributions to the development of this book by their enthusiastic and critical feedback as well as their continuous encouragement. I can only say that they made the effort very much worthwhile. I wish to specially thank Miss Jenny L. Forman, who, as a devoted secretary, both encouraged me in the writing of the book and diligently undertook the typing of the manuscript, during all phases of its development. She also meticulously and patiently typed the final manuscript and assisted in proofreading. Special thanks are extended to Mr. Donald Z. Shutters, who skillfully rendered all the original illustrations. I also wish to express my appreciation to all the authors and publishers who kindly permitted the reproduction of the borrowed illustrations. I would like to thank the National Institutes of Health for their generous support of my research, mentioned in the book. Finally, I extend sincere thanks and appreciation to the capable staff of W. B. Saunders Company for their enthusiasm, continued assistance and cooperation during the publication of this book.

ESMAIL KOUSHANPOUR

CONTENTS

Chapter 1

INTRODUCTION TO THE RENAL-BODY FLUID REGULATING SYSTEM

All cells of the body are bathed by a fluid, called the interstitial fluid, which provides the *internal environment* of the cells. Both volume and composition of the interstitial fluid must remain within narrow limits, or malfunctions result. Abnormal volumes of vascular and interstitial fluids impair cardiovascular function, and abnormal composition of interstitial fluid impairs cell function. The relevant concentrations include those of electrolytes, hydrogen ions, metabolic waste products, and even water (osmotic effects).

Numerous *disturbing factors* tend to upset both the volumes and composition of these body fluids. These include water ingestion, deprivation, or loss; electrolyte ingestion, deprivation, or loss; fortuitous fluxes of acid or alkali; and the metabolic production of waste products or the administration of toxic substances.

Clearly, there must be *active regulation* to maintain the vital constancy of the internal environment in the face of such disturbing factors. The system, in fact, has two compensating components subject to regulatory control. One is the *G.I. (gastrointestinal) system*, which can appropriately adjust intakes (thirst, appetite, etc.). The other, on which we shall focus in this book, is the *kidney*, which can appropriately adjust outputs. In the renal-body fluid regulating system, the kidney plays much the same compensating role as the bone marrow does for the hemoglobin regulator, or the lung for the blood gas regulator.

A FLOW-DIAGRAM OF THE RENAL-BODY FLUID REGULATING SYSTEM

We can acquire an initial orientation by examining a flow-diagram of this system in the steady state of normality, as shown in Figure 1-1, which identifies the major fluid compartments of the body and the principal channels of influx and efflux. Briefly, the flow-diagram specifies the pathways of material flow into and out of a subsystem, depicted by a *box*, where material transformation may take place. The material flow into and out of each subsystem is shown by an *arrow*

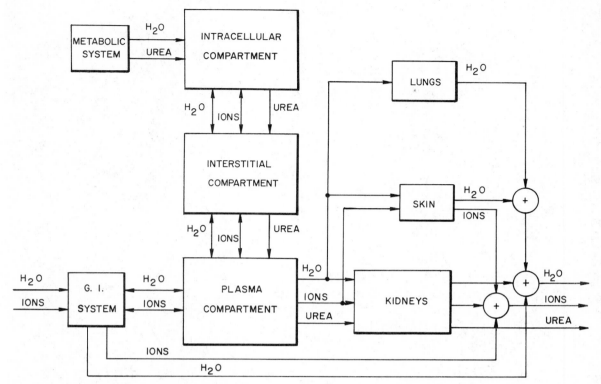

Figure 1-1. Flow-diagram of the normal renal-body fluid regulating system.

entering or leaving the box, on the same or opposite sides. In contrast, the *functional diagram* depicts the cause and effect, the input-output relationships for one or many subsystems and the factors influencing their functional relationships. Thus, such a diagram serves as a basis for a quantitative and eventually a mechanistic description of the system. For a detailed treatment of both the flow-diagram and functional diagram, which are liberally employed whenever appropriate in this book, the interested reader is referred to the materials in Appendix A.

You are already familiar with the *plasma* compartment, which comprises a volume of about 3.2 liters in a healthy 70 kg man. Since the plasma circulates throughout the body, it provides the medium for transporting water and solutes from influx to efflux channels, and for exchanging water and solutes with the largely uncirculated interstitial fluid compartment.

The *interstitial* compartment, of about 8.4 liters, is shown to have a two-way exchange with the plasma. This occurs in the tissue-exchanger, i.e., the systemic capillaries, where partially deproteinized plasma escapes into the interstitium from the arterial end of the capillary, and is then reabsorbed into the blood in the venous end of the capillary. The mechanism of this two-way exchange is *filtration*. The exchange fluxes amount to about 4.5 liters/min, so that 3.2 liters

of plasma are turned over every 0.7 min, and the 8.4 liters of interstitial fluid every 1.9 min. In the steady state, the escape and
reabsorption rates are equal, but in a transient state they may be
temporarily unequal, thus yielding a net *shift* of fluid from one compartment to the other.

The large *intracellular* fluid compartment of about 23.1 liters is
also shown to have a two-way exchange with the interstitial compartment. In the steady state, these two-way fluxes for water are
enormous, but they are much smaller for ions whose penetration of the
cell wall is subject to severe constraints. Water is exchanged by
passive diffusion, and the ions by *diffusion* and/or *active transport*.
In transient states, the two-way fluxes of water may be temporarily
unequal, thus yielding a net *shift* of water between the two compartments. The mechanism for such shifts is *osmosis*. Since the cells
also constitute a *source* for metabolic water and waste products, such
as urea, the metabolic system makes an extra one-way flux for water,
and a one-way flux for urea, which also moves by simple diffusion.

We thus see that the three major fluid compartments, which represent body stores of water and ions, are all dynamic turnover pools.
Only the circulating plasma is subject to extracorporeal influxes and
effluxes, but the interstitial and intracellular compartments can respond quickly, though more or less passively, to changes in the volume
and composition of the plasma.

The main channel for *influxes* of water and solutes into body
fluids is ingestion via the G.I. tract. On the average, these influxes amount to about 2.5 liters of water and 7.0 g of NaCl per day.
To these must be added the 0.3 liters of metabolic water (from oxidation of nutrients) and 30 g of metabolic urea (from deamination of
amino acids) per day. In the steady state these influxes are matched
by equal *effluxes* of 2.8 liters of water and 7.0 g of NaCl and 30 g of
urea per day. Of the four channels for these effluxes, the kidneys
are by far the most important, for they eliminate 1.5 liters of water,
6.2 g of NaCl, and essentially all the urea. There is also some loss
of water through the respiratory tract, and small losses of water and
ions via feces and skin. The water loss by these extrarenal routes
amounts to about 1.3 liters in 24 hours.

Clearly, any temporary inequality between total influxes and
total effluxes will alter the volume and/or composition of the critical body fluid compartments. In the present context, all influx and
efflux channels, *except* the renal, constitute possible disturbance
forcings, to which the kidneys respond by making compensatory adjustments of their own controlled effluxes.

BASIC BIOPHYSICAL CHEMISTRY

Before proceeding further, we must review some basic biophysical
chemistry.

The *concentrations* of substances in body fluids are expressed in
several ways, each with special applications:

1. *Volume %*, e.g., milliliters of substance per 100 ml of fluid.

This is often used for blood gases, and for the water content of body fluids. For example, plasma contains 94 vol% of water, but red cells only 72 vol%.

2. *Weight %*, e.g., grams of solute per 100 ml of fluid. This mixed weight/volume unit is still widely used. Plasma proteins average 7 g/100 ml of plasma and hemoglobin 35 g/100 ml of red cells. These proteins largely account for the different water contents of cells and plasma.

3. *Molar concentration*, e.g., millimoles per liter (mM/L) of fluid. "Normal" or "physiological" saline solution contains 0.9 g% NaCl, which is $(9 \times 10 \ g/L)/(58.5 \ g/mole \times 1000 \ millimoles/mole) = 154$ mM/L. Note that molecular weight of NaCl is 58.5

4. *Equivalent concentration*, e.g., milliequivalents per liter (mEq/L) of fluid. The equivalent weight (or combining weight) is defined as the atomic, radical, or molecular weight divided by valence:

$$1 \ mole \ of \ urea \ = 1 \ equivalent$$
$$1 \ mole \ of \ NaCl \ = 1 \ equivalent$$
$$1 \ mole \ of \ CaCl_2 = 2 \ equivalents$$
$$1 \ mole \ of \ Na_2SO_4 = 2 \ equivalents$$

In the case of electrolytes, the sum of negative charges must equal the sum of positive charges. Since ion valence corresponds to ion charges, the sum of anion equivalents will equal the sum of cation equivalents. For this reason, the ions of body fluids are best expressed in mEq/L.

5. *Osmolar concentration*, e.g., milliosmoles per liter (mOsm/L) of fluid. Osmolality is defined as the number of moles multiplied by the number of dissociating ions:

$$1 \ mole \ urea \qquad = 1 \ osmole$$
$$1 \ mole \ Na^+Cl^- \qquad = 2 \ osmoles$$
$$1 \ mole \ Ca^{++}Cl^-Cl^- = 3 \ osmoles$$
$$1 \ mole \ Na^+Na^+SO_4^{=} = 3 \ osmoles$$

The *colligative* properties of a solution (freezing point depression, boiling point elevation, potential osmotic pressure, etc.) are functions of osmolar concentrations. The normal osmolar concentration of plasma is about 290 ± 10 mOsm/L. Normal saline (0.9 g%, 154 mM/L, 154 mEq/L) has an osmolality of 308 mOsm/L, and therefore is not *iso-osmolar* with plasma. The above were all expressed as "bulk" concentrations, i.e., quantities per unit volume of fluid bulk. Sometimes it is more meaningful to use "water" concentrations, i.e., quantities per unit volume of only the water portion of the fluid. The conversion is simply:

$$"Water" \ concentration = \frac{"Bulk" \ concentration}{Volumetric \ fraction \ of \ H_2O \ in \ the \ fluid} \qquad (1-1)$$

Thus, the lower the water content of a fluid the more the "water" concentration exceeds the "bulk" concentration. We shall make these distinctions in the following way:

"Bulk" Concentration	*"Water" Concentration*
g%	g% in H_2O
mM/L (Molar)	mM/L H_2O (Molal)
mEq/L	mEq/L H_2O
mOsm/L (Osmolar)	mOsm/L H_2O (Osmolal)

Table 1-1 lists the major plasma electrolytes and their concentrations expressed in different units.

Osmosis is the flow of water across a membrane from a solution on one side to a solution on the other side, the latter containing a higher osmolality of solutes to which the membrane is impermeable. The water moves from the higher to the lower concentration of *water* just like a diffusion process. But since the water is the *solvent*, and not just a dissolved solute, the water flows as a convection process, analogous to filtration.

The dependency of osmosis on solute concentration is related to the change in the *chemical potential* of water caused by addition of solute. The chemical potential or molal free energy for pure water (μ) is defined as the ratio of a change in total free energy of water (ΔF_{H_2O}) to a change in the number of moles of water (Δn_{H_2O}), at constant ambient temperature and pressure. Expressed mathematically,

$$\mu = \frac{\Delta F_{H_2O}}{\Delta n_{H_2O}} \qquad (1-2)$$

It so happens that the chemical potential of water in a solution is lower than that of pure water. Therefore, when a solution is separated from pure water by a membrane (permeable only to water), a chemical potential difference between the two sides develops. This difference in chemical potential can be abolished by at least three processes. (1) The free distribution of solutes on both sides of the membrane. This has the effect of equalizing the chemical potential of water on both sides. However, this is not possible if the membrane is permeable only to water. (2) The diffusion of water through the membrane, thereby equalizing the chemical potentials on both sides. (3) The application of mechanical pressure to the solution in order to increase its chemical potential to the level equal to that for pure water. The mechanical pressure thus applied is called the *osmotic pressure* and is a measure of the difference between the chemical potential of the solution and that of pure water.

The osmotic pressure of a solution as defined above is a measure of the lowering of the chemical potential of pure water by the addition of solute. Since the lowering of the chemical potential depends only on the number of solute particles added, the osmotic pressure depends on the number of particles in that solution and not on their size or weight.

If the solution on one side is pure water and that on the other side is one *osmolal* strength of a completely impermeable solute, the osmotic pressure that develops is 22.4 atmospheres, or 17,024 mm Hg. Normal saline of 308 mOsm/L H_2O thus has a *potential* osmotic pressure

TABLE 1-1

Conversion of Plasma Electrolyte Concentrations to mEq/L, or mg%

Electrolytes	Calculated as	Atomic Weight	Valence	Equiva- lent Weight	Conversion Factors (mEq/L from mg%: DIVIDE; mg% from mEq/L: MULTIPLY)	Plasma Concentration (normal ranges) mg/100 ml	mEq/L
CATIONS							
Sodium	Sodium	23	1	23	2.3	310-335	136-145
Potassium	Potassium	39	1	39	3.9	14-21.5	3.5-5.5
Calcium	Total Calcium	40	2	20	2.0	9-11	4.5-5.5
Magnesium	Magnesium	24	2	12	1.2	1.8-3.6	1.5-3.0
ANIONS							
Bicarbonate	CO_2 Content			22.26	2.2	53-75(av. 62) vol%	24-33(av. 28)
Bicarbonate	CO_2 Combining Power			22.26	2.2	53-78(av. 65) vol%	24-35(av. 30)
Chloride	Chloride	35.5	1	35.5	3.5	350-375	98-106
Chloride	Sodium Chloride	58.5	1	58.5	5.8	570-620	98-106
Phosphate	Phosphorus	31.0	1.8	17.2	1.7	2-4.5	1.2-3.0
Sulfate	Sulfur	32.0	2	16.0	1.6	0.5-2.5	0.3-1.5
Protein	Protein				0.41	6-8 grams	14.6-19.4

The phosphate is calculated as phosphorus, with a valence of 1.8. The reason for this is that at normal pH of the extracellular water, 20 per cent of the phosphate ions are in a form with one sodium equivalent (NaH_2PO_4), and 80 per cent are in a form with two sodium equivalents (Na_2HPO_4). The total valence is therefore $(0.2 \times 1) + (0.8 \times 2) = 1.8$.
[From Goldberger, E. (1975).]

of 5244 mm Hg. We say potential, for osmotic pressure that can actually develop depends not only on osmolality, but also on the permeability characteristics of the membrane system used.

The membranes of body cells have permeability constraints, such that NaCl cannot pass through the membrane, although H_2O can easily pass. Hence, cells with an intracellular concentration of impermeable solutes of 154 mOsm/L H_2O and a concentration of impermeable solutes of 154 mOsm/L H_2O in the interstitial fluid are in *osmotic equilibrium*, so that there is no osmotic flow, or shift of water, between them. A solution of impermeable solute having an osmolal concentration of 154 mOsm/L H_2O is said to be an isotonic solution. A solution of 154 mOsm/L H_2O of a *permeable* solute, such as urea, is *iso-osmolar*, but *not isotonic*, for it will not develop an osmotic pressure across the cell membrane.

Whenever the intracellular fluid is exposed to hypertonic (or hypotonic) interstitial fluid, water will flow out of (or into) the cells until the osmolality becomes equal again on both sides. In short, any inequality of impermeable osmolal concentrations can be rectified only by the osmotic shift of water into or out of the cells. Or, to say the same thing another way: *All changes in intracellular fluid volume* (except growth, of course) *are the result of changes in the osmolality of the interstitial fluid*.

The normal efflux channels already identified vary in the osmolality of their fluids. For example, the pulmonary efflux consists of water *vapor*, with zero osmolality. Skin efflux, even in heavy sweating, is hypotonic. Effluxes from the G.I. tract (vomiting and diarrhea, for example) are generally isotonic. Since the kidneys must be able to compensate for both hypo- and hypertonic fluxes, it is not surprising to find that urine osmolality may be adjusted, as needed, from 1/6 isotonicity to 4 times isotonicity.

TYPICAL FORCINGS AND RESPONSES OF THE RENAL-BODY FLUID REGULATING SYSTEM

The disturbance forcings which produce water and electrolyte imbalances include fortuitous *gain* of fluids via the influx channels, fortuitous *loss* of fluids through the efflux channels, and combinations of these. In practice, most of these forcings occur intermittently and are usually short-lived. Hence, they are properly called *pulse* forcings,[*] rather than step forcings, and are followed by *recovery*. The compensatory response of the kidneys, therefore, is to *accelerate* the recovery process and thereby speed up the restoration of volumes and compositions of body fluids toward normal.

Since fortuitous fluid gained or lost may contain different proportions of water and electrolytes, the above forcings are subclassified as *isotonic, hypotonic*, or *hypertonic* forcings. Thus, on the influx side, we may have fortuitous gain of isotonic,

---

[*]See Appendix A for classification of forcings and their characteristics.

hypotonic, or hypertonic fluids, and on the efflux side, we may have fortuitous loss of isotonic or hypotonic fluids. The fortuitous loss of hypertonic fluid occurs only in patients with the syndrome of inappropriate secretion of antidiuretic hormone (SIADH), which will be discussed in Chapter 3.

Table 1-2 summarizes the responses of the renal-body fluid regulating system to the forcings just described. For each forcing, the deviation from normal is indicated by (+) for increase, (-) for decrease, and (0) for no change. The direction of water shift between the extracellular (interstitial plus plasma compartments) and intracellular compartments is indicated by an horizontal arrow (→ or ←).

INFLUXES

A. ISOTONIC. Oral intake or parenteral infusion of a large volume of isotonic saline increases the plasma volume, causing secondary transfer of fluid into the interstitium. The net result is a uniform expansion of the extracellular fluid volume. Since the ingested fluid is isotonic, there is no change in osmolality of the interstitial fluid and hence no net osmotic shift of water into or out of the cells. These characteristic changes in the body fluid compartments produced by fortuitous isotonic fluid influx are termed *isotonic hydration*. Unless otherwise specified, both "tonicity" and "hydration" refer to the extracellular fluid compartment.

The kidneys respond to this extracellular volume expansion by increasing their excretion of both salt and water, producing an increase in urine volume (diuresis). This controlled diuresis rapidly returns the extracellular volume back to normal.

B. HYPOTONIC. Ingestion of a large volume of plain water increases the plasma volume and dilutes plasma osmolality. Fluid then shifts from the plasma into the interstitium. This increases the extracellular volume and decreases its osmolality *(hypotonic hydration)*. The reduced interstitial osmolality causes osmotic shift of water into the cells, causing them to swell and diluting their osmolality. This is called *water intoxication* of cells. The kidneys respond by increasing the excretion of a dilute urine (reduced osmolality), thereby returning the intracellular and extracellular volumes and osmolalities back to normal.

C. HYPERTONIC. Oral or parenteral intake of large amounts of hypertonic fluid increases plasma volume and osmolality. This causes osmotic shift of water into the plasma from the interstitium and diffusion of salt in the opposite direction. The net result is an increase in the volume and osmolality of the extracellular fluid *(hypertonic hydration)*. This induces osmotic shift of water out of the cells, thus reducing their volumes but increasing their osmolality. The kidneys respond by excreting a concentrated urine, thereby restoring the normal state.

TABLE 1-2

Changes from Normal in Fluid Compartments and Controlled
Renal Effluxes in Response to Typical Forcings

Forcings	Effects on Fluid Compartments						Renal Effluxes	
	Extracellular		Water Shift	Intracellular		Terminology	Vol.	Osmolal.
	Vol.	Osmolal.		Vol.	Osmolal.			
1. Influxes								
a. Isotonic	+	0	0	0	0	Isotonic Hydration	+	0
b. Hypotonic	+	−	↑	+	−	Hypotonic Hydration	+	−
c. Hypertonic	+	+	↓	−	+	Hypertonic Hydration	+	+
2. Effluxes								
a. Isotonic	−	0	0	0	0	Isotonic Dehydration	−	+
b. Hypotonic	−	+	↓	−	+	Hypertonic Dehydration	−	+

EFFLUXES

Since the kidneys can only moderate the effects of abnormal effluxes, *correction requires adjustment of influxes*.

A. ISOTONIC. Abnormal loss of water and electrolytes in isotonic concentration leads to reduced extracellular volume, but no change in intracellular volume or tonicity (*isotonic dehydration*). This may occur with hemorrhage, plasma loss through burned skin, and G.I. fluid losses (vomiting and diarrhea, for example). In all these conditions, the kidneys respond by conserving both salt and water.

B. HYPOTONIC. Heavy loss of hypotonic sweat leads to a decrease in extracellular volume and an increase in its osmolality. This will induce osmotic shift of water from cells into the interstitium. The net result is cellular dehydration accompanied by extracellular *hypertonic dehydration*. The kidneys respond by conserving water and excreting salt.

The foregoing flow-diagram analysis reveals *three* important operational features of the renal-body fluid regulating system: (1) The *renal system* plays a central role in maintaining the constancy of the internal environment, a direct consequence of stabilizing the volume and composition of the circulating blood; (2) since the *blood* is an integral part of the extracellular fluid compartment, its regulation is indispensable to the ultimate regulation of the volume and composition of body fluids; and (3) the function of the renal regulator is partly modified by other organ systems.

With this general background serving as the framework, let us now proceed with a systematic analysis and synthesis of the renal-body fluid regulating system, beginning with a consideration of the body fluids component.

PROBLEMS

1-1. Calculate the osmolar concentration (mOsm/L) and the osmotic pressure (mm Hg) exerted by:
   a. 0.9 g% saline solution (MW = 58.5).
   b. 1.8 g% urea solution (MW = 60).

1-2. Calculate the number of grams of glucose (MW = 180) required to make a glucose solution *iso-osmotic* with the solutions (a) and (b) above.

1-3. Calculate the mM/L, mEq/L, and mOsm/L in a liter solution of each of the following solutes:
a. 180 g of urea.
b. 175.5 g of sodium chloride.
c. 90 g of glucose.

1-4. Calculate the osmolality of a 2.5 liter solution containing 7 g salt. Note that this solution represents the daily intake of water and salt via the G.I. system.

1-5. Calculate the osmolality of a 1.5 liter solution containing 7 g salt and 30 g of urea. Note that this solution represents the daily excretion of water, salt, and urea by the kidney.

REFERENCES

1. Gamble, J. L.: *Chemical Anatomy, Physiology and Pathology of Extracellular Fluid. A Lecture Syllabus.* 6th ed. Harvard University Press, Cambridge, Mass., 1967.

2. Goldberger, E.: *A Primer of Water, Electrolytes and Acid-Base Syndrome.* 5th ed. Lea & Febiger, Philadelphia, 1975.

3. Benson, S. W.: *Chemical Calculations.* John Wiley & Sons, Inc., New York, 1954.

4. Hammett, L. P.: *Introduction to the Study of Physical Chemistry.* McGraw-Hill Book Co. Inc., New York, 1952.

Chapter 2

BODY FLUIDS:
NORMAL VOLUMES
AND COMPOSITIONS

We have just learned that the kidneys play a major role in stabilizing the volume and composition of body fluids. To proceed further, we must acquire a basic understanding of fluid and electrolyte balance, a subject which is of great clinical importance.

Postoperative patients, patients with severe vomiting, diarrhea, or excessive sweating, and patients with edema, shock, diabetic coma, or adrenocortical insufficiency all present problems in fluid and electrolyte balance. This chapter provides essential information concerning the methods of measurement and the normal distribution of volumes and compositions of body fluids as a necessary background for understanding the dynamics of their exchange under normal and abnormal conditions.

METHODS OF MEASUREMENT

The *volumes* of various body fluid compartments have been measured by application of the *dilution principle*. In theory, using this method, we can measure the volume of any fluid compartment if we have a test substance that upon injection into the compartment will penetrate it homogeneously without being excreted in urine. In practice, we inject a known quantity of a test substance into the compartment and allow it to penetrate uniformly; we then measure its concentration in a sample drawn from the compartment. The penetrated volume is then calculated from the rearranged definition of concentration:

$$\text{Penetrated volume} = \frac{\text{Known quantity of injected substance}}{\text{Measured concentration of substance}} \quad (2-1)$$

In applying this method to measure the volume of various body fluid compartments in intact subjects, the test substance, usually injected into the plasma, may penetrate into one or more other

compartments as well as be excreted by the kidneys. Consequently,
the plasma concentration of the test substance decreases continuously,
making it difficult to apply the dilution principle in the standard
form. To overcome this difficulty, two test procedures have been
devised, depending on the known renal excretion rate of the test
substance. Regardless of which procedure is used, the test substance
employed should (a) not be toxic, (b) distribute uniformly within the
compartment of interest, (c) not be metabolized during the test
period, and (d) not alter the volume of the compartment being
measured.

　　1. *Single dose injection method* is used for substances with slow
renal excretion rate. In this procedure, when a known quantity of a
test substance is injected into the plasma, two factors determine its
subsequent plasma concentration: renal excretion and possible
penetration into other compartment(s). When a substance which
penetrates into other compartment(s) has achieved uniform distribution,
the rate of decrease in its plasma concentration will, thereafter, be
constant and equal to renal excretion rate.

　　In practice, to find the volume of a body fluid compartment by
this method, a known quantity of a test substance is injected
intravenously and its plasma concentration is then determined at
several successive time intervals. The logarithm of the plasma
concentration is then plotted against time, as illustrated in Figure
2-1.

　　To find the volume of the compartment(s) into which the test
substance has penetrated, we must determine the plasma concentration
which would have been obtained had the test substance penetrated
uniformly and instantaneously throughout the compartment(s) without
being excreted by the kidneys. This *instantaneous* concentration is
obtained by extrapolating the linear portion of the curve, which
reflects constant renal excretion rate, back to zero. Dividing the
quantity of test substance initially injected by this concentration
yields the volume of the compartment(s) penetrated by the test
substance.

　　A detailed discussion of the mathematical basis of the dilution
principle and its applications are given in Appendix B.

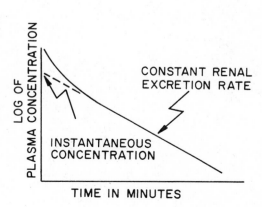

Figure 2-1. Time course of
plasma concentration of a test
substance following a single
dose injection.

2. *Constant-infusion equilibrium method* is used for substances with rapid renal excretion rate. In this procedure, we first inject a large dose of the test substance to increase its plasma concentration. Then, more test substance is slowly infused at a rate matching its renal excretion rate. As a result of this maneuver, changes in plasma concentration of the test substance will be due only to its penetration into other body fluid compartment(s). Once the substance has uniformly penetrated throughout the compartment(s), its plasma concentration should remain constant, at which time the infusion is stopped. Then the urine is collected, until all the test substance which was in the body at the time the infusion was ended has been excreted. This represents the quantity of the test substance which was retained in the body and yielded the plasma concentration at the time the infusion was stopped. Dividing this quantity by the plasma concentration yields the volume of the compartment(s) into which the test substance has penetrated uniformly.

The *compositions* of various body fluid compartments have also been measured by dilution principle. The *concentrations* of various substances present in the accessible body fluid compartments, such as plasma, are measured directly by chemical analysis. However, the concentrations of solutes in the non-accessible compartments, such as interstitial space, are measured indirectly by using dilution principle. This method involves measuring the quantity of *exchangeable* solute in the body and the corresponding volume which contains this solute. Then, by partitioning both quantity and volume between the accessible and non-accessible compartments, the solute concentration in the non-accessible compartment(s) may be determined.

The *exchangeable* quantity of any solute, such as sodium, is measured by introducing a tracer amount of labelled (radioactive) sodium, Na^* (measured in counts per minute, cpm), and then determining its *specific activity* in the plasma, Na^{**}/Na (cpm/ml/mEq), after an adequate equilibration period. Na^{**} is the quantity of labelled sodium (cpm/ml) in a sample of plasma drawn for analysis and Na is the total number of mEq of sodium (labelled plus unlabelled) per milliliter of that sample as determined by chemical analysis. Then, using the dilution principle, the total number of milliequivalents of exchangeable sodium in the body is given by,

$$\text{Exchangeable Na (mEq)} = \frac{\text{Amount of labelled Na injected (cpm)}}{\text{Specific activity of Na in plasma (cpm/mEq)}}$$

$$= \frac{Na^*}{Na^{**}/Na} \tag{2-2}$$

VOLUMES OF BODY FLUID COMPARTMENTS

TOTAL BODY WATER

The total body water in intact man has been measured using three test substances: *antipyrine* and its derivatives, *deuterium oxide* (D_2O), and tritiated water (HTO). Because of the ease of measurement and the rapid rate of distribution, antipyrine has become the substance of choice.

Total body water, as measured by antipyrine, constitutes about 70% of body weight at birth and falls to about 60% of body weight within the first two years of life. This is due to a large extracellular volume which decreases gradually with growth as a result of three factors: (1) an increase in the number of cells; (2) an increase in the size of those tissues with greater intracellular water, such as muscle; and (3) an increase in the amount of body fat.

In adults, total body water, measured by antipyrine, averages about 42.0 liters (60% of body weight) in male and 35.0 liters (50% of body weight) in female. Similar values have been obtained with D_2O and HTO as test substances.

The distribution, by tissues, of the total body water is given in Table 2-1. Note that most of the body water is distributed in muscle (32% of body weight), skin (13%), and blood (7%), with very little in skeleton (3.5%) and adipose tissues (0.01%).

The total body water varies with sex. This variation is due principally to the amount of *body fat*, which is normally about 15% of the body weight. Since fatty tissue contains less water per unit weight, an obese individual has relatively less water than a lean person. In women, after puberty, the total body water per unit of body weight is less compared to that for men. This is due to a greater quantity of fat in women and is related to the blood levels of female sex hormones.

The normal variation in the total body water from person to person is due primarily to variation in *body fat*. In both sexes, the ratio of the total body water to the body weight varies inversely with the amount of fatty tissues. However, the percentage of water in a lean body mass is essentially constant at 73%. (The *lean body mass* is defined as 15% bone, 10% fat, and 75% tissue.) This constancy is the basis of the following empirical formula (Pace and Rathbun, 1945) for determining the percentage of excess fat:

$$\% \text{ Excess fat} = 100 - \frac{\% \text{ water}}{0.732} \times 100 \qquad (2\text{-}3)$$

Another method for determining the quantity of stored fat is to measure the total body specific gravity (sp. gr.). The specific gravity of a substance is defined as the weight of the substance in air divided by the difference between the weight in air and the weight

TABLE 2-1

Distribution of Water and Kinetics of Water Movement in
Various Tissues of a 70 kg Man

Tissues	Per Cent Body Weight	Per Cent Water	Water in Tissues as % Body Weight	Liters of Water	Time for D_2O Equilibration (Minutes)
Muscle	41.7	75.6	31.53	22.10	38
Skin	18.0	72.0	12.96	9.07	120–180
Blood	8.0	83.0	6.64	4.65	RBC 1/60
Skeleton	15.9	22.0	3.50	2.45	120–180
Brain	2.0	74.8	1.50	1.05	
Liver	2.3	68.3	1.57	1.03	10–20
Intestine	1.8	74.5	1.34	0.94	Gastric Juice 20–30
Adipose Tissues	+10.0	10.0	0.01	0.70	
Lungs	0.7	79.0	0.55	0.39	
Heart	0.5	79.2	0.40	0.28	
Kidneys	0.4	82.7	0.33	0.25	
Spleen	0.2	75.8	0.15	0.10	
Total Body	100.0	62.0	60.48	43.40	180

Column 3 of the Table was obtained by multiplying column 1 by column 2 and dividing by 100.
Column 4 of the Table was obtained by multiplying column 3 by 70 kg and dividing by 100.
[Modified from Ruch, T. C., and Patton, H. D. (1974). Water values were taken from Skelton, 1927; D_2O Equilibration values were taken from Edelman, 1952.]

in water. The specific gravity of human fat is 0.918. This value is
much lower than the specific gravity of bone (1.56) or other tissues
(1.06). Since in very lean individuals the upper limit of the
specific gravity is 1.10, a specific gravity of less than 1.10 can be
attributed to an increase in the body fat content. Using the values
of 0.918 and 1.10 as the lower and upper limits of specific gravity,
Rathbun and Pace (1945) have derived the following empirical formula
for determining the percentage of excess fat from the total body
specific gravity in man:

$$\% \text{ Excess fat} = 100 \ (\frac{5.548}{\text{sp. gr.}} - 5.044) \qquad (2\text{-}4)$$

Equations 2-3 and 2-4 describe two different methods of
determining the percentage of excess body fat. Hence, setting them
equal to each other yields another equation relating the percentage
of the total body water to the specific gravity:

$$\% \text{ Water} = 100 \ (4.424 - \frac{4.061}{\text{sp. gr.}}) \qquad (2\text{-}5)$$

This equation can be used to predict from the whole body specific
gravity both the fat and water contents with a reasonable degree of
accuracy.

Using Equations 2-3 and 2-5 we can obtain a graphical relation
of the percentages of the total body water and the excess fat to the
body specific gravity. This is illustrated in Figure 2-2. It is
evident that the variation in body fat is the chief determinant of
the total body specific gravity.

It should be noted that both Equations 2-3 and 2-5 describe a
rectangular hyperbola displaced along the principle Y-axis. However,
for the range of specific gravity values plotted, the linear plots in
Figure 2-2 represent a very small segment of the hyperbola.

Total body water is subdivided into two major compartments
separated by the cell membrane: the intracellular and extracellular
fluid compartments. The extracellular compartment is divided into
two subcompartments separated by the capillary membrane: (a)
intravascular fluid or blood plasma, and (b) *interstitial fluid,*
including lymph, fluids in the dense connective tissues, cartilage,
and bone, and cavity fluids. The latter, also called *transcellular
fluid,* comprises the digestive, cerebrospinal, intraocular, pleural,
peritoneal, and synovial fluids.

The volumes of these fluid compartments can be measured in the
intact subject by virtue of the fact that antipyrine and heavy water
will diffuse freely throughout the total body water, thiocyanate
throughout the extracellular fluid only, and certain large molecular
dyes (T-1824) throughout the blood plasma only. By injecting known
quantities of these substances intravenously, the volumes of the
separate compartments can be calculated approximately from their

resulting concentration in the blood plasma, by the dilution principle.

Table 2-2 summarizes the distribution of body water in a 70 kg healthy young man. The entries corresponding to the capitalized headings are the normal values obtained by application of the dilution principle. For convenience and purposes of comparison, the values are compiled under three categories: entries in column 1 give the volume of total body water and its distribution in each compartment; entries in column 2 give the volume of water in each compartment as a percentage of body weight; and entries in column 3 give the volume of water in each compartment as a percentage of total body water.

EXTRACELLULAR VOLUME

The extracellular volume is very difficult to measure, due to the unavailability of a test substance that does not penetrate the cells. There is no known substance which will remain extracellular and distribute rapidly and uniformly throughout the plasma, interstitial, dense connective tissue, cartilage, bone, and transcellular fluids. Furthermore, the differing rates of equilibration of a test substance in these widely different tissues have made it difficult to interpret the results of dilution tests and led to the confusion of the anatomical space with the "physiological" quantities.

Because of these difficulties, it has become necessary to measure the volume distribution of a specific substance and refer to

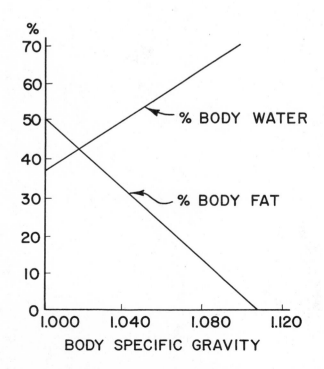

Figure 2-2. Relation of percentage of total body water and excess fat to body specific gravity.

TABLE 2-2

Body Water Distribution in a Healthy 70 kg Young Man

Compartments	Total Volume (liters)	% of Body Water	% of Total Body Water
TOTAL BODY VOLUME (TBV) (by antipyrine method)	42.0	60.0	100.0
TOTAL EXTRACELLULAR VOLUME (ECV) (a) Fast ECV (by rapid equilibration of inulin or radioactive sulfate)	11.6	16.5	27.5
(b) Slow ECV (by slow equilibration of thiocyanate)	18.9	27.0	45.0
PLASMA VOLUME (V_p) (T-1824 method)	3.2	4.5	7.5
INTERSTITIAL VOLUME (V_I) (Fast ECV minus V_p)	8.4	12.0	20.0
Dense connective tissue and cartilage volume	3.2	4.5	7.5
Inaccessible bone volume	3.2	4.5	7.5
Transcellular fluid volume	1.0	1.5	2.5
TOTAL INTRACELLULAR VOLUME (ICV) (TBV minus slow ECV)	23.1	33.0	55.0

[Values taken from data of Edelman, I. S., and Leibman, J. (1959).]

it as, for example, the *inulin space*, if the test substance happens to be inulin.

Two general types of test substances may be used to measure the volume distribution of the extracellular compartment: (1) saccharides, such as inulin, sucrose, and mannitol, and (2) ions, such as thiosulfate, sulfate, thiocyanate, chloride, bromide, and sodium. Because of different rates of penetration of these test substances into the various components of the extracellular space, two phases can be distinguished. One is a *fast-equilibrating phase*, with a half-time of 20 minutes or less, representing the penetration into plasma and interstitial spaces. The other is a *slow-equilibrating phase*, with a half-time of 5 to 9 hours, representing the penetration into the remaining extracellular compartments.

The *extracellular volume* ranges from about 12 liters, determined from fast-equilibrating phase, using inulin or radioactive sulfate as tracer, to 19 liters, determined from slow-equilibrating phase, using thiocyanate as a tracer. The former value includes only plasma and interstitial volumes, while the latter value includes these volumes plus the volumes of fluids in the dense connective tissue and cartilage. In the present context, we shall use the volume distribution of *thiocyanate* as a measure of the total extracellular volume (slow ECV, Table 2-2), which constitutes about 27% of the body weight.

PLASMA VOLUME

Plasma volume may be measured using two methods: (1) plasma albumin or globulin labelling by dye (T-1824) and radioactive iodine (I^{131}), and (2) red cell labelling using isotopes of phosphorus (P^{32}) and chromium (Cr^{51}). In both methods, using the dilution principle, the volume distribution of the labelled protein or cells is determined. In the case of red cell labelling the plasma volume is determined after correcting for the hematocrit. The plasma volume estimated by T-1824 labelled protein, in a healthy young man, averages about 3.2 liters, representing about 7.5% of the total body water.

INTERSTITIAL VOLUME

Interstitial volume, including lymph, can be determined from fast-equilibrating phase with inulin as tracer, after correcting for the plasma volume. The estimated water content in this compartment averages about 8.4 liters, which is equal to 12% of the body weight.

DENSE CONNECTIVE TISSUE AND
CARTILAGE VOLUMES

Dense connective tissue and cartilage fluids differ from interstitial fluids in that they equilibrate very slowly with test substances used to measure the extracellular volume. The water content of cartilage and dense connective tissues has been estimated to be 3.2 liters, or about 4.5% of body weight.

TRANSCELLULAR FLUID VOLUME

Transcellular fluid is not a simple transudate; its composition differs from that of a simple ultrafiltrate (protein-free fraction) of plasma. Of the various components of the transcellular fluids mentioned earlier, the intraluminal gastrointestinal water constitutes the largest fraction; it is about 7.5 ml per kg of the body weight. The volume of cerebrospinal fluid is about 2.8 ml and that of bile is about 2.1 ml per kg of body weight. The total volume of the transcellular compartment is estimated to be 1.0 liter or about 1.5% of body weight.

INTRACELLULAR VOLUME

The volume of intracellular water can only be measured as a difference between the total body volume (TBV) and the extracellular volume (ECV). Hence, any error in the measurement of these quantities will introduce substantial error in the final estimate of the total intracellular volume. The intracellular volume is estimated to be about 23.1 liters or 55% of the total body water.

COMPOSITIONS OF BODY FLUID COMPARTMENTS

Distribution of water within the various body fluid compartments ultimately depends on the quantities of ions in these compartments. Hence, any disturbance in body fluid distribution is always accompanied by displacement of electrolytes. Therefore, to understand the causes of fluid and electrolyte imbalance and to plan corrective therapeutic measures, it is imperative to have a basic understanding of the normal distribution of electrolytes among various compartments.

Like water, anions and cations are distributed between the extra- and intracellular fluid compartments. The principal cations of the extracellular fluid, in the order of amount present, are sodium, potassium, calcium, and magnesium, and the chief anions are chloride, bicarbonate, and phosphate. The major intracellular cations are potassium, sodium, magnesium, and calcium, and the chief anions are phosphate, chloride, sulfate, and bicarbonate.

Table 2-3 summarizes the relative distribution of the electrolyte concentrations in plasma, interstitial, and intracellular fluids. It is apparent that the sum of the concentrations of the cations is equal

TABLE 2-3

Electrolyte Content of Body Fluid Compartments

Electrolyte	Intravascular (IVF)		Interstitial (ISE)	Intracellular (ICF)
	mEq/L of plasma*	mEq/L of water†	mEq/L of water	mEq/L of water
Cations				
Sodium	142	153.0	147.0	10
Potassium	5	5.4	4.0	140
Calcium	5	5.4	2.5	5
Magnesium	3	3.2	2.0	27
Total Cations	155	167.0	155.5	182
Anions				
Bicarbonate	27	29.0	30.0	10
Chloride	103	111.0	114.0	25
Phosphate	2	2.2	2.0	80
Sulfate	1	1.1	1.0	20
Organic Acids	6	6.5	7.5	--
Proteinate	16	17.2	1.0	47
Total Anions	155	167.0	155.5	182

*A plasma water content of 93% was used in the calculations.
†Gibbs-Donnan factors used were 0.95 for monovalent anions and 1.05 for monovalent cations.
[Values taken from Gamble, J. L. (1967), and Edelman, I. S., and Leibman, J. (1959).]

to the sum of the concentrations of the anions in each body fluid compartment, making the solution electrically neutral.

The entries for water concentration of different solutes were calculated using Equation 1-1 by assuming that the plasma is 93% water by weight.

A close examination of this table reveals that the intracellular fluid consists essentially of a solution of K and PO_4 ions, while the extracellular fluid consists essentially of a solution of Na and Cl ions. In addition, the intravascular and intracellular fluids contain proteins, whose concentration influences the distribution of ions, and hence water, between the various body fluid compartments. To illustrate this effect of protein, the intravascular ions are expressed in both "bulk" and "water" concentrations, while the interstitial and intracellular ions are expressed in "water" concentration. Note that regardless of units used to express the ionic concentration, the sum of the concentrations of the cations is equal to the sum of the concentrations of the anions in each body fluid compartment, making the solution electrically neutral.

Further study of this table reveals several important features of electrolyte concentration and distribution between the various body fluid compartments.

A. The extracellular cations have higher "water" concentrations in the plasma (IVF) than in the interstitial fluid (ISF). This difference is due to the plasma proteins, which are negatively charged (anions) at normal blood pH and which normally do not cross the capillary membrane. As a result, the impermeable protein anions bind some positively charged ions (sodium, potassium, etc.), yielding a higher "water" concentration of these ions in the plasma. Consequently, there will be unequal distribution of diffusible cations across the capillary wall, such that the *product* of the diffusible cations and anions will be equal on both sides (to maintain electrochemical neutrality). This unequal distribution of cations due to impermeable proteins is called the *Gibbs-Donnan effect*.

The essence of the *Gibbs-Donnan principle* may best be explained by the example illustrated in Figure 2-3. Initially, a solution of

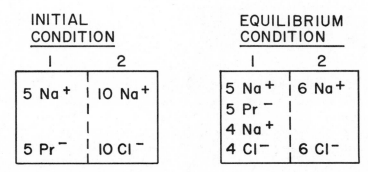

Figure 2-3. A theoretical scheme showing the effect of protein upon the distribution of diffusible anions and cations. [Redrawn from Pitts, R. F. (1974).]

sodium proteinate, Na^+Pr^-, is separated from a saline solution, Na^+Cl^-, by a semi-permeable membrane that is permeable to Na^+ and Cl^-, but impermeable to protein, Pr^-. To simplify the presentation, we assume that the volumes of the two compartments will remain constant as the diffusible ions distribute between the two sides in accordance with their concentration gradients. Hence, any induced osmotic changes in the volumes will be ignored.

Since the initial concentration gradient for Cl^- is greater than that for Na^+, the rate of net movement of Cl^- from side 2 to side 1 will momentarily exceed that of Na^+. Because the membrane is impermeable to Pr^-, the transfer of Cl^- will lead to a momentary increase in the negative ions on side 1. This will generate an electrostatic force on side 1 that will induce a net transfer of Na^+ from side 2 to side 1, thereby making the rate of diffusion of both ions equal. Since Cl^- moves along its concentration gradient, but against the electrical potential gradient, the *work* required to move one equivalent of Cl^- is given by

$$\text{Work} = R \cdot T \cdot \log \frac{[Cl^-]_1}{[Cl^-]_2} - F \cdot E \qquad (2\text{-}6)$$

where R is the gas constant, T is absolute temperature, F is faraday constant, E is the electrical potential difference between the two sides, and $[Cl^-]_1$ and $[Cl^-]_2$ are the chloride concentrations on sides 1 and 2, respectively. Likewise, since Na^+ moves against its concentration gradient, but along the electrical potential gradient, the work required to move one equivalent of Na^+ is given by

$$\text{Work} = R \cdot T \cdot \log \frac{[Na^+]_1}{[Na^+]_2} - F \cdot E \qquad (2\text{-}7)$$

At equilibrium, no work is done by the system, and therefore the sum of the two work equations must be zero. Hence, setting Equations 2-6 and 2-7 equal, and cancelling terms, we get:

$$[Na^+]_2 \cdot [Cl^-]_2 = [Na^+]_1 \cdot [Cl^-]_1 \qquad (2\text{-}8)$$

This equation defines the Gibbs-Donnan rule, which states that, at equilibrium, the *products of the diffusible ions on both sides of the membrane are equal*.

To maintain electroneutrality in each compartment, the sum of anion concentrations (ions with net negative charges, such as Cl^- and Pr^-) must be equal to the sum of cation concentrations (ions with net positive charges, such as Na^+). This may be expressed as

$$[Na^+]_1 = [Cl^-]_1 + [Pr^-]_1 \qquad\qquad (2\text{-}9)$$

$$[Na^+]_2 = [Cl^-]_2 \qquad\qquad (2\text{-}10)$$

Substituting for $[Na^+]_2$ in Equation 2-8 its equivalent from Equation 2-10, we obtain

$$[Cl^-]_2^2 = [Na^+]_1 \times [Cl^-]_1 \qquad\qquad (2\text{-}11)$$

From Equation 2-9 it is evident that some of the sodium ions on side 1 are associated with chloride and some with protein anions. Hence, $[Na^+]_1$ in Equation 2-11 is clearly greater than $[Cl^-]_1$. Equation 2-11 states that the product of two unequal quantities is equal to a square of a quantity. Therefore, if we represent the left side of Equation 2-11 by a rectangle and the right side by a square, it would be easy to show that the sum of the sides of a rectangle is greater than the sum of the sides of a square of equal area. Hence, in terms of the sum of the concentrations, Equation 2-8 may be written as

$$[Na^+]_1 + [Cl^-]_1 > [Na^+]_2 + [Cl^-]_2 \qquad\qquad (2\text{-}12)$$

This inequality is due to the presence of protein anions in the plasma. Thus, presence of protein results in an *increase* in the concentration of diffusible cations and a *decrease* in the concentration of diffusible anions, on the side containing the protein (side 1), compared with the side lacking it. Furthermore, since the sum of the diffusible ions is greater on the side containing the protein (Equation 2-12), the *osmolality* of this side will also be greater, compared with the side lacking protein. The total osmotic pressure on the side containing protein is called the *oncotic pressure*. It is the sum of the protein osmotic pressure and the osmotic pressure of the obligated (bound) cations.

   B. The electrolyte content of the intracellular fluid (ICF) markedly differs from that of the extracellular fluid both in the prevalent ionic species and in the total quantity of ions. First, in the intracellular fluid K and Mg have replaced Na and Ca as the cations, and PO_4 and SO_4 ions have replaced Cl as anions. Also, there is a reduction in the cellular bicarbonate and a marked increase in the cellular proteinate concentrations. Second, the total "water" concentration of the intracellular constituents is much greater compared with that of intravascular or interstitial compartments. This difference is due to impermeable proteins (Gibbs-Donnan effect) which maintain an osmotic equilibrium between a virtually protein-free solution (interstitial fluid) and the intracellular fluid separated by the cell membrane, which is impermeable to proteins but permeable to water and all other solutes.

   C. Despite a high concentration of Na in the ISF, Na concentration in ICF is low, whereas the reverse condition holds for

K ions. Similarly, despite high concentration of Cl and HCO_3 ions in ISF, the concentration of these ions is low in the ICF. Despite leakage of Na into and K out of the cells, the Na-K concentration gradients across the cell membrane are maintained both by active transport and as a consequence of asymmetrical permeability of the cell membrane to K and Na ions and the differing cellular mechanisms involved for their transport. These cellular transport mechanisms have been classified according to whether the net movement of the ion is along or against an electrochemical potential gradient, or whether the transport requires expenditure of cellular energy, or both. Accordingly, three major transport mechanisms have been identified: (1) simple diffusion, (2) convection, and (3) carrier-mediated. The latter is further subdivided into (a) facilitated diffusion and (b) active transport.

> (1) *Simple Diffusion*. A number of substances, such as urea, creatinine, and other organic solutes of small molecular weight, are transported across the cell membrane by simple diffusion. For a given substance, the rate of transport by diffusion is directly proportional to the *concentration gradient* of the substance across the membrane. No expenditure of cellular energy is required for this type of transport.

> (2) *Convection*. Osmotic flow of water may *entrain* some solutes and carry them through a porous membrane. This type of solute transport is called convection. The smaller the molecular weight, the greater would be the ease of its transport by convection. Like simple diffusion, no expenditure of cellular energy is required for this type of transport.

> (3) *Carrier-mediated*. Ions, especially sodium and potassium, and some important metabolites, such as glucose and amino acids, are transported across the cell membrane by carrier-mediated mechanisms. The major characteristic of this type of transport is a temporary binding of the transported solutes to the carrier molecules or binding sites within the membrane.

>> (a) *Facilitated diffusion* involves solute transport by a finite number of membrane sites along the concentration gradient. An important feature of this type of transport is that as the solute concentration gradient increases, the available binding sites will be *saturated*, so that the rate of transport approaches an asymptote. Furthermore, some expenditure of cellular energy is required for this type of transport. The relationship between the rate of solute transport ($\dot{T}_X{}^*$) and solute concentration ([X]) is defined by a right-rectangular hyperbola of the form,

---

[*]Pronounced T-dot sub x, where dot over T denotes rate of change with respect to time; see also Appendix A.

$$\dot{T}_X = \frac{\dot{T}_{max} \cdot [X]}{[X] + K_m}$$

(2-13)

where [X] is the solute concentration, $\dot{T}_{max}$ is the maximum rate of transport (the asymptote when $\dot{T}_X$ is plotted against [X]), and K_m is the substrate concentration yielding half the maximum rate of transport.

(b) *Active transport* is defined as the movement of solutes *against* the electrochemical gradient, exhibiting saturation at high solute concentration and requiring expenditure of cellular energy. Like facilitated diffusion, the rate of transport asymptotically approaches a maximum as the solute concentration increases.

A more detailed description of these cellular transport mechanisms is given in Chapter 7.

Since changes in plasma concentration of Na, K, Cl, and HCO_3 ions and proteins are often used as clinical guides to understanding the causes of fluid and electrolyte imbalance as well as to evaluating the success of therapy, a basic understanding of their normal distribution and factors affecting them is in order.

SODIUM

Nearly all of the exchangeable sodium resides in the extracellular compartment. The exchangeable sodium pool is much higher in infant, compared to that in the adult, a finding compatible with the high total body water observed in the infant.

The combined plasma and interstitial fluids contain about 60% of the total exchangeable sodium. The latter is about 70% of the total body sodium, which consists of about 58 mEq/kg of body weight (Table 2-4). Since these fluids account for 70% of the sodium lost during acute sodium depletion, their functional significance cannot be underestimated.

In short, the relative size of the sodium pool of these compartments is subject to considerable variations with disease. For example, in patients with liver, heart, or kidney disease the edema that occurs constitutes a 20 to 100% increase in the total exchangeable sodium pool. Therefore, these diseases impose a considerable displacement and translocation of sodium among various body fluid compartments and reflect serious disturbances in the mechanisms involved in maintaining normal distribution.

TABLE 2-4

Comparative Distribution of Body Sodium, Potassium and Chloride
Among Fluid Compartments in a Healthy Young Man

Compartments	mEq/kg of Body Weight			% of Total Body		
	Na	K	Cl	Na	K	Cl
Plasma	6.5	0.2	4.5	11.2	0.4	13.6
Interstitial-lymph	16.8	0.5	12.3	29.0	1.0	37.3
Dense connective tissue and cartilage	6.8	0.2	5.6	11.7	0.4	17.0
Exchangeable bone	8.0	-	-	13.8	-	-
Total bone	25.0	4.1	5.0	43.1	7.6	15.2
Transcellular	1.5	1.0	1.5	2.6	1.0	4.5
Total exchangeable extracellular	39.6	-	-	68.3	-	-
Total extracellular	56.6	5.5	28.9	97.6	10.4	87.6
Total body	58.0	53.8	33.0	100.0	100.0	100.0
Total intracellular	1.4	48.3	4.1	2.4	89.6	12.4

[Values taken from Edelman, I. S., and Leibman, J. (1959).]

POTASSIUM

The bulk of body potassium is distributed within the intracellular compartment (Table 2-4), especially muscle cells. Nearly 90% of the total body potassium is exchangeable. In contrast to Na, this exchangeable potassium pool remains constant up to adulthood. However, its distribution is subject to considerable variations with disease. In chronic illness, the potassium loss may be as high as 25% of the total body potassium. These losses are at the expense of intracellular stores, while the extracellular potassium concentration is maintained relatively constant. However, a disturbance in extracellular pH could bring about an acute distortion of the extracellular potassium content. This response is the basis of the dissociated metabolic acidosis and will be considered later.

CHLORIDE

Normally, the chloride content of the extracellular fluid constitutes about 40% of the total exchangeable chloride (Table 2-4). Its distribution and metabolism are influenced by the same factors which stabilize the body content of sodium.

In acid-base disturbance, plasma chloride may vary independently of plasma volume. Thus, hyperchloremia often is seen in certain metabolic acidoses, and hypochloremia often is present in patients with either metabolic alkalosis or respiratory acidosis. Renal regulation of body chloride will be considered later.

BICARBONATE

Bicarbonate content of the body depends on two factors: (1) the metabolic cellular production of carbon dioxide (MR_{CO_2}), and (2) the relative excess of fixed cations, such as Na, K, Ca, and Mg over fixed anions, such as Cl, SO_4, PO_4, and proteinates. Therefore, the size of the bicarbonate pool is determined by the difference between the sum of the fixed cations and the sum of the fixed anions. Any cation excess, imposed by the formation of alkali within the body, is balanced by the hydration of carbon dioxide and the subsequent formation of bicarbonate ions. Conversely, any anion excess imposed by the liberation of acid in the body is balanced by the conversion of the latter to carbon dioxide and water. The carbon dioxide thus formed is eliminated by the lungs. Therefore, the bicarbonate pool is labile and its size is regulated by the respiratory and renal systems. The details of these regulatory mechanisms will be considered later.

PROTEIN

The important plasma proteins from the standpoint of body fluid regulation are albumin and globulin. *Albumin* is the smaller molecule and is present in greater concentration. It is manufactured exclusively by the liver. Albumin plays an important role in the maintenance of the plasma volume. It influences the distribution of the diffusible anions of plasma and binds certain cations such as calcium. A low plasma albumin concentration reflects a low plasma protein concentration. Failure of hepatic function and/or excessive loss of albumin in urine are common explanations for a decreased plasma albumin concentration.

Globulin fraction is subdivided into three components:

1. α_1- and α_2-fractions include the iron-binding globulins, serum esterases, and angiotensinogen.

2. β-globulin fraction contains lipoproteins, including cholesterol, phosphatide, fatty acid, and Vitamin A.

3. γ-globulin fraction includes immune substances, such as are formed in response to infectious hepatitis and measles, and also includes many other antibodies that develop as one grows from infancy to maturity. Included in this fraction are the various factors concerned in the coagulation of blood, including prothrombin, antihemophilic globulin, and fibrinogen.

The origins of some of the plasma protein fractions are obscure. However, immune globulins are thought to be derived in part from lymphoid tissues and the reticuloendothelial system. Fibrinogen and prothrombin are largely derived from the liver, although some fibrinogen may also be formed in bone marrow. Certain other globulins are likewise hepatic in origin.

The normal plasma protein concentration is about 7 g/100 ml of plasma. Of the total plasma proteins, albumin fraction amounts to 4.4 g and globulin fraction is 2.6 g, giving an albumin/globulin (A/G) ratio of 1.67. The critical plasma protein concentration for normal body fluid distribution is about 5.5 g%. In nephrotic syndrome, in which there is excessive albuminuria (> 3.5 g/day) the A/G ratio may fall to 0.84 and even lower. At such low plasma protein concentration there would be a marked distortion of water and electrolyte distribution in the body fluid compartments. Details of the cardiovascular and renal compensatory mechanisms involved will be discussed later.

Finally, it should be pointed out that the distribution of anions and cations within the body fluid compartments exhibits both daily fluctuation and variation with age. Among the cations, the plasma sodium concentration varies slightly with age. Extracellular potassium levels are distinctly high in the infant with gradual decline in concentration with age. Calcium levels are comparable in different age groups, but rise slightly with age. In the case of anions, both chloride and bicarbonate levels vary with age, with a definite sex difference occurring in healthy young adults; the chloride concentration is lower in males and the bicarbonate concentration lower in females. However, there is no apparent sex difference in infants with respect to the concentration of these two ions. The plasma concentration of inorganic phosphate varies with age, being higher just after birth and declining steadily with age. The concentrations of various proteins are low in infants and gradually rise with age.

Because of day-to-day fluctuations of the plasma electrolytes, even during fasting, the stability of the electrolyte concentration in the body fluids is only relative, so that there is an oscillation of the plasma electrolytes under normal conditions.

PROBLEMS

2-1. 100 ml of deuterium oxide (D_2O) in isotonic saline was injected intravenously into a normal man weighing 90 kg. After an equilibration period of 2 hours the concentration of D_2O in plasma water was 0.2%. The urinary, respiratory and cutaneous losses of D_2O were averaged to be 0.4% of the administered dose. Calculate (a) the total body water as a percentage of the body weight, (b) the percentage of excess fat, (c) the amount of excess fat in kilograms, and (d) the total body specific gravity.

2-2. 10 mg of thiocyanate per kg of body weight was injected into a 70 kg subject. Thirty minutes later a sample of plasma was drawn and urine was collected. The concentration of thiocyanate in plasma was 4.6 mg%, and the total amount of thiocyanate excreted was 30 mg. Calculate the thiocyanate space as a percentage of body weight.

2-3. A 70 kg patient received an intravenous dose of radioactive sodium having an activity of 42×10^5 counts/min (cpm). After allowing adequate time for equilibration, a sample of plasma drawn had an activity of 2×10^2 cpm/ml of plasma and a total plasma sodium content (labelled plus unlabelled) of 0.145 mEq/ml. If the urinary loss of radioactive sodium amounts to 2×10^5 cpm, calculate the exchangeable sodium per kg of body weight.

2-4. In an attempt to determine the extracellular volume of an 80 kg patient, 7 g of inulin was injected intravenously and the plasma concentration was subsequently measured at successive time intervals. The values obtained are reproduced in the table on the next page. Calculate (a) the volume of the extracellular space measured by inulin, and (b) the rate of renal excretion of inulin after it is uniformly distributed in the compartment(s).

Time Blood Sample Taken (min)	Inulin Plasma Concentration (mg%)
12	81
18	70
34	42
47	41
62	32
93	24
123	21
183	17
242	13
302	9
364	8
423	7
485	5

2-5.   A test substance not metabolized in the body is infused at a constant rate of 90 mg/min. After 4 hours, the plasma concentration attained a steady state value of 85 mg%. Calculate the volume distribution of the test substance.

2-6.   List *four* essential properties of any substance which would make it suitable as an agent for measuring the volume of a body fluid compartment.
   a.   _____
   b.   _____
   c.   _____
   d.   _____

2-7.   In an 80 kg patient the total body water as measured by deuterium oxide was 60% of the body weight, the inulin space was 20% of the body weight, and the total solute content was 22,800 milliosmoles. Calculate (a) the amount of excess fat in this patient, and (b) the osmolality of the extracellular fluid.

2-8.   The most prevalent diffusible cation and anion of the extracellular fluid are (a) _____, and (b) _____. The most prevalent diffusible cation and anion of the intracellular fluid are (c) _____, and (d) _____. An important plasma protein required for maintenance of normal plasma volume is (e) _____. The large total body water in an infant prior to age 2 is due to (f) _____. The percentage of the total body water in the infant decreases with growth. This is believed to be due to three processes: (g) _____, (h) _____, and (i) _____.

REFERENCES

1. Deane, N.: Methods of study of body water compartments. In: *Methods in Medical Research*. A. C. Corcoran (Ed.), Vol. V. Year Book Medical Publishers, Inc., Chicago, 1952.

2. Deane, N., and Smith, H. W.: The distribution of sodium and potassium in man. *J. Clin. Invest. 31*:197-199, 1952.

3. Edelman, I. S.: Exchange of water between blood and tissues. Characteristics of deuterium oxide equilibration in body water. *Am. J. Physiol. 171*:279-296, 1952.

4. Edelman, I. S., James, A. H., Brooks, L., and Moore, F. D.: Body sodium and potassium. IV. The normal exchangeable sodium, its measurement and magnitude. *Metabolism 3*:530-538, 1954.

5. Edelman, I. S., and Leibman, J.: Anatomy of body water and electrolytes. *Am. J. Med. 27*:256-277, 1959.

6. Früs-Hansen, B.: Changes in body water compartments during growth. *Acta Paediatr. 46*(Suppl. 110):1-68, 1957.

7. Gamble, J. L.: *Chemical Anatomy, Physiology and Pathology of Extracellular Fluid. A Lecture Syllabus.* 6th ed. Harvard University Press, Cambridge, Mass., 1967.

8. Goldberger, E.: *A Primer of Water, Electrolytes and Acid-Base Syndrome.* Lea & Febiger, Philadelphia, 1965.

9. Manery, J. F.: Water and electrolyte metabolism. *Physiol. Rev. 34*:334-417, 1954.

10. Pace, N., and Rathbun, E. N.: Studies on body composition. III. The body water and chemically combined nitrogen content in relation to fat content. *J. Biol. Chem. 158*:685-691, 1945.

11. Pitts, R. F.: *Physiology of the Kidney and Body Fluids.* 3rd ed. Year Book Medical Publishers, Inc., Chicago, 1974.

12. Rathbun, E. N., and Pace, N.: Studies on body composition. I. The determination of total body fat by means of the body specific gravity. *J. Biol. Chem. 158*:667-676, 1945.

13. Ruch, T. C., and Patton, H. D.: *Physiology and Biophysics.* 20th ed. W. B. Saunders Co., Philadelphia, 1974.

14. Schultz, A. L., Hammarsten, J. F., Heller, B. I., and Ebert, R. V.: A critical comparison of the T-1824 dye and iodinated albumin methods for plasma volume measurement. *J. Clin. Invest. 32*:107-112, 1953.

15. Skelton, H.: The storage of water by various tissues of the body. *Arch. Intern. Med. 40*:140-152, 1927.

16. Solomon, A. K.: Equations for tracer experiments. *J. Clin. Invest. 28*:1297-1307, 1949.

17. Walser, M., Seldin, D. W., and Grollman, A.: An evaluation of radiosulfate for the determination of the volume of extracellular fluid in man and dogs. *J. Clin. Invest. 32*:299-311, 1953.

Chapter 3

BODY FLUIDS: TURNOVER RATES AND DYNAMICS OF FLUID SHIFTS

In the previous chapter, we learned about the normal volumes and compositions of body fluids and their distribution between various compartments. With this background, we are now in a position to consider the dynamics of fluid balance and the factors controlling their turnover, distribution and shift between body fluid compartments.

EXTERNAL FLUID EXCHANGE

Maintenance of the normal balance of volume and composition of body fluids depends on the regulation of the influx and efflux quantities. Recalling the flow diagram of the renal-body fluid regulating system in Chapter 1, we see that the exchange of fluid between the body and the environment, or the *external fluid exchange*, occurs through several channels. On the influx side, the G.I. and metabolic systems are the only avenues of normal fluid intake. On the efflux side, fluids leave the body via the G.I. system, lungs, skin, and kidneys. Let us now examine the functional characteristics of each of these influx and efflux routes.

G. I. SYSTEM

The G.I. system plays a dual role in fluid and electrolyte homeostasis. It is the most important source of fluid influx as well as providing a route for fluid efflux. Oral intake is the primary source of water and electrolytes; daily ingestion normally is 2.5 liters of water and 7 g of salt. Including the metabolic water, the daily fluid turnover for a healthy young man is approximately 2.8 liters. In addition, over 8 liters of fluids are secreted into and reabsorbed from the G.I. system daily. This is more than twice the total plasma volume and is equal to more than half of the total volume of extracellular fluid. These secretions are all isotonic with the blood plasma but vary somewhat in composition. Also, about 1000 mEq of sodium is secreted daily into the G.I. tract. This represents about one third of the total exchangeable sodium and about six times the daily dietary intake of sodium.

Minor daily fluctuations in body weight are largely due to slight variations in the hydration of the body, particularly the extracellular fluid volume. In a 24 hr period, in addition to intake, a considerable amount of fluid is exchanged between the G.I. tract and the extracellular compartment. The fluid turnover in the G.I. tract amounts to 20 to 25% of the total body water. Hence, alteration in normal fluid intake and abnormal losses of G.I. secretions could precipitate profound changes in water and electrolyte balance. For instance, excessive loss of G.I. secretions, as in diarrhea or vomiting, rapidly decreases the volume of extracellular water, with concomitant loss of sodium, potassium, and associated anions. This results in a fall of the extracellular crystalloid osmotic pressure, a decrease in the plasma volume and eventual disruption of cellular function. For these reasons, abnormal loss of fluids from the G.I. system leads to rapid alteration in fluid balance and must be replaced promptly.

METABOLIC SYSTEM

Oxidation of foodstuffs provides a secondary but important source of water. The ordinary mixed diet will yield approximately 300 ml of metabolic water in 24 hr. Of the various constituents of the diet, oxidation of 100 g each of protein, fat, and starch yields 41 g, 107 g, and 55 g of water, respectively, whereas oxidation of 100 g of alcohol yields 117 g of water.

In addition to water, the metabolic system yields urea, a nontoxic product of protein metabolism, and toxic wastes which are eliminated by the kidneys.

SKIN AND LUNGS

Skin plays a highly important role in temperature regulation-- a function which, on occasion, may lead to considerable losses of fluids. Hence, the fluid efflux from the skin poses as a disturbance forcing in the renal-body fluid regulating system.

A nonperspiring young man in basal state loses approximately 30 g of water per hour by insensible perspiration. This, together with the water lost from the lungs, constitutes the *insensible loss* of water. A healthy nonperspiring adult in a resting state will have an insensible moisture loss of 800 to 1400 ml/24 hr, depending upon body surface area and metabolic rate. Feverish states will increase the insensible loss of moisture according to the extent to which metabolic rate is augmented. The greater the surface area in relation to mass, the greater will be the relative turnover of fluid in relation to the total fluid content of the body. For example, the daily turnover of fluid by a baby will represent a far higher proportion of its total body water than for an adult. The small reserve in comparison to the large daily turnover of the infant explains why dehydration may develop so rapidly at this time in life.

Sensible sweat is a distinctly hypotonic solution, with a salt concentration ranging from 10 to 70 mEq/L of H_2O. Thus, moderate sweating tends to deplete body water in excess of salt depletion. However, with continuous activity, the loss of sodium and chloride may reach proportions detrimental to normal body fluid homeostasis. Persons doing hard labor in a hot environment may lose 10 to 12 liters of hypotonic fluid per 24 hours. The excessive salt lost during hard labor may lead to a condition called *heat stroke*. If the lost fluid is replaced with salt-free water, another condition, known as *water intoxication*, may develop.

KIDNEYS

Normally, the kidneys excrete about 1500 ml of *hypertonic* urine in 24 hours. This represents about 60% of the normal daily fluid turnover. In addition, the kidneys excrete 30 g of urea per day which is produced from deamination of amino acids. The obligatory minimal daily urine volume, for normal kidneys which must excrete an average load of solutes, is approximately 500 ml. Adding this volume to about 1 liter of daily insensible water loss yields a minimal daily *obligatory* water loss of 1.5 liters. Thus, to maintain normal fluid balance a minimum daily fluid intake of 1.5 liters is necessary.

The ability of the kidney to adjust its excretion of water and solutes makes this organ the most important of all the avenues of fluid efflux. Unlike the G.I. system, skin, and lungs, the primary function of the kidneys is to conserve water and electrolytes, thereby stabilizing the volume and composition of body fluids. For instance, in diarrhea and vomiting, the G.I. system fails to reabsorb the secreted fluids and to retain the ingested fluids. During dehydration of any degree, the skin and lungs continue to lose water by vaporization. In fact, in acidosis the increased rate and depth of breathing result in considerable water loss by vaporization. In contrast, in the face of sodium depletion or lack of intake, the kidneys virtually cease excreting this ion. Similarly, in water deprivation, the kidneys excrete the urinary solutes in the smallest possible volume of water. In short, by adjusting its excretion rate of water and electrolytes the kidney actively stabilizes the body stores of these substances and indirectly stabilizes body fluid homeostasis.

One way to assess this ability of the kidneys to adjust their excretion rate is to measure urine *osmolality*. The most direct method of measuring osmolality is by an osmometer, an instrument which measures the freezing point depression of the sample and relates it to osmolality. However, because such an instrument is not widely available, the ease of measuring specific gravity has made it a commonly used substitute clinical test.

Specific gravity of urine relates the weight of equal volumes of the urine in question and distilled water under standard conditions. Hence, it reflects the weight of the solute in the urine and is not a true measure of the number of solute particles present (osmolality), as would be obtained by measurement of freezing point depression or vapor pressure elevation. Nevertheless, the specific gravity correlates with the osmolality and so it is a useful clinical tool. It indicates the quantity of water relative to solute removed, thus providing a means of testing the concentrating and diluting ability of the kidney.

Figure 3-1 shows the relationship between the specific gravity and urine osmolality. Note that the relationship is not linear and that, at a given osmolality, there is considerable variation in the measured specific gravity. However, to obtain a useful correlation between these two quantities, the mean values read from this graph were fitted by least-squares method to the following equation:

Urinary specific gravity =

$$1.000 + [25 \times 10^{-6} \times (\text{Urinary osmolality, mOsm/L})] \qquad (3\text{-}1)$$

Thus, if the urinary specific gravity is known, we can estimate the total urinary solute output (osmolality) from this equation.

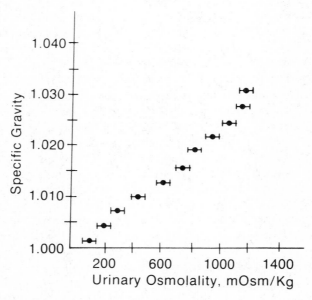

Figure 3-1. Relationship between urinary specific gravity and osmolality. [From Chapman, W. H., Bulger, R. E., Cutler, R. E., and Striker, G. E. (1973).]

For example, suppose that the average urinary specific gravity in a 24 hr urine sample is 1.020 and that the 24 hr urine output is 1200 ml. Then, the total urinary solute output would be 800 mOsm/L x 1.2 L/24 hr = 960 mOsm/24 hr.

INTERNAL FLUID EXCHANGE

The continuous flow and turnover of water and solutes between the circulating blood and the metabolizing cells is called the *internal fluid exchange*. The circulation of this internal fluid takes place across two separate membranes, each with its own specialized exchange processes. *First*, there is an enormous bidirectional flow of water and solutes, with each cardiac output, across the *capillary membrane*, between the plasma and interstitial compartments. This is called the *capillary fluid exchange*. The capillary filtrate thus formed is the source of the interstitial circulation. *Second*, there is an enormous bidirectional flow of water and solutes across the *cell membrane*, between the interstitial and intracellular compartments. This is called the *cellular fluid exchange*. Although both of these exchange processes operate concomitantly to serve the needs of various cells and tissues, the *mechanisms* and forces involved in each process are different and have different origins. Let us now consider these two exchange processes and their mechanism of operation.

CAPILLARY FLUID EXCHANGE

In the steady state, defined as unchanging fluid balance between the plasma and interstitial compartments, water and electrolytes move continuously between the two compartments, in both directions and at equal rates. This total fluid exchange flux has two components: (a) an enormous bidirectional *diffusive* flux of water and electrolytes, and (b) a small bidirectional *convective* (filtration) flow of fluid.

The diffusive flux of fluid is estimated at 120 L/min. This means that the 3.2 liters of plasma water is turned over once every 1.6 sec by this process alone. The *turnover time* for the 8.4 liters of interstitial water is about 4.1 sec! It is this enormous diffusive flux that allows the plasma and interstitial fluids to reach diffusion equilibrium in the capillary exchanger--a condition so necessary for the respiratory gases.

This bidirectional diffusive flow depends primarily on the physical properties of the capillary wall and the size of the solute molecules. The lipid-soluble substances, such as O_2 and CO_2, can diffuse freely across the entire surface of the capillary membrane. However, only 0.2% of the capillary surface is available for diffusion of water and lipid-insoluble molecules, such as Na, Cl, urea, and glucose. Because of the high turnover rate of both the lipid-soluble and lipid-insoluble molecules, a *sieving process* has been suggested as a mechanism of exchange. The limiting factors in the sieving process are thought to be the *size of the molecules*, the *size of the capillary pores*, and the *rate of water filtration*. Under normal physiological conditions, it appears that both diffusion and the sieving process account for the high rate of exchange.

In contrast, the bidirectional filtration flow of water and solutes across the capillary is small, only about 16 ml/min. This means that the plasma water is turned over once every 200 minutes and the interstitial water once every 525 minutes by this process alone. It is the circulation of this capillary transudate that provides the essential nutrients for the maintenance of the normal cellular metabolism. Although both diffusive and convective fluxes occur concomitantly, the physiological significance of the filtration flow is of special interest, because it is primarily concerned with volume *shift* between the intra- and extravascular fluid compartments. Whenever the bidirectional components of this flow are *unequal*, a transient is initiated which will shift fluid flow from one compartment to the other. This transient may lead to a new steady state, in which the two fluid volumes have changed, but are no longer changing. Such shifts of fluid are important in stabilizing the more critical blood volume, at the expense of the interstitial volume, as occurs in hypo- and hypervolemia. If this fluid shift mechanism is disturbed, the interstitial volume may become abnormally large, a condition called *edema*. For these reasons, we shall now examine in more detail the mechanisms of volume shift by filtration in the steady state of normality.

As illustrated in Figure 3-2, the capillary bed consists of two anatomically and functionally distinct components (Zweifach and Intaglietta, 1968): (1) a thoroughfare or arteriovenous (A-V) channel, providing a direct communication between arteriole and venule, thereby serving as physiological *shunts* that bypass the capillaries but provide a ready source of blood commensurate with tissue needs for oxygen and nutrients; and (2) a number of parallel true capillaries, with an average length of 0.5 to 1 mm, branching off the arterial end (also called *metarteriole*) of the A-V channel, thereby providing a *potential* surface for fluid exchange between the blood and the interstitial space. As shown, the metarteriolar wall just proximal to the branching of capillaries has a small cuff of smooth muscles called *precapillary sphincters*, whose periodic opening and closing causes an intermittent flow of blood through the capillary bed. At rest, the capillary blood flow velocity is about 1 mm/sec, allowing sufficient time for equilibration of water and solute concentrations across the capillary membrane.

As a consequence of this anatomical arrangement, the turnover of fluid across the capillary wall, in the steady state, is determined by: (a) the cardiovascular *hemodynamics*, which determine the A-V hydrostatic and oncotic pressure differences, (b) the *temporal* or periodic opening and closing of the precapillary sphincters, which determine the volume of blood flowing through the capillary exchanger, and the *number* and membrane *permeability* of the *spatially* distributed parallel capillaries which may participate in the filtration exchange,

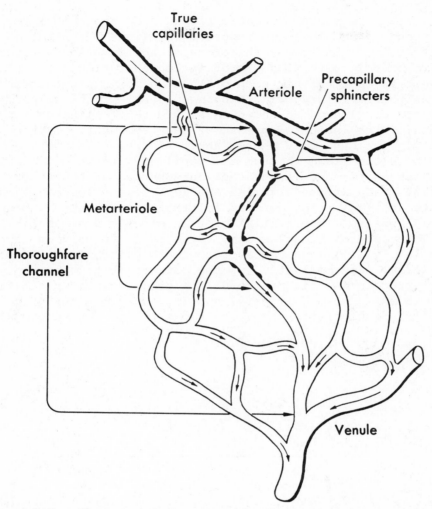

Figure 3-2. Structural details of a capillary bed. [From Deane, N. (1966).]

and (c) the *lymphatic system*, which plays a significant role in returning plasma proteins from interstitium back to the circulating plasma. Let us now consider how each of these factors influence the fluid shift by filtration across the capillary.

HEMODYNAMIC FACTORS

(1) MECHANISM OF TISSUE FLUID FORMATION. The net shift of fluid by filtration across the capillary and its steady state distribution between the intra- and extravascular compartments as first described by Starling (1896) depend, in part, on the algebraic sum of *four*

pressures: (1) the capillary hydrostatic pressure, P_c; (2) the interstitial hydrostatic pressure, P_i; (3) the capillary protein oncotic pressure, π_c; and (4) the interstitial protein oncotic pressure, π_i. The protein *oncotic pressure* is the sum of the protein osmotic pressure and the osmotic pressure of the bound cations (Gibbs-Donnan effect). This is why the protein oncotic pressure increases disproportionately with plasma protein concentration.

To get a "feel" of how each of these hemodynamic factors influences the capillary fluid exchange, consider the simplified diagram of a capillary bed shown in Figure 3-3. Although, in reality, the values of the indicated pressures vary somewhat, for ease of presentation, we have only chosen their mid-range values.

As the blood flows through the capillary, outward filtration of fluid causes a decrease in the capillary hydrostatic pressure from a value of 34 mm Hg at the arterial end (P_a) to a value of 17 mm Hg at the venous end (P_v). The outward filtration is further enhanced by a relatively constant interstitial protein oncotic pressure (π_i) of 4 mm Hg. Thus, in the steady state, there is a net driving force of 21 mm Hg (34 - 17 + 4) which favors outward filtration of fluid across the capillary. Concomitantly, as the outward filtration proceeds, the capillary protein oncotic pressure (π_c) progressively rises from a value of 28 mm Hg at the arterial end (π_a) to a maximum value near the mid-capillary region. As the blood flows toward the venous side, the

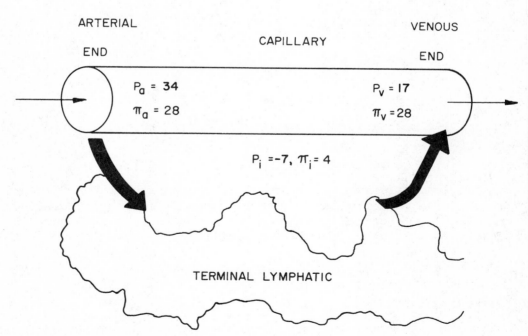

Figure 3-3. A schematic diagram of a capillary bed. [Redrawn and slightly modified from Deane, N. (1966).]

elevated π_C causes an inward filtration of fluid, thereby restoring π_C to its arterial value by the time the blood reaches the venous end. Thus, in the steady state, the capillary protein oncotic pressure provides a net reabsorptive force of 28 mm Hg, favoring inward filtration of fluid back to the blood. The magnitude of this oncotic pressure, primarily due to plasma albumin and globulin, is small compared to the 5100 mm Hg pressure developed by the crystalloids of plasma. However, in contrast to crystalloids, because proteins normally do not cross the capillary wall in large amounts, the physiological significance of the plasma protein oncotic pressure is out of proportion to its small value.

In the steady state, the algebraic sum of the forces favoring outward and inward filtration yields a value of -7, which is exactly equal to the interstitial hydrostatic pressure (P_i) of -7 mm Hg required to balance the other forces. The physiological significance of this negative interstitial hydrostatic pressure will be discussed later in this chapter.

Thus, we see that as the blood enters the arterial end of an exchanging capillary, the algebraic sum of all the hydrostatic pressures (34 + 7 + 4 - 28) yields an *effective outward filtration pressure* (ΔP) of 17 mm Hg, which forces a protein-poor fluid out of the capillary into the interstitium. As this *outward filtration* continues, the capillary hydrostatic pressure falls while its protein oncotic pressure rises. By the time the blood reaches the venous end of this capillary, the effective filtration pressure has *reversed* its direction, so as to force the interstitial fluid back into the capillary. This hydrostatic pressure reversal accounts for the return of 90% of the filtered fluid back into the blood. The remaining 10% is returned to the circulation via the lymphatic system, whose function is discussed below. Thus, if 16 ml/min is filtered out in the arterial half of the capillaries, about 14.5 ml/min is reabsorbed in the venous half; the remaining 1.5 ml/min is returned to the blood via the lymphatic system.

What factors give rise to this effective filtration pressure, and which influence its direction reversal along the capillary? The effective filtration pressure is the algebraic sum of several pressures acting in opposite directions, which are either hydrostatic or colloid osmotic (oncotic) in origin. The main hydrostatic pressure is the capillary blood pressure.

What are the components of this effective pressure, and why does its direction (algebraic sign) reverse along the capillary? The pressure component that acts in the direction of *outward filtration* is *hydrostatic* in origin; it is a *net* hydrostatic pressure defined as the excess of the intracapillary pressure (34 mm Hg) over the smaller (negative) interstitial fluid pressure (-7 mm Hg). This net pressure (41 mm Hg) decreases as the blood pressure decreases along the length of the capillary. The pressure component that acts in the direction of *inward filtration*, or absorption, is *oncotic* (colloid osmotic) in origin; it, too, is a net pressure defined as the excess of plasma oncotic pressure (28 mm Hg) over the smaller interstitial fluid oncotic pressure (4 mm Hg). This net pressure (24 mm Hg) increases along the capillary, as a result of outward filtration of protein-poor filtrate.

We now have two oppositely directed net pressures, whose algebraic sum produces the effective pressure. The net *hydrostatic, filtration* pressure decreases along the capillary, while the net *oncotic, absorptive* pressure increases along the capillary. Toward the arterial end, the excess of filtration over absorption pressures induces outward filtration; toward the venous end, the excess of absorption over filtration pressure induces inward filtration, or absorption. In the steady state, the filtration rate and the absorption and lymphatic return rates are equal, so that no shift of fluid volume between plasma and interstitium occurs.

An important factor contributing to this fluid balance is the protein oncotic pressure of the plasma proteins. As mentioned above and illustrated in Figure 3-4, the plasma protein oncotic pressure (π_p) increases disproportionately with plasma protein concentration ($[Pr]_p$). [The equation fitted to the data in Figure 3-4 is valid for rat as well as human plasma (Allison et al., 1972).] The physiological significance of this nonlinear relationship is that at low plasma protein concentration, such as exists in the interstitial fluids, the oncotic pressure increases linearly with protein concentration. However, at normal plasma protein concentration the oncotic pressure rises markedly with small increases in protein concentration.

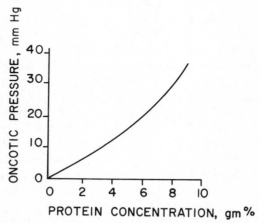

Figure 3-4. Relationship of plasma protein oncotic pressure to plasma protein concentration. Data were fitted, via least-squares forced through the origin, to the following equation:

$$\pi_p = 2.1[Pr]_p + 0.16[Pr]_p^2 + 0.009[Pr]_p^3$$

[Redrawn from Landis, E. M., and Pappenheimer, J. R. (1963).]

Hence, because of this nonlinear relationship, loss of protein-free fluid from the plasma results in a greater rise in oncotic pressure and thus a greater inward filtration force than would be expected. Conversely, the gain of fluid would have a greater effect in diluting the plasma and in reducing the oncotic pressure than would be expected.

From the foregoing analysis, we see that the net shift of fluid from plasma into the interstitium, designated as $\dot{Q}_{p \to i}$, is largely determined by the magnitude of the net filtration forces, ΔP (the algebraic sum of the hydrostatic pressure and protein oncotic pressures). This relationship may be expressed as,

$$\dot{Q}_{p \to i} = k_f(P_c - P_i - \pi_c + \pi_i) = k_f \Delta P \qquad (3-2)$$

where k_f is the capillary filtration coefficient and the other symbols have already been defined. From this relationship, it is evident that any factor which causes an increase in the capillary hydrostatic pressure or a decrease in the plasma protein concentration, and hence in π_c, favors increased outward filtration (from plasma to interstitium). Likewise, any factor which causes a decrease in P_c or an increase in π_c tends to reduce outward filtration, and hence increases inward filtration (from interstitium into plasma).

(2) PRESSURE-FLOW RELATIONSHIP IN A CAPILLARY. To appreciate further the influence of changes in pressures and resistances of the arteriole and venule on the capillary pressure, and hence capillary filtration, consider the idealized capillary model shown in Figure 3-5. According to this scheme, the magnitude of the capillary hydrostatic pressure (P_c) assuming a normal plasma and tissue protein oncotic pressure and tissue hydrostatic pressure, is determined by the arterial (P_a) and venous (P_v) pressures and their respective resistances to blood flow. This dependence may be expressed

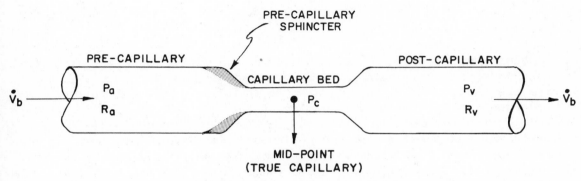

Figure 3-5. An idealized scheme of the pre-capillary, capillary, and post-capillary vascular tree.

quantitatively if we first write defining equations for pre- and post-capillary resistances (R_a and R_v, respectively), and then combine these equations to obtain a defining equation for P_c.

The pre-capillary resistance, analogous to Ohm's law in electricity, may be defined as the ratio of the hydrostatic pressure drop across the pre-capillary vessel to the blood flow, $\dot{V}_b$:

$$R_a = \frac{P_a - P_c}{\dot{V}_b} \tag{3-3}$$

A similar equation may be written for the post-capillary resistance:

$$R_v = \frac{P_c - P_v}{\dot{V}_b} \tag{3-4}$$

Combining Equations 3-3 and 3-4, eliminating the $\dot{V}_b$ term and solving for P_c, we get:

$$P_c = \frac{\dfrac{R_v}{R_a} P_a + P_v}{1 + \dfrac{R_v}{R_a}} \tag{3-5}$$

From this equation, it is evident that for given arterial and venous pressures, the mean capillary hydrostatic pressure depends on the ratio of the post-capillary to pre-capillary resistances to blood flow. Rearranging Equations 3-3 and 3-4, in terms of P_c, yields:

$$P_c = P_a - R_a \dot{V}_b \tag{3-6}$$

$$P_c = P_v + R_v \dot{V}_b \tag{3-7}$$

Equations 3-6 and 3-7 have the form of a linear equation in which P_c is the dependent variable, $\dot{V}_b$ is the independent variable, R_a and R_v are the slope, and P_a and P_v are the ordinate-intercept which become equal to P_c when $\dot{V}_b$ is zero.

Using the theoretical Equations 3-6 and 3-7, Pappenheimer and Soto-Rivera (1948) estimated the capillary hydrostatic pressure in the isolated perfused hindlimbs of cats and dogs by *isogravimetric* method. The experimental procedure consisted of stepwise elevation of the venous pressure to compensate for the stepwise decrement in the arterial pressure, caused by outward fluid filtration, until the limb

weight remained constant. When this was achieved, there were no
further pressure drops across the pre-capillary, capillary, and
post-capillary vasculatures, and therefore no changes in flow. Hence
the arterial and venous pressures became equal to the capillary
hydrostatic pressure. This pressure was called the *isogravimetric*
capillary pressure, P_{iso}. Since during the isogravimetric state there
was presumably no net shift of fluid across the capillary membrane,
P_{iso} was equal to the sum of all pressures opposing outward fluid
filtration. Hence, Equation 3-2 may be written as

$$Q_{p \rightarrow i} = k_f (P_c - P_{iso}) \tag{3-8}$$

where $P_{iso} = (P_i + \pi_c - \pi_i)$ and k_f has already been defined.

Experimentally, Pappenheimer and Soto-Rivera (1948) altered the
blood flow into the perfused hindlimb by varying the arterial pressure
followed by compensatory adjustment of the venous pressure until the
limb weight became constant. The value of P_c was then estimated from
P_{iso} by plotting changes in the arterial or venous pressures against
the changes in blood flow. They found that a change in venous
pressure of 0.5 mm Hg caused a detectable effect on fluid movement
across the capillaries, while a similar fluid shift could be seen
only after a 2 to 4 mm Hg change in the arterial pressure.
Furthermore, the capillary pressure was found to be more sensitive
to a change in venous pressure than to a change in arterial pressure.
Also, the post-capillary resistance (R_v) was independent of the
changes in the blood flow, while the pre-capillary resistance (R_a)
increased monotonically as the blood flow decreased. In addition,
the isogravimetric method allowed measurement of the capillary
filtration coefficient (k_f).

Figure 3-6 summarizes the effects of the hemodynamic factors on
the net fluid shift across the capillary membrane. It depicts the
net fluid movement, i.e., filtration or absorption, as a function of
the hydrostatic pressure gradient across the capillary membrane. We
see that both fluid filtration and absorption are directly
proportional to the difference between the calculated mean capillary
blood pressure and the isogravimetric capillary pressure. The
filtration coefficient, obtained from the slope of the plotted
regression line, was 0.014 ml per 100 g tissue per mm Hg change in
capillary blood pressure. The constancy of this filtration
coefficient at low and high capillary pressures indicated that, under
these conditions, the capillary porosity and surface area were not
influenced by blood pressure. These findings have recently been
confirmed by applying a similar method to the hindlimbs of rats
(Renkin and Zaun, 1955).

(3) SIGNIFICANCE OF NEGATIVE INTERSTITIAL PRESSURE. The finding
that the isogravimetric capillary pressure equals the sum of all
pressures opposing filtration was based on the assumption that the
interstitial hydrostatic pressure remained unchanged and was
unaffected by the experimental forcings. This, however, was found

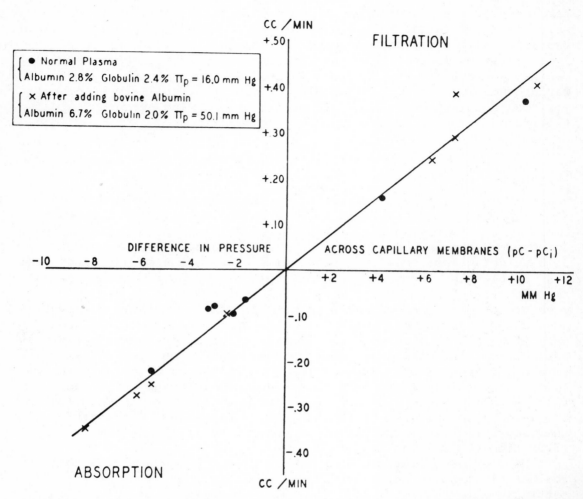

Figure 3-6. Relation of net fluid shift in perfused hind limb of cat to the difference between mean capillary hydrostatic pressure, pC, and the sum of all pressures opposing filtration, pC_i (= P_{iso}). [From Pappenheimer, H. R., and Soto-Rivera, A. (1948).]

not to be the case by Guyton (1963, 1965) who was able to measure the interstitial pressure directly in similar experiments. Guyton found that, contrary to expectations, the interstitial pressure was not normally positive, but rather ranged between -6 to -7 mm Hg, and rose to positive values only in edematous conditions. He also observed that the interstitial pressure was markedly influenced by intravenous fluid infusion as well as changes in arterial and venous pressures.

To ascertain the physiological significance of the normally observed negative (sub-atmospheric) interstitial pressure, Guyton determined the pressure-volume relationship of the interstitial space as follows. He perfused the isolated hindlimbs of dogs with 10% Dextran (a plasma volume expander), while simultaneously measuring the changes in the interstitial pressure and hindlimb weight. The interstitial pressure was measured via a needle catheter inserted into previously implanted perforated plastic spheres. Then, assuming that changes in limb weight reflect changes in the interstitial volume, Guyton constructed pressure-volume curves for the interstitial space. Figure 3-7 depicts such a curve, which is extrapolated to humans from data obtained in dogs. The slope of such a curve, defined as the ratio of the incremental increase in interstitial volume (ΔV) to incremental increase in interstitial pressure (ΔP), depicts the interstitial *compliance* ($\Delta V/\Delta P$). We can see that the interstitial compliance is quite low at normal negative interstitial pressures, but it increases markedly as the interstitial pressure rises to positive values.

The pressure-volume curve, thus obtained, reveals two distinct operating regions for the interstitial space: (1) a low compliance region representing the normal pressure-volume changes, and (2) a high compliance region reflecting the adaptive behavior of the interstitial

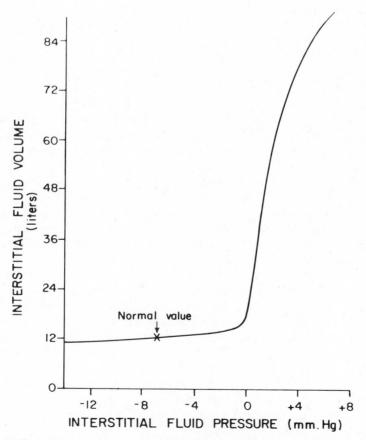

Figure 3-7. Pressure-volume curve of interstitial spaces. The curve is extrapolated to humans from data obtained in dogs. [From Guyton, A. C. (1971).]

space to abnormal pressure-volume changes.

According to Guyton, the normally negative interstitial pressure serves two important physiological functions: (1) it creates a partial vacuum environment which serves to hold the different body tissues together, thereby complementing connective tissue function. When interstitial pressure increases to positive values, fluid accumulates in the interstitial spaces with subsequent edema formation. (2) It also serves to minimize the tissue space across which the nutrients and metabolic waste must traverse. Since nutrient-metabolic waste exchange between blood and cells occurs primarily by diffusion, the compactness of tissue spaces will enormously enhance this exchange.

TEMPORAL AND SPATIAL FACTORS

The periodic opening and closing of the precapillary sphincters produces phasic changes in capillary hydrostatic pressure, allowing the plasma oncotic pressure to predominate intermittently. Hence, an increase in the period during which sphincters are closed, tends to decrease capillary blood pressure relative to capillary oncotic pressure. The resulting hydrostatic pressure gradient favors inward filtration of fluid from the interstitial space to the intravascular compartment. Conversely, an increase in the period during which sphincters are open favors outward filtration of fluid into the interstitium.

At least three conditions are known to *increase* the period during which the sphincters are *closed*: (1) hemorrhage, (2) sympathetic stimulation, and (3) epinephrine injection. The net effect of each of these stimuli is to increase fluid *absorption* into the capillary, thereby producing *hemodilution*, as manifested by a reduced hematocrit.

At least three conditions are known to *increase* the period during which the sphincters are *open*: (1) a rise in body temperature above normal, (2) direct trauma, such as surgery, and (3) prolonged anoxia. The net effect of each of these stimuli is to increase outward filtration of fluid into the interstitium, thereby producing *hemoconcentration*, as manifested by an elevation of hematocrit.

In short, any factor that alters the arteriolar pressure or interferes with free venous outflow affects the process of fluid exchange. Thus, arteriolar dilation or venous obstruction favors filtration from the intravascular to the interstitial compartment. The force which opposes this outward filtration, when protein oncotic pressure is constant, is the interstitial hydrostatic pressure. This pressure depends on the lymphatic flow, the amount of interstitial fluid, the volume of the interstitial space, and the permeability of the capillary membrane. The abnormal operation of any of these factors favors the accumulation of edema fluid.

LYMPHATIC SYSTEM

The lymphatic system provides a normal route for the return of the plasma proteins which have been filtered out of the capillary back into the blood. The amount of proteins leaking out of the capillary in 24 hours is estimated to be equal to that in the circulating blood itself. The normal passage of plasma proteins (both albumin and globulin) through the capillary wall is very important for cellular metabolism and for defense against infection. Impairment of lymphatic drainage leads to excessive fluid accumulation in the interstitial space, with high protein content. A rise in interstitial protein concentration may also result from damage to capillary endothelium from burns or hypoxia.

The normal leakage of a small but potentially significant amount of protein into the interstitial space yields a filtrate protein concentration of about 0.2 to 0.4 g%. This is somewhat less than the interstitial protein concentration of about 2 g% and the lymph protein concentration of about 4 g%. This interstitial protein concentration yields an oncotic pressure of about 4 to 5 mm Hg. Depending on the protein concentration, the interstitial oncotic pressure ranges from a low value of 0.1 mm Hg in the limb interstitium to a high value of 5 mm Hg in the interstitial fluids of intestine and liver (Mayerson, 1963).

The quantity of proteins in the interstitial space is determined by the extent of the lymphatic flow, normally about 100 ml/hr at rest. The progressive accumulation of protein in the interstitial space increases the oncotic pressure, causing an expansion of the interstitial volume at the expense of a reduced fluid absorption by the capillary. The expansion of interstitial volume increases the interstitial hydrostatic pressure, forcing the interstitial fluid into the lymphatic channels, carrying with it the excess accumulated plasma proteins. The overall effect is the restoration of the capillary hydrodynamics to normal. In short, an increase in the tissue fluid proteins increases the rate of lymph flow, and this, by washing the proteins out of the tissue spaces, automatically returns the interstitial protein concentration back to the normal low level.

The lymphatic drainage is increased by factors which elevate either the interstitial hydrostatic pressure (P_i) or the lymphatic flow rate. The interstitial pressure may be increased by one or a combination of the following: (1) an increase in the capillary hydrostatic pressure (P_c); (2) a decrease in the plasma protein oncotic pressure (π_c); and (3) an increase in the permeability of the capillary wall. The lymphatic flow rate may be increased by the action of lymphatogogues--substances which increase lymphatic flow rate. There are two general classes of lymphatogogues: (a) any extracellular expanding agent such as isotonic saline or glucose solution, and (b) histamine and similar substances which cause dilation of the arterioles and contraction of the venules. Thus, lymphatogogues increase the lymphatic flow rate secondary to their effects on the interstitial hydrostatic pressure.

CEREBROSPINAL FLUID

The cerebrospinal fluid, an important component of the transcellular fluid, has at least two main functions: (1) it provides a medium of exchange for nutrients and wastes between brain and blood; and (2) it regulates the volume of the cranium by manipulating its own volume in response to changes in brain blood volume.

The total volume of the cerebrospinal fluid is about 100 to 150 ml in man. Its composition resembles that of protein-free plasma, but has a somewhat lower concentration of the important plasma crystalloids. The cerebrospinal fluid is formed primarily by *secretion* from the blood at the choroid plexuses, at a rate of 20 ml/hr or about 500 ml/day. About 4/5 of this secreted fluid is absorbed via the cerebral arachnoid villi, which are finger-like projections, and most of the rest via the spinal villi. The mechanisms of absorption are *filtration* and *osmosis*.

Due to its osmotic effect, *saline infusion* markedly influences the rate of secretion and absorption of the cerebrospinal fluid. For instance, intravenous infusion of *isotonic* saline causes a temporary rise of the cerebrospinal fluid pressure, which, along with the dilution of plasma proteins, promotes cerebrospinal fluid formation. Similarly, infusion of *hypotonic* saline raises the cerebrospinal fluid pressure, but decreases both the plasma oncotic (dilution of proteins) and crystalloid osmotic (hypotonic salt) pressures. The net effect is the osmotic flow of water from plasma into the cerebrospinal fluid and brain cells. Thus, there would be prolonged rise in the cerebrospinal fluid pressure, a rise in the intracranial pressure and a swelling of the brain. In contrast, infusion of *hypertonic* saline causes a marked fall in the cerebrospinal fluid pressure, a fall in the intracranial pressure, and shrinking of the brain. These effects are the direct consequence of the elevated plasma crystalloid osmotic pressure following hypertonic saline infusion.

Clinically, hypertonic solutions of mannitol or urea are usually infused to lower the abnormally elevated intracranial pressure caused, for instance, by cerebral tumor. Such treatment helps to restore consciousness, relieve headache, and reduce the swelling of the optic disc.

Abnormal elevation of the intracranial pressure may also occur as a result of excessive accumulation of the cerebrospinal fluid due to obstruction of the outflow. Such a pathological fluid accumulation is called *hydrocephalus*. The cause of obstruction may be intra- or extravascular, and it may be fatal if it is not diagnosed and treated promptly.

EDEMA STATE

Edema is defined as the excessive accumulation of fluid in the interstitial space. The immediate cause of edema is an abnormal balance in the hydrostatic and oncotic pressures across the capillary wall. Such an imbalance may result from (1) an abnormal increase in the capillary hydrostatic pressure, as a result of venous obstruction, (2) an abnormal decrease in the plasma protein concentration and hence oncotic pressure, caused by a decrease in intake or synthesis and/or increased renal loss, and (3) an abnormal accumulation of proteins in the interstitial space, due to increased capillary permeability to proteins and/or obstruction of lymphatic return. As a result of any of these factors or their combinations, the rate of outward filtration of water and solutes from the plasma would exceed the rate of their absorption from the interstitium.

Edema may be formed in both extracellular and intracellular compartments. *Extracellular edema* is the usual way in which extra fluid accumulates in the body. This accumulation represents retention of both water and sodium chloride, as an isotonic solution. Both the interstitial and intravascular compartments share in this increase. The distribution of the extra fluid between the intra- and extravascular compartments will depend, in part, upon the normal functioning of the cardiovascular and renal systems as well as the hemodynamic factors operating across the capillary wall. Hence, altered cardiac, renal, hepatic, or endocrine function may be of primary importance in the etiology of edema state.

Retention of fluid without corresponding retention of extracellular electrolytes (NaCl) will lead to an increase in both intra- and extracellular fluids. Intracellular edema is poorly tolerated. Loss of adrenal function or an excess of vasopressin predisposes one to *intracellular edema*. Infusion of electrolyte-poor fluids into anuric or electrolyte-depleted patients may also cause intracellular edema.

Clinically, formation of edema is usually accompanied by an abnormal elevation of the net hydrostatic pressure (ΔP) due to (1) reduced protein synthesis and hence reduced π_C, as in liver cirrhosis and (2) reduced plasma protein concentration and hence reduced π_C, caused by excessive renal protein excretion, as in nephrotic syndrome, or by plasma volume expansion, as in cardiac and renal failures. In all these cases, edema is self-limiting: with the establishment of a new steady state, water and electrolyte exchange may be normal even though the extracellular fluid volume is increased.

CELLULAR FLUID EXCHANGE

The continuous, rapid bidirectional flow of water between the interstitial and intracellular compartments depends on the transcellular *osmolar concentration* gradient and *cellular metabolism*. However, for a given metabolic rate, the net rate of water flow from the interstitium into the cells, designated as $\dot{W}_{i \to c}$, is largely determined by the difference between the cellular ($[Os]_c$) and interstitial ($[Os]_i$) osmolalities:

$$\dot{W}_{i \to c} = k_c([Os]_c - [Os]_i) \qquad (3\text{-}9)$$

where k_C is the cell membrane permeability coefficient. Thus, an increase in the osmolality of the intracellular fluid above that of the interstitial fluid causes a net shift of water into the cell. Conversely, an increase in the interstitial osmolality results in a net transfer of water out of the cell. These osmotic shifts of water between the intra- and extracellular fluid compartments are relative, and an equilibrium may be established in disease states in which both compartments become hypertonic or hypotonic compared to normal.

Cellular metabolism could upset the osmotic equilibrium between the intra- and extracellular fluid compartments. Intracellular water is mobilized when cellular constituents are metabolized. As the amount of cellular proteins and electrolytes decreases so does the capacity of the cell to hold water. It has been estimated that for every mEq of potassium mobilized, 6 g of intracellular water are liberated, while mobilization of 1 g of protein liberates 3 g of intracellular water. Glycogen, like protein, holds three times its weight of water, whereas fat holds one tenth its weight of water. These values refer to the "preformed" water and must not be confused with the water derived from oxidation of food.

DISTURBANCES IN FLUID AND ELECTROLYTE BALANCE

As mentioned in Chapter 1, the various disturbance forcings affecting the renal-body fluid regulating system may be classified as (1) those which alter the normal *influx* and hence impose a *load* on the system and (2) those which affect the normal *efflux* and therefore result in abnormal *loss* from the system. Additionally, any of these disturbances may involve changes in either *volume*, *composition*, *distribution,* or a combination of these, leading to states of *hydration* or *dehydration* of different tonicities in the various body fluid compartments. The underlying causes include either (a) the failure to maintain a normal ratio between the influx and efflux or (b) the failure of the influx-efflux organs, or both of these.

Clinically, disturbances in body fluid distribution may result from one or a combination of several conditions:

1. *Cardiac failure.* The manifestations of altered fluid distribution may vary, depending on what part of the heart has failed. Fluid tends to leave the intravascular compartment or to be unequally distributed between lungs, viscera, and extremities.

2. *Altered permeability of the capillary wall.* This may result from surgical shock or burns. Plasma volume decreases due to loss of plasma proteins, and fluid tends to accumulate in the interstitial space.

3. *Reduced plasma protein oncotic pressure.* Marked reduction in plasma albumin concentration may result from either reduced protein intake or decreased synthesis, as in liver cirrhosis, or increased urinary excretion, as in nephrotic syndrome, or a combination of these. In all cases, the reduced plasma oncotic pressure favors outward filtration of fluid into the interstitium, thereby producing extracellular edema.

4. *Interference with venous return or lymphatic drainage.* Obstruction of venous and/or lymphatic return of fluid back to the cardiovascular system causes accumulation of fluid in the interstitial space at the expense of the intravascular volume.

In order to understand the underlying causes of the *disturbances* in the quantity and distribution of body fluid which occur clinically, the following facts must be kept in mind:

1. *Water can freely penetrate the cell membrane in either direction.* Hence, distilled water admitted to the body is distributed throughout all fluid compartments.

2. *In general, electrolytes (Na, K, Cl, etc.) cannot penetrate normal cell membranes in either direction.* (There are several notable exceptions to this general rule, which may be disregarded for present purposes). Hence, isotonic saline injected intravenously remains entirely extracellular.

3. *Normally, all fluid compartments are isotonic with each other.* Water can freely diffuse between compartments, thus preventing long-lasting anisotonicity.

4. *Osmotic adjustments can be accomplished only by a shift of water.* This follows from the fact that *only water* is freely diffusible. Hence, if hypertonic saline is injected intravenously, water leaves the cells to dilute the extracellular fluid to isotonicity.

5. *The quantity of Na in the body largely determines the volume of extracellular fluid.* Water will be added to or subtracted from the extracellular fluid until its Na concentration is rendered isotonic with the cells.

6. *The protein oncotic pressure of the plasma largely determines the relative volumes of the intravascular and interstitial fluids.* If the plasma proteins are decreased, fluid will escape into the interstitial spaces, producing edema.

Pathological states may arise from deficiencies or excesses in *total* body water. For example, dehydration easily results from restriction of fluid intake. Excess fluid given intravenously may cause cardiac embarassment, as well as peripheral, pulmonary, and cerebral edema.

Of equal importance are pathological states which arise from *improper distribution* of fluid between the various compartments. For example, a *rapid* shift of plasma into the interstitial spaces leads to secondary shock; if the shift occurs so gradually that plasma volume can be maintained by the water and salt intake, clinical edema results.

It is not so widely appreciated that maldistribution of fluid and dehydration can result from a primary electrolyte depletion as well as from a primary water depletion and that such conditions cannot be corrected by measures which fail to restore proper electrolyte balance. In general, water is never lost without electrolytes, nor electrolytes without water, although the relative proportions lost may vary, depending upon the condition responsible. Hence, in treating disturbances of fluid balance, one should bear in mind several factors: (1) the water requirements, (2) the electrolyte requirements, (3) the acid-base balance requirements, and (4) the blood protein oncotic pressure requirements.

Failure to consider all these factors may at times be disastrous. For example, the administration of large amounts of water by mouth to a patient who is both demineralized and dehydrated as a result of excessive sweating will dilute the extracellular fluid, cause excessive cellular hydration and precipitate nausea, vomiting, muscular cramps, and cerebral edema. Also, intravenous administration of saline solution to a patient in secondary shock will not restore the plasma volume because the saline, lacking protein oncotic pressure, cannot be retained intravascularly and merely adds to the edema.

The widespread use of intravenous fluid in clinical practice necessitates an understanding of the possible dangers involved in this form of therapy. Such dangers may arise from several sources, for example, the use of incompatible blood, contamination with pyrogens, etc. The rate at which intravenous fluid can safely be given will vary with the state of hydration of the patient, the efficiency of his myocardium, and the nature of the fluid.

When large quantities of fluid are rapidly introduced into the venous system, several compensatory mechanisms work to prevent an excessive rise in circulating blood volume and venous pressure. These include:

1. Storage in the blood reservoirs of the skin, spleen, liver, and splanchnic area. This fluid is retained in the intravascular compartment, but the increased capacity of the vascular system produced by dilation of these reservoir areas prevents an excessive rise in venous pressure.

2. Storage in the interstitial and/or intracellular compartment. Isotonic saline solution is limited to the extracellular compartment. Hypotonic solutions may increase intracellular water. Excessive accumulation of interstitial fluid constitutes edema, and this may occur in the skin, lungs, brain, or abdominal viscera. Hypertonic solutions pull water into the intravascular compartment and produce a greater rise in blood volume and venous pressure than do isotonic solutions given at the same rate.

3. Passage into the intestinal lumen, pleural cavity, or peritoneal cavity.

4. Excretion by the kidneys.

If fluid is given so rapidly that the operation of these compensatory mechanisms cannot prevent the venous pressure from rising to a critical level of about 25 to 30 cm H_2O, death will occur from the acute cardiac decompensation as the heart dilates beyond its physiological limit. If the myocardium were weak to begin with, a lesser rise in venous pressure would precipitate decompensation. This indicates caution in administering intravenous fluids to patients with damaged hearts.

If the fluid is not given rapidly enough to exceed the capacity of the compensatory mechanisms, acute cardiac decompensation may be avoided, but death may occur from pulmonary or cerebral edema if enough fluid is given.

Obviously, a patient whose body fluids are depleted by acute dehydration, shock, or hemorrhage will tolerate much more rapid rates of fluid infusion than one in whom the water content and distribution is essentially normal to begin with.

We conclude this chapter by examining in some detail the response of the renal-body fluid regulating system to some common forcings resulting from oral or parenteral fluid adminstration or loss. Depending on whether excessive fluid enters or leaves the body, the overall response is classified as hydration or dehydration, respectively.

HYDRATION

Hydration, or fluid and salt retention, results from an excessive influx of water and sodium chloride. Once in the blood, these substances diffuse uniformly between the vascular and interstitial compartments, but no salt enters the intracellular compartment. The final effects depend on the volume, the amount of salt, and the route and rate of administration.

ISOTONIC HYDRATION

Rapid oral intake or intravenous infusion of 2 liters of isotonic saline results in about 10% increase in plasma volume, a decrease in plasma protein oncotic pressure, due to dilution of protein concentration, and an increase in both arterial and venous pressures. The resulting increase in the capillary hydrostatic pressure and decrease in protein oncotic pressure lead to an increase in the effective filtration pressure (ΔP) and eventual shift of fluid from plasma to interstitial compartment. However, because the administered fluid is isotonic, there will be no change in *crystalloid* (nonprotein solutes) osmotic pressure, and hence no change in the intracellular volume. The expansion of the *extracellular volume* leads to increased urinary excretion of salt and water (diuresis), which eliminates about half of the added load in about 4 hours. The remaining fluid is excreted gradually during the next few days.

Infusion of a large volume of isotonic saline at a rate which exceeds urinary excretion results in fluid retention or edema. Fluid retention may also result from either depressed renal excretion of salt and water (renal failure) or excessive expansion of vascular and interstitial volumes (congestive heart failure and hepatic cirrhosis). A more detailed account of renal function in these disease states will be presented in Chapter 13.

HYPOTONIC HYDRATION

An oral intake of 2 liters of water, especially on an empty stomach, is rapidly absorbed into the blood. This results in about 10% increase in plasma volume, but only a 3% fall in the crystalloid osmotic pressure, and a smaller decrease in protein oncotic pressure. The increase in the plasma volume elevates the capillary hydrostatic pressure which along with the reduced crystalloid osmotic and protein oncotic pressures lead to a shift of water from plasma into the interstitial compartment.

Concomitantly, because the interstitial crystalloid osmotic pressure is higher relative to that of plasma, electrolytes, namely NaCl, will diffuse from the interstitial compartment to the plasma. However, in terms of the overall effect, the rate of movement of water from plasma to interstitium is much faster and more important than the diffusion of electrolytes in the opposite direction.

The net effect of water intake is a decrease in the osmolality of the extracellular fluid, thus disturbing the normal volume and osmolality balance between the intra- and extracellular compartments. Owing to the fall in the crystalloid osmotic pressure of the extracellular fluid, water enters the cells. Therefore, the final effect of the ingested water is an increase in the total body water and a decrease in the crystalloid osmotic pressure.

To preserve normal water and electrolyte balance the kidneys begin to eliminate the excess ingested water approximately 30 minutes after its intake. The water diuresis reaches its peak in about 1 hour, then declines and is virtually over in about 3 hours.

HYPERTONIC HYDRATION

Oral intake of large amounts of salt or intravenous infusion of an hypertonic saline solution leads to an increase in the plasma crystalloid osmotic pressure. The rise in plasma osmolality causes water to flow from the interstitium into the plasma, thereby initially increasing plasma volume. Concomitantly, the increase in plasma salt concentration causes NaCl to diffuse into the interstitium. The net result is a uniform increase in the crystalloid osmotic pressure of the extracellular compartment without a change in the volume. The increase in the extracellular fluid osmolality causes water to flow out of the cells, which eventually decreases the intracellular and increases the extracellular volumes.

The renal response to this salt retention is an increase in NaCl excretion spread over several hours. This slow rate of renal excretion is due to inability of the kidneys to eliminate urine having a salt concentration in excess of 450 to 500 mEq/L (roughly three times normal). A survivor of a shipwreck, in a raft at sea, faces a similar danger of salt retention should he choose to drink the sea water; depending on the salt concentration, drinking of the sea water to quench thirst leads eventually to cellular dehydration and death.

DEHYDRATION

Dehydration, or fluid and salt depletion, involves both the extracellular and intracellular fluids in the majority of instances. Like hydration, the final effects of fluid and salt depletion depend on the volume of fluid, the amount of salt, and the route and rate of loss.

ISOTONIC DEHYDRATION

Loss of water and electrolytes in isotonic concentration leads to extracellular isotonic dehydration. Examples of isotonic dehydration with reduced extracellular volume include hemorrhage, plasma loss through burned skin, starvation, and gastrointestinal fluid loss, including G.I. bleeding. Since in all of these conditions insensible and fecal losses of water and electrolytes occur, the kidneys are the only organs which can moderate the effects of fluid loss by conserving salt and water. In fact, in all these cases, renal excretion of salt and water is reduced markedly. However, because of the limited ability of the kidneys and the necessity of excreting a minimum urine volume (about 400 to 500 ml/day), an attempt must be made to replace the fluids and electrolytes lost.

HYPOTONIC DEHYDRATION

Hypotonic dehydration results from efflux of hypertonic fluid. This condition occurs only in patients with the syndrome of inappropriate secretion of antidiuretic hormone (SIADH). This hormone increases the rate of water reabsorption from the distal and collecting tubules of the nephron. The mechanism of this action will be detailed in Chapter 11.

This syndrome is characterized by excessive retention of water, which persists despite a concomitant reduction in the osmolality of the extracellular fluid. Clinical findings include (1) hyponatremia along with plasma hypo-osmolality; (2) continued renal excretion of sodium; (3) a markedly below normal urine osmolality, but less than maximally dilute; and (4) normal renal and adrenal functions. For a further discussion of the pathophysiology of this syndrome and its treatment, the reader is referred to the excellent paper of Bartter and Schwartz (1967).

HYPERTONIC DEHYDRATION

Hypertonic dehydration may be produced by efflux of hypotonic fluid, such as in severe sweating. This results in an increased plasma crystalloid osmotic pressure, which causes water to move by osmosis from cells to interstitium to plasma. If the dehydration is too severe, this induced osmotic flow of water into the plasma may not be sufficient to prevent the onset of circulatory failure.

Renal response to severe sweating is a marked decrease in water excretion, thereby producing a very concentrated urine. To aid the kidneys in their efforts, ingestion or intravenous infusion of hypotonic saline or oral intake of water along with salt tablets is helpful.

Deviations from normal in volume and osmolality of the intra- and extracellular compartments, the direction of fluid shift, and the controlled renal excretion in response to the above forcings (with the exception of hypertonic dehydration) are given elsewhere (Table 1-2).

REPRESENTATION OF FLUID SHIFT:
DARROW-YANNET DIAGRAM

A convenient method of depicting the changes in volume and osmolality of the extra- and intracellular fluid compartments in response to the above forcings is the use of the classic *Darrow-Yannet diagram*. The procedure consists of representing each of the fluid compartments by a rectangle, whose width and height indicate, respectively, the volume and osmolality of that compartment. Also, to illustrate the comparative effects of a forcing on a given compartment and the possible interaction between compartments, the rectangles representing the extra- and intracellular compartments are placed side by side.

Figure 3-8 shows such a diagram, depicting changes from normal in

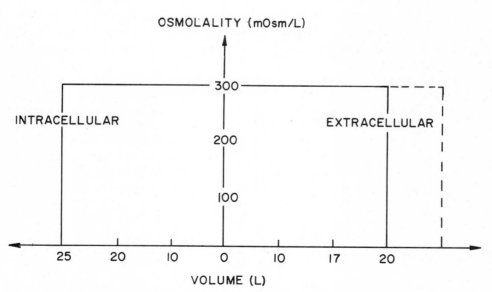

Figure 3-8. Schematic representation of changes from normal in the volume and osmolality of the extra- and intracellular fluid compartments after intravenous infusion of isotonic saline. [Modified from Darrow, D. C., and Yannet, H. (1935).]

the extra- and intracellular fluid compartments following intravenous infusion of a large volume of isotonic saline solution. In this diagram, solid lines represent the normal pattern of fluid distribution, whereas the dashed lines indicate changes from normal in the fluid distribution in response to the forcing. Note also that the area of the rectangle, for each compartment, represents the total milliosmoles of solutes in that compartment:

$$\text{Area (mOsm)} = \text{Volume (L)} \times \text{Osmolality (mOsm/L)} \qquad (3\text{-}10)$$

This expression is useful when determining the direction of fluid shift as well as the final steady state values of the volume and osmolality of the compartment.

To gain experience in using such a diagram, solve problems 3-3 and 3-4 following this chapter, by showing with a Darrow-Yannet plot the change in volumes and osmolalities of the extra- and intracellular fluid compartments after each forcing.

SUMMARY

The materials presented thus far have revealed four important operational features of the renal-body fluid regulating system. (1) The kidneys play a central role in maintaining the constancy of the internal environment, a direct consequence of stabilizing the volume and composition of the extracellular fluid. (2) Since the *blood volume* is an integral part of the extracellular compartment, its regulation is indispensable to homeostasis. (3) On the input side, we could exercise some degree of control over the rate of fluid intake, both orally and parenterally. (4) However, on the output side, the kidneys are the only system which can control the rate of fluid loss; the extrarenal losses, both gastrointestinal and insensible, would presumably occur with little or no control.

In clinical practice, you will be confronted with a more challenging and difficult problem, notwithstanding its enormous reward. You must deduce the causes from the effects and diagnose disease from the symptoms. The keenness of such a deductive effort will depend, in large part, on your knowledge of the various factors affecting the distribution of body fluids and the renal and extrarenal mechanisms involved in maintaining the normal water and electrolyte balance.

Let us now proceed to detail these mechanisms, beginning with an overview of the renal system.

PROBLEMS

3-1. The total solute excreted in a 24 hr urine sample is 1200 milliosmoles. Calculate the total 24 hr excreted urine volume that has to contain this amount of solute if the average urine specific gravity were (a) 1.015, (b) 1.020, and (c) 1.035.

3-2. A patient was given 620 g of human serum albumin over a period of 16 days. Analysis of urinary nitrogen excreted revealed that 468 g of exogenous albumin was metabolized. Other laboratory data showed that the plasma volume rose from 3.86 liters to 4.29 liters; plasma albumin concentration rose from 3.86 to 5.11 g%; total plasma protein rose from 6.54 to 7.63 g%; total circulating plasma albumin rose from 149 to 219 g; and hematocrit fell from 47.5 to 41.7%. Calculate the amount of unmetabolized exogenous albumin in (a) the plasma and (b) the interstitial fluids.

3-3. Consider a 70 kg man whose total body water is 60% of his body weight. If the ratio of the intracellular volume (V_C) to extracellular volume (V_E) is 1.47, and the initial osmolar concentration ([Os]) is 300 mOsm/L, calculate the final osmolar concentration and volume of each of the two compartments after the following forcings, assuming no renal excretion:
a. Infusion of 300 ml of a 15 g% saline solution.
b. Infusion of 2 liters of a 0.9 g% saline solution.
c. Infusion of 4 liters of a 5 g% glucose solution.

3-4. Calculate the final volume and osmolality (equivalent to NaCl) of the extracellular and intracellular compartments after the following forcings.
a. Severe sweating resulting in the loss of 3 liters of water having a NaCl concentration of 75 mEq/L.
b. Oral ingestion of 3 liters of hypertonic saline having a concentration of 450 mEq/L.
c. Oral intake of 2 liters of plain water.
In these calculations assume the following initial normal values: Intracellular volume (V_C)   = 30 liters.
                 Extracellular volume (V_E)   = 15 liters.
                 Plasma osmolality $[Os]_p$ = 300 mOsm/L.
                 Plasma sodium concentration $[Na]_p$ = 150 mEq/L.

3-5. The accompanying table presents deviations from normal findings for five patients.
a. In the first column, enter your choice of an appropriate forcing combination (isotonic, hypotonic, or hypertonic, and efflux or influx; for example, isotonic influx) that accounts for the findings.

   b. In the last column, enter the name of one condition (or
       disease) which is characterized by the findings.
   Definition of symbols used:
   V_p = Plasma volume
   $[Na]_p$ = Plasma sodium concentration
   $[Pr]_p$ = Plasma protein concentration
   Ht   = Hematocrit
   $[Na]_u$ = Urinary sodium concentration

Patient	Forcings	V_p	$[Na]_p$	$[Pr]_p$	Ht	$[Na]_u$	Condition or Disease
1	_____	+	0	−	−	+	_____
2	_____	−	+	+	+	+	_____
3	_____	+	+	−	−	+	_____
4	_____	−	0	+	+	−	_____
5	_____	+	−	−	−	−	_____

3-6. Briefly explain the role of proteins in the differential
      distribution of anions and cations between plasma and
      interstitial fluid compartments.

3-7. Briefly discuss the current concepts of tissue fluid formation
      and list the forces involved and their modes of operation.

3-8. State concisely why the effective plasma protein oncotic
      pressure increases disproportionately as the plasma protein
      concentration increases.

3-9. Define edema and briefly discuss the various conditions which
      precipitate edema formation.

3-10. Define osmosis, osmolality, and osmotic pressure.

REFERENCES

1. Allison, M. M., Lipham, E. M., and Gottschalk, C. W.: Hydrostatic
    pressure in the rat kidney. *Am. J. Physiol. 223*:975-983, 1972.

2. Bartter, F. C., and Schwartz, W. B.: The syndrome of
    inappropriate secretion of antidiuretic hormone. *Am. J. Med.
    42*:790-806, 1967.

3. Chapman, W. H., Bulger, R. E., Cutler, R. E., and Striker, G. E.: *The Urinary System, An Integrated Approach.* W. B. Saunders Co., Philadelphia, 1973.

4. Darrow, D. C., and Hellerstein, S.: Interpretation of certain changes in body water and electrolytes. *Physiol. Rev. 38*:114-137, 1958.

5. Darrow, D. C., and Yannet, H.: The change in the distribution of body water accompanying increase and decrease in extracellular electrolyte. *J. Clin. Invest. 14*:266-275, 1935.

6. Deane, N.: *Kidney and Electrolytes.* Prentice-Hall, Inc., Englewood Cliffs, N. J., 1966.

7. Elkinton, J. R., and Danowski, T.: *The Body Fluids: Basic Physiology and Practical Therapeutics.* The Williams & Wilkins Co., Baltimore, 1955.

8. Guyton, A. C.: A concept of negative interstitial pressure based on pressures in implanted perforated capsules. *Circ. Res. 12*:399-414, 1963.

9. Guyton, A. C.: Interstitial fluid pressure. II. Pressure-volume curves of interstitial spaces. *Circ. Res. 16*:452-460, 1965.

10. Guyton, A. C.: *Textbook of Medical Physiology.* W. B. Saunders Co., Philadelphia, 1971.

11. Guyton, A. C., Coleman, T. G., and Granger, H. J.: Circulation: overall regulation. *Ann. Rev. Physiol. 34*:13-46, 1972.

12. Landis, E. M., and Pappenheimer, J. R.: Exchange of substances through the capillary walls. In: *Handbook of Physiology.* Vol. 2, Sec. 2, *Circulation.* Edited by W. F. Hamilton and P. Dow. Washington, D. C., American Physiological Society, 1963, pp. 961-1034.

13. Mayerson, H. S.: Physiologic importance of lymph. In: *Handbook of Physiology.* Vol. 2, Sec. 2, *Circulation.* Edited by W. F. Hamilton and P. Dow. Washington, D. C., American Physiological Society, 1963, pp. 1035-1073.

14. Pappenheimer, H. R., and Soto-Rivera, A.: Effective osmotic pressure of the plasma proteins and other quantities associated with the capillary circulation in the hind limbs of cats and dogs. *Am. J. Physiol. 152*:471-491, 1948.

15. Renkin, E. M.: Capillary blood flow and transcapillary exchange. *Physiologist 9*:361-366, 1966.

16. Renkin, E. M., and Zaun, B. D.: Effects of adrenal hormones on

capillary permeability in perfused rat tissues. *Am. J. Physiol. 180*:498-502, 1955.

17. Starling, E. H.: On the absorption of fluids from the connective tissue spaces. *J. Physiol. 19*:312-326, 1896.

18. Zweifach, B. W., and Intaglietta, M.: Mechanics of fluid movement across single capillaries in the rabbit. *Microvasc. Res. 1*:83-101, 1968.

Chapter 4

AN OVERVIEW OF THE RENAL SYSTEM

The primary function of the renal system is to stabilize the volume and electrolyte concentration of the extracellular fluid, and indirectly those of the intracellular fluid compartment, by forming urine. Specifically, the kidneys:

1. Conserve water and osmoles normally present in the body.

2. Conserve the major electrolytes of body fluids, especially sodium, potassium, bicarbonate, and chloride ions.

3. Eliminate excess water, electrolytes (especially hydrogen ions), and osmoles resulting from fortuitous influxes.

4. Eliminate metabolic waste products of which the body is the source and toxic materials which may gain access to the body.

The functional unit of the kidney is the *nephron*, of which there are 1.25 million per kidney. A representative nephron, shown in Figure 4-1, consists of two major components: (1) a *renal corpuscle* or *ultrafilter*, comprising a tuft of glomerular capillaries and Bowman's capsule, and (2) a *renal tubule* or *tubular exchanger*, composed of a sequence of a proximal tubule, a loop of Henle, and distal and collecting tubules.

The mechanism of operation of the nephron consists of three processes:

1. First, the renal corpuscle forms a large volume (about 180 L/24 hr) of essentially protein-free *filtrate*, having the same osmolar concentration of all the crystalloids as that in the aqueous phase of plasma. The filtrate thus formed contains all the plasma solutes regardless of whether they are to be conserved or eliminated.

2. The renal tubules then *selectively* process this filtrate. Approximately 99% of the filtered water (178.5 L/24 hr) is conserved, allowing only 1.5 L/24 hr to be excreted in urine. The filtered crystalloids are selectively conserved by *two* tubular exchange processes: (a) *reabsorption* from tubules into the blood of those substances that the body needs, and (b) *secretion* from blood into the tubules of those substances which must be eliminated from the body.

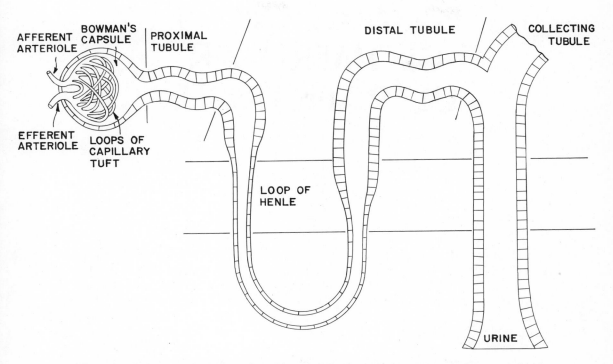

Figure 4-1. A schematic diagram of a representative nephron.

3. The renal tubules also selectively conserve the total quantity of filtered water and osmoles, thereby adjusting *urine osmolality* to the body needs.

We will examine each of these processes in detail in the ensuing chapters.

Chapter 5

FORMATION OF GLOMERULAR ULTRAFILTRATE

The normal human kidneys receive a *blood* flow of about 1200 ml/min, which, assuming a hematocrit (Ht) of 45%, corresponds to 660 ml/min *plasma* flow. At the same time, the glomerular ultrafilter forms 125 ml/min of glomerular filtrate. The *filtration fraction*, defined as the ratio of the glomerular filtration rate (GFR) to renal plasma flow (RPF), is thus 125/660 = 0.19. This means that 19% of the entering plasma volume is removed as filtrate. Note that the filtration fraction refers to the bulk volume of fluids, not to their solutes, and only to the filtration stage.

The filtrate thus formed is essentially protein-free, containing all the crystalloids in the same osmolar concentration as that in the aqueous phase of plasma, except for a small difference due to the Gibbs-Donnan effect. The mechanism of glomerular ultrafiltration is similar to that for tissue fluid formation described in Chapter 3. Hence, for ultrafiltration to occur, sufficient energy, supplied by the cardiovascular system, is required to develop (1) an *osmotic force* (π) to separate proteins from the plasma, and (2) an *hydrostatic force* (P) to overcome the frictional resistance of the ultrafilter membrane to filtrate flow. Since the ultrafiltrate separates primarily proteins, the magnitude of the required *osmotic force* is small and equal to the plasma protein oncotic pressure in the glomerular capillaries (π_g). The magnitude of the *hydrostatic force* on the other hand, is large and equal to the difference between the glomerular capillary blood pressure (P_g) and the interstitial pressure in Bowman's capsule and connected tubules (P_i). Thus, for a given ultrafilter permeability, the glomerular filtration rate (GFR) bears a direct and positive relationship to the algebraic sum of these forces or the effective filtration force (ΔP_f):

$$GFR = k_g(P_g - P_i - \pi_g) = k_g \cdot \Delta P_f \qquad (5-1)$$

where k_g is the *filtration coefficient* (an expression of fluid permeability of the ultrafilter membrane) and is expressed in ml/min per mm Hg. This relationship is depicted diagrammatically in Figure 5-1.

From this relationship, we see that the rate of formation of glomerular filtrate depends on two factors: (1) the *structural* characteristics of the ultrafilter and the permeability of its filtering membranes, symbolized by k_g, and (2) the *hemodynamics* of blood supplying the nephron, symbolized by ΔP_f. Let us examine the role of each and the factors influencing their functions.

STRUCTURAL AND FUNCTIONAL CHARACTERISTICS OF THE RENAL ULTRAFILTER

The renal ultrafilter consists of (1) an inner layer of endothelial cells lining the glomerular capillary wall, (2) a layer of noncellular basement membrane, and (3) a layer of epithelial cells making up the Bowman's capsule, continuous with the cuboidal cells of the tubules. The interstitial space between these layers is occupied by a syncytium of *mesangial* cells. Figure 5-2 shows an electron micrograph of the structural components of the renal ultrafilter.

The endothelial and epithelial cell membranes each have a thickness of about 400 Angstrom units ($\overset{\circ}{A} = 10^{-8} cm$), while the basement membrane has a thickness of about 3250 $\overset{\circ}{A}$ in humans (Jorgensen and Weis Bentzon, 1968) and about 1250 $\overset{\circ}{A}$ in mice (Rhodin, 1955). Thus, the plasma filtrate must pass through two relatively thin layers and the thick basement membrane.

Both the vascular endothelial and capsular epithelial layers are permeable to water and crystalloids. The basement membrane is believed to be a hydrated gel with limited permeability, restricting the passage of plasma colloids (proteins and lipids).

Functionally, the filtration coefficient (k_g) is determined by three factors: (1) The *pore size* of the three membranes making up the ultrafilter. (2) The *spatial* alignment of the passing molecules and

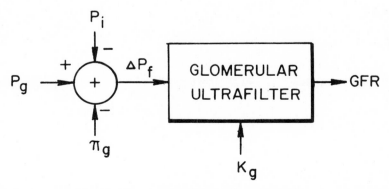

Figure 5-1. A functional diagram of glomerular ultrafiltration.

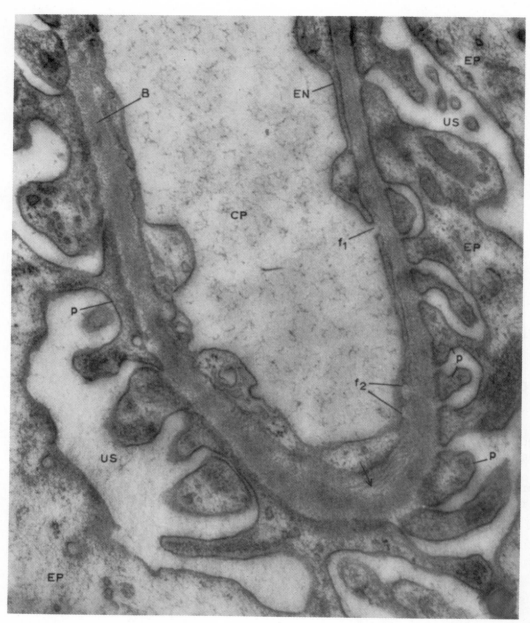

Figure 5-2. Electron micrograph of a glomerular capillary loop of the rat, showing endothelium (EN) with fenestrae (f_1, f_2), basement membrane (B), epithelium (EP) with podocytes (p), capillary lumen (CP), and urinary space (US). [From Farquhar, M. G., Wissig, S. L., and Palade, G. E. (1961).]

membrane pores and their geometric relationships. This is called *steric hindrance*. (3) The *shearing forces* arising from sliding of molecules past the pore walls, slowing down their motion. This is called *viscous drag*. For charged molecules, due to steric hindrance, the rate of penetration is inversely proportional to the size of the molecule relative to pore size. For viscous drag, the rate of penetration is also inversely proportional to pore size, due to the stationary layer of fluid lining the pores. Thus, the greater the ratio of the diameter of the molecule to pore size, the greater is the viscous drag.

As defined by Equation 5-1, GFR is proportional to the effective filtration force (ΔP_f) required to overcome the frictional resistance of the ultrafilter to filtrate flow. From structural and physical considerations given above, it is apparent that the magnitude of these *frictional forces* are a function of the size, number, and spatial distribution of pores making up the ultrafilter. Although electron microscopic studies have not yet succeeded in defining a clear-cut anatomical basis for these pore-like properties of the ultrafilter, physiological studies of the glomerular sieving of various solutes have yielded estimates of the effective pore size, their spatial distribution, and functional characteristics. The following analysis of estimation of pore size of glomerular capillary is adapted from Pappenheimer (1953).

To simplify the analysis, Pappenheimer made two assumptions. *First*, the filtrate flow through the ultrafilter has a *laminar* profile. This implies a linear velocity gradient along the glomerular capillary with maximum velocity occurring at mid-length. *Second*, the ultrafilter has N parallel pores through which the filtrate flows. Incorporating these assumptions into Equation 5-1, we obtain

$$GFR = \frac{N\pi r^4}{8\eta x} \cdot \Delta P_f \qquad (5-2)$$

where r is the pore radius, η is the filtrate viscosity, x is the ultrafilter thickness, and the other terms have already been defined. Equation 5-2 is named after *Poiseuille*, who derived it for flow through cylindrical tubes.

Since the total cross-sectional area of the pores (A_p) is equal to $N\pi r^2$, Equation 5-2 may be written as

$$GFR = \frac{A_p \cdot r^2}{8\eta x} \cdot \Delta P_f \qquad (5-3)$$

Comparing Equations 5-3 and 5-1 yields

$$K_g = \frac{A_p \cdot r^2}{8\eta x} \qquad (5-4)$$

This equation states that the ultrafilter permeability or filtration coefficient (K_g) is directly proportional to the square of the pore radius and total cross-sectional area, and inversely proportional to filtrate viscosity and ultrafilter thickness. Thus, any factor that alters these parameters has an adverse effect on the ultrafilter permeability. However, because radius appears as a square quantity, its changes have a far greater effect on K_g than those of the other parameters.

To estimate pore size, we may reaarange Equation 5-4 as follows,

$$r = \sqrt{\frac{\sqrt{8\eta K_g}}{A_p/x}} \qquad (5-5)$$

For artificial membranes, such as collodion or cellophane, the filtration coefficient (K_g), the total cross-sectional area (A_p), and the membrane thickness (x) can be readily determined. However, in the case of the glomerular membrane of the normally functioning kidney, measurement of these parameters is not practical. Therefore, to estimate pore size of the ultrafilter membrane, under *in vivo* conditions, a modification of Equation 5-5 has been used.

It is an experimental fact that the rate of diffusion (passage) of a molecule through a membrane in comparison to its rate of free diffusion through water is proportional to the pore area. If K_S is the coefficient of free diffusion of a substance S in water, $\Delta[S]$ is the difference in the concentration of S on the two sides of the membrane, and dS/dt is the rate of passage of S through the membrane with a surface area A_p and thickness x, then, according to the Fick diffusion equation:

$$\frac{dS}{dt} = K_S \cdot A_p \frac{\Delta[S]}{x} \qquad (5-6)$$

Substituting for A_p/x in Equation 5-5 its equivalent from Equation 5-6, we obtain the following equation for pore radius,

$$r = \sqrt{\frac{8\eta \cdot K_g \cdot K_S \cdot \Delta[S]}{dS/dt}} \qquad (5-7)$$

To apply this equation to a living glomerular capillary membrane, we must determine K_S, dS/dt, and $\Delta[S]$. Although quantities K_S and dS/dt are difficult to assess, it is relatively easy to measure the difference in concentration, $\Delta[S]$, on the two sides of the membrane. The ease of measuring $\Delta[S]$, coupled with the knowledge that certain small molecular weight proteins, such as myoglobin or egg albumin, when infused intravenously are partially filtered by the ultrafilter, provided the basis for using the following modified diffusion equation called the *molecular sieving equation*:

$$\frac{[S]_f}{[S]_p} = \frac{1 + \dfrac{K_S}{GFR} \cdot \dfrac{8\eta K_g}{r^2}}{\dfrac{1 + 2.4\, a/r}{2(1 - a/r)^2 - (1 - a/r)^4}} + \frac{K_S}{GFR} \cdot \frac{8\eta K_g}{r^2} \qquad (5\text{-}8)$$

where $[S]_f$ is the concentration of S (myoglobin or egg albumin) in the filtrate, $[S]_p$ is the plasma concentration of S, r is the pore radius, and (a) is the Einstein-Stoke radius of S—that is, the radius of a sphere which would diffuse at the same rate as molecules of S. This equation takes into account the effects of steric hindrance and viscous drag on protein filtration. It has been used to measure the number and pore size of muscle capillary membrane as well as to characterize the glomerular ultrafilter of intact animals and man. For details of derivation of Equation 5-8, the reader is referred to Pappenheimer's paper (1953).

To solve Equation 5-8 for pore radius (r) and to apply it to a living glomerular membrane, we must evaluate the terms $[S]_f/[S]_p$, K_S, K_g, (a), and GFR. The values of K_S and (a) for myoglobin and egg albumin, as well as their filtrate to plasma concentration ratios, $[S]_f/[S]_p$, have been determined (Table 5-1). Note that the larger the substance, the smaller is the ratio of its filtrate to plasma concentration. The glomerular filtration rate (GFR) can also be readily measured (see Chapter 6). Thus, simultaneous solution of

TABLE 5-1

Relationships Among Molecular Weight, Molecular
Dimensions, and Glomerular Sieving of Solutes

Substance	Molecular Weight (grams)	Radius from Diffusion Coefficient (K_g) (Angstroms)	$\dfrac{[S]_f}{[S]_p}$
Water	18	1.0	1.0
Urea	60	1.6	1.0
Glucose	180	3.6	1.0
Sucrose	342	4.4	1.0
Inulin	5200	14.8	0.98
Myoglobin	17,000	19.5	0.75
Egg Albumin	43,500	28.5	0.22
Hemoglobin	68,000	32.5	0.03
Serum Albumin	69,000	35.5	<0.01

Equation 5-8 for myoglobin and egg albumin provides two equations, permitting evaluation of the two unknowns, namely, filtration coefficient (K_g) and pore radius (r).

The functional characteristics of the glomerular capillaries, as determined by Equation 5-8, are summarized in Table 5-2. Because many simplifying assumptions were made in calculating the table entries, their absolute values should be regarded with some reservations. Nevertheless, these quantitative data have portrayed a revealing picture of the glomerular membrane and have provided an insight into the nature of cellular processes involved in the formation of the filtrate. Recognizing the importance of the effective filtration forces (ΔP_f), the present analysis has emphasized the role of two intermembrane diffusive and flow forces in the formation of filtrate, namely, *diffusion* and *filtration* or *bulk flow*. A detailed consideration of these and other renal transport processes is given in Chapter 7.

HEMODYNAMICS OF GLOMERULAR FILTRATION

The glomerular filtration rate depends largely on the blood pressure-flow relationship in the glomerular capillaries. The capillary circulation, in turn, is determined by the blood supply of the nephron. Since the latter is an integral component of the renal circulation, a review of the intrarenal blood supply is essential to an understanding of the hemodynamics of glomerular filtration.

BLOOD SUPPLY OF THE KIDNEY

Each kidney receives its blood supply from a single renal artery, which usually divides into ventral and dorsal branches before entering the hilus (Fig. 5-3). Each branch divides into a number of interlobar arteries, passing between calyces and penetrating the renal tissues between the pyramids. The interlobar arteries, at the

TABLE 5-2

Functional Characteristics of Glomerular Capillaries

Total glomerular capillary area	5500-15,000 cm^2/100 g kidney
Total capillary pore area (A_p)	500-1000 cm^2/100 g kidney
Functional pore area	1/10-1/20
Pore diameter ($2r$)	70-100 $\overset{\circ}{A}$
Pore length (x)	400-600 $\overset{\circ}{A}$
Filtration coefficient (K_g)	1.9-4.5 ml/min/mm Hg/100 g kidney

[Modified from Pappenheimer, J. R. (1955).]

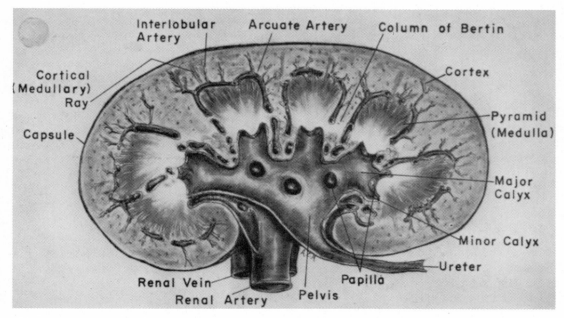

Figure 5-3. Coronal section of the kidney showing gross structure and vascular supply. (From Allen, A. C.: *The Kidney: Medical and Surgical Diseases.* 2nd ed. New York, Grune & Stratton, 1962. Used by permission.)

corticomedullary border, bend around the base of the medullary pyramids to form the arch-like arcuate arteries. From the arcuate arteries, the interlobular arteries arise at right angles, in turn giving rise to short pre-glomerular arterioles known as the afferent arterioles, which supply blood to the nephron. Each afferent arteriole breaks up into from 20 to 40 capillary loops grouped into from 5 to 8 lobules. This capillary tuft is known as the glomerulus. The glomerular capillaries combine to form the post-glomerular arteriole, known as the efferent arteriole. Insofar as the glomerular capillaries are concerned, the kidney is the only organ in which true capillaries are fed and drained by arterioles. The efferent arteriole, in turn, gives rise to the peritubular capillary network, which pervades the tubules of the nephron. These capillaries will eventually combine to form the venules, which in turn become the interlobular veins, the arcuate veins, the interlobar veins, and the renal vein.

There is an elaborate network of lymphatic vessels in the cortex, but none in the medulla. The lymphatic vessels accompany and surround the interlobar, arcuate, and interlobular arteries. A second lymphatic plexus underlies the kidney capsule. There are no lymphatics in the glomerulus. With this background, let us now focus on the hemodynamics of blood flow in the glomerular capillaries.

HEMODYNAMICS OF BLOOD FLOW IN
GLOMERULAR CAPILLARIES

As depicted in Figure 5-4, the afferent arteriole is the only source of blood supply to the glomerular capillaries. The latter consists of 20 to 40 capillary loops arranged in parallel. This anatomical configuration allows for rapid blood flow through the glomerulus and provides maximum capillary surface area for filtration. After passing through the capillaries, the blood leaves through the efferent or post-glomerular arteriole. Accordingly, in the steady state, the glomerular filtration rate (GFR) is equal to the difference between the volume of blood flowing into ($\dot{V}_{in}$) and out of ($\dot{V}_{out}$) the glomerular capillaries:

$$GFR = \dot{V}_{in} - \dot{V}_{out} \tag{5-9}$$

The magnitude of these inflow and outflow volumes depend primarily on the *blood pressure* in the afferent (P_a) and efferent (P_e) arterioles and their respective *resistances* R_a and R_e. The arteriolar resistances are determined by the degree of constriction of smooth muscles in the pre- and post-glomerular arterioles.

Assuming that the locus of glomerular capillary resistance, R_g, is midway between R_a and R_e, the magnitude of $\dot{V}_{in}$ is then determined by the pressure gradient ($P_a - P_g$) across the two resistances R_a and R_g in series:

$$\dot{V}_{in} = \frac{P_a - P_g}{R_a + R_g} \tag{5-10}$$

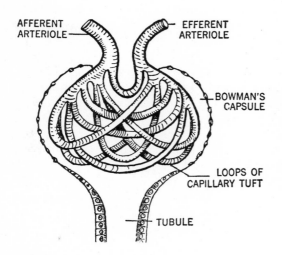

AFFERENT ARTERIOLE

EFFERENT ARTERIOLE

BOWMAN'S CAPSULE

LOOPS OF CAPILLARY TUFT

TUBULE

Figure 5-4. Structural details of renal corpuscle. (From Best, C. H., and Taylor, N. B.: *The Physiological Basis of Medical Practice.* 6th ed. Copyright 1955, The Williams & Wilkins Company, Baltimore.)

where P_g is the blood pressure in the glomerular capillaries, and the denominator is the algebraic sum of the two resistances in series.

Similarly, an expression for $\dot{V}_{out}$ in terms of the appropriate pressures and resistances would be

$$\dot{V}_{out} = \frac{P_g - P_e}{R_g + R_e} \qquad (5\text{-}11)$$

Since potential changes in R_g are infinitesimal as compared to those in R_a and R_e, Equations 5-10 and 5-11 may be further simplified by dropping the R_g terms.

Substituting the simplified Equations 5-10 and 5-11 into Equation 5-9, and consolidating the fractions, we get:

$$GFR = \frac{P_a - P_g}{R_a} - \frac{P_g - P_e}{R_e} \qquad (5\text{-}12)$$

Since P_g decreases from an initial value equal to P_a to a final value equal to P_e, if we assume a linear decrease, its value at midway in the glomerulus would be $P_g = (P_a + P_e)/2$. Substituting this in Equation 5-12, we get:

$$GFR = \frac{1}{2}\left\{\frac{P_a - P_e}{R_a} - \frac{P_a - P_e}{R_e}\right\} \qquad (5\text{-}13)$$

Equation 5-13 reveals that, insofar as the hemodynamics of the glomerular circulation are concerned, the magnitude of GFR is determined by blood pressures and resistances of the afferent and efferent arterioles. Thus, a step increase in P_a, assuming the other parameters remain unchanged, increases GFR, while a step increase in R_a decreases GFR. In contrast, a step increase in R_e increases GFR. It should be remembered that these alterations in GFR are mediated by induced changes in P_g.

Needless to say, normally changes in P_a and P_e are related to changes in systemic arterial (P_{AS}) and venous (P_{VS}) blood pressures. Hence, for a given intrarenal resistance, a step increase in P_{AS} causes a proportional increase in P_a and eventually in GFR. Conversely, a step increase in P_{VS} induces a proportional increase in P_e, thereby reducing GFR.

Changes in plasma protein concentration, and hence plasma protein oncotic pressure (π_p) markedly influence GFR. This effect is mediated by changes in π_g. As ultrafiltration proceeds, π_g increases from an initial value equal to the protein oncotic pressure in the afferent arteriole (π_a) to a final value equal to that in the efferent arteriole (π_e). Since π_a is nearly identical to the plasma protein oncotic pressure in the systemic blood (π_p), changes in π_g may be expressed in terms of π_p:

$$\pi_g = \left(\frac{RPF}{RPF - GFR} \right) \pi_p \qquad (5\text{-}14)$$

Equation 5-14 is an example of the application of the law of conservation of mass to plasma proteins. It states that for a given renal plasma flow (RPF) and π_p, the incremental increase in π_g is proportional to GFR. Thus, changes in GFR, resulting from pathological alterations in glomerular hemodynamics or ultrafilter permeability, have a profound influence on protein homeostasis as well as on the normal functioning of the renal tubules.

As defined earlier (Equation 5-1), the glomerular filtration rate depends on the permeability of the renal ultrafilter and the algebraic sum of the hydrostatic and protein oncotic pressures prevailing across its membranes. The magnitude of these pressures in mammalian kidneys have been estimated by various methods. The best quantitative values are obtained by "micropuncture techniques." Briefly, the procedure involves puncturing surface glomeruli with glass micropipettes, having an outer diameter of 6 to 10 μ. The glomeruli are identified under stereomicroscope with illumination provided by passing a high intensity light through a rod of fused quartz.

Using the above procedure along with a servo-nulling micropipette transducer, the hemodynamic forces involved in the ultrafiltration have been measured directly by three groups of investigators. The values are summarized in Table 5-3.

An unexpected finding in two of these studies (Brenner et al., 1971; Andreucci et al., 1971) was that the effective filtration pressure (ΔP_f) decreased from the values given in the table at the

TABLE 5-3

Forces Involved in Glomerular Ultrafiltration in Rat

Mean systemic arterial pressure, $\overline{P}_{AS}$	110-130 mm Hg
Glomerular capillary pressure, P_g	45-52 mm Hg
Interstitial pressure in Bowman's capsule, P_i	8-15 mm Hg
Net hydrostatic pressure, $(P_g - P_i)$	35-37 mm Hg
Glomerular protein oncotic pressure, π_g	18-26 mm Hg
Effective filtration pressure, ΔP_f	10-18 mm Hg
Filtration coefficient, K_g $\quad 3.0 \times 10^{-5} - 7.5 \times 10^{-5}$	(ml/min·mm Hg)/
	cm^2 cap. surface

[Data from Brenner et al. (1971), Andreucci et al. (1971), and Allison et al. (1972).]

arteriolar end of the glomerulus to zero at the efferent end of the glomerulus. Another important finding (Andreucci et al., 1971) was that the changes in single nephron GFR (SNGFR) were proportional to those of effective filtration pressure after ureteral obstruction and mild or massive plasma volume expansion by intravenous saline infusion, suggesting no significant change in glomerular permeability under these conditions. Furthermore, Brenner and associates (1971) found that the systemic arterial pressure fell an average of 51% by the time the blood reached the glomerulus. A second pressure drop occurred between the glomerulus and the efferent arteriole. Thus, as shown in Figure 5-5, and in consistence with Equation 5-13, the major drop in the intrarenal vascular pressure occurs on either side of the glomerular capillary bed.

The foregoing analysis reveals that the formation of the glomerular filtrate depends on the structural and permeability characteristics of the ultrafilter membrane and the hemodynamic factors that determine the effective filtration pressure. Thus, any factor that alters either of these variables will have a profound influence on GFR. The following are some examples of factors affecting ΔP_f and hence GFR:

1. *Elevation of systemic arterial pressure,* following intravenous fluid infusion, leads to an increase in P_a, P_g, and hence ΔP_f, which increases GFR.

2. In *hemorrhagic shock,* when the blood pressure falls below 50 mm Hg, *anuria* results. This is due to a marked reduction in P_g and

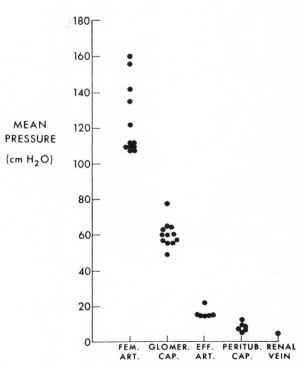

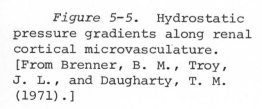

Figure 5-5. Hydrostatic pressure gradients along renal cortical microvasculature. [From Brenner, B. M., Troy, J. L., and Daugharty, T. M. (1971).]

hence GFR. If blood is reinfused, arterial blood pressure will rise, thereby increasing GFR and restarting urine formation.

3. Elevation of *ureteral pressure* or *intrapelvic pressure,* due to obstruction or stone formation, leads to an increase in tubular interstitial pressure, thereby decreasing ΔP_f and hence GFR.

4. *A rise in renal venous pressure* leads to distention of the venules and the capillaries. The resulting rise in the capillary blood pressure compresses adjacent tubules until pressure in them equals that in the capillaries. The net result is a decrease in ΔP_f and hence in GFR.

5. *A decrease in plasma protein concentration,* which might occur in protein deficiency, starvation, cirrhosis of the liver (decreased protein synthesis), or nephrotic syndrome (increased urinary loss of proteins) is expected to decrease π_g, thereby increasing ΔP_f and hence GFR. However, this expected increase in GFR may not occur in early stages of the diseases. An explanation might be that the reduced plasma protein concentration in these conditions tends to have a much greater effect in the systemic circulation, where it reduces the effective circulating blood volume, due to edema formation. Therefore, the effect of decrease in π_g on GFR will be somewhat blunted by a parallel reduction in P_g, secondary to reduced plasma volume (Deane, 1966).

COMPOSITION OF THE GLOMERULAR ULTRAFILTRATE

Chemical analyses of the glomerular filtrate fluid (f), collected by micropuncturing the early portions of the proximal convoluted tubules, have revealed that it is *iso-osmotic* and *isotonic* with the similarly collected protein-free plasma fluid (P) from the glomerulus (Windhager, 1968).

The ultrafiltrate, as described above, is virtually a protein-free solution. It consists of about 94 per cent water by volume and 6 per cent solutes. It contains two types of solutes: electrolytes and nonelectrolytes. Table 5-4 compares the concentration of important electrolytes in the ultrafiltrate with that of plasma. Note that there is a slight but significant difference in the concentration of cations and anions in the plasma and ultrafiltrate. This difference, as explained in Chapter 2, is due to the retention of protein anions on the plasma side. The ratio of anion or cation concentration of filtrate to that of plasma is called the Gibbs-Donnan ratio. Since proteins are negatively charged at normal hydrogen ion concentration, the Gibbs-Donnan ratio for cations is less than unity, and that for anions is greater than unity. Typically, the Gibbs-Donnan ratios for the most prevalent cations and anions of the plasma and filtrate, namely, sodium and chloride, are 0.95 and 1.05, respectively.

TABLE 5-4

A Comparison of Electrolyte Concentration in
Plasma and Ultrafiltrate

Electrolytes	Plasma Concentration (mEq/L)	Ultrafiltrate Concentration (mEq/L)	Gibbs-Donnan Ratio
Cations			
Sodium	142	135.0	0.95
Potassium	4	3.8	0.95
Calcium	5	2.5	0.50
Magnesium	3	1.5	0.50
	154	142.8	
Anions			
Chloride	103	108.0	1.05
Bicarbonate	27	28.4	1.05
Phosphate	2	2.0	1.00
Sulfate	1	1.0	1.00
Organic Acids	5	5.0	1.00
Proteins	16	0.0	0.00
	154	144.4	

REGULATION OF GLOMERULAR FILTRATION RATE

Experimental observations (reviewed by Thurau [1964] and Harvey [1964]) have shown that GFR increases linearly as the renal arterial pressure is increased from 20 to 90 mm Hg. However, when the renal arterial pressure is raised beyond 90 mm Hg, GFR remains constant. Similarly, RPF increases linearly when renal arterial pressure is raised from 10 to 70 mm Hg, but remains constant as the pressure is varied from 70 to 190 mm Hg. However, in contrast to GFR, RPF increases again as the pressure is raised beyond 190 mm Hg. This constancy of GFR and RPF when renal arterial pressure is varied from 90 to 190 mm Hg, shown in Figure 5-6, is called *autoregulation*. It has been observed in *denervated* and *isolated* kidneys during blockade of ganglia, and even in the absence of red blood cells. This intrinsic regulation of renal circulation is believed to be a means of stabilizing both the renal blood flow and glomerular filtration rate in the face of changes in the renal arterial pressure. The mechanism of this autoregulation may best be understood if we relate the renal blood flow (RBF), the driving renal arterial pressure (P), and the renal arterial resistance (R) by the equation RBF = P/R.

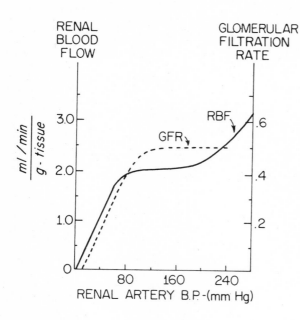

Figure 5-6. Steady state levels of renal blood flow (RBF) and glomerular filtration rate (GFR) as a function of perfusion pressure in denervated, blood-perfused kidney. Note the relative independence of pressure exhibited by flow and GFR. (Redrawn from Shipley and Study, *Amer. J. Physiol. 167*:676-688, 1951.)

Thus, referring to Figure 5-6, at pressure values below 70 mm Hg, renal blood flow is a positive linear function of pressure, while the renal resistance remains constant. At pressure values ranging from 70 to 190 mm Hg, the resistance becomes a positive linear function of pressure, while the flow increases very little. Since over such a pressure range the GFR is unchanged, the increase in resistance with increasing pressure is attributed to the increase in the resistance of the *afferent arteriole*. This pressure-flow relationship is one aspect of renal autoregulation. The other aspect is that when blood pressure exceeds 190 mm Hg, the filtration fraction (GFR/RPF) falls as the renal plasma flow increases.

The *adaptive* changes in the resistance of the afferent arteriole are directly related to the degree of vasoconstriction of the smooth muscles lining the walls of these vessels. That this is the mechanism by which constancy of GFR and RBF is maintained at normal blood pressure is supported by three lines of evidence:

1. Direct micropuncture measurement of glomerular capillary blood pressure (P_g) with simultaneous blood pressure recordings (Windhager, 1968) have shown that:

    (a) Up to a mean systemic arterial blood pressure ($\overline{P}_{AS}$) of 90 mm Hg, P_g is a positive linear function of $\overline{P}_{AS}$.

    (b) As the $\overline{P}_{AS}$ is varied between 90 and 190 mm Hg, P_g remains constant.

These findings are summarized in Figure 5-7.

2. The adaptive increase in the intrarenal resistance which follows an increase in the renal perfusion pressure is attributed to the contraction of the smooth muscle lining the walls of the afferent arterioles. This concept is the basis of the *myogenic theory* of renal autoregulation.

In support of this theory, Thurau and Kramer (1959) found that

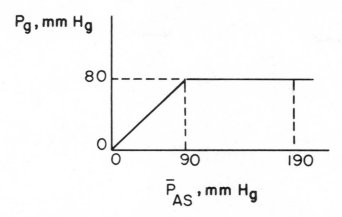

Figure 5-7. Relationship between glomerular capillary blood pressure (P_g) and mean systemic arterial pressure ($\overline{P}_{AS}$) over the range where renal blood flow is autoregulated.

paralysis of these muscles by papaverine (a smooth muscle relaxant) abolished renal autoregulation. They observed that, normally, a step change in renal arterial pressure in the range from 90 to 190 mm Hg, resulted in an immediate increase in renal blood flow followed by a phasic return to its initial value. However, following papaverine infusion, the same step change in pressure resulted in an immediate increase in the renal blood flow, which leveled off at the high value without any phasic response, indicating the loss of autoregulation.

   3. Recent studies, reviewed by Guyton et al. (1964), Vander (1967), and Davis (1971), have provided strong evidence in support of two other theories for an intrarenal, local feedback mechanism regulating GFR. This regulating system consists of a specialized structure within the nephron, called the *juxtaglomerular apparatus*. Before we can proceed to describe the function of this system, a brief review of its morphology is in order.

   MORPHOLOGY OF JUXTAGLOMERULAR APPARATUS. The distal convoluted tubule juxtaposes with the afferent arteriole as it penetrates the cortical tissues. The arteriolar endothelial cells and the tubular epithelial cells in the area of contact undergo a series of complex morphological changes, giving rise to the juxtaglomerular apparatus with three distinct cell types (Fig. 5-8):
   (a) <u>Granular Cells</u>. These are the differentiated smooth muscle cells in the media of the afferent arteriole (Barajas and Latta, 1967). They are believed to be the site of synthesis, storage, and release of renin (a "neutral" protease and a potential pressor enzyme).
   (b) <u>Macula Densa Cells</u>. These are the specialized tubular epithelial cells that mark the transition from the thick ascending limb of the loop of Henle (the pars recta of the distal tubule) to the pars convoluta of the distal tubule. These cells are closely associated anatomically with the granular cells. They are sensitive to the

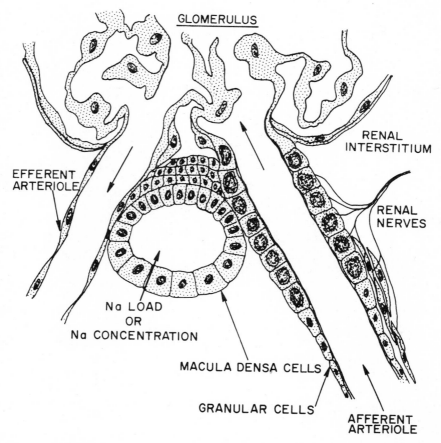

Figure 5-8. The structure of the renal ultrafilter and the juxtaglomerular apparatus. (Modified from Davis, J. O.: What signals the kidney to release renin? *Circ. Res. 28*:301-306, 1971. By permission of The American Heart Association, Inc.)

osmolality and the quantity of filtered sodium (sodium load) remaining in the fluid leaving the loop of Henle.

    (c) <u>Mesangial Cells</u>. These are the interstitial cells in contact with both the granular and macula densa cells.

    The regulation of GFR by the juxtaglomerular apparatus has been the subject of considerable investigation since its endocrine function was first suggested by Goormaghtigh (1945). Of the several theories advanced to date to explain the autoregulation of GFR (Renkin and Gilmore, 1973), that proposed by Thurau and associates (1967) has received the most attention. They proposed that the macula densa cells function as a part of an intrarenal feedback mechanism to regulate GFR. The support for this concept, known as the *macula densa theory* of renin release, has come from experiments in rats in which the distal tubules of single nephrons were perfused with solutions of different compositions. Thurau and co-workers (1967) found that in renin-rich kidneys (produced by sodium-free diet) perfusion of distal tubule with a solution of 150 and 300 mM NaCl resulted in a high incidence of proximal tubular collapse, which was taken as an indication of diminished GFR. Perfusion of the distal tubules with a sodium bromide solution produced similar results. However, perfusion with a solution of choline chloride or isotonic mannitol had little effect. Assuming that the perfused solution had reached the macula densa cells, these findings suggest that these cells are sensitive only to changes in sodium concentration of the tubular fluid and not to osmolality. The above response was almost completely abolished in rats with renin-depleted kidneys (produced by substituting isotonic saline for drinking water). These findings have recently been confirmed by additional experiments (Cooke et al., 1970; Schnermann et al., 1970).

The essence of the macula densa theory as it pertains to the present discussion may be summarized as follows.

A high concentration of sodium in the fluid passing by the *macula densa cells* stimulates the granular cells, presumably via the mesangial cells, to release renin into the adjacent afferent arteriolar blood. This enzyme combines with its substrate *angiotensinogen* (found chiefly in the α_2-globulin fraction of plasma) to form angiotensin I. This substance is readily converted into the potent vasopressor substance angiotensin II (Ng and Vane, 1967; Gocke et al., 1969). The increase in angiotensin II level in the adjacent afferent arteriolar blood causes constriction of the afferent arteriole, thereby reducing P_g and hence GFR. In this manner, changes in GFR manifested by changes in the sodium load and monitored by the macula densa cells, are kept within normal limits through this mechanism.

It should be noted that the above sequence of events is believed to operate at the individual nephron level. However, a recent microperfusion study of the loop of Henle and macula densa in rats (Morgan, 1971) has disputed the control of individual nephron GFR by the macula densa. Morgan found that the glomerular filtration rate of an individual nephron was remarkably independent of changes in the volume flow or composition of fluid bathing the macula densa cells. In view of his and other findings cited earlier, Morgan suggests that although changes in the sodium concentration at the macula densa may be the stimulus for renin release, its effects are not at the individual nephron level. The renin so released may enter the surrounding interstitium by diffusion, where it enhances local synthesis of angiotensin II and the eventual constriction of the afferent arterioles in that region. In this manner, changes in sodium concentration at the macula densa bring about a local negative feedback control of glomerular filtration rate in a few nephrons.

We may conclude that although the mechanism of renin release as a consequence of changes in sodium concentration in the tubular fluid at the macula densa is as yet unresolved, the involvement of the macula densa-renin-angiotensin system in a negative feedback control of GFR has not been disputed. A more detailed treatment of the physiological significance of the macula densa theory and its possible role in the renal-body fluid regulating system will be presented in Chapter 12.

Due to their strategic location, the juxtaglomerular (JG) cells also act as "volume" receptors by sensing the changes in blood flow in the afferent arteriole via the *granular cells*. This aspect of JG cell function has led to the formulation of the *baroreceptor theory* of renin release (Tobian, Tomboulian, and Janecek, 1959). Therefore, these cells play an important role in the extrarenal feedback mechanism regulating the volume and composition of the fluid entering and leaving the kidney, and hence the entire body fluids. This role of JG cells will be considered in Chapter 12.

From the foregoing discussion it is evident that the glomerular filtration rate and the various factors affecting it play a key role in the ultimate renal regulation of body fluids. To fully understand the changes in GFR and its effects on renal functions, it is imperative to measure its value in normally functioning kidneys. Since measurement of GFR, based on Equation 5-1, poses numerous technical problems and is impractical in clinical practice, we shall resort to an empirical method of measuring GFR, based on the dilution principle. A description of the application of this principle in determining GFR, RPF, and tubular functions is given in Chapter 6.

PROBLEMS

5-1. In each of the following circumstances, if you expect glomerular filtration rate to increase, mark (+), if you expect it to decrease, mark (−), and if you expect no change to occur, mark (0).
   a. A rise in blood pressure at the glomerulus. _____
   b. Increased crystalloid osmotic pressure of the blood plasma. _____
   c. A marked decrease in the concentration of proteins in the blood plasma. _____
   d. Constriction of the afferent arteriole to the glomerulus. _____
   e. An intravenous injection of isotonic sucrose. _____
   f. An intravenous injection of epinephrine sufficient to raise the blood pressure. _____
   g. Coffee intake. _____

5-2. If the plasma concentration of sodium is 144 mEq/L and that for chloride is 100 mEq/L,
   a. Calculate the ultrafiltrate concentration of sodium if its chloride concentration is 110 mEq/L.
   b. Calculate the Gibbs-Donnan factor for both sodium and chloride.

5-3. Rank as higher or lower the difference between the capillary hydrostatic (P_C) and protein oncotic (π_C) pressures ($P_C - \pi_C$) in the lungs and kidneys relative to that in the G.I. system. Briefly indicate the physiological benefits of your choice.

5-4. Complete the following table by indicating the steady state deviation from normal (+ for increase; - for decrease; and 0 for no change), for the items listed to each forcing.
$\overline{P}_{VS}$ = mean systemic venous pressure.
$\overline{P}_{AS}$ = mean systemic arterial pressure.
GFR = glomerular filtration rate.
π_p = plasma protein oncotic pressure.
R_a = pre-glomerular capillary resistance.
R_v = post-glomerular capillary resistance.

Forcings	$\overline{P}_{VS}$	$\overline{P}_{AS}$	GFR	π_p
a. Infusion of 2 liters of isotonic saline.				
b. Venous hemorrhage equal to 20% of blood volume.				
c. Infusion of 2 liters of plasma.				
d. A step increase in R_a.				
e. A step increase in R_v.				

REFERENCES

1. Allen, A. C.: *The Kidney: Medical and Surgical Diseases*. 2nd ed. Grune & Stratton, New York, 1962.

2. Allison, M. E., Lipham, E. M., and Gottschalk, C. W.: Hydrostatic pressure in the rat kidney. *Am. J. Physiol. 223*: 975-983, 1972.

3. Andreucci, V. E., Herrera-Acosta, J., Rector, Jr., F. E., and Seldin, D. W.: Effective glomerular filtration pressure and single nephron filtration rate during hydropenia, elevated ureteral pressure, and active volume expansion with isotonic saline. *J. Clin. Invest. 50*:2230-2234, 1971.

4. Barajas, L., and Latta, H.: Structure of the juxtaglomerular apparatus. *Circ. Res.* Vols. *20* and *21*(Suppl. 2):79-89, 1967.

5. Best, C. H., and Taylor, N. B.: *The Physiological Basis of Medical Practice.* 6th ed. The Williams & Wilkins Co., Baltimore, 1955.

6. Brenner, B. M., Troy, J. L., and Daugharty, T. M.: The dynamics of glomerular ultrafiltration in the rat. *J. Clin. Invest. 50*: 1776-1780, 1971.

7. Cooke, C. R., Brown, T. C., Zacherle, B. J., and Walker, W. G.: Effect of altered sodium concentration in the distal nephron segments on renin release. *J. Clin. Invest. 49*:1630-1638, 1970.

8. Davis, J. O.: What signals the kidney to release renin? *Circ. Res. 28*:301-306, 1971.

9. Deane, N.: *Kidney and Electrolytes.* Prentice-Hall, Inc., Englewood Cliffs, N. J., 1966.

10. Farquhar, M. G., Wissig, S. L., and Palade, G. E.: Glomerular permeability: I. Ferritin transfer across the normal glomerular capillary wall. *J. Exp. Med. 113*:47-66, 1961.

11. Gocke, D. J., Gerter, J., Sherwood, L. M., and Laragh, J. H.: Physiological and pathological variations of plasma angiotensin II in man. Correlation with renin activity and sodium balance. *Circ. Res. 24*(Suppl. 1):131-146, 1969.

12. Goormaghtigh, N.: Facts in favor of an endocrine function of renal arterioles. *J. Pathol. Bacteriol. 57*:392-393, 1945.

13. Guyton, A. C., Langston, J. B., and Navar, B.: Theory of renal autoregulation by feedback at the juxtaglomerular apparatus. In: *Autoregulation of Blood Flow.* Edited by P. C. Johnson. *Circ. Res. 15*(Suppl. 1):187-197, 1964.

14. Harvey, R. B.: Effects of adenosine triphosphate on autoregulation of renal blood flow and glomerular filtration rate. In: *Autoregulation of Blood Flow.* Edited by P. C. Johnson. *Circ. Res. 15*(Suppl. 1):178-182, 1964.

15. Jorgensen, F., and Weis Bentzon, M.: The ultrastructure of the normal human glomerulus. *Lab. Invest. 18*:42-48, 1968.

16. Morgan, T.: A microperfusion study of influence of macula densa on glomerular filtration rate. *Am. J. Physiol. 220*:186-190, 1971.

17. Ng, K. K. F., and Vane, J. R.: Conversion of angiotensin I to angiotensin II. *Nature 216*:762-766, 1967.

18. Ochwadt, B.: Relation of renal blood supply to diuresis. *Prog. Cardiovas. Dis. 3*:501-510, 1961.

19. Pappenheimer, J. R.: Passage of molecules through capillary walls. *Physiol. Rev. 33*:387-423, 1953.

20. Pappenheimer, J. R.: Über die Permeabilität der Glomerulummembranen in der Niere. *Klin. Wochschr. 33*:362-365, 1955.

21. Pitts, R. F.: *Physiology of the Kidney and Body Fluids.* 3rd ed. Year Book Medical Publishers, Inc., Chicago, 1974.

22. Renkin, E. M., and Gilmore, J. P.: Glomerular filtration. In: *Handbook of Physiology*, Sec. 8, *Renal Physiology.* Edited by J. Orloff and R. W. Berliner. Washington, D. C., American Physiological Society, 1973, pp. 185-248.

23. Rhodin, J.: Electron microscopy of the glomerular capillary wall. *Exp. Cell Res. 8*:572-574, 1955.

24. Schnermann, J., Wright, F. S., Davis, J. M., v. Stackelberg, W., and Grill, G.: Regulation of superficial nephron filtration rate by tubuloglomerular feedback. *Arch. Ges. Physiol. 318*: 147-175, 1970.

25. Shipley, R. E., and Study, R. S.: Changes in renal blood flow, extraction of inulin, glomerular filtration rate, tissue pressure and urine flow with acute alterations of renal artery blood pressure. *Am. J. Physiol. 167*:676-688, 1951.

26. Thurau, K.: Renal hemodynamics. *Am. J. Med. 36*:698-719, 1964.

27. Thurau, K., and Kramer, K.: Weitere untersuchungen zur myogen Natur der Autoregulation des Nierenkreislanfes. *Arch. Ges. Physiol. 269*:77-93, 1959.

28. Thurau, K., Schnermann, J., Nagel, W., Horster, M., and Wohl, M.: Composition of tubular fluid in the macula densa segment as a factor regulating the function of the juxtaglomerular apparatus. *Circ. Res. 21*(Suppl. 2):79-89, 1967.

29. Tobian, L.: Relationship of juxtaglomerular apparatus to renin and angiotensin. *Circulation 25*:189-192, 1962.

30. Tobian, L., Tomboulian, A., and Janecek, J.: Effect of high perfusion pressures on the granulation of juxtaglomerular cells in an isolated kidney. *J. Clin. Invest. 38*:605-610, 1959.

31. Vander, A. J.: Control of renin release. *Physiol. Rev. 47*:359-382, 1967.

32. Windhager, E. E.: *Micropuncture Technique and Nephron Function.* Appleton-Century-Crofts, New York, 1968.

Chapter 6

RENAL CLEARANCE: MEASUREMENTS OF GLOMERULAR FILTRATION AND RENAL BLOOD FLOW

In a limited sense the function of the kidney is to remove excess water and solutes as well as waste products of metabolism from the circulating plasma. To accomplish this, the renal corpuscle makes a copious ultrafiltrate of the renal plasma flow (RPF), which subsequently is modified both in volume and composition by tubular reabsorption and secretion, yielding a small volume of hypertonic urine. Accordingly, the final volume and composition of the excreted urine depends largely on the volume of plasma filtered at the glomerulus (GFR) and the fraction which escaped filtration (RPF-GFR) and was subsequently processed by the tubules.

It is of particular interest to know whether the urinary excretion of a given substance is due to ultrafiltration, secretion, reduced reabsorption, or a combination of these. Furthermore, it is of practical value to know in what segments of the nephron each of these tubular processes has occurred and to what extent each process determines the final amount of a given substance excreted in the urine. Such information not only provides a sound basis for understanding the normal functioning of the kidney, it also gives an insight into delineating the possible causes of abnormal kidney function, diagnosing the disease, and assessing the success of the therapy as well as the final prognosis.

Renal plasma flow and GFR as well as tubular functions are readily measured by the application of the dilution principle. However, before describing the specifics of the method we need to learn two important associated concepts.

PERMEABILITY RATIO

As described in Chapter 5, the composition of the glomerular filtrate is largely determined by the permeability of the ultrafilter. Small molecular size substances, such as electrolytes, glucose, and urea, which can freely pass through the ultrafilter membranes will have the same concentrations in the ultrafilter and plasma. On the other hand, substances with sufficiently large molecular size, such as plasma proteins and lipids, will not freely pass through the ultrafilter. Therefore, their concentrations in the ultrafiltrate will be less than that in plasma. A convenient way to measure the functional permeability of the ultrafilter for a given substance (x) is to compare its concentration in the ultrafiltrate ($[x]_f$) with its "bulk" concentration in the arterial plasma ($[x]_p$). Such a comparison may be called the *permeability ratio* for that substance, designated by symbol K_x, and defined by Equation 6-1,

$$\text{Permeability Ratio } (K_x) = \frac{\text{Filtrate Concentration } ([x]_f)}{\text{Plasma Concentration } ([x]_p)} \quad (6\text{-}1)$$

Certain endogenous and exogenous substances used to study renal function are often bound to plasma proteins. Since only the free (unbound) portion can pass through the ultrafilter membranes, the filtrate concentration will be less than the plasma concentration. For these substances the permeability ratio is less than one.

It should be remembered that the use of plasma permeability ratio is meaningful only when the substance is confined to the plasma. Also, remember that the whole blood permeability ratio, a sometimes useful quantity, will tend to vary with the hematocrit, depending on whether the substance penetrates red blood cells or not.

EXTRACTION RATIO

The kidney removes varying fractions of the total quantity of a substance brought to it by the blood, as the arterial plasma makes one transit through the renal vasculature (Fig. 6-1, upper panel). The ratio of the quantity of a substance excreted in urine to the total quantity brought to the kidney by the arterial plasma inflow is called the *extraction ratio*, symbolized E_x, and defined by Equation 6-2:

$$\text{Extraction Ratio } (E_x) = \frac{\text{Quantity Excreted in Urine}}{\text{Total Quantity Brought to Kidney}}$$

$$= \frac{\dot{V}_u [x]_u}{\dot{V}_{pa} [x]_{pa}} \quad (6\text{-}2)$$

where $\dot{V}_{pa}$ and $\dot{V}_u$ are the renal arterial plasma and urine volume flows in ml/min, and $[x]_{pa}$ and $[x]_u$ are the renal arterial plasma and urinary concentrations of substance x in mg/ml, respectively.

For different substances E_x may have values ranging from 0 (not excreted at all, such as plasma proteins) to 1.0 (completely excreted). If E_x for a substance is zero, it means that the kidney excretes none,

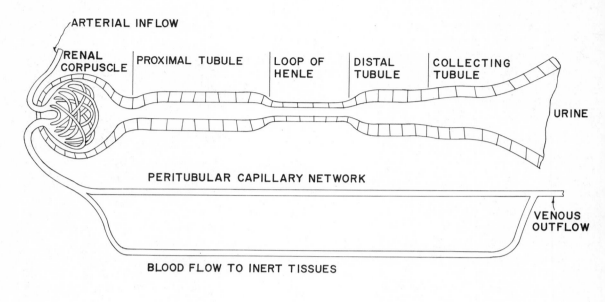

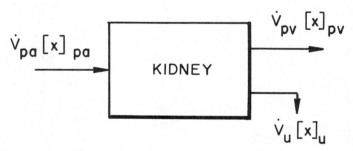

Figure 6-1. Upper panel, a schematic diagram of a representative nephron and its blood supply. *Lower panel*, a schematic diagram of input-output mass flow through the kidney.

and the renal venous plasma outflow would have a higher concentration than the arterial plasma inflow (because of the concentrating effect of forming an x-free glomerular filtrate). On the other hand, if E_x for a substance approaches unity, it means that the kidney excretes all of it, leaving a zero concentration in the venous plasma outflow.

Experimental measurement of E_x, using Equation 6-2, is not always easy, for one of the terms in the denominator ($\dot{V}_{pa}$) may not be known, although the other three terms can be measured directly. But the equation may be written in another form, taking advantage of the fact that what appears in the urine must have disappeared from the blood, as illustrated in Figure 6-1 (lower panel), so that

$$\dot{V}_u[x]_u = \dot{V}_{pa}[x]_{pa} - \dot{V}_{pv}[x]_{pv} \qquad (6-3)$$

where $\dot{V}_{pv}$ and $[x]_{pv}$ are the renal venous plasma outflow and concentration of substance x, respectively.   Substituting Equation 6-3 for the numeratory of Equation 6-2 yields:

$$E_x = \frac{\dot{V}_{pa}[x]_{pa} - \dot{V}_{pv}[x]_{pv}}{\dot{V}_{pa}[x]_{pa}} = 1 - \frac{\dot{V}_{pv}[x]_{pv}}{\dot{V}_{pa}[x]_{pa}} \qquad (6\text{-}4)$$

Now, if we can find a substance whose concentration in the venous outflow is zero ($[x]_{pv} = 0$), Equation 6-4 reduces to:

$$E_x = 1.0 \qquad (6\text{-}5)$$

Such a substance is very useful, for it can be used to measure the arterial plasma inflow, $\dot{V}_{pa}$.   But, to anticipate, it is known that $\dot{V}_{pa}$ is usually about 660 ml/min (Chapter 5), whereas $\dot{V}_u$ is normally 1 to 3 ml/min.   Hence, $\dot{V}_{pv}$ is about 99.7% of $\dot{V}_{pa}$, allowing us to set $\dot{V}_{pa} = \dot{V}_{pv}$ with negligible error.   Substitution of this equality excludes all flow terms and reduces Equation 6-4 to:

$$E_x = \frac{[x]_{pa} - [x]_{pv}}{[x]_{pa}} \qquad (6\text{-}6)$$

This equation provides a practical means of measuring the extraction ratio with reasonable accuracy, specially if E_x approaches unity.

It should be remembered that the plasma extraction ratio is meaningful only if the substance is confined to the plasma.   Also, keep in mind that the whole blood extraction ratio is meaningful for a substance that is present in cells as well as plasma, but will tend to vary with the hematocrit.

RENAL CLEARANCE:
MEASUREMENT OF PLASMA VOLUME FLOW

Formation of urine ultimately involves the tubular reabsorption of water and solutes from the ultrafiltrate as it passes through the various nephron segments and secretion of selected solutes into tubules from the blood supplying these segments.   Since the ultrafiltrate is virtually protein-free plasma, then, in the final analysis, it is the total plasma supplying the nephron which is the source of any substance excreted into the urine.   Moreover, if a large quantity of a substance is excreted into the urine, it follows that a large fraction of the total plasma volume supplying the nephron and containing that substance must have been processed to yield the quantity excreted.   Consequently, it is of interest to know the *volume of plasma which contains the same quantity of the substance as is excreted in urine in one minute*.   The volume of plasma flowing into the kidney per minute and containing this substance is called the *plasma flow* for that substance. Note that its value may range from zero, for a substance not excreted in the urine, to a value equal to the actual renal plasma flow, for a substance which is completely removed from blood by the kidney.

In practice, to measure the plasma flow of any substance, we inject it intravenously continuously, so as to maintain a *steady* plasma level throughout the period. While the plasma level is steady, we collect urine over a specified number of minutes, and then determine the urinary concentration of the substance. The plasma concentration is also measured on a blood sample drawn in the middle of the urine collection period.

If $[x]_u$ is the urinary concentration of substance x in mg/ml and $\dot{V}_u$ is the urine flow in ml/min, then $[x]_u\dot{V}_u = E_x$ is the urinary *excretion rate* of this substance in mg/min. Now, if $[x]_p$ is the plasma concentration of x, the ratio of the urinary excretion rate to plasma concentration ($[x]_u\dot{V}_u/[x]_p$) yields the volume of plasma which contains the same quantity of substance x as is excreted in the urine in one minute. It is thus expressed in ml/min. We shall designate this plasma flow by the symbol $\dot{V}_x$, where subscript x is a reminder that the plasma flow thus measured represents that fraction of the total renal plasma flow (RPF = $\dot{V}_p$) from which the substance has been cleared:

$$\dot{V}_x = \frac{[x]_u\dot{V}_u}{[x]_p} \qquad (6-7)$$

If the extraction ratio for a substance x as it passes through the kidney is 1, i.e., $[x]_{pv} = 0$ which according to Equation 6-4 implies that $[x]_{pa}\dot{V}_{pa} = [x]_u\dot{V}_u$, then its plasma flow ($\dot{V}_x$) is a measure of the *true* renal plasma flow ($\dot{V}_p$); if the extraction ratio is other than 1, it is only a *virtual* or apparent measure of renal plasma flow.

The plasma flow of a substance, thus measured, is also called renal *clearance* of that substance, and defined as the virtual volume of the plasma from which a given substance is removed per minute. Thus, renal clearance is an empiric measure of the ability of the kidney to remove a substance from the blood plasma.

The clearance formula which is widely used is somewhat different in appearance from Equation 6-7. Therefore, to maintain continuity with the literature we shall write the above clearance equation in terms of the classical notations:

$$C_x = \frac{U_x V}{P_x} \qquad (6-8)$$

where U_x and P_x are the urinary and plasma concentrations of substance x in mg/ml, respectively, V is the urine flow in ml/min, and C_x is the clearance of substance x in ml/min.

Having thus described, in general terms, the meaning of renal plasma flow and the procedure for measuring it, we are now ready to apply this concept to determine the glomerular filtration rate, the renal plasma flow, and blood flow, as well as tubular functions.

MEASUREMENT OF GLOMERULAR FILTRATION RATE (GFR)

The plasma flow or clearance of a substance as such provides no information about the mechanisms by which the kidney removes that substance from the plasma. The substance may have been removed by ultrafiltration, tubular reabsorption, or secretion, or a combination of these. To determine the magnitude of each process, it is necessary to measure GFR and RPF.

For any blood solute (x) which passes the glomerular ultrafilter, but is not created or destroyed by the kidney, nor secreted or reabsorbed by the renal tubule, a *filtrate-urine* mass balance must apply to the passage of filtrate through the tubule. This simply means that the rate of influx of x into the filtrate must equal its rate of efflux into the final urine. Since these fluxes may be expressed as the product of a volume flow ($\dot{V}$) and a concentration ([x]) we may write this filtrate-urine mass balance as follows:

$$\dot{V}_f [x]_f = \dot{V}_u [x]_u \qquad (6-9)$$

where the subscripts refer to filtrate and urine. Simple rearrangement yields a *dilution principle* formula for calculating filtrate volume flow:

$$\dot{V}_f = \dot{V}_u [x]_u / [x]_f \qquad (6-10)$$

which simply states that dividing the solute by its concentration yields the solvent. Note the similarity of this equation with Equation 6-7.

This formula is not yet suitable for practical use, because of difficulty in measuring $[x]_f$. But the latter can be determined indirectly by making use of the permeability ratio (K_x), defined as the ratio of filtrate concentration to arterial plasma "bulk" concentration:

$$K_x = [x]_f / [x]_{pa} \qquad (6-11)$$

Now, if x is not metabolized by peripheral tissues, its superficial venous plasma concentration ($[x]_p$) will be the same in arterial plasma as in venous plasma from any superficial (nonrenal) vein. Hence,

$$[x]_p = [x]_{pa} = [x]_{pv} \qquad (6\text{-}12)$$

Substituting Equations 6-11 and 6-12 into Equation 6-10 yields a practical formula for plasma flow ($\dot{V}_p$):

$$\dot{V}_p = \dot{V}_u [x]_u / K_x [x]_p \qquad (6\text{-}13)$$

It has been found that *inulin*, a fructo-polysaccharide (MW = 5200), is a nontoxic substance which is not metabolized by tissues (hence $[In]_{pv} = [In]_{pa}$), and is neither created nor destroyed (Gutman et al., 1965). Also, it is neither secreted nor absorbed by the tubules (hence the filtrate-urine mass balance is valid), and has a *known* and *constant* K_x of 1.06 ("bulk"). When expressed in "water" concentration units, the K_x is unity, meaning that inulin has equal "water" concentration in plasma and filtrate. Hence, the practical formula for measuring the glomerular filtration rate is:

$$GFR = \dot{V}_{In} = \frac{\dot{V}_u [In]_u}{1.06 [In]_p} \qquad (6\text{-}14)$$

where $[In]_u$ and $[In]_p$ are the inulin concentrations in the urine and plasma, respectively, and $\dot{V}_{In}$ is the fraction of renal plasma flow which contains the same amount of inulin as is excreted in urine in 1 min.

In order for $\dot{V}_{In}$ to be a true measure of the glomerular filtration rate, in addition to the above requirements, its value must be *constant* and *independent* of inulin plasma concentration. This implies that the inulin excretion rate must be directly proportional to, and a linear function of, inulin plasma concentration. These relationships are summarized graphically in Figure 6-2. Since inulin fulfills all of these requirements, its clearance is a true measure of GFR.

In practice, to measure GFR from inulin clearance, we inject inulin intravenously continuously until its plasma concentration maintains a steady state. At this time, a timed sample of urine is collected (for measuring $\dot{V}_u$ and $[In]_u$), and midway through this period a venous blood sample is taken (for measuring $[In]_p$).

To illustrate the calculation, consider the following inulin clearance data obtained from a patient: urine volume, $\dot{V}_u = 60$ ml/hr; urine concentration of inulin, $[In]_u = 100$ mg%; and plasma inulin concentration, $[In]_p = 1$ mg%. Before we can use Equation 6-14 to calculate the glomerular filtration rate in this patient, it is convenient to convert the units for these data to those expressed in this equation. Thus, we may express volume of urine excreted per minute rather than per hour, and urine and plasma inulin

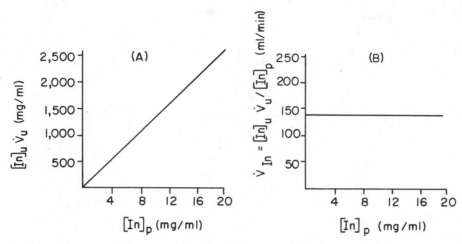

Figure 6-2. Relationship of the excretion rate (*A*) and clearance (*B*) of inulin to plasma concentration. [Redrawn from Pitts, R. F. (1974).]

concentrations in mg/ml rather than mg%. Carrying on these conversions yields: $\dot{V}_u$ = 60 ml/hr = 60 ml/60 min = 1 ml/min; $[In]_u$ = 100 mg% = 100 mg/100 ml = 1 mg/ml; and $[In]_p$ = 1 mg% = 1 mg/100 ml = 0.01 mg/ml. Now, substituting these values into Equation 6-14, we get:

$$GFR = \dot{V}_{In} = \frac{1 \text{ ml/min} \times 1 \text{ mg/ml}}{0.01 \text{ mg/ml} \times 1.06} = 93.4 \text{ ml/min} \qquad (6\text{-}15)$$

If, as is customary, we omit the K_{In} value of 1.06 from the above equation, we get a value of 100 ml/min for GFR in this patient.

In a healthy young man, inulin clearance yields an average value of 118 ml/min for GFR. You will find this normal value elsewhere cited as 125 ml/min (actually 125 ml/min/1.73 m^2 body surface area), because the K_{In} of 1.06 is usually omitted from the Equation 6-14. The use of K_{In} would be more logical, however, since the fundamental principle of the method estimates *filtrate* concentration from the plasma ("bulk") concentration.

The glomerular filtration varies with body size and age. GFR is low in newborn (Winberg, 1959) due to prominent visceral epithelial cell layers enfolding the glomerular capillary membrane. The GFR does not assume adult characteristics until one to three years after birth. Its value decreases in very old people, even in the absence of renal disease (Davies and Shock, 1950).

It should be clear that the tubular system must reabsorb most of the 118 ml/min of glomerular filtrate to have only 1 to 3 ml/min of final urine. This large GFR is remarkably constant. Although it is subject to pathological variations, the kidneys do not adjust its rate as a means of compensating for disturbances affecting the renal-body fluid regulating system. Furthermore, as far as solutes are concerned, glomerular filtration is essentially *nonselective* (except for proteins and lipids), and *non-adjustable*. The controlled, compensatory processes of the kidney reside in the tubular system.

PARTITION OF TOTAL RENAL CLEARANCE

In general, the total excretion rate of a substance x ($[x]_u \dot{V}_u$) by the kidney is the algebraic sum of three processes: (1) the rate at which the substance is delivered to the tubules by glomerular filtration; (2) the rate at which it is absorbed by the tubules; and (3) the rate at which additional amount of the substance is added to the tubular fluid by secretion. The quantity of the substance filtered at the glomerulus is called *filtered load* ($\dot{F}_x$). It is equal to the product of the glomerular filtration rate (GFR), the arterial plasma concentration of the substance ($[x]_p$), and the permeability ratio for that substance (K_x). The net rate of excretion due to tubular transport ($\dot{T}_x$) per minute is determined by whether the substance is absorbed or secreted. Since secretion of a substance into the tubular lumen represents an *addition* to the amount already filtered, it may be designated by $+\dot{T}_x$. Conversely, because absorption of a substance represents a *reduction* in the amount already filtered, it may be designated by $-\dot{T}_x$. Using these notations, the total rate of excretion of a substance may now be expressed as

$$[x]_u \dot{V}_u = GFR[x]_p K_x \pm \dot{T}_x \qquad (6\text{-}16)$$

Dividing the above equation by the plasma concentration ($[x]_p$), we obtain an expression which partitions the plasma flow for that substance ($\dot{V}_x$) into the fraction processed by filtration and that processed by tubular transport:

$$\dot{V}_x = \frac{[x]_u \dot{V}_u}{[x]_p} = GFR \cdot K_x \pm \frac{\dot{T}_x}{[x]_p} \qquad (6\text{-}17)$$

Note that each term in this equation has a dimension of volume flow (ml/min). Therefore, Equation 6-17 represents another definition for the total clearance of a substance in terms of the glomerular and tubular components:

$$\text{Total Clearance} = \frac{\text{Glomerular}}{\text{Clearance}} \pm \frac{\text{Tubular}}{\text{Clearance}} \qquad (6\text{-}18)$$

If the kidney removes a substance from the plasma by filtration only (such as inulin), the tubular clearance is zero and the excretion rate will be proportional to the plasma concentration.

If the clearance of a substance involves filtration and either tubular absorption or secretion, then the magnitude of its tubular clearance depends on the plasma concentration and the tubular transport capacity for absorption or secretion. The rate of tubular transport (T_x) at a given plasma concentration depends on the kind of substance being transported. For the present discussion, the overall tubular transport--either secretion or absorption--may be classified according to whether the renal tubular cells have a *maximum tubular transport capacity (Tm_x)* for the particular substance or not. The maximum tubular transport capacity implies that as long as the plasma concentration is below the *threshold concentration* which saturates the transport process, all of the filtered quantity of the given substance is absorbed or a maximal fraction of the quantity of the substance entering peritubular capillaries (which escaped filtration) is secreted. The quantitative aspects of this classification of the renal transport mechanism will be considered in Chapter 9. For the present purpose of understanding the influence of the tubular clearance on the overall clearance, we choose those substances, such as glucose (filtered and absorbed) and para-aminohippurate (filtered and secreted), for which the renal tubular cells have a maximum transport capacity. Accordingly, Equation 6-17 becomes

$$\dot{V}_x = GFR \cdot K_x \pm \frac{\dot{Tm}_x}{[x]_p} \qquad (6\text{-}19)$$

The total clearance of a substance which is removed from the renal plasma by both filtration and tubular secretion decreases as the plasma concentration increases. This is because the right-hand side of Equation 6-19 represents the algebraic sum of a constant quantity ($GFR \cdot K_x$) and a varying quantity ($\dot{Tm}_x/[x]_p$). Since the value of $\dot{Tm}_x$ (amount of the substance transported maximally per minute) is constant for a given substance, then the tubular clearance ($\dot{Tm}_x/[x]_p$) decreases as $[x]_p$ increases. Therefore, at a high plasma concentration the total clearance of a substance which is either absorbed (glucose) or secreted (para-aminohippurate, or PAH) asymptotically approaches the glomerular filtration rate or the inulin clearance. In the case of glucose, which is filtered and subsequently absorbed maximally in the proximal tubule, the tubular clearance increases as the plasma concentration increases. At a very high plasma concentration, the total clearance *increases* and asymptotically approaches the inulin clearance. In contrast, for a substance such as PAH, which is filtered and maximally secreted in the proximal tubule, at high plasma concentration the total clearance *decreases* and asymptotically approaches the inulin clearance. The relation of total clearance of PAH ($\dot{V}_{PAH}$) and glucose ($\dot{V}_G$) to that of inulin ($\dot{V}_{In}$) at high plasma PAH and glucose concentrations in man are illustrated graphically in

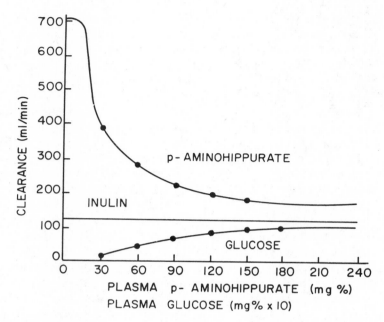

Figure 6-3. Relation of clearances to plasma concentrations of p-aminohippurate, glucose and inulin. [Redrawn from Pitts, R. F. (1974).]

Figure 6-3.

The glomerular filtration rate is defined as the volume of plasma filtered per minute and not as the volume of plasma water. Since plasma is 93 to 94% water by weight and 6 to 7% solutes, including proteins, the volume of water filtered is approximately 93 to 94% of the GFR. The normal variations in urine flow are due to changes in water absorption and not to the glomerular filtration rate. Approximately 60 to 80% of the filtered water is absorbed in the proximal tubules. This is called *obligatory* water absorption. The remaining 20 to 40% is absorbed in variable quantities mainly in the distal and collecting tubules. This is called *non-obligatory* or *facultative* water absorption and is regulated by the antidiuretic hormone (ADH). In the presence of normal plasma ADH concentration, most of this water is absorbed, reducing the urine flow to about 1 to 3 ml/min. The upper limit of facultative water absorption is determined by the osmotic activity of the non-absorbed solutes in the tubular urine.

CLINICAL MEASUREMENT OF GLOMERULAR FILTRATION RATE

In most patients with suspected renal disease, for whom frequent assessment of glomerular filtration rate is required for both diagnosis and a guide to prognosis, it is clinically impractical to measure the inulin clearance. This technical difficulty in measuring renal function by inulin clearance in clinical situations, plus the ease and rapidity required to assess renal function in disease, has prompted a continuous search for suitable endogenous substances whose clearances approximate that of inulin. Of the various potential endogenous substances whose clearance might be of diagnostic value, the endogenous urea and creatinine clearances have received most attention.

Although historically the endogenous urea clearance was the test of choice (Van Slyke, 1941), in recent years it has been largely replaced by the endogenous creatinine clearance (Hopper, 1962). Therefore, to better appreciate the potential value of the endogenous creatinine clearance in assessing renal malfunction, in this section we shall discuss the clearance of both of these substances and delineate their advantages and shortcomings.

ENDOGENOUS UREA CLEARANCE

Urea, the nitrogenous product of protein metabolism, is, apart from water, the chief constituent of urine. It is freely filtered at the glomerulus, and approximately 40% of it is reabsorbed from the tubular fluid by back-diffusion. Therefore, its clearance accounts for only 60% of the true GFR, as measured by the inulin clearance.

The tubular reabsorption rate of urea depends largely on the urine flow. The greater the urine flow, the smaller is the urea reabsorption rate by back-diffusion and the greater is its renal clearance. At urine flow above 2 ml/min, urea reabsorption rate diminishes markedly and its renal clearance approaches that of inulin. Therefore, at very high urine flow, urea clearance gives an approximate measure of GFR.

In practice, urea clearance is determined by measuring urea excretion rate during one hour and then drawing a blood sample at the halfway point of urine collection. Thus, urea clearance gives the volume of plasma which contains the same amount of urea as is excreted in urine in 1 hour (not 1 min).

The results of the urea clearance are expressed as per cent of normal. The endogenous urea clearance measured in man varies between 64 and 99 ml/min/1.73 m^2 body surface area, when urine flow is greater than 2 ml/min. A urea clearance of 74 ml/min is considered 100% of maximal urea clearance, yielding a normal range of 86 to 132%. A urea clearance of 70 to 80% of normal cannot always be considered low, particularly if the adult individual is small.

If it becomes necessary to perform the urea clearance in patients with a urine flow below 2 ml/min, the so-called standard urea clearance (C_s) may be calculated. The standard urea clearance is an empirically derived formula (Smith, 1951) which states that the clearance of urea changes in proportion to the square root of the urine flow, when the latter is below 2 ml/min:

$$\text{Standard Clearance } (C_S) = \frac{U\,V}{P} \tag{6-20}$$

The standard urea clearance in normal man determined at a urine flow of 1 ml/min is 54 ml/min. It should be noted that the standard clearance defined by Equation 6-20 is no longer a "clearance" as defined earlier, but rather a mathematical attempt to correct for the variation in urea excretion rate, when urine flow is below 2 ml/min. Hence, the standard urea clearance cannot be compared to clearances performed in the same individual at other urine flow rates.

Since the renal clearance of urea, at urine flow rates above 2 ml/min, depends primarily on the glomerular filtration rate, it will be reduced in those situations in which the GFR may be reduced in the absence of parenchymal renal disease; i.e., heart failure, severe dehydration, or shock. The endogenous urea clearance is low in the newborn, becomes normal by about 2 years of age, and again declines in the aged to approximately 50 to 60% of normal in the ninth decade of life.

Despite its earlier clinical use, the endogenous urea clearance is now largely replaced by the endogenous creatinine clearance, which is described below. This is because there are at least three major limitations in the routine clinical application of the endogenous urea clearance as a measure of GFR. First, since the rate of urea production is variable, its blood level changes in response to dietary protein intake, hepatic function, catabolic processes, and gastric hemorrhage. Second, renal excretion of urea depends on GFR and the rate of tubular reabsorption by back-diffusion. The reabsorption rate is found to be related directly to the urine flow rate. And third, at low urine flow rates (less than 2 ml/min) the clearance values obtained are inaccurate, even when the correction formula (Equation 6-20) is used. In contrast, creatinine is not reabsorbed and its renal excretion rate is not related directly to urine flow.

ENDOGENOUS CREATININE CLEARANCE

In a creatinine-free diet, muscle creatinine and phosphocreatinine are the only source of urinary creatinine. Since normally the muscle mass is relatively constant, the creatinine turnover is also relatively constant. This constancy is reflected in the stable plasma concentration and urinary excretion of creatinine. In addition, unlike urea, the endogenous creatinine clearance does not depend on urine flow rate or the dietary protein intake.

Creatinine, when given intravenously, is freely filtered at the glomerulus and is also secreted by the tubules. Hence, like PAH, creatinine clearance at normal plasma concentration (0.64 to 1.1 mg%) is substantially greater than inulin clearance. However, at high plasma concentration (in excess of 100 mg%), creatinine clearance asymptotically approaches inulin clearance. This is believed to be a consequence of the existence of maximal tubular secretion rate $\dot{T}m$ for creatinine. In man, $\dot{T}m$ for creatinine is about 13 mg/100 ml GFR.

Endogenous creatinine clearances for normal subjects varying in age from 19 to 52 years are listed in Table 6-1.

Since 1940, endogenous creatinine clearance has become a widely accepted measure of glomerular filtration rate. It was shown then by Steinitz and Türkland (1940) and subsequently by Brod and Sirata (1948) that the renal excretion of endogenous creatinine was largely dependent on the glomerular filtration rate and that its renal clearance closely approximated that of inulin in both normal subjects and those with impaired renal function.

Although inulin clearance is generally accepted as the most accurate method of measuring GFR, the techniques required are complicated to perform and therefore useful only as a research tool. The endogenous creatinine clearance, on the other hand, is not subject to these practical limitations and therefore is well suited for general clinical use. The simplicity, and the advantages and shortcomings of the routine clinical application of the endogenous creatinine clearance, compared to inulin and urea clearance methods, have been well documented (Tobias et al., 1962; De Wardener, 1958).

As pointed out by these authors, for practical clinical purposes endogenous creatinine clearance has been found to be equal to inulin

TABLE 6-1

Serum Creatinine Concentration and Endogenous Creatinine Clearance in 78 Normal Men and 24 Normal Women

	Men		Women	
	Serum Creatinine Concentration (mg%)	Creatinine Clearance (ml/min)	Serum Creatinine Concentration (mg%)	Creatinine Clearance (ml/min)
Range	1.0-1.6	72.0-141.0	0.8-1.4	74.0-130.0
Mean	1.274	105.4	1.09	95.4
Standard Error	0.014	1.57	0.03	3.67
Standard Deviation	0.122	13.9	0.145	18.0

[From Hopper, J., Jr. (1951).]

clearance, both as a diagnostic test and as a prognostic guide. Furthermore, when performed at regular intervals, endogenous creatinine clearance was found to be a sensitive test over an unusually wide range of renal damage, especially in following the prognosis of patients with advanced renal insufficiency. The main disadvantage is that the normally low plasma concentration of endogenous creatinine plus the presence of significant amounts of nonspecific chromogen in the plasma makes the measurement of the endogenous plasma creatinine concentration somewhat imprecise (Relman and Levinsky, 1963).

MEASUREMENT OF RENAL PLASMA FLOW (RPF)

For any (noncreated, nondestroyed) blood solute (x) a *blood-urine* mass balance must apply to each single passage of the blood through the kidneys. This simply means that the arterial influx must equal the sum of venous and urinary effluxes (Fig. 6-1). This balance is valid regardless of the degree of glomerular filtration, of tubular secretion or absorption, and of whether the substance has access to red blood cells or is confined to the plasma.

Of more practical interest is the *plasma-urine* mass balance, which is valid *only* if the solute is confined to the plasma phase of blood. This mass balance may be written by rearranging Equation 6-3 as:

$$\dot{V}_{pa}[x]_{pa} = \dot{V}_{pv}[x]_{pv} + \dot{V}_{u}[x]_{u} \qquad (6\text{-}21)$$

In the case of mass balance for volume flows, it turns out that the plasma flows are enormous compared to the ultimate urine flow, so that we can equate the arterial and venous plasma flows to the renal plasma flow ($\dot{V}_p$) and write, with only a fraction of a per cent error,

$$\dot{V}_p = \dot{V}_{pa} = \dot{V}_{pv} \qquad (6\text{-}22)$$

Substituting Equation 6-22 into Equation 6-21 yields a simplified mass balance expression:

$$\dot{V}_p[x]_{pa} = \dot{V}_p[x]_{pv} + \dot{V}_u[x]_u \qquad (6\text{-}23)$$

Simple rearrangement now yields a Fick principle formula for calculating the *renal plasma flow*:

$$\dot{V}_p = \frac{\dot{V}_u [x]_u}{[x]_{pa} - [x]_{pv}} \qquad (6\text{-}24)$$

This equation states that analogous to measuring the cardiac output from the ratio of the oxygen consumed to the arteriovenous oxygen concentration difference, the renal plasma flow may be determined from the ratio of the excretion rate of a substance (x) to its renal arteriovenous concentration difference. The arteriovenous concentration difference is a measure of the amount of substance (x) removed from each milliliter of plasma as it perfuses the kidney. Therefore, the ratio of the excretion rate to the arteriovenous concentration difference gives the total volume of plasma which contains the same quantity of substance x as is excreted in urine in 1 min.

There are at least two difficulties in measuring renal plasma flow in man by the application of the Fick principle. *First*, the renal venous outflow ($\dot{V}_{pv}$) is not equal to the renal arterial inflow ($\dot{V}_{pa}$), as required by the Fick principle. This inequality is due to a small but significant urine flow, which may be negligible if $\dot{V}_u$ is small. *Second*, it is impractical in clinical medicine to procure a renal venous blood sample in man. However, if the urine flow is small and the extraction ratio (E_x) for the test substance is very high (i.e., $[x]_{pv} \to 0$), the Fick equation (Equation 6-24) then reduces to the clearance equation for that substance.

In practice, the assumption that $\dot{V}_u$ is small (hence, $\dot{V}_{pa} = \dot{V}_{pv}$) has a less serious effect on the accuracy of calculation of RPF from Fick equation than the substitution of superficial venous blood sample for the renal venous blood sample. However, the difficult sampling of renal venous blood can be avoided by using the extraction ratio (E_x), defined earlier (Equation 6-2) as the fraction of the arterial influx that the kidneys excrete. This is simply the ratio of two terms in Equation 6-23:

$$E_x = \frac{\dot{V}_u [x]_u}{\dot{V}_p [x]_{pa}} \qquad (6\text{-}25)$$

If we replace $\dot{V}_u [x]_u$ in this equation by the difference between the arterial influx and venous efflux (Equation 6-22), we obtain an expression, analogous to Equation 6-6, which excludes all flow terms:

$$E_x = \frac{[x]_{pa} - [x]_{pv}}{[x]_{pa}} = \frac{[x]_p - [x]_{pv}}{[x]_p} \qquad (6\text{-}26)$$

The second form of Equation 6-26 replaces the superficial venous plasma for the arterial plasma sample, a valid substitution if substance x is not metabolized by nonrenal tissues. With this formula we can experimentally search for a substance having a *known* and *constant* E_x.

Substituting Equation 6-26 into Equation 6-24 yields a practical clearance formula for measuring renal plasma flow:

$$\dot{V}_p = \frac{\dot{V}_u [x]_u}{E_x [x]_p} = \frac{\dot{V}_x}{E_x} \qquad (6\text{-}27)$$

where $\dot{V}_x$ is the renal clearance of substance x.

It has been found that para-aminohippurate (PAH) is a nontoxic substance which is not metabolized by nonrenal tissues. Furthermore, PAH is neither created nor destroyed by the kidney and it is confined to plasma (making the plasma-urine mass balance valid). In addition, within certain plasma concentrations (1 to 10 mg%), extraction ratio of PAH is nearly constant between 0.70 to 0.90 in dogs and 0.85 to 0.95 in man (Smith, 1951), revealing that it is both readily filtered and also secreted by renal tubules. Hence, the particular formula for measuring *renal plasma flow* (RPF) from the clearance of PAH is:

$$RPF = \frac{\dot{V}_u [PAH]_u}{0.9 [PAH]_p} = \frac{\dot{V}_{PAH}}{0.9} \qquad (6\text{-}28)$$

where 0.9 is the average PAH extraction ratio in man. Since PAH is primarily secreted by the proximal tubules, its renal clearance ($\dot{V}_{PAH}$) without correcting for the extraction ratio yields an approximate measure of the cortical renal plasma flow.

The PAH clearance method (Equation 6-28) yields an average RPF for healthy young man of 660 ml/min. By also measuring the hematocrit (Ht), the plasma flow may be converted to *renal blood flow*, RBF:

$$RBF = \frac{RPF}{1 - Ht} \qquad (6\text{-}29)$$

The normal hematocrit of 0.45 thus yields a normal RBF of 1200 ml/min, which, it can be seen, is 20% of the total resting cardiac output of 6.0 L/min.

FILTRATION FRACTION

The fraction of renal plasma flow which is filtered through the glomeruli is called the *filtration fraction* (FF). This is estimated from the ratio of inulin clearance to PAH clearance.

$$\text{Filtration Fraction} = \frac{\text{Glomerular Filtration Rate, ml/min}}{\text{Renal Arterial Plasma Flow, ml/min}}$$

$$= \frac{\dot{V}_{In}}{\dot{V}_{PAH}} = \frac{\dot{V}_{In}}{\dot{V}_{p}} \tag{6-30}$$

The filtration fraction in man normally varies from 16 to 20%.

The filtration fraction as defined above may be regarded as the *glomerular extraction ratio*. The overall extraction ratio of any substance was defined earlier (Equation 6-2) as the fraction of the total quantity brought to the kidney which is excreted in the urine. The quantity brought to the kidney is equal to the product of the plasma concentration and the renal arterial plasma flow, i.e., $[x]_p \dot{V}_p$. The quantity removed by the kidney is equal to the quantity excreted in the urine, i.e., $[x]_u \dot{V}_u$. Therefore, the overall extraction ratio, assuming permeability ratio of unity, will be:

$$\text{Extraction Ratio} = E_x = \frac{[x]_u \dot{V}_u}{[x]_p \dot{V}_p} \tag{6-31}$$

Equation 6-31 may also be written as

$$E_x = \frac{[x]_u \dot{V}_u}{[x]_p} \cdot \frac{1}{\dot{V}_p} = \frac{\dot{V}_x}{\dot{V}_p} \tag{6-32}$$

This latter equation shows that the extraction ratio for a substance is equal to the fraction of the renal arterial plasma flow ($\dot{V}_p$) which is cleared of that substance ($\dot{V}_x$).

Knowing the filtration fraction and extraction ratio, we can determine the manner by which the kidney processes a given substance. The ratio of the filtration fraction (Equation 6-30) to extraction ratio (Equation 6-31) provides such information:

$$\frac{FF}{E_x} = \frac{\dfrac{\dot{V}_{In}}{\dot{V}_p}}{\dfrac{[x]_u \dot{V}_u}{[x]_p \dot{V}_p}} = \frac{\dot{V}_{In}[x]_p}{[x]_u \dot{V}_u} \tag{6-33}$$

This equation states that the ratio of the *filtration fraction* to the *extraction ratio* is equal to the ratio of the *filtered load* ($\dot{V}_{In}[x]_p$) to the *excretion rate* ($[x]_u \dot{V}_u$) of that substance. It may be used to estimate *net* rates of secretion or absorption of a substance. Therefore, a ratio of 1 implies that the net excreted rate is equal to the quantity filtered per minute. A ratio less than 1 implies that net secretion has occurred.

Note that Equation 6-33 gives only the net rates of secretion and absorption, respectively. The fact that there is net absorption does not rule out secretion, and vice versa.

CLEARANCE RATIO

A closer look at Equation 6-33 reveals that the right-hand side of this equation, when inverted, is merely a ratio of the clearance of a substance ($\dot{V}_x$) to that of inulin ($\dot{V}_{In}$). Clearance of a substance relative to that of inulin can also provide an approximate index of the manner by which that substance is processed by the kidneys. If a substance is filtered and subsequently secreted by the tubules, its renal clearance is greater than that of inulin. However, if the substance is filtered and then is subsequently absorbed by the tubules, its renal clearance would be less than that of inulin. In either case, if the secretion and absorption processes involve a *saturable* type of mechanism, i.e., maximum tubular transport, then, as the plasma concentration of either substance is increased, the renal clearance of the substance approaches that of inulin (see Fig. 6-3).

PARTITION OF RENAL BLOOD FLOW

Normal renal function is dependent upon normal renal circulation. Acute reduction in renal blood flow is often accompanied by a marked alteration of function, which may lead to oliguria and renal insufficiency. The resulting acute derangements in function are due to abnormal changes in renal hemodynamics and maldistribution of blood flow within the kidney. In the normal kidney, changes in renal blood flow and its distribution between the *cortex* and *medulla* have profound influence on the ability of the kidney to concentrate or dilute urine and hence on the rate of excretion of salt and water.

To understand the magnitude of these changes in intrarenal circulation and the regions of the kidney affected by the redistribution of renal blood flow, a knowledge of normal distribution of renal blood flow is necessary. The conventional clearance techniques described earlier in this chapter provide an overall measure of GFR and RPF. As such, these measurements provide little information about the distribution of blood between the cortex and medulla.

The widely used method for measurement of distribution of renal blood flow in man is the inert gas isotope "washout" technique. Briefly, the procedure (Thornburn et al., 1963) involves injecting a small bolus of saline saturated with radioactive krypton (Kr^{85}) or xenon (Xe^{133}) rapidly into the renal artery. The lipid-soluble gas diffuses so rapidly across the capillary membranes that the renal tissue is saturated almost instantaneously. The removal of the isotope from the tissue is thus limited by the rate of blood flow in the capillaries supplying these tissues. The disappearance of the radioactive isotope can be monitored by placing an external detector over the kidney. Since the method is non-invasive, requiring no blood or urine sample, it can be used in oliguric patients.

The disappearance curve of radioactive krypton from the kidney follows a complex exponential, which has been analyzed into four components, each representing blood flow in a region of the kidney (Fig. 6-4). These components have been localized in the dog by autoradiographs and shown to represent blood flow through (I) outer cortex, (II) inner cortex and outer medulla, (III) vasa recta and inner medulla, and (IV) perirenal and hilar fat.

Briefly, the procedure for analyzing the disappearance curve into its components involves extrapolating the linear portion of the exponential curve, shown by a heavy black line in Figure 6-5, back to zero time. The resulting line gives the disappearance curve for component IV. Subtracting this curve from the original curve yields another exponential. Extrapolating the linear portion of this curve back to zero time, yields the disappearance curve for component III. Repeating the subtraction and extrapolation processes once more yields a third exponential curve, which can be resolved into two linear lines, representing disappearance curves for components II and I, respectively. The blood flow for each component is determined by a method similar to that outlined in Chapter 2 (see also Appendix B) for measurement of body volume and composition. The results are assembled in the table within Figure 6-5. On the average, the cortical renal blood flow constitutes about 80% of the total, while blood flow in the outer medulla and inner medulla represent about 10% and 5%, respectively.

In addition to partitioning the total renal blood flow into different regions, these measurements have provided evidence for the rate of blood flow in the vasa recta. As indicated by the value at half-time ($t_{1/2}$) (Fig. 6-5), the blood flow in these vessels is indeed very slow, a condition which is ideally suited for the maintenance of high solute concentration observed in the medullary region in the antidiuretic state (see Chapter 11).

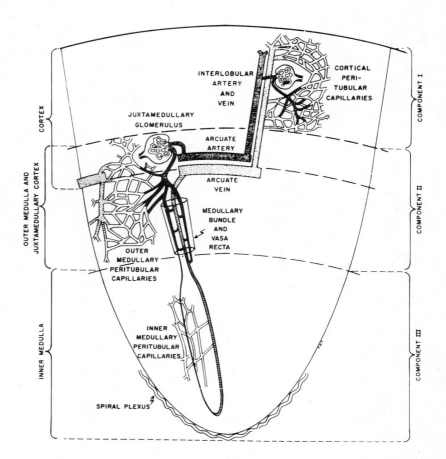

Figure 6-4. A schematic illustration of renal circulation in the dog. (From Thornburn et al.: Intrarenal distribution of nutrient blood flow determined with Krypton[85] in the unanesthetized dog. *Circ. Res. 13*:290-307, 1963. By permission of The American Heart Association, Inc.)

The differences in the rate of blood flow in the cortex and medulla, as indicated by differences in half-time, are of more than academic interest. They reflect differences in the rate of blood flow in the capillaries supplying the *cortical* and *juxtamedullary* nephrons (see Chapter 11 for further details). On the average, cortical nephrons account for absorption of nearly 60 to 80% of the filtered volume and its dissolved solutes. Since cortical blood flow is fairly rapid, tubular absorption in the cortical nephrons is markedly influenced by alterations in blood flow and hydrostatic and plasma colloid oncotic pressures in the peritubular capillaries supplying these nephrons. Thus, it has been shown that an increase in the capillary hydrostatic pressure depresses tubular absorption, while an increase in the capillary plasma oncotic pressure facilitates tubular absorption of the filtrate in the proximal tubules of the cortical nephrons (Windhager et al., 1969).

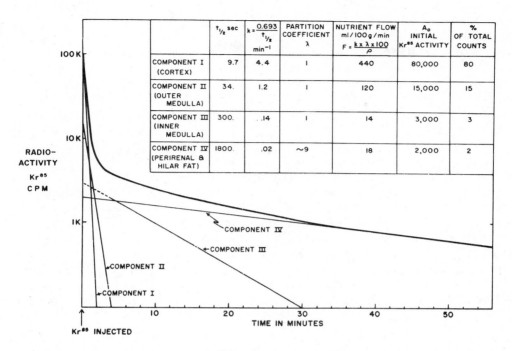

	$t_{1/2}$ sec	$k = \dfrac{0.693}{t_{1/2}}$ min^{-1}	PARTITION COEFFICIENT λ	NUTRIENT FLOW ml/100g/min $F = \dfrac{k \times \lambda \times 100}{\rho}$	A_0 INITIAL Kr^{85} ACTIVITY	% OF TOTAL COUNTS
COMPONENT I (CORTEX)	9.7	4.4	1	440	80,000	80
COMPONENT II (OUTER MEDULLA)	34.	1.2	1	120	15,000	15
COMPONENT III (INNER MEDULLA)	300.	.14	1	14	3,000	3
COMPONENT IV (PERIRENAL & HILAR FAT)	1800.	.02	~9	18	2,000	2

Figure 6-5. A typical Kr[85] disappearance curve following injection of the isotope into renal artery. (From Thornburn et al.: Intrarenal distribution of nutrient blood flow determined with Krypton[85] in the unanesthetized dog. *Circ. Res. 13*:290-307, 1963. By permission of The American Heart Association, Inc.)

In contrast, because of the complexity of the vascular supply of the juxtamedullary nephrons, blood flow through these nephrons is quite variable. Since these nephrons are the final common pathway for urine formation, changes in blood flow rates and capillary hydrostatic and plasma oncotic pressures in these regions will alter urinary volume and composition (Barger and Herd, 1973). For example, in saline diuresis, both GFR and blood flow through the cortex are increased. But due to elevated capillary hydrostatic pressure, absorption of sodium and water from the proximal tubule is depressed (Earley and Friedler, 1965). As a result, a greater volume of filtrate is delivered to the more distal segment of the nephron for final processing. Despite the fact that blood flow in the medullary regions is reduced in diuresis, significant amounts of the filtered sodium and water will escape absorption by the distal segments of the nephron, accounting for the solute washout observed in diuresis (Barger and Herd, 1973).

The opposite response of the cortical and medullary blood flows observed in saline diuresis suggests a possible functional separation of the blood supply to these two intrarenal regions. This possibility has recently been confirmed by Slotkoff and his associates (1968), who found that the distribution of radioiodine (I[131]) labelled Diodrast within the cortex and medulla followed two parallel pathways. Hence, changes in the blood flow to one region may not necessarily be followed by changes in the other region.

A similar blood flow pattern has been observed in other diuretic states, e.g., diabetes insipidus, mannitol diuresis, and after administration of diuretic agents, such as furosemide and ethacrynic acid (Chapter 11). On the other hand, in conditions leading to salt retention, such as congestive heart failure, the cortical blood flow is reduced while the medullary blood flow is increased (Sparks et al., 1972). In acute renal failure, cortical blood flow is even more severely reduced, while the medullary blood flow is relatively well maintained (Barger, 1966).

Mechanisms regulating renal blood flow and its intrarenal distribution are very complex. There is considerable evidence that sympathetic innervation of the renal vessels plays an important role in such a regulation (Davis, 1971). However, as alluded to earlier in Chapter 5, there is increasing evidence suggesting that the humoral factors, such as angiotensin, ADH, adrenal steroids, and prostaglandins, play an even greater role in regulation of intrarenal blood supply and distribution (Lee, 1970).

PROBLEMS

6-1. Complete the following table by making the appropriate calculations:

Table 1

Substance	Total Plasma Conc. (mg%)	Permeability Ratio (K_x)	Filtrate Conc. (mg%)
a. Inulin	80.0	1.0	
b. Phenol Red	1.0	0.2	
c. Na p-aminohippurate		0.8	4.0
d. Diodrast iodine	2.0		1.5

6-2. Complete the following table by making the appropriate calculations:

Table 2

Substance	$[x]_{pa}$ (mg%)	$[x]_{pv}$ (mg%)	$[x]_{pa} - [x]_{pv}$ (mg%)	E_x
a. Inulin	50	40		
b. Glucose	100			0
c. Diodrast iodine	4	0		
d. Na p-aminohippurate	4			1.0
e. Creatinine		15		0.25

6-3. What must the renal venous concentration be when the extraction ratio is 1? _____

6-4. What single concentration measurement will be equal to the renal arteriovenous difference for a substance with an extraction ratio of 1? _____

6-5. Complete the following table by making the appropriate calculations:

Table 3

	Plasma Inulin Conc. (mg%)	Urine Inulin Conc. (mg/ml)	Urine Volume Flow (ml/min)	Inulin Filtered (mg/min)	GFR (ml/min)
a.	565	260	2.8		
b.	380	160	3.0		
c.		110	2.5		120
d.		112	2.0		125
e.	85		2.3	110	
f.	50		2.3	70	

6-6. Calculate the renal plasma flow from the following data obtained with Na p-aminohippurate:
   a. Plasma concentration = 5 mg%
   b. Urine concentration = 14.6 mg/ml
   c. Urine flow = 2.4 ml/min
   d. Assume PAH extraction ratio = 0.9

6-7. If hematocrit is 0.55, calculate the total renal blood flow.

_____

6-8. If the cardiac output is 4 L/min, calculate the percentage of the total cardiac output which passes through the kidney.

_____

6-9. Using the average value for glomerular filtration rate from Table 3, calculate the filtration fraction. _____

6-10. Using the value for renal plasma flow which you calculated in the Problem 6-6, calculate the quantity of inulin (mg/min) brought to the kidney in each of the six experiments in Table 3. Record your results in Table 4 below:

Table 4

Experiments	Total Inulin Brought to Kidney (mg/min)	Extraction Ratio
a.		
b.		
c.		
d.		
e.		
f.		

6-11. Calculate the extraction ratio of each of these six inulin experiments and enter the results in Table 4 above.

6-12. The filtration fraction may be regarded as a glomerular extraction ratio for plasma, i.e., it is the ratio of the volume of plasma removed by the ultrafilter to the total volume brought to it.
   a. If a substance has a permeability ratio of 1 and is neither reabsorbed nor secreted by the tubules, which of the following relationships would hold? (Check correct one).
       (1) Extraction Ratio = Filtration Fraction _____.
       (2) Extraction Ratio > Filtration Fraction _____.
       (3) Extraction Ratio < Filtration Fraction _____.
   b. If a substance has a permeability ratio less than 1 and is neither reabsorbed nor secreted by the tubules, which of the relationships of 6-12a. would hold? _____
   c. If a substance has a permeability ratio of 1 and is partially reabsorbed by the tubules, which of these relationships would hold? _____
   d. If a substance has an extraction ratio greater than the filtration fraction, what process must be involved in its excretion? _____

6-13. What requirements must a substance meet in order for its plasma clearance to equal the glomerular filtration rate? _____

6-14. What requirements must a substance meet in order for its plasma clearance to equal the rate of renal plasma flow? _____

6-15. If a substance has a plasma clearance greater than the glomerular filtration rate, what process must be concerned in its excretion? _____

6-16. If a substance has a plasma clearance less than the glomerular filtration rate, what are two possible explanations in terms of fundamental renal excretory processes?

a. _____

b. _____

6-17. If RPF is 700 ml/min, calculate the extraction ratios corresponding to the following plasma clearances.

Table 5

Substance	Plasma Clearance (ml/min)	Extraction Ratio
a. Na p-aminohippurate	700	
b. Phenol Red	400	
c. Creatinine	180	
d. Inulin	130	
e. Glucose	0	

6-18. Construct a graph with extraction ratios (0 to 1.0) as abscissae and plasma clearance (0 to 700 ml/min) as ordinates. Plot the data from Table 5.

a. From your graph, what plasma clearance would be found for substances having the following extraction ratios?

$E_x = 0.8$; $\dot{V}_x = $ _____

$E_x = 0.4$; $\dot{V}_x = $ _____

$E_x = 0.2$; $\dot{V}_x = $ _____

6-19. The data listed below may be described by a double exponential curve of the form,

$$y(t) = A e^{-k_1 t} + B e^{-k_2 t}$$

Time, t (min)	$[x]_p$ (mg%)
5	50.0
10	41.9
15	36.0
20	32.0
25	28.0
30	24.8
35	22.0
40	19.5
45	17.5
50	16.1
60	13.2

Calculate (a) the parameters A, B, k_1, and k_2, and (b) the time constant for each exponential component (see Appendix B).

6-20. Renal function studies in a patient produced the following data:

Clearance of inulin   80 ml/min
Plasma concentration of Z   25 mg%
Urine concentration of Z   12 mg/ml
Urine flow rate   5 ml/min

Assume permeability ratio for substance Z is 1.0.
a. Is the substance Z absorbed or secreted? Compute it.
b. Compute the filtered load of the substance Z.

6-21. In a patient the GFR = 130 ml/min, RPF = 700 ml/min, and permeability ratio for glucose = 1.0. Complete the table below by calculating the following:
1. Quantity of glucose filtered, mg/min.
2. Quantity of glucose absorbed, mg/min.
3. Total quantity of glucose brought to the kidney, mg/min.
4. Plasma clearance of glucose, ml/min.
5. Extraction ratio for glucose.

	Plasma Glucose (mg%)	Urinary Loss of Glucose (mg/min)	Glucose Filtered (mg/min)	Total Glucose Brought to Kidney
a.	100	0		
b.	500	275		

	Plasma Clearance of Glucose	Extraction Ratio of Glucose	Glucose Absorption Rate
a.			
b.			

6-22. Select by number from the list at the right the *items* called for by each of the statements at the left.

a. To calculate the glomerular filtration rate _____.

b. To calculate the rate of plasma flow to the peritubular capillaries _____.

c. To calculate Tm of substance x _____.

1. Urine flow rate.
2. Renal plasma flow rate.
3. Urine inulin concentration.
4. Urine PAH concentration.
5. Urine concentration of x.
6. Plasma concentration of inulin.
7. Plasma PAH concentration.
8. Plasma concentration of x.

d. To calculate the clearance of substance x _____.
e. To determine whether substance x is secreted or reabsorbed _____.
f. To calculate the osmolar clearance _____ (see Chapter 11).

9. Glomerular filtration rate.
10. Solute-free water clearance.

6-23. The following data were obtained in a patient subjected to renal function tests:

Plasma concentration of sodium = 140 mEq/L
Urine concentration of sodium = 120 mEq/L
Plasma concentration of glucose = 400 mg%
Urine concentration of glucose = 25 mg/ml
Urine flow rate = 4 ml/min
Inulin clearance = 100 ml/min
PAH clearance = 500 ml/min

Assume permeability ratio = 1.0 for sodium and glucose. Also assume extraction ratio of 1.0 for PAH. Using these data, calculate the following:
a. Filtered load of sodium _____
b. Rate of reabsorption of sodium _____
c. Maximum tubular transport capacity for glucose _____
d. Plasma concentration at which glucose transport is just maximal _____
e. Filtration fraction _____

6-24. What is the osmolar concentration (osmolality) of blood urea when BUN (blood urea nitrogen) is 100 mg%. Assume that nitrogen constitutes 47% of urea molecule and that the molecular weight of urea is 60.

6-25. The intravenous infusion of a substance raised its plasma concentration to 145 mg%. If the concentration of the substance in the renal vein is 0.55 mg/ml, *calculate* (a) the amount of the substance removed by the kidney, and (b) the extraction ratio of this substance.

6-26. If the inulin clearance is 120 ml/min and the maximum tubular transport of glucose (Tm_G) is 360 mg/min, *calculate* (a) the plasma glucose concentration at which glucose is absorbed maximally, and (b) the amount of glucose excreted in the urine when the plasma glucose concentration is 130 mg%.

6-27. Substances X, Y, and Z are freely permeable across the glomerular membrane. They are not stored, formed, or destroyed by the kidney tissue. The following data are obtained from a normal subject.

Substance	Plasma Concentration (mg/ml)	Urine Concentration (mg/ml)
X	1.0	300
Y	5.0	300
Z	10.0	300
Inulin	10.0	600

In the table below, indicate the renal processing of which of these three substances (X, Y, and Z) most closely resembles that for the substances listed below. Place the appropriate letter (X, Y, or Z) in the space provided.

Substance	Renal Processing Resembles That of:
a. _____	Glucose
b. _____	Para-aminohippurate
c. _____	Urea
d. _____	Inulin

6-28. Using clearance technique, describe explicitly how you can determine whether a substance if filtered, reabsorbed, or secreted by the kidney.

REFERENCES

1. Barger, A. C.: Renal hemodynamic factors in congestive heart failure. *Ann. N. Y. Acad. Sci. 139*:276-284, 1966.

2. Barger, A. C., and Herd, J. A.: Renal vascular anatomy and distribution of blood flow. In: *Handbook of Physiology*, Sec. 8, *Renal Physiology*. Edited by J. Orloff and R. W. Berliner. Washington, D. C., American Physiological Society, 1973, pp. 249-313.

3. Brod, J., and Sirota, J. H.: Renal clearance of endogenous "creatinine" in man. *J. Clin. Invest. 27*:645-654, 1948.

4. Davis, J. O.: What signals the kidney to release renin? *Circ. Res. 28*:301-306, 1971.

5. Davies, D. F., and Shock, N. W.: Age changes in glomerular filtration rate, effective renal plasma flow, and tubular excretory capacity in adult males. *J. Clin. Invest. 29*: 496-507, 1950.

6. De Wardener, H. E.: *The Kidney: An Outline of Normal and Abnormal Structure and Function*. Little, Brown and Co., Boston, 1958.

7. Earley, L. E., and Friedler, R. M.: Changes in renal blood flow and possibly the intrarenal distribution of blood during the natriuresis accompanying saline loading in the dog. *J. Clin. Invest. 44*:929-941, 1965.

8. Gutman, Y., Gottschalk, C. W., and Lassiter, W. E.: Micropuncture study of inulin absorption in the rat kidney. *Science 147*:753-754, 1965.

9. Hopper, J., Jr.: Creatinine clearance: simple way of measuring kidney function. *Bull. Univ. Calif. Med. Center 2*:315-324, 1951.

10. Lee, J. B.: Prostaglandins. *Physiologist 13*:379-397, 1970.

11. Pilkington, L. A., Binder, R., De Haas, J. C. M., and Pitts, R. F.: Intrarenal distribution of blood flow. *Am. J. Physiol. 208*:1107-1113, 1965.

12. Pitts, R. F.: *Physiology of Kidney and Body Fluids*. 3rd ed. Year Book Medical Publishers, Inc., Chicago, 1974.

13. Pomeranz, B. H., Birtch, A. G., and Barger, A. C.: Neural control of intrarenal blood flow. *Am. J. Physiol. 215*:1067-1081, 1968.

14. Ravel, R.: *Clinical Laboratory Medicine*. 2nd ed. Year Book Medical Publishers, Inc., Chicago, 1973.

15. Relman, A. S., and Levinsky, N. G.: Clinical examination of renal function. In: *Diseases of the Kidney*. Edited by M. B. Strauss and L. G. Welt. Little, Brown and Co., Boston, 1963.

16. Slotkoff, L. M., Eisner, G. M., and Lilienfield, L. S.: Functional separation of renal cortical-medullary circulation: Significance of Diodrast extraction. *Am. J. Physiol. 214*: 935-941, 1968.

17. Smith, H. W.: *The Kidney--Structure and Function in Health and Disease*. Oxford, New York, 1951.

18. Sparks, H. V., Kopald, H. H., Carriere, S., Chimoskey, J. J. E., Kinoshita, M., and Barger, A. C.: Intrarenal distribution of blood flow with chronic congestive heart failure. *Am. J. Physiol.* *223*:840-846, 1972.

19. Steinitz, K., and Türkland, H.: Determination of glomerular filtration by endogenous creatinine clearance. *J. Clin. Invest.* *19*:285-298, 1940.

20. Thornburn, G. D., Kopald, H. H., Herd, J. A., Hollenberg, M., O'Morchoe, C. C. C., and Barger, A. C.: Intrarenal distribution of nutrient blood flow determined with Krypton[85] in the unanesthetized dog. *Circ. Res.* *13*:290-307, 1963.

21. Tobias, J. G., McLaughlin, R. F., Jr., and Hopper, J., Jr.: Endogenous creatinine clearance. *New Eng. J. Med.* *266*:317-323, 1962.

22. Ullrich, K. J., Kramer, K., and Boylan, J. W.: Present knowledge of the countercurrent system in the mammalian kidney. *Progr. Cardiovasc. Dis.* *3*:395-431, 1961.

23. Van Slyke, D. D.: Renal function tests. *New York State J. Med.* *41*:825-833, 1941.

24. Winberg, J.: 24-hour true endogenous creatinine clearance in infants and children without renal disease. *Acta Paediat.* *48*:443-452, 1959.

25. Windhager, E. E., Lewy, J. E., and Spitzer, A.: Intrarenal control of proximal tubular reabsorption of sodium and water. *Nephron* *6*:247-259, 1969.

Chapter 7

BIOCHEMICAL BASIS OF TUBULAR TRANSPORT

The ultrafiltrate, as it traverses the various nephron segments, undergoes considerable modifications both in volume and composition. The small volume of the excreted urine is largely due to reabsorption of nearly all of the ultrafiltrate, both solutes and water, along with addition of some important solutes by tubular secretion.

Although mechanisms of renal tubular transport differ, depending on the particular solutes involved, certain transport mechanisms are common to both reabsorption and secretion processes. In Chapter 5, those mechanisms related to the formation of the glomerular ultrafiltrate were described. Here we shall expand on those concepts by a systematic examination of the principles of transport across the cell membrane. These ideas should provide the basis for understanding the mechanisms of renal tubular reabsorption and secretion of solutes and water, to be discussed in Chapters 8 and 9.

CLASSIFICATION OF CELLULAR TRANSPORT

The mechanism of transport of solutes and water across the cell membrane has been the subject of extensive theoretical and experimental studies. Without attempting to examine the details or resolve the controversies (Wilbrandt and Rosenberg, 1961), we shall consider those principles which have both been well documented and widely used by renal physiologists.

As mentioned in Chapter 2, translocation of solutes and water across the cell membrane may be classified into *three* categories: (1) transport by convection, bulk flow, or filtration; (2) transport by simple (passive) diffusion; and (3) carrier-mediated transport. The last category is further subdivided into (a) facilitated diffusion and (b) active transport.

The characteristics and the forces involved in solute and water transport by filtration have already been described (Chapter 5).

However, since a sound understanding of the theoretical basis of diffusion is fundamental to comprehension of the concept of carrier-mediated transport, a repetition of the diffusion concept is necessary. Therefore, let us begin this section with a description of the principles of simple or passive diffusion and then examine the characteristics and rules governing the carrier-mediated transport and its subdivisions.

SIMPLE OR PASSIVE DIFFUSION

In Chapter 2, diffusion was defined as the translocation of solutes and water across a porous membrane, permeable to both, along their respective chemical and electrical gradients until equilibrium is reached. The diffusion rate (dS/dt) for either solute or solvent is given by Fick's equation:

$$\frac{dS}{dt} = -K_S \cdot A_P \frac{\Delta [S]}{X} \qquad (7\text{-}1)$$

The diffusion rate in moles/sec/cm^2 is often referred to as the *flux density* and designated by the symbol J. The product term ($K_S \cdot A_P$) is denoted by D and called *diffusion coefficient*; it is measured in cm^2/sec. $\Delta [S]/X$ is the change in concentration with distance (membrane thickness) and is called *concentration gradient*. The negative sign, added here on the right side of Equation 7-1, indicates that the flux moves in a direction opposite to that of an increasing concentration. Incorporating these new notations, Equation 7-1 becomes:

$$J = -D \frac{\Delta [S]}{X} \qquad (7\text{-}2)$$

The operational significance of the various terms in Equation 7-2 is illustrated schematically in Figure 7-1. The negative sign in the equation is represented by the arrow drawn within the membrane, connecting the line indicating the level of concentration of S on the two sides of the membrane ($[S]_1$ and $[S]_2$, respectively).

Diffusion across many biological membranes involves flux through finite distance of a membrane thickness (X). Hence, incorporating membrane thickness into the diffusion coefficient yields a more meaningful and easily measurable index of membrane permeability. The new index is called *permeability coefficient* (k_p), and is defined by Equation 7-3:

$$k_p = \frac{D}{X} \qquad (7\text{-}3)$$

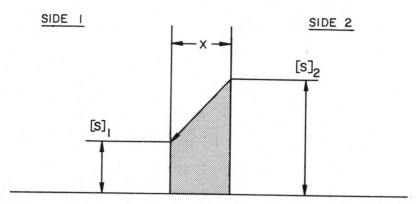

Figure 7-1. A scheme depicting diffusion Equation 7-2. $[S]_1$ and $[S]_2$ represent the concentration of S on the two sides of the membrane with thickness X, respectively.

Incorporating k_p into Equation 7-2 yields:

$$J = -k_p([S]_2 - [S]_1) \qquad (7-4)$$

where the terms in the parentheses represent the concentration difference $\Delta[S]$. Expanding Equation 7-4, we obtain an expression relating net flux (J) across the membrane to the difference between the influx and efflux:

$$\text{Net flux} = -k_p \cdot [S]_2 + k_p \cdot [S]_1 \qquad (7-5)$$

where $-k_p \cdot [S]_2$ represents the flux *into* and $+k_p \cdot [S]_1$ the flux *out of* the membrane, as indicated by the *minus* and *plus* signs, respectively.

From Equation 7-4 it is evident that if simple diffusion is the mechanism by which a solute is transported across the membrane, then the net flux is linearly and directly proportional to the difference in the solute concentrations on the two sides. In such a case, solute concentration would be the only factor limiting the net flux. However, if the solute transport involves mechanisms other than or in addition to diffusion, then the net flux is not linearly related to the concentration difference. Such a *nonlinear* relationship exemplifies a *carrier-mediated* type of transport, in which case both solute and carrier concentrations on the two sides of the membrane will be the factors limiting the net flux.

Although many conceivable relationships between the net flux and the solute concentration exist, we have selected three for consideration. The choice was dictated by (a) the ease of handling the theoretical treatment of the concepts, and (b) more importantly, the wide usage of these relationships in studying transport characteristics of biological membranes. Figure 7-2 presents the relationship of *reaction rate*, a factor related to net flux, to solute concentration for two transport mechanisms: (a) *simple diffusion* and (b) *carrier-mediated transport*, represented by *right-rectangular hyperbola* and *sigmoid* (S-shape) curves. Having already characterized transport by simple diffusion, let us now consider the carrier-mediated transport.

CARRIER-MEDIATED TRANSPORT

The concept of membrane as a porous barrier, evolved from diffusion studies, assumed a cell membrane with static structures designed to protect cellular constituents. However, recent extensive studies (Wilbrandt and Rosenberg, 1961) have necessitated a drastic change in this simple concept. The cell membrane is now believed to consist of a *dynamic structure* with the ability to regulate, through its internal machinery, the transport of solute across it.

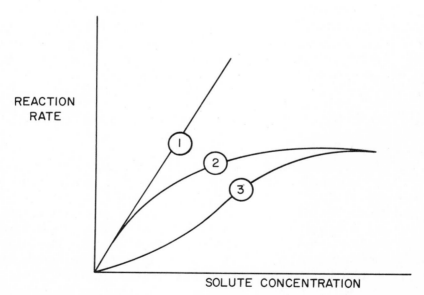

Figure 7-2. The relation of reaction rate to solute concentration for three types of transport: (1) simple diffusion; (2) carrier-mediated transport with fixed amount of carrier, represented by the right-rectangular hyperbola; and (3) carrier-mediated transport with variable amounts of carrier, represented by the sigmoid curve.

According to the most popular current concept, translocation of solutes across the membrane involves a temporary binding to parts of the membrane. If this binding is not rigidly fixed within the membrane and the solute-membrane complex can in some way move through the membrane, the transport is called *carrier-mediated*. This concept, although still hypothetical, has provided a powerful means of explaining many qualitative and quantitative aspects of cellular transport.

Carrier-mediated transport involves two types of chemical reactions, namely, *unimolecular* and *bimolecular* reactions. Since understanding the kinetics of carrier-mediated transport is ultimately related to an understanding of kinetics of these reactions, we shall begin this section with a quantitative description of the kinetics of these two types of reactions.

UNIMOLECULAR REACTIONS

The simplest chemical reaction involves the conversion of one molecule (A) into another (B). In chemical terminology, molecule A is called the *reacting substance* and B the *product*.

The rate of conversion of substance A into B, called *rate constant (K)*, is determined by the quantity of substance A reacting or B produced by the reaction per unit time. This idea is symbolized in Equation 7-6:

$$A \xrightarrow{K} B \qquad (7\text{-}6)$$

According to the principle of chemical-reaction kinetics, the rate of a chemical reaction (conversion of A to B in Equation 7-6) is proportional to the product of concentrations of the reacting substances. Applying this principle to the above reaction, we obtain:

$$[\dot{A}] = -K \qquad (7\text{-}7)$$

where $[\dot{A}]$ is the rate (dot over the bracketed quantity) of change of concentration of A per unit time. The negative sign indicates that the quantity of reacting substance decreases as the product is formed.

The rate of change of the reacting substance ($[\dot{A}]$) may or may not depend on the concentration of the reacting molecule ($[A]$). If $[\dot{A}]$ is *independent* of $[A]$, then the chemical reaction is called a *zero-order* reaction, and is described by the rate Equation 7-7. However, if $[\dot{A}]$ *depends* on $[A]$, then the chemical reaction is called a *first* or *higher-order* reaction, depending on the *sum of exponents* of the concentration factor which appear in the rate equation. For example, if the conversion of A into B is an *irreversible first-order* chemical reaction, then it can be described by the following rate equation,

$$[\dot{A}] = -K[A] \tag{7-8}$$

Chemically, the rate constant K is a measure of the probability of conversion of A into B, and is defined by the following equation:

$$K = Ze^{-\dfrac{E_a}{RT}} \tag{7-9}$$

where Z is the frequency of collisions of molecules of A and $e^{-E_a/RT}$, called *Boltzman's constant*, is the fraction of molecules of A with kinetic energy greater than the activation energy (E_a) required to initiate the conversion. Activation energy is measured in calories per mole. R is the molar gas constant in cal/deg/mole and T is the absolute temperature in degrees Kelvin. Addition of a catalyst or an enzyme lowers the activation energy.

Often it is convenient to express the increase in reaction rate occurring as a function of temperature. The term Q_{10} has been employed to describe the relative increase in velocity for a rise in temperature of 10 degrees centigrade.

To get an insight into the meaning of rate constant K, we have plotted (Fig. 7-3) the change in concentration of the reacting substance with time, during a chemical reaction. As shown, the concentration changes exponentially with time ($[A]_t$) reaching a value equal to 37 per cent of the original concentration ($[A]_{t=0}$) in one time constant (τ). The slope of the exponential curve is equal to the rate constant K, which is the reciprocal of the time constant (see Appendices A and B for further meaning of τ).

In the case of *reversible first-order* chemical reactions, not only the reactant A is converted into the product B, but also B is converted into A, as shown by the following reaction:

$$A \underset{K_2}{\overset{K_1}{\rightleftharpoons}} B \tag{7-10}$$

where K_1 is the rate constant for the conversion of A into B (*forward reaction*) and K_2 is the rate constant for the conversion of B into A (*backward or reverse reaction*).

According to the principles of chemical reaction kinetics, the net rate of change in reactant concentration with time ($[\dot{A}]$) is determined by the algebraic sum of the forward and backward reactions:

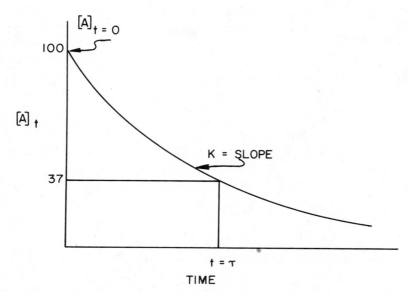

Figure 7-3. Time-course of change in the concentration of the reacting substance. $[A]_{t=0}$ is the original concentration and $[A]_t$ is the concentration at any other time during the reaction. They are related by the exponential equation $[A]_t = [A]_{t=0}e^{-Kt}$.

$$[\dot{A}] = -K_1[A] + K_2[B] \qquad (7\text{-}11)$$

where $-K_1[A]$ represents the fractional decrease and $+K_2[B]$ the fractional increase in $[\dot{A}]$. At equilibrium, $[\dot{A}] = 0$, and Equation 7-11 becomes,

$$-K_1[A]_{eq} + K_2[B]_{eq} = 0 \qquad (7\text{-}12)$$

The subscript *eq* indicates that these are concentrations at equilibrium. From Equation 7-12 we get:

$$\frac{[B]_{eq}}{[A]_{eq}} = \frac{K_1}{K_2} = K_{eq} \qquad (7\text{-}13)$$

where K_{eq} is the equilibrium constant of the reaction.

In any chemical reaction, the rate of change of the total free energy of the system (ΔF) depends on the change in the free energy of the reactants and products. Since K_{eq} is a measure of this latter quantity, it is related to ΔF by the following equation:

$$\Delta F = -RT \ln K_{eq} \tag{7-14}$$

where ln is the logarithm to the base e or the natural logarithm, and R and T were already defined. Taking advantage of rules for logarithm ($\ln = \log_e = 2.3 \log_{10}$), Equation 7-14 may be written in a more convenient form:

$$\Delta F = -2.3 \, RT \log K_{eq} \tag{7-15}$$

where $\log_{10}$ is the logarithm to the base 10. The negative sign indicates that the reaction occurs spontaneously. This happens if the numerical value of K_{eq} is greater than zero. If the value of K_{eq} is less than zero, ΔF will be positive, which means that energy must be expended in converting the reactants into the product.

Having thus delineated the fundamental laws of chemical kinetics for unimolecular reactions, let us now apply them to some physiologically important bimolecular reactions.

BIMOLECULAR REACTIONS

The simplest bimolecular reaction is one involving combination of two molecules to form a third one. Such a reaction may be illustrated by the following equation:

$$A + B \underset{K_2}{\overset{K_1}{\rightleftharpoons}} AB \tag{7-16}$$

where A and B are the reactants, AB is the product, K_1 is the rate constant for the forward reaction, and K_2 is the rate constant for the reverse reaction. At equilibrium, the rate constant for the formation of product is given by:

$$K_{eq} = \frac{K_1}{K_2} = \frac{[AB]}{[A] \cdot [B]} \tag{7-17}$$

A high value of K_{eq} indicates a high *affinity* (association) of A for B to form the product AB. Conversely, the equilibrium rate constant for the reverse reaction--conversion of product to reactants--is given by the equation:

$$K_m = \frac{K_2}{K_1} = \frac{[A] \cdot [B]}{[AB]}$$ (7-18)

where K_m is the dissociation constant and is a measure of the extent of the *binding* of A to B to form AB. The value of K_m is given by the reciprocal of K_{eq}. Thus, the greater the binding of the reactants, the smaller is the K_m (but the greater is the K_{eq}), and the greater would be the formation of the product.

Bimolecular reactions are the most common steps in any chain of complex chemical reactions occurring in biological systems. Because of this strategic position, they play a key role in any carrier-mediated transport. Basic to such a transport mechanism is the interaction of the so-called *substrate*--either a hormone, a neurochemical transmitter, or a drug--with a *carrier* substance, which in some circumstances may be replaced by a *receptor* or an *enzyme*. It is this carrier-substrate or enzyme substrate interaction which constitutes the core of most chemical reactions in biological systems, including the carrier-mediated transport.

To understand the mechanism of such a transport scheme and the factors affecting its efficiency, a rigorous mathematical treatment of the kinetics of the enzyme-substrate interaction is necessary. Such a formulation was first described by *Michaelis and Menten*. In this section, we shall first detail their formulation and then apply the concepts to the drug-receptor interactions which have a profound physiological and pharmacological significance in renal tubular transport of solutes. For an extensive treatment of this subject, consult the reviews by Bodansky (1959), Frieden (1964) and Christensen (1975).

THE MICHAELIS-MENTEN FORMULATION OF ENZYME-CATALYZED REACTIONS

Suppose we are interested in the effect of substrate concentration on the rate at which the substrate is converted into products, in a chemical reaction involving an enzyme or carrier. For simplicity, let us assume that at the start of the reaction only the substrate (S) and the enzyme (E) are present. As the reaction proceeds, a certain amount of S combines with E to form an enzyme-substrate complex (ES). The latter will then undergo appropriate chemical changes to yield the products (P) plus the enzyme to be reused in further conversion of the substrate. These two chemical reactions may be represented as follows:

$$S + E \underset{K_2}{\overset{K_1}{\rightleftharpoons}} ES \underset{K_4}{\overset{K_3}{\rightleftharpoons}} E + P$$ (7-19)

Applying the laws of chemical-reaction kinetics, the relationship between the rate of product formation ($[\dot{P}]$) and the substrate concentration ($[S]$) may be described by the following equations:

$$[\dot{ES}] = K_1[E]_f[S] + K_4[E]_f[P] - (K_2 + K_3)[ES] \tag{7-20}$$

$$[\dot{P}] = K_3[ES] - K_4[E]_f[P] \tag{7-21}$$

$$[E]_t = [E]_f + [ES] \tag{7-22}$$

where subscripts t and f stand for *total* and *free*, respectively.

Since at steady state, $[\dot{ES}] = 0$, and assuming that the rate constant $K_4 = 0$ (irreversible dissociation of ES), and the substrate concentration $[S]$ is much greater than $[ES]$, Equation 7-20 may be simplified to:

$$K_1[E]_f[S] = (K_2 + K_3)[ES] \tag{7-23}$$

Substituting for $[E]_f$ its equivalent expression from Equation 7-22 and rearranging terms, $[ES]$ may be expressed by the following equation:

$$[ES] = \frac{[E]_t \cdot [S]}{[S] + \dfrac{K_2 + K_3}{K_1}} \tag{7-24}$$

Chemically, the rate of formation of the product ($d[P]/dt = [\dot{P}]$) is given by the velocity of reaction yielding the product ($v = dP/dt$). Incorporating this fact into Equation 7-21 and assuming that $K_4 = 0$ (irreversible dissociation of ES), Equation 7-21 may be expressed as:

$$v = K_3[ES] \tag{7-25}$$

If we assume further that at high substrate concentration all of the enzyme is bound to the substrate, then $[E]_f = 0$ and $[E]_t = [ES]$. Consequently, at high substrate concentration the rate of product formation is maximal and hence the velocity of reaction becomes maximum. Therefore, at high substrate concentration Equation 7-25 becomes

$$\left(\frac{dP}{dt}\right)_{max} = V_{max} = K_3 [E]_t \qquad (7\text{-}26)$$

where V_{max} is the maximum velocity. Now multiplying both sides of Equation 7-24 by K_3 and replacing equivalent terms by v (Equation 7-25) and V_{max} (Equation 7-26), we obtain the following important equation relating the reaction velocity to substrate concentration in an enzyme-catalyzed reaction:

$$v = \frac{V_{max} \cdot [S]}{[S] + \dfrac{K_2 + K_3}{K_1}} \qquad (7\text{-}27)$$

where the rate constant terms in the denominator are collectively called Michaelis constant (K_m) and defined by the equation:

$$K_m = \frac{K_2 + K_3}{K_1} \qquad (7\text{-}28)$$

Hence, Equation 7-27 becomes:

$$v = \frac{V_{max} \cdot [S]}{[S] + K_m} \qquad (7\text{-}29)$$

Assuming that the rate constant K_2 is much greater than K_3, then Equation 7-28 gives the dissociation constant of the enzyme-substrate complex:

$$K_m = \frac{K_2}{K_1} = \frac{[S] \cdot [E]}{[ES]} \qquad (7\text{-}30)$$

The reciprocal of Michaelis constant ($1/K_m$) is a measure of the affinity of the enzyme for the substrate.

Solving Equation 7-29 for K_m and rearranging, we get:

$$K_m = [S]\left(\frac{V_{max}}{v} - 1\right) \qquad (7\text{-}31)$$

When the reaction is half completed, that is, $v = 1/2\ V_{max}$, Equation

7-31 becomes

$$K_m = [S] \qquad\qquad (7\text{-}32)$$

That is, K_m is numerically equal to the substrate concentration at which half-maximum velocity of reaction is obtained. K_m also has the dimension of concentration (moles/liter).

Equation 7-29 describes a *rectangular hyperbola*, where v is the dependent variable, [S] is the independent variable, K_m is the slope and V_{max} is the asymptote. Figure 7-4 shows the hyperbolic relation of the velocity to the substrate concentration. Note that at high substrate concentration the velocity approaches a maximum.

Experimentally, it is possible to estimate K_m by determining the concentration at half-maximum velocity. However, because of the hyperbolic relationship between velocity and substrate concentration, the estimate is only approximate. The result can be improved enormously if we transform Equation 7-29 into a form which yields a straight line. This transformation is called *Lineweaver-Burk* double-reciprocal:

$$\frac{1}{v} = \frac{K_m}{V_{max}} \cdot \frac{1}{[S]} + \frac{1}{V_{max}} \qquad\qquad (7\text{-}33)$$

Equation 7-33 is of the form $y = a + bx$, where $1/v = y$, $1/[S] = x$, $1/V_{max} = a$ or the y-intercept, and $K_m/V_{max} = b$ or the slope. Therefore, when $1/v$ is plotted against $1/[S]$, a straight line results (Fig. 7-5). At infinite substrate concentration, when $1/[S] = 0$, from Equation 7-33 we get $1/v = 1/V_{max}$ (that is, the intercept on the velocity (ordinate) axis yields the value for the maximal velocity). At infinite velocity, when $1/v = 0$, the intercept on the concentration (abscissa) axis gives the value for the dissociation constant of the

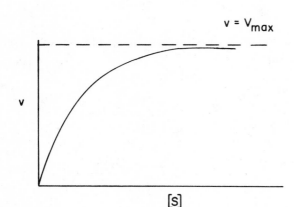

Figure 7-4. Hyperbolic relation of reaction velocity to substrate concentration.

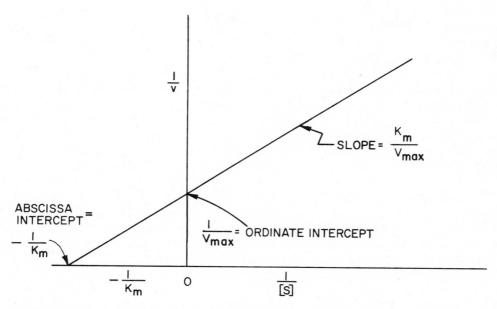

Figure 7-5. Lineweaver-Burk plot of the reaction velocity against substrate concentration.

enzyme-substrate complex, $1/K_m = -1/[S]$.

The enzyme-catalyzed reactions are influenced by a number of factors, including temperature, pH, and inhibitors. Let us briefly consider the effects of each.

A. EFFECTS OF TEMPERATURE. When enzyme-catalyzed reactions are studied over a range of temperatures, it is commonly observed that the velocity of reaction passes through a maximum (optimum). This temperature is not well defined and may vary with the pH, substrate concentration, purity of preparation, activators, or inhibitors present, etc. The failure to give proportionate increases in reaction rate at higher temperatures is due to inactivation (either reversible or irreversible) of the catalyst. As in other chemical reactions at low temperatures (before inactivation), a relationship between reaction velocity (v) and the temperature is given by the Arrhenius equation (Equation 7-34):

$$v = E_o e^{-\frac{E_a}{RT}} \tag{7-34}$$

where E_o is the minimum or threshold activation energy and E_a, R, and T have already been defined.

B.   EFFECTS OF pH.   When enzyme-catalyzed reactions are studied over a range of pH, under otherwise standardized conditions, it is also commonly observed that the rate passes through a maximum.   This phenomenon, like the effects of temperature, can be adequately explained by inactivation of the enzyme.   Usually the curve depicting the pH effects is monophasic, but like the optimum temperature, the optimum pH is not a fundamental constant of each enzyme but may vary with the temperature, concentration and type of buffer cofactor and substrate concentration.   The decrease from optimal enzyme activity often follows a bell-shaped curve--like an acid-base dissociation curve.   In any particular case, however, the effects of pH on catalysis could be due to ionization of the substrate, or the enzyme.

C.   ACTION OF INHIBITORS.   It is often observed that various compounds inhibit a particular enzyme-catalyzed reaction.   It is possible from a knowledge of chemistry and kinetics to characterize the relative effectiveness of the inhibitor as well as to obtain information concerning the mechanism of inhibition.
Inhibitors generally fall into three categories:
1.   Competitive Inhibitors.   They are often structurally related to the substrate and compete for it with the enzyme.   Presumably inhibition occurs by combination of the inhibitor with the same enzyme site which binds with the substrate during the catalytic process. In this type of inhibition, K_m but not V_{max} is affected.   Hence, increasing the substrate concentration reverses the inhibition.   A Lineweaver-Burk plot of reaction velocity as a function of competitive inhibitor and substrate concentrations is shown in Figure 7-6.   Note that increasing the inhibitor concentration affects both K_m and slope.

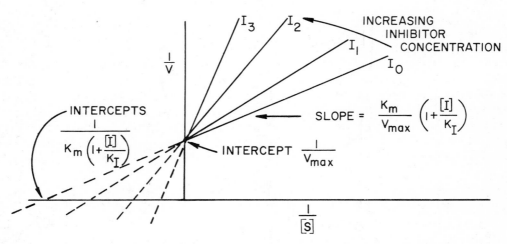

Figure 7-6.   Lineweaver-Burk plot of the reaction velocity against substrate concentration in the presence of a competitive inhibitor.

The general equation describing this type of inhibition is:

$$\frac{1}{v} = \frac{K_m}{V_{max}} \left(1 + \frac{[I]}{K_I} \right) \frac{1}{[S]} + \frac{1}{V_{max}} \qquad (7\text{-}35)$$

where $[I]$ is the inhibitor concentration and K_I is the rate constant for the dissociation of the enzyme-inhibitor complex.

2. Uncompetitive Inhibitors. They influence V_{max} but not the slope, K_m/V_{max}. In this case an increase in substrate concentration does not overcome the inhibition. Presumably the mechanism of inhibition involves combination with the enzyme-substrate complex, although the same type of inhibition would be produced from an essentially irreversible combination of enzyme with inhibitor, yielding a catalytically inactive complex. Uncompetitive inhibitors are very frequently specific for a particular enzyme or group of enzymes. A Lineweaver-Burk plot of uncompetitive type inhibition yields typical curves shown in Figure 7-7. The general equation describing this type of inhibition is:

$$\frac{1}{v} = \frac{K_m}{V_{max}} \cdot \frac{1}{[S]} + \left(1 + \frac{[I]}{K_I} \right) \frac{1}{V_{max}} \qquad (7\text{-}36)$$

3. Noncompetitive Inhibitors. They affect V_{max} but not K_m. These inhibitors do not compete with the substrate for the enzyme, and at a constant inhibitor concentration, the extent of inhibition is the

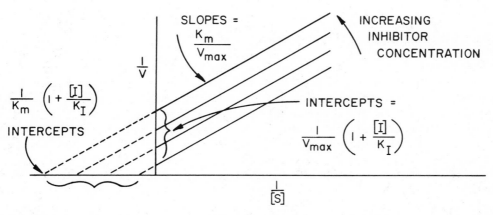

Figure 7-7. Lineweaver-Burk plot of the reaction velocity against substrate concentration in the presence of an uncompetitive inhibitor.

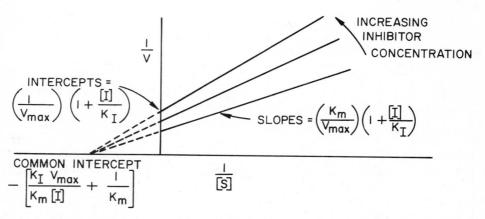

Figure 7-8. Lineweaver-Burk plot of the reaction velocity against substrate concentration in the presence of a non-competitive inhibitor.

same at all substrate concentrations. Inhibitors which react with functional groups (SH, OH, COOH, NH_2, etc.) and many types of reagents which alter protein structure with consequent denaturation fall into this category. A Lineweaver-Burk plot of noncompetitive inhibition is shown in Figure 7-8. The general equation which describes this type of inhibition is:

$$\frac{1}{v} = \left(1 + \frac{[I]}{K_I}\right)\left(\frac{K_m}{V_{max}} \cdot \frac{1}{[S]} + \frac{1}{V_{max}}\right) \tag{7-37}$$

THE DRUG OR HORMONE-RECEPTOR INTERACTION

The action of various drugs or hormones on target tissues is believed to be a consequence of a series of complex chemical reactions beginning with the interaction of, for example, the hormone (H) with a receptor site (R). The hormone-receptor complex (HR) thus formed will then initiate a series of complex chemical reactions within the target tissues, leading eventually to the emergence of the desired response.

Figure 7-9 presents a block diagram of some of the steps involved in drug or hormone-receptor interaction, as revealed by recent elaborate studies (Sutherland et al., 1968). The receptor is represented by a box in the left, with hormone concentration ([H]) as the input and the hormone-receptor complex concentration ([HR]) as the output. In this scheme, it is assumed that the hormone combines with one receptor and that all receptors are identical. The two arrows impinging at the bottom of the box are the indirect forcings, and more

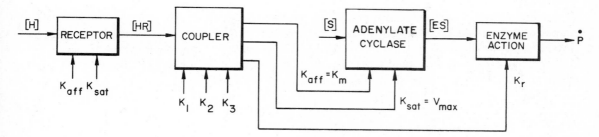

Figure 7-9. A schematic diagram showing possible steps involved in drug- or hormone-receptor interactions.

specifically may be called the *properties* of the receptor box. As such, for a given hormone concentration (input) the receptor properties determine the magnitude of the hormone-receptor complex concentration (output). The first property (K_{aff}) denotes the *relative affinity* of the hormone for the receptor. It is analogous to the reciprocal of the Michaelis constant (K_m). The second property (K_{sat}) denotes the *maximum number of receptors occupied* by the hormone when its concentration is infinite. It is a measure of the receptor binding capacity and is analogous to V_{max}. Accordingly, the concentration of the hormone-receptor complex ([HR]) depends not only on the hormone concentration but also on the two receptor properties (K_{aff} and K_{sat}).

Analogous to the Michaelis-Menten formulation of the kinetics of the enzyme catalyzed reactions, we may write an equation relating the output of the receptor box ([HR]) to the input ([H]) and receptor properties (K_{aff}) and K_{sat}):

$$[HR] = \frac{K_{sat} \cdot [H]}{K_{aff} + [H]} \tag{7-38}$$

The next box, called the *coupler*, represents the physical or chemical coupling of the hormone-receptor complex, formed on the outside surface of the target cell membrane. The three arrows, designated as K_1, K_2, and K_3, impinging at the bottom of the coupler box, represent the properties of the coupler. They influence the reactions depicted by the next two boxes, as discussed below.

The enzyme involved in the chemical reaction represented by box three is *adenylate cyclase*; it breaks two phosphate groups from the adenosine triphosphate or ATP yielding a cyclic form of the adenosine 3',5'-monophosphate (c-AMP). In the block diagram, the ATP concentration in the cell is represented by [S], which is the substrate upon which adenylate cyclase acts, and the rate of production of c-AMP as $\dot{P}$, which is related to the final tissue response. Substantial experimental evidence indicate that the response induced by the hormone is directly related to the rate of formation of c-AMP.

As shown in the diagram, the rate of production of c-AMP ($\dot{P}$) is directly related to the concentration of the enzyme-substrate complex, [ES]. In accordance with the Michaelis-Menten concept of enzyme kinetics, we may relate [ES] to the substrate concentration ([S]) and the two enzyme properties (K_m and V_{max}) as follows:

$$[ES] = \frac{1}{K_r}\left(\frac{V_{max} \cdot [S]}{K_m + [S]}\right) \tag{7-39}$$

where K_r represents the rate of conversion of ES to the product and is analogous to K_3 in Equation 7-19. The rate of formation of the product ($\dot{P}$) may be related to [ES] by the equation

$$\dot{P} = K_r[ES] \tag{7-40}$$

As indicated by the block diagram, through the coupler, the hormone-receptor complex influences the formation of both ES and c-AMP. In the absence of precise information, these relationships may be represented by the following three linear equations:

$$K_m = K_1[HR] \tag{7-41}$$

$$V_{max} = K_2[HR] \tag{7-42}$$

$$K_r = K_3[HR] \tag{7-43}$$

Incorporating these relationships into the Equation 7-39 and then substituting the results into Equation 7-40 yields an expression relating the rate of formation of the product ($\dot{P}$) or the ultimate tissue response to the hormone concentration ([H]):

$$\dot{P} = \left(\frac{K_2[S]}{K_2 + [S]}\right)\left(\frac{K_{sat} \cdot [H]}{K_{aff} + [H]}\right) \tag{7-44}$$

Assuming that there is a large and constant supply of the substrate S (that is, ATP) within the cell, then, according to

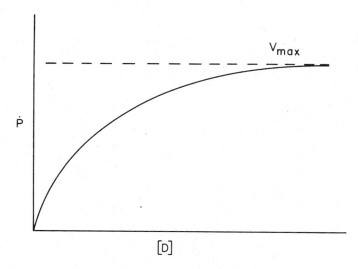

Figure 7-10. The dose-response relationship of a typical drug.

Equation 7-44, the rate of formation of the product or the response is a hyperbolic function of the hormone or drug concentration, as depicted in Figure 7-10. Because the first portion of this graph rises very steeply, the effect of drug concentration on the rate of product formation may be better displayed by plotting $\dot{P}$ against the logarithm of the drug concentration. Such a plot yields a *sigmoid* or S-shape curve, as shown in Figure 7-11. In this plot, the rate of product formation at maximal drug concentration is called the *intrinsic activity*. This is the conventional method used by pharmacologists to represent the *dose-response* relationship for a drug, which has also been widely adopted by biochemists.

FACILITATED DIFFUSION

Facilitated diffusion represents a type of carrier-mediated transport. It differs from *free diffusion* in two respects: (a) facilitated diffusion leads to equilibration, rather than accumulation, of the substrate; and (b) its efficiency depends on both the substrate and carrier concentrations and their interactions.

Experimental analyses of substrate transport, particularly in red blood cells (Britton, 1964) have revealed that the kinetics of facilitated diffusion is strongly analogous to that of enzyme-catalyzed chemical reactions. Keeping this in mind, certain characteristics common to carrier-mediated transport and facilitated diffusion in particular may be listed as follows:

1. The transport mechanism is saturated at high substrate concentration.

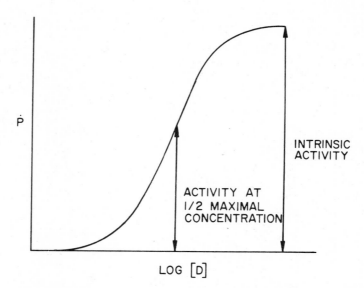

Figure 7-11. Conventional plot of the dose-response relationship of a typical drug.

2. There are both structural specificity and affinity of the carrier for the substrate.

3. Presence of a second substrate (B) competitively inhibits the transport of the first (A), such that the two fluxes are not additive $(J_A + J_B > J_{A+B})$.

4. With near saturation of carrier-substrate interactions, the flux is proportional to the reciprocal of the difference in substrate concentration $(J_A \simeq 1/\Delta[A])$.

5. Under similar conditions, substrate flux is inversely related to carrier affinity $(J_A \simeq K_m)$. This relationship holds with either fixed or mobile receptor sites or carriers.

6. The concentration gradient of one substrate may cause uphill transport of another substrate. This is called *counter transport*, not active transport, and can occur only with mobile carrier.

7. Addition of one substrate will increase the flux of another substrate, depending upon their affinities for the carrier. This is called *competitive acceleration*.

The kinetics of the carrier-mediated transport is much more complex than that for the enzyme-catalyzed chemical reactions. This is, in part, due to the fact that conversion of the substrate to the products is not irreversible. Recognizing this, Rosenberg and Wilbrandt (1963) formulated a quantitative description of the carrier-mediated transport by applying the Michaelis-Menten concepts of enzyme kinetics using the following assumptions:

1. Substrate (S) is transported through the membrane as a complex (SC) with the carrier (C).

2. Rates of substrate movement are proportional to the

difference in the substrate-carrier complex at the two sides of the membrane ($J_S \simeq [SC_1] - [SC_2]$).

3. Carrier and carrier-substrate complex have the same diffusion coefficient in the membrane (though it may be greater than that for substrate alone).

4. There is a fixed amount of the carrier within the membrane, so that $[C]_t = [C]_f + [SC]$, where $[C]_t$ and $[C]_f$ are the total and free carrier concentrations, respectively.

5. There is a chemical equilibrium between the substrate and carrier at each membrane interface, as expressed by Equation 7-45:

$$K_{CS} = \frac{[S][C]_f}{[SC]} \tag{7-45}$$

where K_{CS} is the dissociation constant for the substrate-carrier complex. Also, the equilibrium time is very rapid relative to the diffusion time.

Figure 7-12 incorporates these assumptions in a scheme for carrier-mediated transport. As shown, combination of the substrate and carrier on side 1 yields a certain concentration of carrier-substrate complex, determined by the equilibrium reaction shown on the left. The substrate then diffuses through the membrane as SC, according to the SC concentration gradient within the membrane. When SC reaches side 2, it dissociates into the substrate and carrier according to equilibrium equations shown on the right. Carrier regeneration on side 2 increases its concentration, resulting in the return of carrier to side 1 according to the carrier concentration gradient. In all these reactions, the diffusion of carrier and carrier-substrate complex is the rate-limiting reaction. The

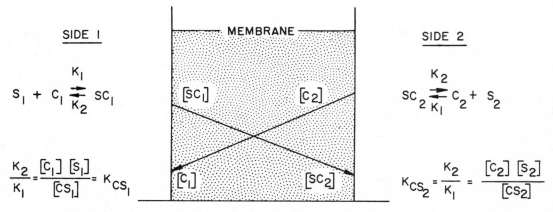

Figure 7-12. A schematic representation of the carrier-mediated transport.

transport process depicted in Figure 7-12 continues as long as the substrate is available.

Having described those features of the carrier-mediated transport common to both facilitated diffusion and active transport, let us now consider quantitatively the distinguishing characteristics of each.

In facilitated diffusion, the affinity between the carrier and substrate is the same on both sides of the membrane. Thus, the dissociation constants for the carrier-substrate complex on both sides are equal: $K_{CS_1} = K_{CS_2}$. This results in rapid equilibration even if

$[SC_1]$ is not equal to $[SC_2]$. Therefore,

$$\frac{[S_1][C_1]}{[SC_1]} = \frac{[S_2][C_2]}{[SC_2]} \tag{7-46}$$

Note that if there is no substrate concentration gradient across the membrane (that is, $[S_1] = [S_2]$), the above equation becomes

$$\frac{[C_1]}{[C_2]} = \frac{[SC_1]}{[SC_2]} \tag{7-47}$$

which states that the substrate-carrier concentration gradient in one direction is equal to the free carrier concentration gradient in the other direction. In such a condition, no substrate transport occurs. Therefore, to have any substrate flux, there must be a substrate concentration gradient.

To explore other factors affecting this type of transport, let us examine the kinetics of facilitated diffusion. For this analysis, we assume that the total carrier concentration will, in the steady state, be the same on the two sides and throughout the area within the membrane:

$$[C]_t = [C]_f + [SC] \tag{7-48}$$

Substituting for $[C]_f$ in Equation 7-45 its corresponding value from Equation 7-48 and solving for $[SC]$ yields:

$$[SC] = [C]_t \left(\frac{[S]}{K_{CS} + [S]} \right) \tag{7-49}$$

The terms in parentheses are a measure of the fraction of total carrier bound to substrate within the membrane. Since substrate can only pass through the membrane in combination with the carrier, then

its flux (J_S) is equal to the substrate-carrier complex flux (J_{SC}).
Both substrate and complex fluxes are proportional to the
substrate-carrier concentration gradient:

$$J_S = J_{SC} = D_{SC}/\zeta \, ([SC_1] - [SC_2]) \qquad (7\text{-}50)$$

where ζ is the membrane thickness, D_{SC}/ζ is the membrane permeability
to the complex, and the term in parentheses is the concentration
gradient of the complex. Expressing the substrate-carrier
concentration on each side of the membrane in terms of total and free
carrier concentrations (Equation 7-48), Equation 7-50 becomes

$$J_S = J_{SC} = (D_{SC}/\zeta \cdot [C]_t) \left(\frac{[S_1]}{K_{CS_1} + [S_1]} - \frac{[S_2]}{K_{CS_2} + [S_2]} \right) \qquad (7\text{-}51)$$

The product term in the first parentheses represents the maximum
substrate flux and the terms in the second parentheses represent the
difference in the fraction of total carrier bound to the substrate on
the two sides of the membrane.

Equation 7-51 may be used to explore the effects of four
conditions on transport by facilitated diffusion.

1. EQUAL SUBSTRATE CONCENTRATION ON BOTH SIDES ($[S_1] = [S_2]$).
In the absence of substrate concentration gradient, the terms in the
second parentheses in Equation 7-51 become zero and hence there will
be no substrate flux ($J_S = J_{SC} = 0$).

2. LOW CARRIER SATURATION. When substrate concentration is
below saturating level, less substrate-carrier complex will be formed.
This means that the value of K_C far exceeds $[S]$ in Equation 7-51.
Hence, if $K_{CS_1} = K_{CS_2} = K_{CS}$, we get:

$$J_S = D_{SC}/\zeta \cdot [C]_t \cdot \frac{1}{K_{CS}} \, ([S_1] - [S_2]) \qquad (7\text{-}52)$$

where $1/K_{CS} = K_m$ is a measure of the affinity between carrier and the
substrate. In this case, substrate flux is largely determined by the
product of total carrier concentration and affinity ($[C]_t \cdot 1/K_{CS}$).
Thus, at low substrate concentration or low carrier saturation,
substrate flux may be approximated by a simple diffusion.

3. HIGH CARRIER SATURATION. At high substrate concentration,
the carrier will be fully saturated, in which case the value of $[S]$
will be much greater than K_{CS}. Assuming that $[S_1]/(K_{CS_1} + [S_1]) = 1$
and $[S_2]/(K_{CS_2} + [S_2]) < 1$, Equation 7-51 becomes

$$J_S = D_{SC}/\zeta \cdot [C]_t \left(1 - \frac{[S_2]}{K_{CS_2} + [S_2]}\right) \qquad (7\text{-}53)$$

It is apparent from this equation that the substrate flux is limited by its concentration on side 2 of the membrane ($[S_2]$). Reducing $[S_2]$, such as might occur if the substrate is removed or metabolized, increases the carrier-substrate concentration gradient thereby increasing substrate flux across the membrane.

4. COMPETITIVE INHIBITION. Suppose there are two substrates, R and S, which can combine with the carrier, C. Then Equation 7-48 will become

$$[C]_t = [C]_f + [CR] + [CS] \qquad (7\text{-}54)$$

Assuming, as before, that the substrate transport is equal to the substrate-carrier complex flux, we can express the relative rate of complex formation in terms of dissociation constant:

$$K_{CS} = \frac{[S][C]}{[SC]} \qquad (7\text{-}55)$$

$$K_{CR} = \frac{[R][C]}{[CR]} \qquad (7\text{-}56)$$

Substituting for [CR] and [CS] in Equation 7-54 their corresponding expressions from Equations 7-55 and 7-56, and expressing the resulting equation in terms of [CS], we obtain

$$[CS] = [C]_t \left(\frac{[S]}{[S] + K_{cs} + R\dfrac{K_{CS}}{K_{CR}}}\right) \qquad (7\text{-}57)$$

Comparison of Equations 7-57 and 7-49 shows the effect of addition of a second substrate (R) on the relative concentration of the complex formed between the carrier and the first substrate ($[CS]$). This effect is determined by the term $R(K_{CS}/K_{CR})$ in Equation 7-57. If the carrier has a greater affinity for R than S, then $R(K_{CS}/K_{CR}) > 1$, in which case an increase in the concentration of R results in a proportional decrease in J_S.

ACTIVE TRANSPORT

In Chapter 2, active transport was defined as the movement of solute against an electrochemical gradient. Unlike facilitated diffusion for which $K_{CS_1} = K_{CS_2}$ and for which there was *equilibration*

of the carrier on both sides of the membrane, active transport is characterized by *inequality* of K_m on both sides and an *uphill* transport. This uphill flow of material (from lower to higher chemical potential) is believed to be coupled to a downhill transport of another material.

Analogous to facilitated diffusion, Rosenberg and Wilbrandt (1963) have made a quantitative treatment of the active transport based on the assumption that there are "asymmetric chemical reactions of a fixed quantity of the carrier between two forms C and Z, differing in their affinities to the substrate. The necessary gradient, then, is maintained by metabolic chemical reactions and the continuous carrier flow is replaced by a metabolically driven carrier cycle."

Figure 7-13 illustrates schematically the essential elements of an uphill transporting carrier system. The basic assumptions are: (1) the membrane contains a fixed total quantity of carrier, cycling between the two forms C and Z, and (2) the two carriers have different affinities for the substrate S, characterized by the Michaelis constants K_{CS} and K_{ZS}, respectively. Furthermore, it is assumed that the carriers are in equilibrium with the substrate, as shown, and can move through the membrane by diffusion, both in the free form (C and Z) and bound to the substrate (CS and ZS). Free substrate cannot pass

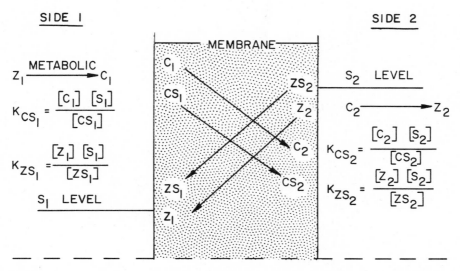

Figure 7-13. A schematic diagram of an uphill transporting carrier system, representing active transport.

through the membrane.

Assuming that the diffusion coefficients (D), for both free and bound carriers are identical, then the total carrier concentration will, in the steady state, be the same on the two sides of the membrane:

$$[C]_t = [C]_f + [Z]_f + [CS] + [ZS] \qquad (7\text{-}58)$$

Since the substrate can only move through the membrane in combination with the carrier, its flux is given by,

$$J_S = J_{CS+ZS} = \frac{D}{\zeta} [C]_t \left([CS_1] + [ZS_1] - [CS_2] - [ZS_2] \right) \qquad (7\text{-}59)$$

Expressing the various carrier-substrate concentration terms in the parentheses in terms of the dissociation equations given in Figure 7-13, Equation 7-59 becomes

$$J_S = \qquad (7\text{-}60)$$

$$\frac{D}{\zeta} [C]_t \left\{ \frac{[S_1]}{[S_1] + K_{CS_1} \left(\dfrac{K_{ZS_1} + K_{ZS_1} \dfrac{[Z_1]}{[C_1]}}{K_{ZS_1} + K_{CS_1} \dfrac{[Z_1]}{[C_1]}} \right)} - \frac{[S_2]}{[S_2] + K_{CS_2} \left(\dfrac{K_{ZS_2} + K_{ZS_2} \dfrac{[Z_2]}{[C_2]}}{K_{ZS_2} + K_{CS_2} \dfrac{[Z_2]}{[C_2]}} \right)} \right\}$$

The above equation can be simplified by replacing as shown:

$$\theta_1 = K_{CS_1} \left(\frac{K_{ZS_1} + K_{ZS_1} \dfrac{[Z_1]}{[C_1]}}{K_{ZS_1} + K_{CS_1} \dfrac{[Z_1]}{[C_1]}} \right) \qquad (7\text{-}61)$$

$$\text{and} \qquad \theta_2 = K_{CS_2} \left(\frac{K_{ZS_2} + K_{ZS_2} \dfrac{[Z_2]}{[C_2]}}{K_{ZS_2} + K_{CS_2} \dfrac{[Z_2]}{[C_2]}} \right) \qquad (7\text{-}62)$$

Then,

$$J_S = \frac{D}{\zeta} [C]_t \left(\frac{[S_1]}{[S_1] + \theta_1} - \frac{[S_2]}{[S_2] + \theta_2} \right) \qquad (7\text{-}63)$$

where θ_1 and θ_2 are equal to the concentration of S_1 and S_2 at half-saturation. They are the "steady-state" constants relating substrate-carrier reactions on the two sides of the membrane.

Equation 7-63, describing the kinetics of the C-Z carrier system, differs from the Equation 7-51 for the equilibrating carrier system or the facilitated diffusion in two respects. First, the Michaelis constants (K_{CS_1} and K_{CS_2}) in Equation 7-51 are replaced by two complex functions (θ_1 and θ_2) containing the Michaelis constants for the two carrier complexes CS and ZS and the concentration ratios of the two carriers on the two sides of the membrane. Second, due to metabolic asymmetry ($[Z_1]/[C_1] \neq [Z_2]/[C_2]$), the functions θ_1 and θ_2 differ.

Finally, there are two conditions which make θ_1 equal to θ_2--that is, transforming the active transport Equation 7-63 into the equilibrating carrier system or the facilitated diffusion. First, if $[Z_1]/[C_1] = [Z_2]/[C_2]$ (i.e., if they are symmetrical metabolic reactions), and second, if the two carriers have equal affinities for the substrate on both sides of the membrane ($K_{CS} = K_{ZS}$).

With these materials serving as the background, we are now ready to consider in Chapters 8 and 9 the mechanisms of renal transport for various solutes present in the ultrafiltrate as well as a quantitative account of those which are finally excreted in the urine.

PROBLEMS

7-1. The following table lists the dose-response data for the action of a drug with and without the presence of an inhibitor.

Drug Concentration (mg/ml)	Response (Arbitrary Units)	
	Without Inhibitor	With Inhibitor
20	25	16
22	26	18
25	28	19
29	29	21
33	32	23
40	34	26
50	37	28
67	40	32
100	45	38
200	50	45

a. Calculate the dissociation constant for the drug-receptor complex.
b. Calculate the dissociation constant for the inhibitor-receptor complex.
c. Indicate the type of inhibitor used.

7-2. On a Lineweaver-Burk transformation of a rectangular hyperbolic process,
a. What is the ordinate intercept a measure of?
b. What is the abscissa a measure of?

7-3. For "carrier-mediated" transport, the net flux of substrate is considered to be *directly proportional* to what?

7-4. Give a descriptive explanation for how a "carrier-mediated" transport could have substrate flux inversely related to substrate-carrier affinity.

7-5. What are the two conditions under which active transport is reduced to facilitated diffusion?
a. _____
b. _____

7-6. The dissociation equilibrium constant between D-mannose and human red blood cells (RBC's) has been estimated as 0.02 M. If the RBC's were allowed to equilibrate in 0.2 M D-mannose solutions, what would be the expected initial flux, expressed as a fraction of the maximum possible flux, of that sugar?

REFERENCES

1. Bodansky, O.: Diagnostic applications of enzymes in medicine. *Am. J. Med.* *27*:861-874, 1959.

2. Britton, H. G.: Permeability of the human red cell to labelled glucose. *J. Physiol.* *170*:1-20, 1964.

3. Christensen, H. N.: *Biological Transport*. 2nd ed. Addison-Wesley Publishing Co., Inc., Reading, Mass., 1975.

4. Curran, P. F., and Schultz, S. G.: Transport across membranes: general principles. In: *Handbook of Physiology*. Vol. 3, Sec. 6, *Alimentary Canal*. Edited by C. F. Code and W. Heidel. Washington, D. C., American Physiological Society, 1968, pp. 1217-1243.

5. Frieden, C.: Treatment of enzyme kinetic data. *J. Biol. Chem.* *239(10)*:3522-3531, 1964.

6. Rosenberg, T., and Wilbrandt, W.: Carrier transport uphill. I. General. *J. Theoret. Biol.* *5*:288-305, 1963.

7. Sutherland, E. W., Robison, C. A., and Butcher, R. W.: Some aspects of biological role of adenosine 3',5'-monophosphate (cyclic AMP). *Circulation* *37*:279-306, 1968.

8. Wilbrandt, W., and Rosenberg, T.: The concept of carrier transport and its corollaries in pharmacology. *Pharmacol. Rev.* *13*:109-183, 1961.

Chapter 8

TUBULAR PROCESSING OF GLOMERULAR ULTRAFILTRATE: MECHANISMS OF ELECTROLYTE AND WATER TRANSPORT

Once the glomerular filtrate is formed, the next major steps in the renal regulation of body fluids occur in the *tubular exchanger*. Here, as the filtrate flows under a hydrostatic pressure head along the various nephron segments, almost all the filtered water and solutes are *reabsorbed* from, while some organic compounds are *secreted* into the tubules, yielding a small, concentrated volume of urine. The final volume and composition of this *excreted* urine will largely depend on the *efficiency* of these two tubular transport processes and their intra- and extrarenal regulation.

Our present knowledge of the mechanisms of tubular processing of the filtrate is primarily due to the development of numerous quantitative methods for the study of renal function. Therefore, a familiarity with the essence of these methods and the scope of their applications should provide a better understanding of the renal mechanisms that they purport to elucidate. Hence, we begin this chapter with a brief description of the various methods used to characterize the renal transport mechanisms involved in the *sequential processing* of the ultrafiltrate and its components.

METHODS OF STUDYING TUBULAR TRANSPORT

While the clearance techniques described in Chapter 6 provided much useful information about the overall performance of the kidney, they have limited value in assessing the sequential processing of the filtrate and its constituents along the various nephron segments. Direct information about the mechanisms of tubular processing of the filtrate and its constituents have been obtained from the application of four widely used methods:

MICROPUNCTURE COLLECTION OF
TUBULAR FLUID

The micropuncture collection and analysis of fluid from single mammalian nephrons was first introduced by Richards and Walker and their collaborators (1937). Since then, this technique has been successfully applied to collect and analyze fluids from the proximal and distal convoluted tubules of the superficial nephrons as well as the medullary segments of the loop of Henle and collecting tubules (Gottschalk and Lassiter, 1967). Recent refinements of these techniques have made it possible to isolate and analyze fluids collected from segments of the nephron previously inaccessible to direct study (Kokko, 1974).

Briefly, the technique involves puncturing, under a stereomicroscope and quartz rod illumination, the desired tubular segment with micropipette, having an outer diameter of 6 to 10 μ. A small volume of tubular fluid (about 1 microliter) is then collected under free flow conditions and analyzed. After collection of the tubular fluid, a dye solution is then injected to mark the punctured site for subsequent determination of its position relative to the glomerulus by microdissection. Such a procedure permits quantitative analysis of the tubular transport process along the length of a given nephron segment.

The tubular concentration of a given solute, thus obtained, at any position along the nephron depends not only on how much of the solute has been reabsorbed, but also on how much water has left the tubular segment. Since we are interested in solute transport, the effect of water movement can easily be eliminated by comparing the ratio of the tubular fluid-to-plasma solute concentration, or simply TF/P, to that of a non-absorbable solute which remains in the tubule, such as inulin. Since for a given collected sample, the tubular volume flow is the same, the TF/P ratios are identical to clearance ratios described in Chapter 6. The rationale for comparing the TF/P ratio of a solute to that of inulin to assess the nature of tubular transport of that solute is as follows.

The quantity of a substance x filtered per minute is given by the product of the glomerular filtration rate (GFR) and the plasma concentration of the substance ($[x]_p$), assuming a permeability ratio of unity,

$$\text{Quantity of x filtered} = \text{GFR} \cdot [x]_p \qquad (8\text{-}1)$$

Similarly, the quantity of a substance x remaining in any tubular segment of the nephron is given by the product of the volume of the filtrate remaining in that segment ($\dot{V}_f$) and the tubular concentration of substance x in that segment ($[x]_f$):

$$\text{Quantity of x remaining} = \dot{V}_f \cdot [x]_f \qquad (8\text{-}2)$$

Thus, at any point along the nephron the difference between the quantity filtered and the quantity remaining in the tubule is the amount of substance x which has been transferred across the tubular cells ($\dot{T}_x$). Therefore, for any nephron segment, we can write a material balance equation relating the quantity filtered to that remaining in the tubule:

$$GFR \cdot [x]_p = \dot{V}_f \cdot [x]_f \pm \dot{T}_x \qquad (8\text{-}3)$$

where the $\pm$ signs indicate whether the solute is secreted ($+\dot{T}_x$) into or reabsorbed ($-\dot{T}_x$) from the tubule. If a substance is neither reabsorbed nor secreted, then $\dot{T}_x = 0$, and Equation 8-3 becomes

$$GFR \cdot [x]_p = \dot{V}_f \cdot [x]_f \qquad (8\text{-}4)$$

Writing Equation 8-4 in terms of the fluid-to-plasma concentration ratios, we get

$$[x]_f/[x]_p = GFR/\dot{V}_f \qquad (8\text{-}5)$$

Analogous equation for inulin yields

$$[In]_f/[In]_p = GFR/\dot{V}_f \qquad (8\text{-}6)$$

where the right hand side of Equation 8-6 is now recognized as the reciprocal fraction of fluid remaining in the tubule, or the so-called *rejection ratio*.

Now, from Equation 8-4, the fraction of a substance x remaining in any tubular segment of the nephron may be expressed as

$$\text{Fraction of x remaining} = \dot{V}_f \cdot [x]_f/GFR \cdot [x]_p \qquad (8\text{-}7)$$

Note that for inulin the value of this fraction is unity. Rearranging Equation 8-7 in terms of the fluid-to-plasma concentrations ratios, we obtain

$$\text{Fraction of x remaining} = \frac{[x]_f/[x]_p}{GFR/\dot{V}_f} \qquad (8\text{-}8)$$

Comparing this equation with Equation 8-6 reveals that the denominator of Equation 8-8 is the same as the fluid-to-plasma concentration ratio for inulin ($[In]_f/[In]_p$). Substituting this ratio in Equation 8-8, the fraction of substance x remaining in the tubular fluid may now be expressed as a ratio of the fluid-to-plasma concentration ratio of the substance to that for inulin:

$$\text{Fraction of x remaining} = \frac{[x]_f/[x]_p}{[In]_f/[In]_p} = \frac{(TF/P)_x}{(TF/P)_{In}} \qquad (8-9)$$

If the TF/P ratio of the solute in question were greater than that for inulin, then the solute must have been secreted into the tubule. If the TF/P ratio for the solute were less than that of inulin, then the solute must have been reabsorbed.

The successful application of micropuncture technique over the past few decades has greatly contributed to the evolution of our present concepts of renal function. Specifically, it has elucidated the renal transport mechanisms for a variety of plasma solutes (Gottschalk and Lassiter, 1973), the renal action of drugs, particularly the diuretics, and the mechanism of concentration and dilution of urine and its modulation by hormones (Wirz and Dirix, 1973). The knowledge thus gained has provided the basis for the present integrated analysis of the regulation of the extracellular volume and osmolality by the renal-body fluid regulating system.

STOP-FLOW MICROPERFUSION

Another powerful method for direct determination of tubular transport is the stop-flow microperfusion of a small tubular segment with a known solution. This procedure, first introduced by Richards and Walker (1937) and later modified by Shipp and associates (1958) and Gertz (1963), is a modification of the free-flow micropuncture collection of the tubular fluid described above.

Briefly, the method involves injecting a small volume of colored mineral oil into the lumen of a renal tubule, and then splitting the oil column in two by the injection of the test perfusate. In this way, the injected test fluid is completely sealed off by oil on both sides, and any subsequent observed changes in the volume and composition of the perfusate are attributed to the activity of the tubular cells to which the fluid was exposed. The injected fluid is usually left in contact with the tubular cells for a known period of time, and then collected and analyzed for any changes in composition. Figure 8-1 illustrates the essence of this technique.

The reabsorptive rate of the injected fluid can be estimated as follows. As the fluid is reabsorbed, the length (L) of the injected fluid column between the oil decreases without visible changes in the tubular diameter. Assuming that the tubular radius does not change, then the fractional change in length (L/L_0) corresponds to the

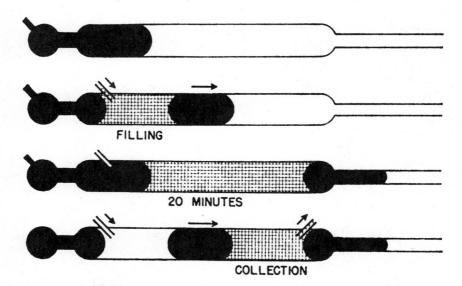

Figure 8-1. Schematic drawing showing technique of stop-flow microperfusion [From Giebisch, G. (1961).]

fraction of fluid volume remaining (V/V_0) where L_0 and V_0 are the initial length and volume, and L and V are the length and volume of the injected fluid at the time of collection. This fractional volume declines exponentially as a function of time:

$$\ln \frac{V}{V_0} = -k \cdot t \qquad (8-10)$$

where k is the *reabsorptive rate constant* per second and t is the time in seconds.

Another way of describing this relationship is the following, adapted from Arrizurieto-Muchnik and his associates (1969).

For a given tubular segment of length (L) and cross-sectional area (πr^2) the reabsorptive rate constant (k) may be expressed as the ratio of reabsorptive rate per unit tubular length ($\dot{R}$) and cross-sectional area (πr^2). Expressed mathematically,

$$k = \frac{\dot{R}}{\pi r^2} \qquad (8-11)$$

If $\dot{R}$ and r remain constant along the length of the tubular segment, then the change in fluid volume per unit time (dV/dt) should be inversely proportional to the initial volume injected:

$$\frac{dV}{dt} = -\frac{\dot{R}}{\pi r^2} \cdot V \tag{8-12}$$

or

$$\frac{dV}{V} = -\frac{\dot{R}}{\pi r^2} \cdot dt \tag{8-13}$$

Integrating Equation 8-13 from t = 0 to t = T, where T is the time required for fluid reabsorption in the *split-oil drop* experiments, we get:

$$\ln \frac{V_t}{V_0} = -\frac{\dot{R}}{\pi r^2} \cdot T \tag{8-14}$$

This equation also holds for the free-flow experiments, where T is defined as the tubular transit time of lissamine green dye, except that $V_0/V_t = [In]_f/[In]_p$ as defined by Equation 8-6, and hence,

$$\ln \frac{[In]_f}{[In]_p} = \frac{\dot{R}}{\pi r^2} \cdot T \tag{8-15}$$

or

$$\frac{\ln \frac{[In]_f}{[In]_p}}{T} = \frac{\dot{R}}{\pi r^2} \tag{8-16}$$

A modification of this method is the flow-through microperfusion of a punctured tubular segment. The procedure involves introducing the perfusate into a tubular lumen through one glass micropipette and recollecting it at a more distal site with a second micropipette. To prevent nonperfusing luminal fluid from contaminating the perfusate, the tubular segments not involved in perfusion are sealed off with oil columns. These methods have yielded extensive quantitative information about the tubular activity on the perfused fluid, such as bidirectional rate of ion movements, and the effects of tubular geometry and volume flow on fluid reabsorption rate.

SHORT-CIRCUIT CURRENT MEASUREMENT

This method, first applied to toad bladder and frog skin (Ussing and Zerahn, 1951), provides a direct quantitative measure of the net active transport of an ion across the cell membrane. Since active transport involves the transport of a solute, such as sodium ion, against an electrochemical gradient, this method provides a direct measure of the magnitude of this transport.

Briefly, the technique involves measuring the electrical current that must be applied to reduce the membrane potential to zero. This applied current, which abolishes the electrical gradient, is called the *short-circuit* current. It has been shown to be a direct measure of the active transport of an ion by the membrane.

Combining the short-circuit current with stop-flow microperfusion techniques, several investigators have studied the characteristics of active transport in isolated nephron segments. The experimental procedure involves splitting the previously injected oil column with small volume of Ringer's solution. Then, a microelectrode, filled with 3 M potassium chloride solution, with tip potential less than 2.5 mV, is inserted into the previously punctured tubule. The potential difference is measured between the luminal electrode and the indifferent electrode placed on the surface. Figure 8-2 shows schematically the technique of electrode placement and measurement of short-circuit current. The interpretation of experimental data thus obtained is analogous to that described for frog skin.

STOP-FLOW ANALYSIS OF TUBULAR URINE IN WHOLE KIDNEY

This technique, often referred to as "the poor man's micropuncture," developed by Malvin and his associates (1958) has provided much valuable information about tubular transport function for a variety of solutes and their site of transport along the

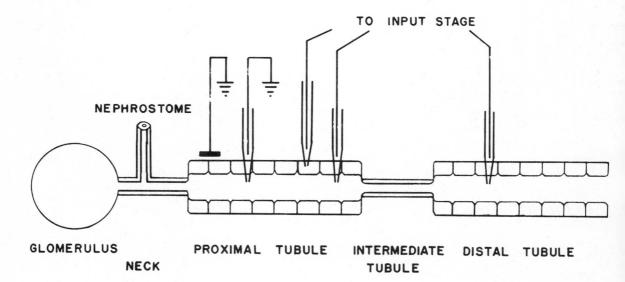

Figure 8-2. Single tubule of *Necturus* nephron showing relation of indifferent and recording microelectrodes to various tubular structures. [From Giebisch, G. (1960).]

nephron. The method is based on the idea that stopping the urine
flow allows the various tubular processes to function at maximum
efficiency. Thus, during acute ureteral occlusion, any substance
which is normally absorbed is continuously absorbed, while any
substance that is secreted will be continuously added to the trapped
urine. In this manner, an exaggerated *concentration profile*, for a
given solute, along the various nephron segments will be established.
After approximately 10 minutes, the occlusion is removed and small
(0.5 ml) serial urine samples are collected. Each sample removed
represents urine trapped in a successively more proximal segment of
the nephron.

The approximate tubular location of each collected sample will be
verified from the analysis of urine-to-plasma concentration (U/P)
ratio of inulin administered prior to occlusion. The tubular
transport will be determined, as before, from the comparison of the
U/P ratio for the solute in question relative to that of inulin.

Figure 8-3 shows the tubular concentration profiles for sodium,
glucose, and PAH as obtained by this method. To eliminate the effect
of variable flow rates during collection, the various solute
concentrations are plotted against the *accumulated* volume of urine
which has appeared since the removal of the clamp. Note that the
concentration of glucose--a substance maximally absorbed--is low in
the more proximal samples, corresponding to 9 to 11 ml on the volume
scale. On the other hand, sodium, which is actively absorbed all
along the nephron, shows an initial decrease in concentration,
followed by an increase, reaching a plateau at about the same time
on the volume scale. In the case of PAH, the maximal urinary PAH

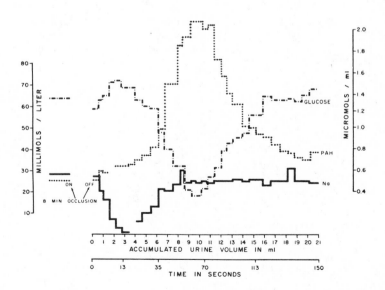

Figure 8-3. Concentration pattern developed for PAH, sodium and
glucose during stop-flow. [From Malvin, R. L., Wilde, W. S., and
Sullivan, L. P. (1958).]

concentration occurs in the same tubular location where glucose concentration is minimal, indicating that PAH is secreted by the proximal tubule.

Accurate localization of tubular transport by the stop-flow experiments in whole kidney is limited by some "smearing" of the solute concentration profile patterns. This is attributed to (1) the mixing of the tubular urine with urine already in the catheter when occlusion is removed, (2) the heterogeneity of the nephron population in the whole kidney, and (3) the glomerular filtration which proceeds (even though to a small extent) during the complete tubular blockade. In addition, the composition of the filtrate issuing from the proximal tubule may be greatly altered as it passes through the distal parts of the nephron. However, this effect is assumed to be small due to rapid tubular flow rate immediately after the clamp is released.

Application of these methods to the study of renal function have verified the existence of the *three* general types of cellular transport described in Chapter 7.

SEQUENTIAL PROCESSING OF THE FILTRATE ALONG THE NEPHRON

Glomerular filtrate undergoes considerable modification of both volume and composition as it flows along the various nephron segments. However, depending on the type of solute present, the tubular processes involved are quite different in each nephron segment, in terms of both the mechanisms of transport and the quantity of the solute and fluid transported. Therefore, to facilitate presentation, we shall consider the tubular processing of the major constituents of the filtrate along three sequential nephron segments: (A) Proximal tubule, (B) loop of Henle, and (C) distal and collecting tubules. Where appropriate, any similarities and differences in the filtrate processing in these segments will be mentioned, and their known physiological significance in relation to body fluid homeostasis will be discussed. Furthermore, to emphasize the importance of correlation between structure and function for each of these nephron segments, a brief description of their morphology will be included.

PROXIMAL TUBULE

MORPHOLOGY

The proximal tubule is divided into an extensively *convoluted* segment (pars convoluta), followed by a *straight* portion (pars recta) which extends into the outer medulla of the kidney. Both segments are composed of a single layer of cuboidal epithelial cells, each having a round nucleus in the middle and a large number of rod-like mitochondria (Fig. 8-4). The *luminal membrane* of these cells is corrugated (hence, the name "brush border"), consisting of a large

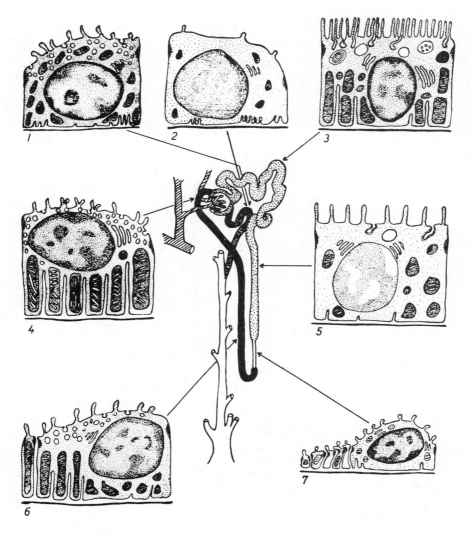

Figure 8-4. Diagram showing the essential features of the cells lining different parts of a typical cortical nephron in mammalian kidney as seen with the electron microscope. (1) Collecting tubule (dark cell); (2) collecting tubule (light cell); (3) proximal convoluted tubule; (4) distal convoluted tubule; (5) pars recta of proximal tubule; (6) thick ascending limb; and (7) thin segments of the loop of Henle. [From Rhodin, J. (1958).]

number of microvilli, thereby increasing the surface area available for cellular transport. The *peritubular membrane* lacks brush border and rests on a *basement membrane*. The presence of a large number of mitochondria is probably related to the energy requirements for the active transport performed by these cells.

GENERAL CHARACTERISTICS OF
FILTRATE TRANSPORT

Numerous micropuncture and microperfusion studies of the proximal tubule in the rat, dog, and monkey, under a great variety of experimental conditions (reviewed by Windhager, 1968; Koushanpour et al., 1971; Giebisch and Windhager, 1973) have established that, as the filtrate flows through this segment: (1) Water is always absorbed in direct proportion to the sum of the osmolar solutes, so that the filtrate-to-plasma osmolality ratio ($[TF/P]_{osm}$) does not change regardless of whether the final urine is more or less concentrated. This phenomenon, shown in Figure 8-5, indicates that the filtrate is reabsorbed iso-osmotically along this segment, meaning that the tubular fluid and reabsorbate have the same osmotic pressure. (2) In the absence of significant amounts of non-absorbable solute (such as mannitol):

(a) Sodium is absorbed in direct proportion to water, so that its tubular fluid-to-plasma molal concentration ratio does not change. This is illustrated in Figure 8-6, where TF/P for sodium and sodium-to-inulin TF/P ratios are plotted on a logarithmic scale as a function of the tubular length.

(b) The osmolar sum of nonsodium solutes is also absorbed in direct proportion to water, although individual solute species may be absorbed in greater (glucose, for example), or lesser (urea, for

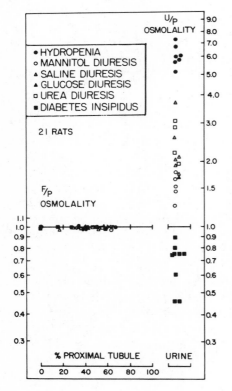

Figure 8-5. Micropuncture data from rats showing iso-osmotic reabsorption of fluid along the proximal convoluted tubule. Note that proximal tubular fluid osmolality relative to plasma water (F/P) remains constant at unity whether the final urine is more concentrated than plasma (hydropenia) or less concentrated than plasma diuresis). [From Gottschalk, C. W. (1961).]

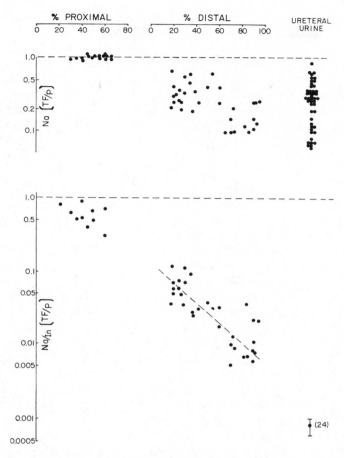

Figure 8-6. Tubular fluid-to-plasma concentration ratios (TF/P) for sodium (upper panel) and sodium-to-inulin (Na/In) (lower panel), plotted on a logarithmic scale, as a function of proximal and distal tubule lengths and in ureteral urine from rats under control conditions. [From Malnic, G., Klose, R. M., Giebisch, G. (1966).]

example) amounts than water.

According to present understanding, the *absorptive mechanisms* for the important constituents of the filtrate are: (1) sodium and potassium are absorbed by an active process, while bicarbonate and chloride ions are transported passively down the electrochemical gradients established by the active transport of sodium and potassium; (2) glucose, amino acids, proteins, inorganic phosphates and sulfates, and uric acids are all transported actively, with characteristic maximum tubular absorptive capacity for each; (3) urea is absorbed by passive diffusion, but not so rapidly enough to attain diffusion equilibrium at each point along the tubule; and (4) the concentration gradients established by active reabsorption of sodium and potassium generate an osmotic force which induces absorption of water by passive diffusion (osmosis) so rapidly as not to depart from osmotic equilibrium.

Since sodium is the most abundant constituent of the filtrate, its tubular absorption is the key to the overall filtrate processing. Thus, any factor that interferes with sodium absorption has an adverse effect on filtrate absorption. Indeed, as we shall see later, interference with sodium absorption is the most common basis for inducing diuresis. Hence, it is important to have a clear understanding of the mechanism of *active sodium reabsorption*.

METHODOLOGICAL BASIS OF ACTIVE ABSORPTION OF AN ELECTROLYTE

As mentioned in Chapter 7, *passive* transepithelial transport of an electrolyte may result from the action of three physical forces: (1) chemical concentration or activity gradients, (2) electrical potential gradients, and (3) convection or solvent drag. The transepithelial transport of the electrolyte not accounted for by these forces was classified as *active* transport. Since an electrical potential gradient always coexists with the active transport of an electrolyte, its measurement is a key to assessing whether the electrolyte is transported actively or not.

To determine the site and magnitude of the active transport of an electrolyte, three types of electrical potential gradients have been measured on single nephrons:

1. The *transepithelial* potential gradient, obtained by recording the electrical potential difference between the tubular lumen and the peritubular interstitial fluid. Comparison of this *measured* electrical potential gradient (PD) with the *theoretical* potential gradient (E) for that electrolyte calculated from the Nernst equation allows one to decide whether an ion is transported actively or not. According to the Nernst equation, if a membrane were permeable to only one type of ion, such as sodium, in the steady state the theoretical transmembrane electrical potential gradient would be a function of the chemical concentration gradient of that ion:

$$E = - \frac{RT}{zF} \ln \frac{[x]_1}{[x]_b} \qquad (8\text{-}17)$$

where z is the valence of the electrolyte, F is the faraday constant, defined as the charge upon one mole of univalent ions (96,500 coulombs/mole), $[x]_1$ and $[x]_b$ are the concentrations of the particular electrolyte in the tubular lumen and blood, respectively, and R and T have already been defined. If measured transepithelial potential gradient is equal to the calculated theoretical gradient (PD = E), then the ion is transported passively, otherwise active transport may be involved.

2. The *transluminal* and *transcellular* electrical potential

gradients, obtained by measuring the electrical potential differences across the luminal and peritubular membranes of single renal tubular cells. Such electrical measurements, in conjunction with ionic concentration gradients across the same membranes, permit one to locate the site of active transport within the cell.

3. The measurement of *short-circuit current*, which, along with the knowledge of net movement (flux) of a given ion, allows one to determine the fraction of the total ion movement which is due to active transport.

Whether an ion is actively transported or not can be determined experimentally by comparing the observed bidirectional fluxes for that ion, and hence their ratio, with the theoretical ratio calculated from Ussing's (1949) flux equation:

$$\frac{J_{l \to b}}{J_{b \to l}} = \frac{[x]_b}{[x]_l} \exp - \frac{zFE}{RT} \qquad (8\text{-}18)$$

where $J_{l \to b}$ is the ion flux from lumen to blood, $J_{b \to l}$ is the ion flux from blood to lumen, and the other terms have already been defined. Note that the value of transepithelial electrical potential gradient (E) used in this equation is calculated from the Nernst equation. Also, in this formulation the effect of solvent drag on ion movement is assumed to be small and hence is not included.

To evaluate Equation 8-18, and hence to determine the mechanism of ion transport, we need to measure simultaneously three quantities: (1) the bidirectional ion flux ratio, $J_{l \to b}/J_{b \to l}$; (2) the chemical concentration gradients for the ion across the cell membranes; and (3) the electrical potential gradient across the cell membranes. If the measured ion flux ratio is equal to the theoretical ratio calculated from Equation 8-18, the ion must be transported passively. If the measured flux ratio exceeds the theoretical ratio, the ion is transported actively. A measured flux ratio less than the calculated ratio indicates that some of the ions do not diffuse freely under the influence of the prevailing transmembrane electrochemical gradients. Such an ion movement, independent of the electrochemical gradients, is called *exchange diffusion*. It is believed to be due to the competition for the carrier by the same ion species present on both sides of the membrane. Hence, exchange diffusion does not contribute to the net ion transport, but results in increased turnover rate.

As mentioned above, the Nernst equation defines the dependency of the transmembrane electrical potential gradient on the transmembrane chemical concentration gradient of an ion, assuming that the membrane is **permeable** only to that ion. As such, the Nernst equation represents a special case of the more general Ussing's flux equation. It is derived by assuming that $J_{l \to b} = J_{b \to l}$, and then rewriting Equation 8-18 in terms of E in logarithmic form:

$$E = - \frac{RT}{zF} \ln \frac{[x]_1}{[x]_b} \qquad (8\text{-}19)$$

Replacing the natural logarithm (ln = $\log_e$) by logarithm to the base 10 (ln = 2.3 log) yields

$$E = -2.3 \frac{RT}{zF} \log \frac{[x]_1}{[x]_b} \qquad (8\text{-}20)$$

At an ambient temperature of $36^\circ C$ and for a univalent ion, the term (2.3 RT/zF) has a value of 60 and is expressed in millivolts (mV). This substitution simplifies Equation 8-20 to:

$$E = -60 \log \frac{[x]_1}{[x]_b} \qquad (8\text{-}21)$$

The fact that the net ion flux across the membrane depends on the prevailing electrochemical gradients (Ussing's equation) and that the generated electrical gradient is a function of the chemical concentration gradient (Nernst equation) have provided the basis for determining the *relative permeability* of the cell membrane to a given ion. The procedure involves measuring the bidirectional flux of that ion from the disappearance rate of the isotope of that ion added to the tubular fluid at zero transepithelial electrical potential gradient induced by short-circuit current. The ion flux is measured in the direction *opposite* to that of the net ion transport--that is, from the backflux--on the assumption that it is passive.

Application of these methods to different segments of the nephron have provided the necessary evidence for determining the mechanisms of tubular transport of the major constituents of the glomerular filtrate.

MECHANISMS OF SODIUM ABSORPTION

Numerous micropuncture, microperfusion, and electrophysiological studies in the mammalian nephron (Seely and Boulpaep, 1971; Giebisch and Windhager, 1973) have revealed the following patterns of electrochemical potential gradients for sodium transport across the proximal tubule epithelial cell and its membrane components:

1. The tubular lumen is always electrically negative with respect to the peritubular fluid. The recorded *transepithelial* electrical potential gradient is about 4 mV, with lumen being negative. Furthermore, the luminal electronegativity is found to be

sodium-dependent; it is abolished when sucrose replaced sodium chloride in a perfused kidney.

2. The cell interior is also electronegative with respect to both the tubular and peritubular fluids. However, the recorded *transluminal* electrical potential gradient is somewhat smaller (about 66 mV, cell interior negative) than the *transcellular* potential gradient (about 70 mV, cell interior negative).

3. The intracellular sodium concentration ($[Na]_c$) is significantly lower (about 40 mEq/L) than that in the tubular fluid ($[Na]_f$) and peritubular fluid ($[Na]_p$) (both concentrations being about 145 mEq/L).

Synthesis of the above electrochemical potential gradients thus obtained yields the following patterns for sodium transport across the two membrane components of the proximal cell. At the *luminal membrane*, there is an electrical potential gradient of about 66 mV (cell interior negative) which favors sodium (a cation) entry into the cell. This electrical force is further complemented by a concomitant concentration gradient for sodium from lumen to cell interior ($\Delta[Na] = 105$ mEq/L). Consequently, sodium enters the cell *down* its electrochemical potential gradients by *passive* diffusion. However, because transluminal sodium transport by this process can not fully account for all the sodium reabsorbed across the proximal epithelial cell, the possibility of participation of a carrier-mediated process (such as facilitated diffusion) cannot be excluded. On the other hand, since the cell interior has a lower sodium concentration than the peritubular fluid, and is also electronegative, it follows that sodium must leave the cell across the *peritubular membrane against* its electrochemical gradients by *active* transport. This conclusion is confirmed by a recent finding that the peritubular membrane contains the sodium-potassium stimulated adenosine triphosphatase (ATPase) enzyme system (Katz and Epstein, 1967), a requirement for active transport. Finally, it has recently been found that transepithelial reabsorption of sodium is a function of the magnitude of the intracellular sodium pool. The size of this pool is determined by the rates at which sodium enters the proximal cell by passive or facilitated diffusion and leaves the cell by active transport. Of these two processes, the active transport component at the peritubular membrane appears to be the rate-limiting process (Crabbe and DeWeer, 1969).

Figure 8-7 summarizes the various components of the electrochemical potential gradients involved in sodium transport across a mammalian proximal tubule cell. As shown, sodium enters the cell by passive (or facilitated) diffusion (depicted by broken arrow) along its electrochemical gradients. Once inside, sodium is then actively extruded against its electrochemical gradients (depicted by solid arrow) across the peritubular membrane into the surrounding interstitial fluid. From there, sodium, along with an anion (such as bicarbonate or chloride) and water pass through the basement and capillary membranes as a result of the prevailing regional hydrostatic and protein oncotic pressure gradients (Lewy and Windhager, 1968). In short, as a result of both passive and active transport processes and

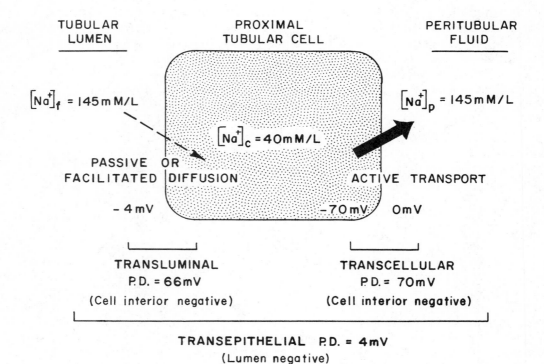

Figure 8-7. A scheme showing the electrical potential difference (P.D.) profile across a mammalian proximal tubular cell and the localization of sites of passive and active sodium transport.

peritubular hydrostatic and oncotic pressure gradients, sodium ions are reabsorbed *iso-osmotically* along the proximal tubule (Fig. 8-5). A more complete description of the mechanism of this iso-osmotic transepithelial sodium transport will be given later in this section.

Besides partitioning the ion transport process into active and passive components, measurement of short-circuit current on single nephrons has provided the basis for correlating the proximal tubule sodium reabsorption with renal oxygen consumption. From such measurements, Kill and associates (1961) have found a stoichiometric relationship between sodium reabsorption and renal oxygen consumption, such that about 20 to 30 Eq of sodium is absorbed per mole of oxygen. Furthermore, it has been established that both renal oxygen consumption and proximal tubule sodium absorption are positive functions of glomerular filtration rate. However, recent attempts to elucidate the biochemical pathways involved by studying the effects of metabolic inhibitors upon active sodium transport in different parts of the nephron have led to the conclusions (1) that the oxygen consumption of renal cortex far exceeds that of medulla, a finding consistent with the enormous amount of sodium and water absorbed in the cortically located proximal and distal tubules, and (2) that although oxygen is necessary for electrolyte transport in the intact kidney, the marked difference in the enzyme patterns of cortical and medullary tissues suggests the existence of some nonconventional energy-consuming metabolic processes (Abodeely and Lee, 1971; Cohen and Barac-Nieto, 1973). This conclusion is confirmed by Weinstein and Klose (1969), who found no change in isotonic sodium reabsorption in the proximal tubule after intraluminal injection of 2,4-dinitrophenol. The absence of any effect by this inhibitor of the ATP mediated metabolic pathway was interpreted to indicate that the energy for sodium reabsorption may be derived directly from the electron transport chain.

POTASSIUM ABSORPTION

Quantitative analyses of electrolyte distribution across the proximal tubule cell membranes have revealed that potassium concentration inside the cell is some 20 to 40 times higher than that in the extracellular fluid. On the other hand, the transcellular gradients for sodium and chloride ions are somewhat less than tenfold. Also, the renal cell membranes are far more permeable to potassium and chloride ions than to sodium ions. This asymmetric ionic permeability of the renal cell membranes is believed to be the primary source generating the observed transmembrane electrical potential gradients. The magnitude of these potentials is related directly to the concentration gradients of potassium and chloride ions across these membranes.

Figure 8-8 (upper left panel) shows a plot, on a logarithmic scale, of the tubular fluid-to-plasma concentration ratios (TF/P) for potassium as a function of tubular length in rat proximal tubule under control conditions. It is evident that potassium TF/P ratios fall consistently below unity, suggesting net transepithelial potassium reabsorption (Malnic et al., 1964). To eliminate the effect of water reabsorption on potassium TF/P ratios and to determine the relative amount of potassium remaining in the tubule and hence not reabsorbed, the potassium TF/P ratios are divided by inulin TF/P ratios in the corresponding micropuncture samples. The resulting potassium-to-inulin (K/In) TF/P ratios on logarithmic scale plotted as a function of tubular length are shown in the lower left panel of Figure 8-8. It is evident that by the time the filtrate reaches 65% of the proximal tubule length, about 70% of the filtered potassium has been reabsorbed (K/In TF/P = 0.3). At least in rat, it has been found that the extent of potassium reabsorption along the proximal convoluted tubule is independent of the metabolic state of the animal.

Since the tubular lumen is electronegative with respect to the peritubular fluid (Fig. 8-7), the transepithelial reabsorption of potassium is believed to be active in nature. Furthermore, because the tubular concentration of potassium ($[K]_f = 4$ mEq/L) is

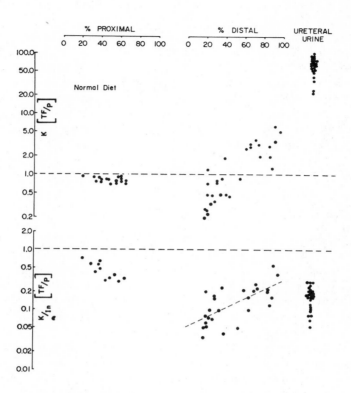

Figure 8-8. Tubular fluid-to-plasma concentration ratios (TF/P) for potassium (upper panel) and potassium-to-inulin (K/In) (lower panel), plotted on a logarithmic scale, as a function of proximal and distal tubule lengths and in ureteral urine from rats under control conditions. [From Malnic, G., Klose, R. M., and Giebisch, G. (1964).]

significantly lower than that in the cell interior ($[K]_C$ = 150 mEq/L), the site of active potassium reabsorption must be at the luminal membrane. This conclusion is strengthened further by the fact that the transcellular electrical potential gradient (measured across the peritubular membrane) is found to be much closer to the equilibrium potential gradient generated by potassium ions (calculated from the Nernst equation) than the electrical potential gradient measured across the luminal cell membrane. However, as we shall see later, the possibility that cellular uptake of potassium across the peritubular membrane may also be active can not be excluded.

CHLORIDE ABSORPTION

Although 40 to 50% of the filtered chloride is reabsorbed along the proximal convoluted tubule in nondiuretic rats, the tubular concentration is found to be considerably higher than that in the

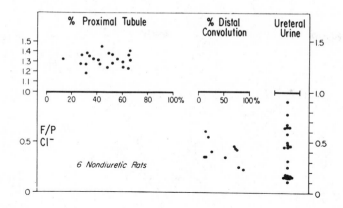

Figure 8-9. Tubular fluid-to-plasma concentration ratios (F/P) for chloride along the proximal and distal convoluted tubules and in ureteral urine from nondiuretic rats. [From Gottschalk, C. W. (1963).]

plasma (Fig. 8-9). This higher tubular chloride concentration is not due to tubular secretion, but rather is postulated to be the result of early and preferential reabsorption of bicarbonate with concomitant fall in the intratubular pH (Kokko, 1974). This preferential bicarbonate reabsorption has been confirmed by recent experiments and, as suggested by Windhager (1974), may "establish favorable chloride concentration gradients so that in the later part of the proximal tubule reabsorption of sodium and water becomes mainly a passive process."

The observed rise in tubular hydrogen ion concentration (low pH) is due to hydrogen ion secretion by the proximal tubule. Considerable evidence exists that this secretory process is located at the luminal cell membrane (Giebisch and Malnic, 1970), raising the possibility that active hydrogen ion secretion may be coupled to passive sodium reabsorption at the same site. However, present evidence indicates that the nature of this hydrogen-sodium exchange is *nonspecific*--that is, sodium ion *per se* is not necessary for hydrogen ion secretion.

The proximal tubular chloride concentration may be lowered in the presence of poorly absorbable anions, such as sulfate (Malnic and De Mello Aires, 1970), and after infusion of carbonic anhydrase inhibitors and mannitol (Cortney, 1969). Furthermore, hypokalemia (as might be developed in potassium deprivation or depletion) elevates tubular chloride concentration while at the same time increases bicarbonate reabsorption (Bank and Aynedjian, 1965). A more detailed discussion of the significance of these findings is presented in Chapter 10.

MECHANISM OF COUPLED SODIUM
AND WATER TRANSPORT

Analysis of tubular fluid-to-plasma concentration ratios for inulin ($[TF/P]_{In}$) along the proximal tubule of nondiuretic rats has revealed a progressive increase in this ratio, reaching a value of about 3 by the end of the convoluted segment (Fig. 8-10). Since inulin is a non-absorbable solute, the rise in its tubular concentration relative to that in plasma ($[TF/P]_{In} > 1$) is taken as evidence of water reabsorption along the tubule. Accordingly, it has been found that in rats, about 60% of the filtered water is reabsorbed by the time the filtrate reaches the end of the proximal convoluted tubule (Giebisch and Windhager, 1964), while in dogs and monkeys only 45% and 30% is reabsorbed, respectively (Bennett et al., 1967, 1968). The percentage of the filtrate volume reabsorbed along the proximal tubule has been found to be relatively constant, under normal physiological conditions. Consequently, fluid reabsorption along

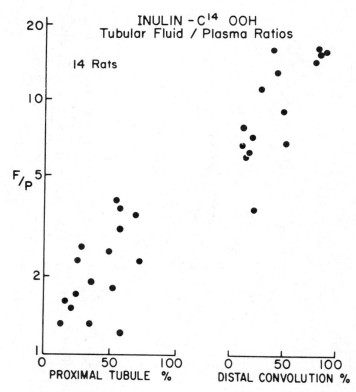

Figure 8-10. Tubular fluid-to-plasma concentration ratios (F/P) for inulin along the proximal and distal convoluted tubules of nondiuretic rats. [From Gottschalk, C. W. (1961).]

this segment is called *obligatory*.

Because the filtrate (solutes and water) is absorbed iso-osmotically along the proximal tubule, as evidenced from $[TF/O]_{osm} = 1.0$ in Figure 8-5, then one would expect a large osmotic force (estimated as 20 mOsm/L) to exist between the tubular lumen and the peritubular capillary blood to account for the observed absorption of such a large fraction of the filtered water. However, osmotic force of such a magnitude has never been found experimentally (Giebisch, 1972).

To resolve this discrepancy between the expected and actually observed osmotic driving force, Giebisch (1969) proposed a model of the renal proximal tubule cell to account for the observed reabsorption of the large quantity of sodium and water along the proximal tubule. Actually, this model is based on a scheme proposed by Curran and MacIntosh (1962) for isotonic transport across the epithelial membrane. Diamond and Bossert (1967) have provided both functional and anatomical evidence in support of this scheme for isotonic reabsorption across the mammalian gallbladder wall.

Figure 8-11 presents schematically the salient features of Giebisch's model. Each renal tubule cell is depicted with two distinct membranes: a *luminal* (apical) and a *peritubular* (basal) membrane. The adjacent cells are connected by a narrowing of the *intercellular space* on the apical side, called the *tight junction*. The space within the tight junction and the larger intercellular space constitute an extracellular compartment within the renal tubular epithelium. As envisioned by this model, this extracellular space is believed to play a key role in the transepithelial reabsorption of sodium and water. The essence of this transepithelial transport may be summarized as follows.

Luminal sodium enters the renal cell along its electrochemical gradient. Once inside, sodium ions are then actively pumped into the intercellular space across its membrane, which is an extension of the peritubular cell membrane. This would lead to accumulation of sodium in the intercellular space, thereby generating a local region of hyperosmolality within the tubular epithelium. The osmotic concentration gradient thus established induces osmotic flow of water into the intercellular space either through the tight junction or across the cell compartment, or both. The accumulated iso-osmotic fluid, owing to the limited expandability of the intercellular space, develops a small but transient hydrostatic pressure gradient along this space, which forces the fluid to move from the apical to the basal side of the intercellular space. This reabsorbate, as suggested by Windhager and his associates (1969), will then cross the basement and capillary membranes by a force determined by the balance of the prevailing regional hydrostatic and protein oncotic pressure gradients.

Giebisch (1969) has presented three arguments in support of the important role played by the intercellular space in the proposed coupled transport of sodium and water:

1. Electrophysiological studies in rat proximal tubule have

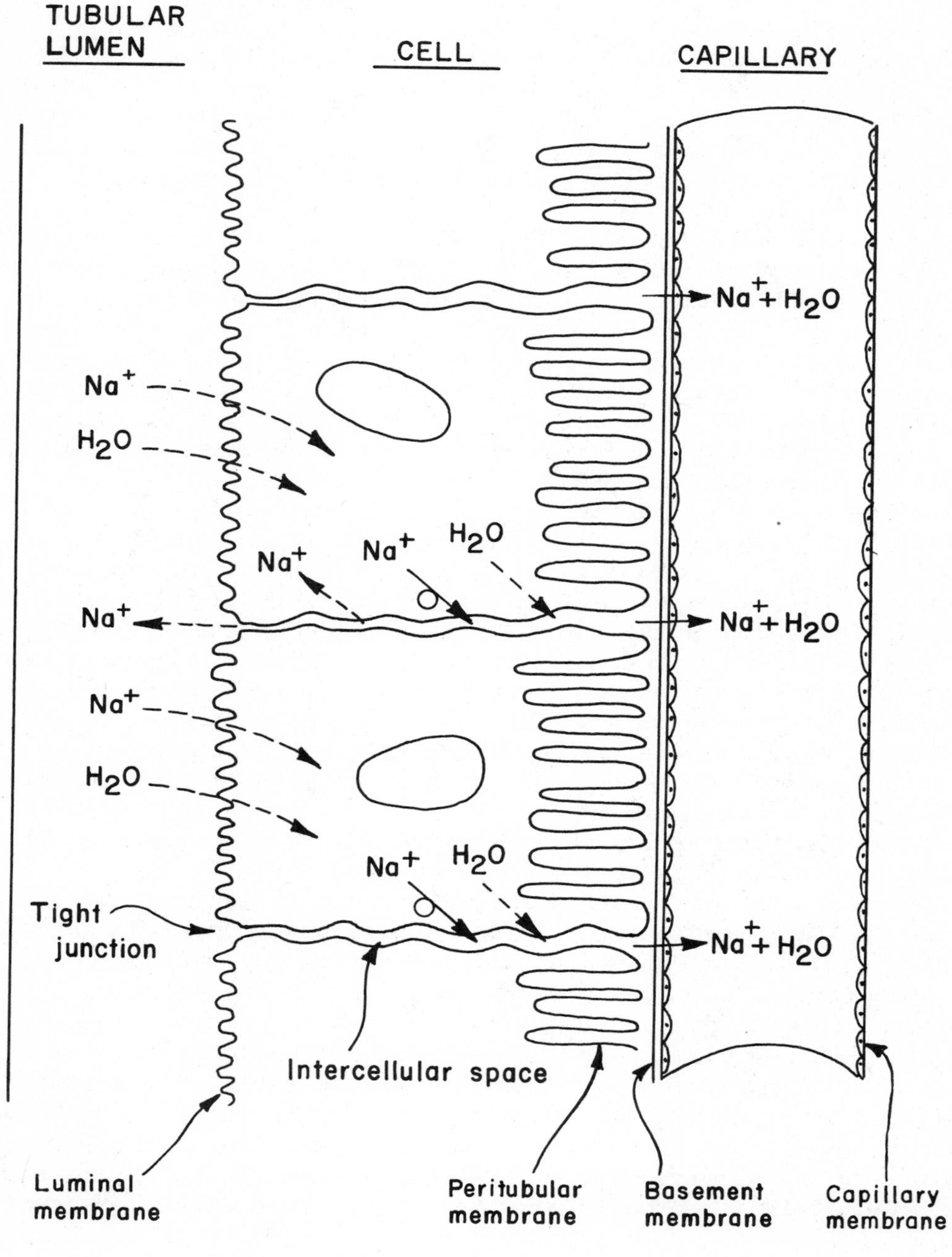

Figure 8-11. A schematic diagram of the renal tubule cell showing transepithelial movement of sodium and water. [Modified from Giebisch, G., and Windhager, E. E. (1973).]

shown that the specific electrical resistance of this tubule is quite low compared to that measured in other epithelial tissues as well as the more distally located nephron segments. This low electrical resistance may be due to one of two properties of the tubular epithelium: (a) the tubular cell membranes have an inherently low electrical resistance; and (b) there are extracellular channels connecting the tubular lumen to the peritubular fluid. Recent experimental evidence supports the latter possibility (Giebisch, 1969).

2. Measurement of ion permeability of the luminal and peritubular membranes of the proximal tubule cell has revealed marked ion selectivity for these membranes (Windhager et al., 1967). For example, it has been found that the peritubular membrane is some 25 times more permeable to potassium than to sodium ions, and some 2.5 times more permeable to potassium than to chloride ions. In contrast, when the permeability properties of the whole proximal tubule cell are measured, such an ion selectivity is not observed. This marked difference between the ion permeability of the proximal tubule cell as a whole and of its individual membranes strongly suggests that other structures besides the cell membranes, namely the intercellular shunts, must account for the ease of sodium and water transport across the proximal epithelium.

3. The above proposed intercellular shunt model can readily explain a number of observations in which experimentally induced changes in the peritubular capillary hemodynamics (namely, changes in peritubular capillary hydrostatic and protein oncotic pressures) have been shown to profoundly influence the net reabsorption of sodium and water in the proximal tubule (Earley and Friedler, 1966; Windhager et al., 1969). A more detailed description of these experiments and their physiological importance is given in the next section.

MECHANISM OF SODIUM-POTASSIUM EXCHANGE
AT THE PERITUBULAR MEMBRANE

Recent evidence strongly suggest that active sodium extrusion from the proximal cell into the peritubular fluid (intercellular space) appears to be coupled to potassium uptake into the tubular cell from the peritubular fluid. Furthermore, it has been found that this sodium-potassium coupling at the peritubular membrane is mediated by a Na-K stimulated ATPase enzyme system (Skou, 1957; Proverbio et al., 1970). On the basis of these and other findings, Whittembury and Proverbio (1970) have advanced the following double-pump hypothesis to describe the active sodium-potassium exchange across the peritubular cell membrane.

As depicted in Figure 8-12, active transcellular (across peritubular membrane) transport of sodium occurs along two separate pathways, each having its own specialized pump. Furthermore, the two transport modes of sodium are affected differently by changes in temperature and inhibitor drugs. Pump A actively transports sodium,

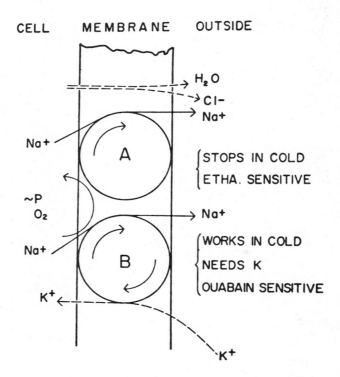

CELL   MEMBRANE   OUTSIDE

Figure 8-12. Schematic representation of the double-pump hypothesis depicting the active sodium-potassium exchange across the peritubular membrane of the renal tubule cell. [From Whittembury, G., and Proverbio, F. (1970).]

coupled with chloride and water, from the cell interior to the peritubular fluid. As shown, the activity of this pump is markedly reduced at low temperature and is inhibited by ethacrynic acid (ETHA), a diuretic drug. Since the activity of this pump affects iso-osmotic absorption of sodium, its role is postulated to be that of regulating the renal cell volume. In contrast, pump B is involved in the active sodium-potassium exchange across the peritubular cell membrane. The activity of this pump is less temperature-sensitive, requires potassium, and is inhibited by ouabain, a cardiac glycoside which inhibits Na-K stimulated ATPase activity. The activity of both pumps is suppressed when oxygen supply is reduced.

REGULATION OF FILTRATE PROCESSING
ALONG THE PROXIMAL TUBULE

Renal regulation of volume and osmolality of body fluid compartments ultimately depends on the capacity of the tubular epithelium of the nephrons to adapt its rate of sodium reabsorption to changes in glomerular load. It is well established that changes in glomerular filtration rate are usually compensated for by parallel changes in tubular reabsorption along the nephron. More explicitly, it has been found that regardless of how GFR is altered, the fraction of filtered sodium reabsorbed by the tubules and that which is not reabsorbed (and therefore excreted), remain constant. This implies that the absolute amounts of both the sodium reabsorbed and not reabsorbed vary in the same direction as the changes in GFR. This parallel relationship between GFR and tubular reabsorption is commonly referred to as the *glomerular-tubular balance*. Since the proximal tubule accounts for the reabsorption of nearly 70% of the filtered sodium, this nephron segment must play a major role in the maintenance of such a balance and it is, therefore, the most prominent regulator of body sodium. Furthermore, inasmuch as renal transport of sodium is not a time-limited process (see Chapter 9), the existence of a glomerular-tubular balance for sodium serves to conserve body stores of sodium and to minimize excessive loss in conditions which produce sodium imbalance.

Numerous studies, reviewed by De Wardener (1973) and Earley and Schrier (1973), have demonstrated that the glomerular-tubular balance is influenced by several factors. Chief among them are (a) changes in tubular concentration of sodium, (b) presence of poorly absorbable solutes, such as mannitol, urea, and sulfate, in the filtrate, (c) changes in hemodynamics of systemic circulation following expansion of intravascular or extracellular volume by fluid infusion, and (d) alterations in Starling forces in the blood perfusing the kidney, particularly at the glomerulus and post-glomerular capillary vasculature. Since the first two exert their effects primarily at the luminal side and the last two at the peritubular side of the renal cell membrane, we shall describe the modes of their actions in accordance with whether they exert their effects on the luminal or peritubular side of the renal cell membrane.

LUMINAL CONTROL OF FILTRATE ABSORPTION

Proximal absorption of sodium and water can be modified by altering the luminal concentration of sodium. This may be done either directly, by changing plasma concentration of sodium, or indirectly, by intravenous infusion of poorly absorbable solutes.

1. EFFECT OF CHANGES IN PLASMA SODIUM CONCENTRATION. It is well established that infusion of hypertonic saline increases plasma sodium concentration, filtered load of sodium, absolute sodium reabsorption by the tubules, and urinary sodium excretion. The available evidence indicates that the induced natriuresis is due to increased plasma sodium concentration and not to changes in GFR, systemic effect of volume expansion or reduction in plasma protein oncotic pressure by dilution. Although micropuncture studies have confirmed that hypernatremia inhibits and hyponatremia stimulates proximal sodium

reabsorption, the tubular mechanisms involved are not well understood.

The possibility that the natriuretic effect accompanying saline infusion is in part due to the dilution of a nonrenal, nonadrenal circulating hormone was first demonstrated by De Wardener and associates (1961). They showed that infusion of isotonic saline in dogs resulted in natriuresis which could not be prevented by either administration of aldosterone or experimental reduction in GFR. Since that study, many investigators have used a variety of experimental models to substantiate the effect of such a natriuretic hormone.

The experimental model that has afforded the best insight into this question is the cross-circulation technique. The procedure involves transfusing blood from the aorta of a donor dog to the aorta of a recipient dog. The blood is then returned from the recipient's inferior vena cava to the inferior vena cava of the donor dog. In this way, hemodynamics and renal response of both dogs to intravenous saline infusion into the donor dog can be studied. The response of the recipient dog to such an infusion has been analyzed to detect the effect of concentration changes of the natriuretic hormone in question (Johnston et al., 1967).

The results of numerous cross-circulation experiments have strongly implied that changes in concentration of a natriuretic hormone are responsible for natriuresis observed after saline infusion or blood volume expansion with iso-oncotic solutions or blood. This conclusion has been confirmed by numerous variations of the original whole animal cross-circulation experiments, including perfusion of isolated kidney with blood from intact donor animal (Tobian et al., 1967) in combination with micropuncture analysis of sodium transport along the nephron.

More recently, Krück (1969) observed a dose-dependent increase in renal sodium excretion without a change in potassium excretion in Na-depleted, fasted rats injected with a urine extract from an orally hydrated normal man. Since urine extract from patients with congestive heart failure failed to produce natriuresis in rats, the author concluded that the absence of a normally present humoral factor is responsible for sodium retention and edema in these patients.

Much research has been done to elucidate the organ(s) which might be the source of this natriuretic hormone. It is now clear that the kidney is not the source of this hormone. Recent experiments have implicated the brain (Lockett, 1966) and liver (Daly et al., 1967) as the possible organs producing this natriuretic hormone. That neither ADH nor oxytocin, both of which are produced by the hypothalamus, is the natriuretic hormone has recently been confirmed (Schrier et al., 1968).

Despite these studies, there is as yet no direct endocrinological proof of the existence of this hormone, even though its inhibitory effect on sodium transport is well documented.

2. EFFECT OF POORLY ABSORBABLE SOLUTES. Numerous micropuncture studies have established that presence of poorly absorbable solutes, such as mannitol, urea, and sulfate, in the filtrate alter the tubular

concentration of sodium, and hence its proximal reabsorption. For example, Giebisch and Windhager (1964) found that during hypertonic mannitol diuresis in rats, TF/P for sodium decreased along the proximal tubule, leading to development of a blood-lumen sodium concentration gradient of 30 to 50 mEq/L by the end of this segment. The final urine was found to be iso-osmotic, with urinary sodium concentration below that in the plasma.

Since tubular fluid remains iso-osmotic relative to plasma during mannitol diuresis, presence of the poorly absorbable mannitol in the tubular fluid obligates osmotic retention of water within the tubule. This would reduce obligatory osmotic flow of water despite active sodium reabsorption along the proximal tubule. As a result, excess tubular water dilutes tubular sodium, decreasing its concentration along this segment, a factor responsible for the observed diminished net transepithelial sodium absorption.

The diuretic effect of urea in the proximal tubule is different from that of mannitol. Urea appears to act directly or indirectly to reduce net proximal sodium reabsorption. This could occur by either a reduction of sodium efflux or an increased backflux of sodium into the lumen. There is no available evidence to suggest any effect of urea on the active component of sodium transport across the proximal epithelium. In the rat, the permeability of the distal tubule to urea is found to be only about one tenth that of the proximal tubule. Furthermore, the urea-induced diuresis and natriuresis appear to depend on the amount of urea administered and occur mainly within the distally located nephron segments. In the dog, only a small fraction of the filtered urea is reabsorbed in the distal tubule (Edwards et al., 1973). Thus, it is possible that even less urea is reabsorbed under the conditions of high-urea load. Thus, the magnitude of urea-induced diuresis and natriuresis was found to be a function of reabsorptive response of the distally located nephron segments.

Because normally the intratubular sodium concentration is the same as that in the plasma, its control is not considered to be the most important mechanism regulating proximal sodium absorption. However, most investigators concur that the most important mechanism is the proportionality that exists between the rate of delivery of fluid into the tubule and the rate of its proximal absorption, in the absence of changes in tubular fluid sodium concentration (Windhager, 1974). Experimental evidence supporting this relationship and the factors which modify it are described next.

PERITUBULAR CONTROL OF FLUID ABSORPTION

Numerous studies have shown that the "peritubular blood environment" and the factors modifying it exert profound influence on the net proximal reabsorption of sodium and water, and hence the glomerular-tubular balance. To elucidate the mechanisms involved and to dissociate the effects of systemic and intrarenal hemodynamic factors, the peritubular environment has been modified using two classes of experimental forcings: (a) alterations in systemic hemodynamics induced by intravenous fluid expansion of extracellular or intravascular volumes; (b) alterations in intrarenal hemodynamics induced by changes in GFR and peritubular Starling forces. Let us now examine the effects of each forcing and the underlying physiological mechanisms.

1. EFFECT OF EXTRACELLULAR VOLUME EXPANSION. It is well established that changes in the extracellular *volume* produce inverse changes in ADH secretion, and hence parallel changes in urine flow. On the other hand, changes in plasma sodium concentration and therefore plasma *osmolality* produce parallel changes in ADH secretion and hence an inverse change in urine flow. It follows that for the volume and osmolality of the extracellular fluid to remain constant, changes in the extracellular volume should influence not only the rate of water excretion, but also the rate of sodium excretion. Thus, as we have seen before, a decrease in the volume of the extracellular fluid, as in hemorrhage, reduces urinary sodium excretion, whereas urinary sodium excretion is increased after infusion of saline or plasma, or blood infusion.

Mechanisms underlying the relationship between the extracellular fluid or blood volume expansion and the urinary sodium excretion have been the subject of considerable investigations. Dirks and associates (1965) were the first to study, by micropuncture, the effect of saline infusion on the proximal tubule sodium reabsorption. They found that the observed natriuresis following saline infusion was the result of depression of proximal sodium reabsorption. The disruption of the glomerular-tubular balance after saline infusion was found to be due, in part, to the induced decrease in the *tubular transit time* subsequent to elevation of GFR. It should be noted that a decrease in the tubular transit time tends to reduce the contact time between the epithelial cells and the filtrate, as the latter flows along the tubule. The net effect is that less time would be available for complete equilibration of tubular fluid with surrounding epithelial cells, and hence a reduced fluid absorption.

Subsequent micropuncture studies, using split-oil drop and microperfusion techniques, have not only confirmed these findings but have also demonstrated that the depression of tubular reabsorption, following the expansion of the extracellular volume, was limited to the proximal tubule and had no effect on the more distally located nephron segments--namely, the loop of Henle and the distal and collecting tubules. For example, micropuncture studies of superficial nephrons in both rats and dogs (Earley and Schrier, 1973) have shown that although saline infusion decreases the fraction of filtered sodium reabsorbed as well as the absolute sodium reabsorption rate in the proximal tubule by about 50%, the urinary excretion is only increased to about 10% of the filtered load. If the response of these nephrons is representative of the nephron population within the kidney, such findings imply that a major fraction of the sodium escaping proximal reabsorption is reabsorbed by the distally located nephron segments. Thus, urinary sodium excretion represents that fraction of the filtered load which has escaped reabsorption by the distal nephron segments.

Landwehr and associates (1967) studied, by micropuncture technique, sodium reabsorption in various segments of rat nephron in response to saline infusion. They found that both the fraction of filtered sodium reabsorbed by the loop of Henle as well as the absolute rate of sodium reabsorption in this segment were increased. However, saline infusion did not alter the absolute rate of sodium reabsorption in the distal convoluted and collecting tubules. Thus, it appears that the extent of urinary excretion of sodium in saline diuresis depends on the extent that the increase in sodium reabsorption (both fractional and absolute) by the loop of Henle compensates for the decrease in sodium reabsorption by the proximal tubule.

That the proximal fluid reabsorption is highly sensitive to the degree of extracellular fluid volume expansion was demonstrated recently be Brenner and Berliner (1969). Using re-collection micropuncture technique (a procedure whereby fluid is collected from the same tubule under both control and experimental conditions) they found an inverse relationship between the fraction of sodium reabsorbed by the proximal tubule and the degree of expansion of the extracellular fluid volume. However, they observed that the fraction of filtered sodium excreted in urine changed little over a wide range of changes in the extracellular fluid volume. Thus, this substantiates the findings cited earlier that the compensatory increase in sodium reabsorption by the distally located nephron segments determines the extent of natriuresis, despite the volume expansion sufficient to depress the proximal sodium reabsorption.

The effect of extracellular volume expansion on proximal reabsorption explains in part the observed normal range in fluid reabsorption (50 to 75%) by this segment, as determined from TF/P inulin ratios. The results, however, are not specific to saline loading. Similar depression of the proximal fluid reabsorption has been found after an expansion of the intravascular volume by hyperoncotic albumin solution (Howards et al., 1968).

Although both extracellular and intravascular volume expansion depress proximal sodium reabsorption, only the former leads to significant natriuresis. Thus, only saline loading appears to compromise the ability of the distally located nephron segments to compensate for the reduced proximal sodium reabsorption. The probable mechanisms for this difference will be discussed later.

2. EFFECT OF CHANGES IN GFR. That the extracellular fluid or intravascular volume expansion produces its natriuretic effects, at least in part, via induced parallel changes in the systemic and renal hemodynamics is well documented. Of particular interest here are those studies which have specifically modified the rate of delivery of sodium to the proximal tubule by changing GFR, thereby altering the balance of Starling forces in the post-glomerular peritubular capillary vasculatures. Experimentally, GFR may be reduced by partial

constriction of the abdominal aorta or renal artery, partial occlusion of the renal vein, and partial obstruction of the ureter. The GFR may be increased by acute expansion of the extracellular volume by intravenous infusion of saline, iso-oncotic solutions, or blood.

As mentioned earlier, an acute increase in GFR, produced by expansion of the extracellular fluid volume depresses proximal sodium reabsorption and hence promotes natriuresis. On the other hand, an acute reduction of GFR by the above three maneuvers has not always produced similar renal responses. Several factors may contribute to the heterogeneity of the response.

Because reduction of GFR induced by partial constriction of renal artery, renal vein, or ureter is mediated by different mechanisms, these maneuvers produce different urinary sodium excretion patterns. To understand the reasons, a brief description of the mechanisms whereby GFR is reduced by these procedures is in order.

Partial constriction of the abdominal aorta or renal artery reduces renal perfusion pressure, thereby reducing the hydrostatic blood pressure at the glomerulus and hence reducing GFR. Partial constriction of the renal vein leads to a retrograde increase in the peritubular hydrostatic pressure, thereby causing partial tubular collapse, which increases the intratubular hydrostatic pressure and reduces GFR. Finally, partial ureteral obstruction increases ureteral pressure which, in turn, leads to an increase in intratubular hydrostatic pressure, thereby reducing GFR. Furthermore, all three procedures are known to produce intrarenal vasodilation. They differ, however, in that aortic constriction and venous occlusion tend to reduce cortical blood flow, while ureteral obstruction elevates total renal blood flow.

Regardless of which procedure was employed, Rodicio and associates (1969) found that in hydropenic (water-deprived rats), acute reduction of GFR increased fractional sodium and water reabsorption in the proximal tubule, suggesting excellent glomerular-tubular balance. This was associated with an induced increase in tubular transit time, a factor which promotes filtrate absorption by increasing the contact and equilibration time of the tubular fluid with the surrounding epithelial cells and the peritubular blood. In contrast, intravenous saline infusion superimposed on the same maneuvers disrupted the glomerular-tubular balance. The mechanism whereby salt load does this is not known. However, other studies (DeWardener, 1973) have shown that although reduction of GFR by partial constriction of the renal artery increased proximal sodium reabsorption and decreased urinary sodium excretion, reduction of GFR by occlusion of renal vein and ureteral obstruction produced opposite effects: reduced proximal sodium reabsorption and increased urinary sodium excretion.

The apparent conflict in these findings may be resolved if we remember the following points:

(a) Changes in GFR produced by these three maneuvers are brought about by different mechanisms. Constriction of renal artery reduces hydrostatic pressure at the glomerular as well as post-glomerular capillaries. The first effect reduces GFR and increases tubular transit time, a factor which favors increased luminal sodium reabsorption. The second effect reduces the balance of hydrostatic-oncotic pressure gradients across the peritubular membrane, thereby increasing peritubular uptake of reabsorbate. The net result of both effects is increased proximal sodium reabsorption.

(b) When GFR is reduced by constriction of the renal vein, although tubular transit time is increased, the hydrostatic-oncotic pressure gradient across the peritubular membrane is also increased. The former effect tends to increase reabsorption, whereas the latter effect tends to decrease reabsorption. The results of the available experiments suggest that the effect of pressure gradient on proximal sodium reabsorption is more important than changes in tubular transit time. Thus, renal vein occlusion was found to decrease proximal sodium reabsorption. However, the compensatory increase in sodium reabsorption by the distally located nephron segments somewhat blunts this effect and reduces urinary sodium excretion.

(c) It should be noted that the effect of changes in GFR may be mediated by both a change in filtration fraction (GFR/RPF) and a change in the balance of hydrostatic-oncotic pressure gradients across the peritubular capillaries.

In summary, an increase in GFR produces a parallel increase in filtration fraction and a secondary increase in the protein oncotic pressure in the post-glomerular capillary vasculature. The former decreases tubular transit time, thereby reducing tubular absorption; the latter increases capillary uptake of reabsorbate, thereby obscuring the extent of the effect of increase in GFR on tubular reabsorption. The compensatory adjustments in renal sodium excretion in response to changes in GFR or sodium load appear to be mediated by changes in reabsorption in both proximal and distal tubules. The mechanism of such a compensatory adjustment involves induced changes in absorption characteristics at the luminal and peritubular membranes.

3. EFFECT OF CHANGES IN RENAL PERFUSION PRESSURE. Changes in renal perfusion pressure bring about parallel changes in sodium excretion rate. However, as described in Chapter 5, changes in mean renal perfusion pressure between 80 and 190 mm Hg (the autoregulatory range) are not accompanied by changes in GFR or RPF (McDonald and DeWardener, 1965).

The mechanism whereby changes in mean arterial pressure bring about parallel changes in sodium excretion has been clarified by a number of recent experiments (Earley and Schrier, 1973). The results of these studies suggest that the natriuretic effect of the increase in mean arterial pressure is due to the transmission of the elevated pressure to the post-glomerular capillary vasculature. At this site, the relative increase in hydrostatic pressure over the protein oncotic pressure decreases the capillary uptake of the reabsorbate by the proximal tubule, thereby increasing urinary sodium excretion (Koch et al., 1968). That an increase in renal perfusion pressure, without an equivalent rise in GFR, depresses tubular reabsorption and produces marked natriuresis has also been well established (Selkurt et al., 1965).

4. INFLUENCE OF INTRARENAL HEMODYNAMICS ON SODIUM TRANSPORT.
The results of numerous recent experiments strongly favor the concept
of intrarenal transcapillary hydrostatic-oncotic pressure gradients
as an important determinant of capillary uptake of reabsorbate along
the proximal tubule and hence sodium transport along the nephron.
This concept best explains a number of experimental results, although
it is based on the assumption that the capillary uptake of the
reabsorbate is the limiting step in the overall filtrate reabsorption
along the nephron.

The major intrarenal hemodynamic variables in such a control of
capillary uptake of reabsorbate are: capillary resistance, capillary
hydrostatic, and capillary oncotic pressures. Thus, any factor which
alters these variables will have a profound influence on the capillary
absorption of the filtrate. For example, vasodilation reduces
capillary uptake, whereas a rise in protein concentration increases
the uptake. Micropuncture studies have localized the site of action
of these intrarenal hemodynamic variables as the proximal tubule.
Furthermore, their effects on tubular reabsorption do not appear to
be mediated by changes in tubular volume. Thus, in keeping with the
proximal cell model depicted in Figure 8-11, changes in intrarenal
hemodynamic variables exert their influence on the uptake of
reabsorbate from the intercellular spaces into the capillary. Hence,
an increase in protein oncotic pressure speeds, while an increase in
hydrostatic pressure retards, the rate of such a fluid uptake.

An important factor modulating the effect of transcapillary
hydrostatic-oncotic pressure gradient on tubular reabsorption is the
glomerular filtration rate. Of more practical interest is the
filtration fraction (GFR/RPF), a factor determining the protein
concentration in the post-glomerular plasma, and hence capillary
absorption.

The results of several experiments have shown that expansion of
blood volume with hyperoncotic solutions depresses proximal sodium
reabsorption, with little change in urinary excretion. This implies
that the increased plasma oncotic pressure, at the peritubular
capillary level, has a lesser effect on reabsorption than the parallel
increase in the hydrostatic pressure induced by expansion of blood
volume. However, when blood volume was expanded to the same degree
by infusion of hypo-oncotic or iso-oncotic solutions, despite the
same degree of depression of the proximal tubule, the urinary sodium
excretion was increased. This difference in urinary sodium excretion
is due to the fact that whereas blood volume expansion depresses
proximal sodium reabsorption, the effect of plasma oncotic pressure is
more pronounced in the distal tubule than in the proximal tubule.

Windhager and co-workers (1969) have provided the most direct
evidence for the effect of peritubular plasma oncotic pressure on
proximal sodium reabsorption. Microperfusing the neighboring
peritubular capillaries with hyperoncotic dextran, they found a
significant increase in proximal sodium reabsorption as measured by
split-oil drop technique. They also found that proximal sodium
reabsorption increased as filtration fraction increased, further
emphasizing the effect of plasma oncotic pressure.

Perhaps the strongest evidence implicating the importance of plasma oncotic pressure on proximal sodium reabsorption is the experiments of Brenner and associates (1969). They found that the proximal sodium reabsorption in rat varies directly with protein concentration of the post-glomerular capillary, whether the latter was altered by bolus infusion of saline, iso-oncotic or hyperoncotic solutions.

With the renal cell model discussed earlier (Fig. 8-11) in mind, Earley and Daugharty (1969) have proposed the scheme shown in Figure 8-13 to describe the intrarenal pathways involved in renal response to volume expansion.

To further illustrate the influence of the intrarenal hemodynamics on the proximal sodium transport, consider the idealized scheme of renal vasculature shown in Figure 8-14, which is an extension of the scheme described earlier (Fig. 3-5).

In this scheme, we have lumped all the intrarenal resistances as the linear combination of three resistances: pre-glomerular resistance (R_a), post-glomerular resistance (R_e), and venular resistance (R_v). P_C and π_C are the hydrostatic and protein oncotic pressures of the peritubular capillary blood. The other terms have already been defined.

Using this model, let us write defining equations for the pressure-flow relationships for the entire kidney and the two components relevant to the present discussion--namely, the glomerulus and the peritubular capillary network.

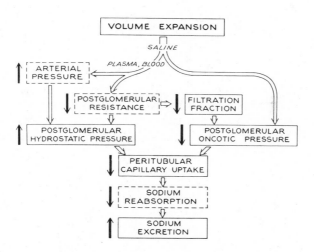

Figure 8-13. A scheme depicting the intrarenal pathways through which extracellular volume expansion may influence sodium excretion. *Open arrows* indicate sequence of events and *solid arrows* indicate the direction of change. Broken lines enclosing some of the factors indicate that the mechanisms mediating the change are unknown. (From Earley, L. E., and Daugharty, T. M. (1969). Reprinted by permission from *The New England Journal of Medicine*, Vol. 281, pp. 72-86, 1969.)

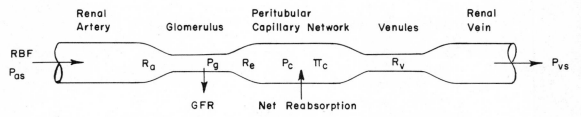

Figure 8-14. A schematic model of renal vasculature.

In accordance with the notions introduced in Chapters 3 and 5, the renal blood flow (RBF) may be defined as the ratio of the hydrostatic pressure drop across the kidney vasculature ($P_{AS} - P_{VS}$) to the linear sum of the three intrarenal resistances. Expressed algebraically:

$$RBF = \frac{P_{AS} - P_{VS}}{R_a + R_e + R_v} \qquad (8-22)$$

Since renal plasma flow equals RBF(1 - Ht), where Ht is the hematocrit, we can rewrite the above equation in terms of RPF:

$$RPF = \frac{P_{AS} - P_{VS}}{R_a + R_e + R_v} (1 - Ht) \qquad (8-23)$$

For a given RPF, the hemodynamics of the post-glomerular peritubular capillary blood is determined by the fraction of RPF which is filtered at the glomerulus, or GFR. The latter was defined earlier by the equation:

$$GFR = \frac{1}{2} \left(\frac{P_a - P_e}{R_a} - \frac{P_a - P_e}{R_e} \right) \qquad (8-24)$$

The filtration fraction, FF, is then given by dividing Equation 8-24 by Equation 8-23:

$$FF = \frac{GFR}{RPF} = \frac{\dfrac{1}{2} \left(\dfrac{P_a - P_e}{R_a} - \dfrac{P_a - P_e}{R_e} \right)}{\dfrac{P_{AS} - P_{VS}}{R_a + R_e + R_v} (1 - Ht)} \qquad (8-25)$$

The hydrostatic blood pressure in the peritubular capillary (P_c) is given by:

$$P_c = \left(\frac{RPF}{1 - Ht} - GFR \right) R_v + P_{VS} \qquad (8-26)$$

where the term in parentheses is the fraction of renal blood flow which has escaped filtration. The protein oncotic pressure in this blood (π_c) is given by:

$$\pi_c = \left(\frac{RPF}{RPF - GFR} \right) \pi_p \qquad (8-27)$$

Finally, the net rate of fluid reabsorption ($\dot{T}_f$) by the peritubular capillary network is given by the difference between the hydrostatic and protein oncotic pressures, with the latter as the major determining force:

$$\dot{T}_f = k_f (\pi_c - P_c) \qquad (8-28)$$

where k_f is the permeability coefficient of the capillary membrane. Thus, an increase in π_c relative to P_c increases $\dot{T}_f$, whereas a relative decrease in π_c reduces $\dot{T}_f$.

Because changes in π_c and P_c are ultimately determined by the renal and extrarenal factors defined by Equations 8-23 and 8-24, in the final analysis the magnitude of $\dot{T}_f$ depends on the influence of the systemic hemodynamics and their effective regulation.

From Equation 8-27 it can be seen that the major factor influencing π_c is the GFR and π_p, independently of changes in RPF. Thus, if π_p and RPF remain constant, changes in π_c and hence capillary uptake of reabsorbate ($\dot{T}_f$) are related to changes in GFR. Furthermore, as shown by Equation 8-26, the effect of P_c on $\dot{T}_f$ will be evident only in the absence of large changes in GFR.

Table 8-1 summarizes the effects of several maneuvers on the intrarenal hemodynamics and the net capillary uptake of the reabsorbate, both predicted by Equations 8-26 to 8-28 and observed by experiments discussed earlier.

TABLE 8-1

Directional Changes in Some Intrarenal Hemodynamics
in Response to Some Selected Forcings

Forcings	Response						
	RPF	GFR	FF	P_c	π_c	$\dot{T}_f$	Tubular-Transit Time
Step increase in P_{VS} (venous occlusion)	−	−	0	+	0	+	+
Step increase in R_v	−	−	0	+	0	−	+
Step increase in R_a	−	−	0	−	0	+	+
Step increase in R_e	−	+	+	−	+	+	−
Step increase in ureteral pressure (ureteral obstruction)	+	−	−	+	−	+	+
Step decrease in P_{AS} (aortic constriction)	−	−	0	−	0	+	+

LOOP OF HENLE

MORPHOLOGY

Anatomically, the loop of Henle consists of three segments:
(1) the pars recta of the proximal tubule; (2) a thin U-shaped loop,
of a smaller diameter than the proximal tubule, which descends into
the renal medulla; and (3) a thick ascending portion constituting the
pars recta of the distal tubule, the next sequential nephron segment.
Figure 8-4 depicts the structural detail of the cells constituting the
different segments of the loop. Functionally, the loop of Henle will
be considered hereafter to consist of a *descending limb* composed of a
short thick segment followed by a long thin segment, and an *ascending
limb* composed of a short thin segment followed by a relatively longer
thick segment. To further emphasize its role in concentration and
dilution of urine, the thick ascending segment has also been referred
to as the *diluting segment*. The significance of this functional
classification will be discussed in Chapter 11.

GENERAL CHARACTERISTICS OF
FILTRATE TRANSPORT

Until recently, the inaccessibility of the medullary portions of
the nephron to direct micropuncture made it virtually impossible to
study the mechanism of sequential processing of the filtrate along the
different segments of the loop of Henle. Our present understanding of
the processing of the filtrate along this segment of the nephron has
proceeded in two successive stages. The first was the extension of
the micropuncture techniques to collection and analysis of fluids
obtained from the tip of the loop and adjacent structures in hamsters.
The resulting information, in conjunction with that previously
obtained about filtrate processing in the late proximal and early
distal convoluted tubules of rats, provided the basic information
regarding the *overall* processing of the filtrate along the loop of
Henle. The second was the application of recent modifications of
microperfusion techniques to isolated segments of rabbit loop of
Henle. This made it possible to study directly the mechanism of
sequential processing of the filtrate along this segment.

To facilitate presentation, we shall begin this section with a
description of the overall processing of the filtrate along the loop.
And, where appropriate, we will incorporate recent findings to provide
an insight into the mechanism of sequential processing within the
loop. A fuller discussion of these findings and their significance
in urine concentration and dilution will be given in Chapter 11.

In 1951, Wirz and co-workers, measuring osmolality of renal
tissue slices in rat by direct cryoscopy, found a progressive increase
in osmolality from corticomedullary junction to the tip of the renal

papillae. Their findings have recently been confirmed by several micropuncture studies which showed that TF/P for inulin was significantly higher in fluid collected from the loop bend than that collected from the late proximal convoluted tubules (Lassiter et al., 1966; Jamison, 1968, 1970; Marsh, 1970). From this evidence, it was suggested that the filtrate becomes progressively hyperosmotic as it flows down the descending limb. The probable mechanism for this increase in osmolality was thought to be either net water reabsorption from or net solute addition to the tubular fluid as it flows along the descending limb.

That the net water abstraction is the mechanism for this increase in tubular fluid osmolality is based on a recent *in vitro* microperfusion study of rabbit descending limb. In a series of experiments, Kokko (1974) not only confirmed the progressive increase in tubular fluid osmolality, but also found that the descending limb cell membranes have a significantly lower passive permeability to sodium and urea compared to that for water. This finding constitutes unequivocal evidence that, at least in rabbit, the increase in osmolality of the filtrate as it flows down the descending limb is due primarily to water abstraction and not to solute addition.

In contrast, as shown in Figure 8-15, micropuncture analysis of the fluid collected from the early distal tubule, and hence that emerging from the ascending limb, was found to be always hypo-osmotic, whether the final urine was concentrated (U/P > 1.0) or not. Since the fluid collected at the loop bend was always hyperosmotic, the hypotonicity of the early distal fluid implied that the filtrate must become progressively dilute as it flows up the ascending limb. The probable mechanism for this decrease in osmolality was thought to be either net solute abstraction or net water addition. The question has been resolved by recent studies of Morgan and Berliner (1968) in rats and Kokko (1974) in rabbits. These investigators found that, in both species, the ascending limb membranes were highly impermeable to osmotic flow of water, but not to passive diffusion of solutes. Their findings constitute unequivocal evidence that the hypotonicity of the fluid emerging from the ascending limb is due primarily to net solute reabsorption and not to net water addition.

A number of recent experiments have clarified the type of solutes reabsorbed along the loop of Henle and the modes of their transport. These are summarized below.

A comparison of TF/P for sodium in the fluid collected from the late proximal and early distal convoluted tubules has revealed that nearly 25 to 40% of the filtered sodium is reabsorbed along the loop of Henle in rodents (Ullrich and Marsh, 1963; Gottschalk, 1964; Jamison et al., 1967; Berliner and Bennett, 1967; Windhager, 1968), while somewhat less is reabsorbed in dogs (Seely and Dirks, 1969) and monkeys (Tanner and Selkurt, 1970). The mode of this sodium reabsorption was assumed to be similar to that in the proximal tubule--namely, by an active mechanism--an assumption which has been questioned by recent findings in the rabbit. Nevertheless, the fact that a large fraction of the filtered sodium is reabsorbed along the loop, plus the finding that sodium chloride and urea are the most

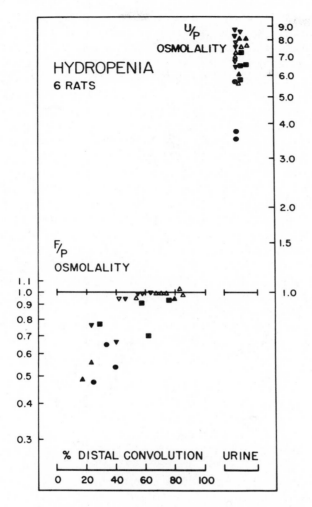

Figure 8-15. Tubular fluid-to-plasma osmolality ratios (F/P) along the distal convoluted tubules and urine-to-plasma osmolality ratios (U/P) from hydropenic rats. Different symbols refer to different rats. [From Gottschalk, C. W. (1961).]

abundant constituents of the filtrate at the loop bend, have led to the suggestion that the hypotonicity of the early distal fluid is due to active sodium and passive urea absorption along the ascending limb.

That active sodium absorption in excess of water might occur along the ascending limb was suggested by Jamison (1968), who analyzed fluid collected by free-flow micropuncture technique, from the rat ascending limb of the loop of Henle. He found a higher TF/P for inulin, a lower osmolality, and a lower sodium-to-inulin TF/P in the ascending limb, compared to those in the adjacent descending limb. Although the observed lower sodium concentration in the ascending limb may imply active absorption of this ion, it does not necessarily prove it. The question of whether sodium is actively reabsorbed or not can only be resolved by simultaneous measurements of both electrical potential (which was not measured in this study) and concentration gradients across the loop segment.

Recent microperfusion studies in the rabbit in which both electrical potential and concentration gradients were measured do not corroborate Jamison's conclusion. Table 8-2 summarizes these results, which indicate that sodium is transported passively, not actively, along the loop. Furthermore, these data indicate that the hypotonicity of the fluid emerging from the ascending limb is due to active chloride absorption along the thick portion and passive sodium and urea absorption along the entire length of this loop segment.

As is evident from the data in Table 8-2, there are striking differences in the modes of electrolyte, urea, and water transport along the loop of Henle, compared to that in the proximal, distal, and collecting tubules.

Compared to the proximal tubule, the transepithelial electrical potential gradient is zero in the descending limb and the thin segment of the ascending limb. This finding, along with the relatively low permeability to passive solute transfer, provides the electrochemical evidence for the proposed passive sodium and urea transport along these loop segments. The relatively high permeability of the descending limb to water suggests that water is absorbed along this segment by osmosis, as a result of the osmotic force generated by passive solute movement.

In contrast, in the ascending limb not only do the modes of electrolytes and water transport differ markedly from that in the descending limb, but also there are significant differences between the thin and thick portions of this segment. This is illustrated by a comparison of the transepithelial electrical gradient and passive solute and water permeability characteristics of these two segments.

The thin ascending segment is characterized by being highly impermeable to osmotic flow of water, permeable to sodium, chloride, and urea, and by having a transepithelial electrical gradient of zero. The latter two features account for the proposed passive mode of solute transport along this segment. On the other hand, the thick ascending segment, though it is highly impermeable to osmotic flow of water, is relatively impermeable to solute and has a transepithelial electrical gradient which is both steeper than that for the proximal tubule (6.7 mV as compared to 5.8 mV) and opposite in sign (lumen positive). The latter two observations provide unequivocal evidence, at least in the rabbit, for active chloride and passive sodium and urea absorption along this segment.

The asymmetric permeability characteristics of the descending and ascending limbs to electrolytes, urea, and osmotic flow of water, described above, have provided the basis for numerous theories advanced to explain the role of the loop of Henle in concentration and dilution of urine. Although details of these theories and our current understanding of the mechanism of urine concentration and dilution are discussed elsewhere (Chapter 11), a brief description of their salient

TABLE 8-2

Transport Characteristics of Various Segments of
Rabbit Nephrons Perfused In Vitro

Nephron Segments	Substance	Passive Permeability ($\times 10^{-5}$ cm/sec)	Measured Transepithelial Electrical Potential, PD (mV)	Mode of Transport
1. Proximal Convoluted Tubule	Sodium	8.1	-5.8 (lumen	Active
	Chloride	3.8	negative)	Passive
	Urea	5.3		Passive
	Water	29-63		Osmosis
2. Descending Limb of Henle's Loop	Sodium	1.6	0	Passive
	Urea	1.5		Passive
	Water	171		Osmosis
3. Thin Ascending Limb	Sodium	24.9	0	Passive
	Chloride	116		Passive
	Urea	6.7		Passive
	Water	0		None
4. Thick Ascending Limb	Sodium	6.3	+6.7 (lumen	Passive
	Chloride	1.1	positive)	Active
	Urea	0.9		Passive
	Water	0		None
5. Distal Convoluted Tubule	Sodium	low	-10 to -45	Active
	Potassium	low	(lumen	Active
	Chloride	low	negative)	Active
6. Cortical Collecting Tubule	Sodium	0.083	-35 (lumen	Active
	Potassium	1.0	negative)	Active (secretion)
	Chloride	4.7		Passive

[From data reported by Kokko, J. P. (1974); Burg, M., and Stoner, L. (1974).]

features here will serve to synthesize our knowledge of the overall processing of the filtrate by this nephron segment.

To facilitate presentation, we begin by considering the filtrate processing along the thick ascending segment. Here, active (chloride) and passive (sodium and urea) reabsorption of solutes, without osmotic flow of water, leads to the development of a local region of hyperosmolality in the surrounding medullary interstitium, at each horizontal level along the ascending limb. The tubular fluid, in turn, becomes hypo-osmotic, at each level, relative to the surrounding medullary interstitium. To maintain tissue isotonicity, the tubular fluid in the descending limb comes to osmotic equilibrium at each level, due to abstraction of water, with the surrounding hyperosmotic interstitium. In so doing, the descending limb fluid becomes progressively hyperosmotic, reaching its maximum value at about the loop bend. The net result is that the fluid emerging from the loop of Henle will be slightly hypo-osmotic relative to that entering the loop. This would lead to a net accumulation of solute within the medullary interstitium, making it hyperosmotic and thereby inducing osmotic absorption of water from the adjacent structures, including the collecting tubules. It is this latter effect that determines the final volume and osmolality of the excreted urine, and hence the extent of its concentration.

From the foregoing considerations, it is evident that any factor that alters solute and water absorption along the loop of Henle will have a profound effect on the magnitude of the osmolality gradient established within the medullary interstitium and hence on the final concentration of the excreted urine. Let us now examine some of these factors.

FACTORS MODIFYING FILTRATE PROCESSING ALONG THE LOOP OF HENLE

Like the proximal tubule, the epithelial cells of the loop of Henle have the ability to adjust their sodium reabsorption rate to the load delivered to this nephron segment. However, in contrast to the proximal tubule, because of the very low permeability of the ascending limb epithelium to osmotic flow of water mentioned above, there is considerable lag between sodium and water reabsorption along the loop. In fact, it has been found (Landwehr et al., 1968) that both sodium and water reabsorption along the loop are flow-rate dependent, with the flow-dependency of water reabsorption being much greater. Their findings are shown in Figure 8-16, which depicts an inverse relationship between the fractional reabsorption of sodium and water loads by the loop of Henle and the flow rate into the loop. The sequence of events thought to be responsible for this inverse relationship may best be explained by considering the effect of reduced GFR on sodium and water reabsorption rate along the loop.

An acute reduction in GFR, and hence in the fluid load entering the loop, will result in an increase in the transit time of fluid through the loop. Because of the relatively low water permeability

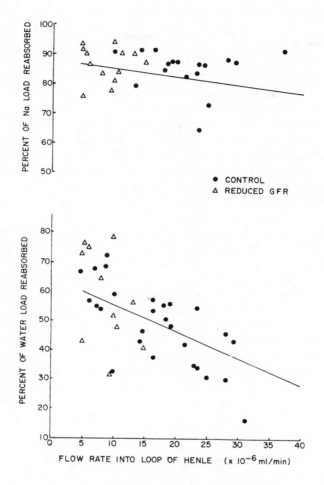

Figure 8-16. Fractional reabsorption of sodium and water by short loops of Henle as a function of flow rate into the loop of Henle during control conditions and after acute reduction of GFR by partial clamping of the renal artery. *Upper panel*, relation between fractional reabsorption of sodium load from the loop of Henle and flow rate entering the loop. *Lower panel*, relation between fractional reabsorption of water load from the loop of Henle and flow rate entering the loop. [From Landwehr, D. M., Schnermann, J., Klose, R. M., and Giebisch, G. (1968).]

of the ascending limb epithelium, the time the fluid is in contact with the epithelial cells will be an important determinant of water absorption. Hence, a reduction in flow rate into the loop will result in a more complete absorption and equilibration of tubular fluid with the surrounding medullary interstitium. Thus, within low physiological flow rates (10 to 15 x 10^{-6} ml/min), the sodium concentration leaving the ascending limb will be inversely related to the flow rate into the loop as well as the GFR (Fig. 8-16).

Although osmotic flow of water along the distal and collecting tubules is known to be affected by blood levels of antidiuretic hormone (ADH), ADH has no effect on water transport along the loop of Henle. Thus, Morgan and Berliner (1968) found, in the absence of ADH, a diffusional permeability for tritiated water (HTO) of 119 x x 10^{-5} cm/sec for the descending limb and less than half of this for the ascending limb and collecting tubule (50 and 45 x 10^{-5} cm/sec, respectively). However, in the presence of ADH, the diffusional permeability in the collecting tubule increased to 87, while ADH had no effect on the permeability of the ascending or descending limb. The net water flux in the descending limb was found to be 10 times that in the ascending limb. As mentioned earlier, these studies, along with those of Kokko (1974), provided the experimental proof for the relative water impermeability of the ascending limb epithelium, a prerequisite for the so-called countercurrent multiplication system for urine concentration and dilution in the loop of Henle.

Finally, the net water and sodium absorption along the loop can also be modified by selective diuretics. For example, furosemide (Clapp and Robinson, 1968) and ethacrynic acid (Goldberg et al., 1964) have been found to reduce, by about 50%, the net sodium and water reabsorption in the loop of Henle. The effects of these diuretics are presumed to be on the ascending limb epithelium. The significance and the probable mechanisms of their action in relation to the urine concentrating role of the loop of Henle will be considered in Chapter 11.

DISTAL AND COLLECTING TUBULES

MORPHOLOGY

The *distal tubule* is shorter than the proximal tubule and is characterized by columnar epithelial cells containing rod-shaped mitochondria. Like the proximal tubule, this nephron segment is divided into a straight portion (the pars recta) lined with somewhat thinner cells with deep luminal interdigitations, and a convoluted portion (the pars convoluta) composed of somewhat thicker cells with fewer luminal interdigitations. Figure 8-4 shows the salient features of the distal tubule and the cells making up its two segments.

The *collecting tubule* is both the longest and the largest portion of the nephron. It is formed by fusion of several distal tubules as they descend into the renal medulla in close proximity to the loop of Henle. On the basis of number of mitochondria, the epithelial cells lining the collecting tubule have been divided into *light* and *dark* cells, the latter cells containing more mitochondria than the former (Fig. 8-4). Several collecting tubules fuse to form the papillary duct of Bellini, through which the urine empties into the renal pelvis.

GENERAL CHARACTERISTICS OF
FILTRATE TRANSPORT

Micropuncture analysis of fluids collected from the accessible portions of the distal and collecting tubules in rats, dogs, and monkeys, and microperfusion of these as well as of the inaccessible segments isolated from rabbits, have established that: (1) Early distal fluid is always hypo-osmotic, becoming iso-osmotic as the filtrate passes through the distal convoluted segment. (2) Sodium is reabsorbed actively and its absorption is enhanced by adrenal mineralocorticoids (aldosterone). However, sodium absorption is adversely affected by changes in tubular flow rate and presence of poorly absorbable solutes in the tubular fluid. (3) Potassium is reabsorbed actively and secreted passively along the distal tubule, while only active reabsorption takes place along the collecting tubules. Furthermore, potassium secretion is enhanced in the presence of aldosterone and reduced in its absence. Whether the distal tubule transports potassium by net reabsorption or net secretion depends on the plasma concentration of this ion and on the metabolic state of the body. (4) Bicarbonate is reabsorbed passively along the electro-chemical gradients generated by sodium and potassium transport. However, chloride is reabsorbed actively against its electrochemical gradient. (5) Water is always absorbed by osmosis, as a result of the osmotic force developed by active and passive solute absorption. Osmotic absorption of water along both segments is enhanced in the presence of antidiuretic hormone (ADH), and is reduced when ADH is absent.

Let us now examine some of the evidence which has delineated the above characteristics of sequential processing of the filtrate along these distally located nephron segments.

FILTRATE OSMOLALITY. As shown in Figure 8-15, the fluid emerging from the ascending limb of the loop of Henle and hence entering the early distal tubule is hypo-osmotic (F/P osmolality ratio less than unity). It remains hypotonic during dehydration, during induced osmotic diuresis, and whether ADH is present or not. However, as this hypotonic fluid passes through the convoluted segment, it gradually becomes iso-osmotic (F/P osmolality ratio approaches unity). But if ADH is absent, the early distal fluid continues to remain hypo-osmotic as it flows along the convoluted segment. During its passage through the collecting tubule, the normally iso-osmotic filtrate becomes progressively hyperosmotic owing to osmotic efflux of water into surrounding hypertonic medullary interstitium. In the absence of ADH, the osmolality of the final urine will be lower than normal.

In the final analysis, the observed osmolality profile is determined by the differential rates of solute and water transport along these distally located nephron segments. Since the major constituents of the filtrate delivered to these segments are sodium, potassium, chloride, and urea, the extent of their tubular processing will largely determine the final volume and osmolality of the excreted urine. Therefore, the remainder of this section will be devoted to a closer examination of the tubular processing of these filtrate components and the factors which modify their transport along these segments.

SODIUM TRANSPORT. As depicted in Figure 8-6, sodium is reabsorbed continuously in the distal tubule, thereby lowering its TF/P ratios below unity all along the length of this segment. Moreover, comparison of TF/P ratios for sodium along the distal and proximal tubules reveals a steep blood-to-lumen concentration gradient for this ion in the distal tubule (TF/P < 1), compared to no gradient in the proximal tubule (TF/P = 1). Furthermore, split-oil drop experiments have shown that sodium reabsorptive rate per unit tubular length in the distal tubule is only one-fourth of that in the proximal tubule. Also, water permeability of the distal epithelial cells was found to be only 40% of that for the proximal tubule, a factor which accounts for the smaller fraction of water load being reabsorbed in the distal segment. These striking differences in reabsorptive rates for sodium and water between the proximal and distal tubules suggest that active sodium and osmotic water reabsorption along the distal tubule require much steeper electrochemical potential gradients. This conclusion is further substantiated by direct measurements of both electrical and chemical gradients in rat (Malnic et al., 1966) and rabbit (Burg and Stoner, 1974) nephrons.

Inspection of the sodium-to-inulin TF/P ratios in the lower panel of Figure 8-6 shows that nearly two-thirds of the filtered sodium is reabsorbed by the time the filtrate reaches the end of the proximal convoluted tubule. Furthermore, sodium reabsorption is about 90% complete by the time the tubular fluid reaches the first 15% of the distal tubular length.

Similar comparison of sodium-to-inulin TF/P ratios between the early and late distal convoluted tubule and ureteral urine reveals that most of the remaining 10% of the filtered sodium is reabsorbed along the distal tubule, with only 1% being reabsorbed along the collecting tubules. Quantitatively, similar reabsorption patterns for sodium have been observed in dogs and monkeys (Giebisch and Windhager, 1973).

The magnitude of sodium reabsorption along the distal tubule may be modified markedly by the presence of poorly absorbable solutes in the tubular fluid and by the rate of tubular volume flow. Lassiter and associates (1964) observed an *inverse* relationship between the tubular concentration of sodium and urea along the distal tubule in nondiuretic rats, concentration of sodium being low and that of urea being high. They attributed this to passive *recirculation* (by back-diffusion) of the urea reabsorbed from the collecting tubule into the loop of Henle, thereby increasing the urea concentration in the fluid entering the distal tubule. In contrast, in *saline diuresis* (induced by intravenous infusion of hypertonic NaCl) urea concentration in the distal tubule was found to be lower and sodium concentration higher, compared to the nondiuretic conditions. These latter findings were attributed to (1) a reduction in sodium reabsorption in the proximal tubule, thereby increasing its concentration in the distal tubule, and (2) a reduction in the recirculation of urea from the collecting tubule into the loop of Henle. Both of these factors tend to reduce urea concentration emerging from the loop of Henle and hence in the distal tubule. The rationale for this conclusion may be stated as follows.

Numerous clearance studies have established that *osmotic diuresis*, induced by intravenous infusion of saline or solutions containing poorly absorbable electrolytes or non-electrolytes, increases urinary excretion of sodium. Micropuncture studies have revealed that the natriuresis results from a suppression of proximal reabsorption of sodium, despite a compensatory increase in sodium reabsorption by the loop of Henle and to a minor extent by the distal and collecting tubules. Consequently, a larger than normal fraction of the glomerular filtrate would reach the distal and collecting tubules. Since urea is reabsorbed by passive diffusion, the high rates of volume flow through the loop of Henle and distal and collecting tubules, caused by diuresis, would reduce the tubular transit time, a factor which prevents the development of a steep urea concentration gradient required for its passive recirculation. As a result, urea concentration in the fluid emerging from the ascending limb of the loop of Henle and hence entering the distal tubule will be lowered. The reduced tubular transit time will also decrease tubular contact time for sodium, a factor which reduces active sodium reabsorption in the distal tubule, thereby increasing its tubular concentration. Accordingly, in saline diuresis, an increase in sodium concentration in the distal tubule is accompanied by a simultaneous decrease in urea concentration. Thus, the extent of normal iso-osmotic reabsorption of the filtrate along the late distal tubule depends on the amount of poorly absorbable solute present in the tubular fluid. Presence of such a solute will induce osmotic retention of water which along with continuous active sodium reabsorption leads to the development of a significant blood-to-lumen concentration gradient for sodium, and the opposite for urea.

Another factor which influences the rate of sodium reabsorption by the distal and collecting tubules is the blood level of the adrenal hormone aldosterone (Lowitz et al., 1969). The fraction of sodium reabsorbed under the influence of this hormone is very small, amounting to only 2% of the filtered sodium. Nevertheless, the continuous loss of this amount of sodium, in the absence of aldosterone, would be fatal if not replaced. The available evidence (see Chapter 11) indicate that aldosterone enhances passive reabsorption of sodium across the luminal cell membrane.

From the foregoing discussion it is clear that, in contrast to the proximal tubule, the distal and collecting tubules can absorb variable amounts of filtrate and its constituents, subject to hormonal intervention. Thus, fluid absorption in these segments is non-obligatory and hence is properly called *facultative*. As we see later, it is the smooth coordination of the adaptive reabsorptive capacity of the loop of Henle along with hormonal control of fluid reabsorption by the distal and collecting tubules which eventually determines the final volume and osmolality of the excreted urine.

POTASSIUM TRANSPORT. Numerous micropuncture studies in most mammalian nephrons have revealed that potassium is the only plasma electrolyte which is both reabsorbed from and secreted into the renal tubules. It has been established further that virtually all of the filtered potassium is actively reabsorbed by the proximal tubule, while the main site for potassium secretion is the distal tubule.

This marked difference in potassium transport pattern between the proximal and distal tubules is well illustrated in Figure 8-8. In the proximal tubule, we see that both the tubular fluid-to-plasma concentration ratios (TF/P) for potassium and the potassium-to-inulin TF/P ratios are clustered below unity, suggesting a net reabsorption of this ion along this nephron segment. This is consistent with the net reabsorption of a large fraction of filtered sodium and water in this segment.

In contrast, in the distal tubule, we see that the TF/P ratios for potassium increase from an initial low value in the early portion to a high value in the late portion, indicating a progressive increase in tubular potassium concentration. This is due to either a net potassium secretion or net reabsorption of water in excess of solute, or both. However, inspection of the potassium-to-inulin TF/P ratios reveal that, although these ratios increase along the distal tubule, they all fall below unity, suggesting a net potassium reabsorption. Despite this, some potassium must have been secreted into the tubules and eventually excreted in the urine, as evidenced by the measurable TF/P ratios in the ureteral samples.

That potassium secretion is confined only to the distal tubule is strongly suggested by the relative decrease in the potassium-to-inulin TF/P ratios in the ureteral urine, compared to those at the end of the distal tubule. This decline in TF/P ratios indicates net potassium reabsorption in the nephron segments beyond the distal tubule--namely, the collecting tubules. However, this conclusion must be considered only tentative, since its proof requires direct measurement of the electrochemical potential gradients across the epithelium of the rat collecting tubules. Furthermore, it is well to remember that the distal samples, yielding the data plotted in Figure 8-8, were collected from the *cortical* (superficial) nephrons which have short loops of Henle, while the ureteral urine samples are an admixture of fluids issued from both cortical and *juxtamedullary* (deep) nephrons which have long loops of Henle. The significance of this and other differences between these two nephron types will be discussed in Chapter 11.

CHLORIDE TRANSPORT. As shown in Figure 8-9, and similarly to sodium, chloride concentration decreases along the distal tubule, reaching a value of about one-fifth of that in the plasma by the end of this segment. Furthermore, comparison of the early and late distal tubular F/P ratios indicates that about 6% of the filtered chloride is reabsorbed along this segment.

Recent micropuncture studies of the isolated rabbit distal tubule have revealed that chloride is reabsorbed actively against its electrochemical gradients (Burg and Stoner, 1974). Despite this, some chloride is excreted in the final urine, as evidenced by the F/P ratios in the ureteral urine samples.

Like sodium, reabsorption of chloride along the distal tubule is adversely affected by the presence of poorly absorbable anions, such as sulfate.

In the collecting tubule, chloride concentration becomes very steep, due not to chloride secretion, but to proportionately more water reabsorption in this segment.

MECHANISM OF POTASSIUM SECRETION

Results of extensive micropuncture studies of the type illustrated in Figure 8-8 have revealed that the distal tubule has the capacity for both net secretion and net reabsorption of potassium, depending on the plasma potassium concentration and the metabolic state of the body. Thus, any maneuver which increases plasma potassium concentration will maximally stimulate net potassium secretion, while any factor which decreases plasma potassium concentration will suppress net potassium secretion. Let us now examine some of the major evidence which provided the basis for our current understanding of the mechanism of potassium secretion by the distal tubules.

Direct measurements of electrochemical potential gradients along the rat distal tubule have revealed that: (1) Both the concentration and the percentage of potassium remaining in the tubular fluid increase, while those for sodium decrease (Fig. 8-17, upper and middle panels). (2) There is a progressive increase in the luminal negativity along the distal tubule (Fig. 8-17, lower panel). This would account for the relative increase in potassium permeability in the second half of the distal tubule, as evidenced by the increased percentage of this ion appearing in that segment. Similar results have been found by Burg and Stoner (1974), who measured transepithelial electrical potential gradients across the isolated rabbit distal tubule (Table 8-2).

This observed *inverse* relationship between the tubular potassium and sodium concentrations together with the reduced reabsorptive rate for sodium along the distal tubule, alluded to earlier, would imply a lowering of the intracellular concentration of sodium. If so, in order to preserve isotonicity within the tubular cell, there must be a compensatory increase in the intracellular concentration of potassium. That this might be the case is strongly implied by the progressive increase in both concentration and percentage of potassium appearing along the distal tubule, a situation favored by a compensatory increase in the intracellular potassium concentration.

The above arguments suggest the possibility of a *one-to-one exchange* as the possible mechanism for sodium reabsorption and potassium secretion at the luminal membrane in the distal tubule.

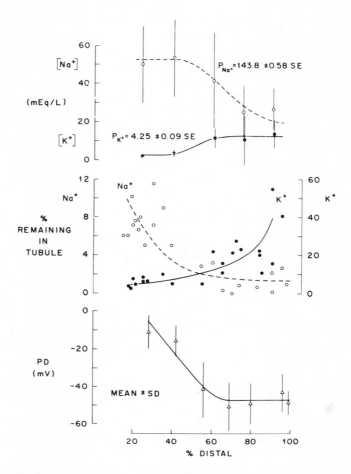

Figure 8-17. Tubular fluid sodium and potassium concentrations, relative rates of sodium reabsorption and potassium secretion (expressed as % remaining), and transepithelial electrical potential difference (PD) along the distal tubule of rat nephron. P_{Na^+} and P_{K^+} are the measured plasma concentration of sodium and potassium, respectively. Vertical bars depict standard deviation (SD) of the plotted data. [From Giebisch, G. and Windhager, E. E. (1973).]

That this is *not* strictly the mechanism of potassium secretion is the conclusion supported by several studies, notably those by Malnic and associates (1966). Since their findings have provided the best experimental evidence for the currently accepted mechanism of potassium secretion, closer examination of their data will facilitate the understanding of the proposed mechanism.

Malnic and co-workers (1966), using micropuncture techniques, made a comprehensive study of sodium and potassium transport along the rat proximal and distal tubules in response to two classes of forcings: (1) Those which modify the *intake* of either potassium or sodium, thereby affecting the cellular uptake of these ions from blood as well as their filtered loads and hence their net tubular transport. (2) Those which alter the *volume flow rate* in the tubules, thereby modifying net tubular reabsorption of sodium and hence secretion of potassium. Their findings, summarized in Figures 8-18 and 8-19, reveal several important characteristics of potassium transport along the rat nephron.

Gross inspection of these figures shows that despite a wide variation in the urinary excretion rates of potassium (Fig. 8-19), the fraction of filtered potassium entering the distal tubule varies but little (Fig. 8-18). This indicates that, regardless of the type of forcing used, the fractions of filtered potassium reabsorbed by the proximal tubule and by the loop of Henle are quite comparable. In other words, even in conditions which caused the urinary excretion rate of potassium to exceed its filtered load, virtually all of the filtered potassium is reabsorbed, and the excreted potassium is primarily of secretory origin. Let us now closely examine the effect of each forcing on potassium transport capacity of the distal tubule and analyze its possible mechanistic significance.

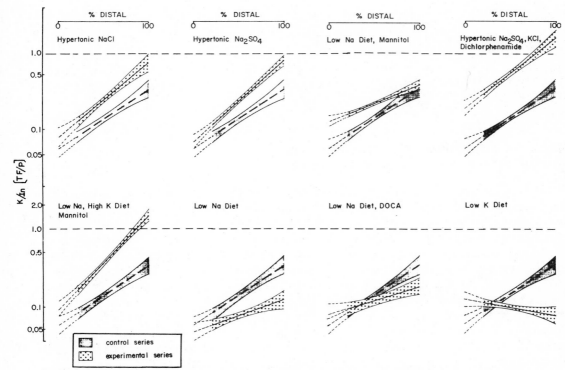

Figure 8-18. Comparison of potassium-to-inulin TF/P ratios along the distal convoluted tubules in rats under various dietary intake regimes and fluid loading. Regression lines were obtained by least-squares method. The width of the area around each regression line represents ±1 standard error. Values between 0 and 20% distal tubular length (dashed lines) were extrapolated. [From Malnic, G., Klose, R. M., and Giebisch, G. (1966).]

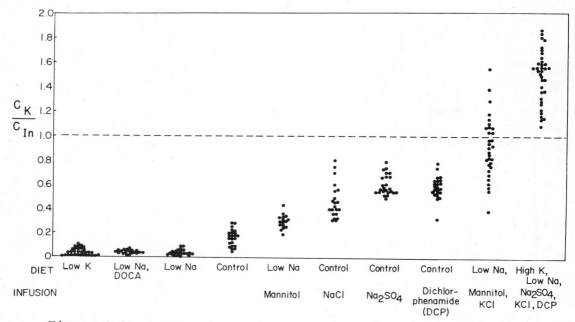

Figure 8-19. Comparison of potassium-to-inulin clearance ratios (C_K/C_{In}) from rats under various dietary intake regimes and fluid loading. [From Malnic, G., Klose, R. M., and Giebisch, G. (1966).]

EFFECT OF ALTERATIONS IN POTASSIUM AND SODIUM INTAKE ON POTASSIUM SECRETION

The effects of reduced dietary intake of potassium and sodium on potassium secretion by the distal tubule are shown in the lower panel of Figure 8-18. In both cases, there is a marked suppression of potassium secretion compared to normal. In the case of low-K diet, reduced plasma concentration of potassium would tend to decrease cellular uptake of potassium, thereby lowering the intracellular concentration of this ion and hence its net secretion. A reduced filtered load of potassium, on the other hand, would tend to increase reabsorption of potassium along the nephron due to longer transport time, and hence decrease its urinary excretion rate. The combined effect of these two mechanisms is to reduce urinary excretion rate of potassium (Fig. 8-19) by maximizing net reabsorption and minimizing net secretion.

In the case of low-Na diet, reduced filtered load of sodium coupled with its continuous active reabsorption in the proximal tubule would tend to lower the concentration of sodium in the fluid entering the distal tubule. Since net sodium reabsorption is always accompanied by net absorption of an anion (to preserve electrical neutrality), the lowered concentration of sodium in the tubular fluid would tend to reduce the luminal negativity. The resulting reduced transepithelial electrical gradient (Fig. 8-17) will tend to decrease net potassium secretion. Thus, as we shall see shortly, any factor that increases the transepithelial electrical gradient across the distal tubule stimulates potassium secretion and inhibits sodium reabsorption by this nephron segment. Likewise, any factor which increases distal tubular concentration of sodium, such as administration of poorly absorbable salts like sodium sulfate, enhances potassium secretion and suppresses sodium reabsorption by this nephron segment. Since sulfate is a poorly absorbable anion, it tends to increase luminal negativity and hence transepithelial electrical gradient, a factor favoring net potassium secretion. This explains why sodium sulfate is a more powerful kaliuretic agent than sodium chloride.

From the foregoing analysis, it follows that excessive dietary intake of potassium and sodium will maximally stimulate potassium secretion by changes opposite to those discussed above and summarized in Table 8-3. These results clearly implicate *electrical coupling* of Na-K rather than a one-to-one exchange as the possible mechanism of potassium secretion by the distal tubule.

Further support for this proposed mechanism comes from those experiments which have used aldosterone and its inhibitors to dissociate sodium reabsorption from potassium secretion. Administration of deoxycorticosterone-acetate (DOCA), a synthetic mineralocorticoid known to induce hypokalemic alkalosis, to rats fed low-Na diet (Fig. 8-18, lower panel) had surprisingly little effect on potassium secretion. Thus, it appears that a low-Na diet tends to protect the animal from the kaliuretic effect of DOCA.

A more striking finding in this respect is the recent observation of Wiederholt (1968). He found that, in adrenalectomized rats treated with aldosterone, administration of actinomycin D inhibited the anti-natriuretic effect of aldosterone but did not impair the ability of the distal tubule to secrete potassium. To anticipate, actinomycin D inhibits DNA-dependent synthesis of RNA (the so-called gene transcription), an intermediate step in aldosterone-dependent sodium reabsorption in the distal tubule (see Chapter 11 for further details). These findings are consistent with the view that a one-to-one Na-K exchange can not account for potassium secretion.

EFFECT OF ALTERATIONS IN THE VOLUME FLOW RATE ON POTASSIUM SECRETION

That the electrical coupling of Na-K may indeed be the mechanism mediating potassium secretion by the distal tubule is further substantiated by a comparative study of those forcings which modify tubular volume flow rate. As depicted in Figure 8-18 (upper panel), intravenous infusion of either hypertonic NaCl or Na_2SO_4 increased the fraction of filtered potassium remaining at the end of the distal tubule. This indicates that *osmotic diuresis* (as the renal effect of

TABLE 8-3

Changes From Normal in Urinary Potassium Excretion and the Possible Renal Mechanisms Involved in Response to Some Typical Forcings

Forcings	Urinary Potassium Excretion	Possible Mechanisms
1. Potassium Intake		
a. High	Increased	Increased cellular uptake of K^+ leads to increased net distal tubular secretion.
b. Low	Decreased	Decreased net secretion due to reduced cellular K^+ uptake.
2. Sodium Intake		
a. High	Increased	Increased net secretion due to increased electrical PD and flow rate in distal tubule (osmotic diuresis).
b. Low	Decreased	Decreased net secretion due to changes opposite to those mentioned above.
3. Hydrogen Ion Balance		
a. Respiratory or Metabolic Alkalosis	Increased	Increased cellular K^+ uptake leads to increased net distal tubular secretion.
b. Acute Respiratory or Metabolic Acidosis	Decreased	Decreased net secretion due to changes opposite to those mentioned above.

TABLE 8-3 (Cont.)

Forcings	Urinary Potassium Excretion	Possible Mechanisms
4. Blood Levels of Aldosterone		
a. High	Increased	Increased distal tubular net secretion due to enhanced cellular K^+ uptake.
b. Low	Decreased	Decreased net secretion due to changes opposite to those mentioned above.
5. Water Balance		
a. Hypertonic Dehydration	Increased	Increased net secretion due to increased cellular K^+ concentration subsequent to dehydration.
b. Hypotonic Hydration	Decreased	Decreased net secretion due to changes opposite to those mentioned above.
6. Administration of Diuretics		
a. Chlorothiazide	Increased	All three diuretics increase flow rates in distal tubule, thereby increasing net secretion.
b. Furosemide	Increased	
c. Ethacrynic Acid	Increased	
d. Mercurials	Decreased	Decreased net secretion due to decreased cellular K^+ uptake.
e. Amiloride	Decreased	Decreased net secretion due in part to reduced electrical PD.

[Modified from Valtin, H. (1973).]

intravenous infusion of these and similar solutions is called) induces kaliuresis, as a result of increased net potassium secretion. The explanation for this finding is as follows. As described earlier, osmotic diuresis depresses proximal tubular reabsorption of sodium and water, thereby increasing the volume of filtrate delivered to the distal tubule as well as its sodium concentration. This high volume flow rate further reduces sodium reabsorption along the distal tubule, resulting in even greater increase in its concentration in this segment. Thus, we see that the net effect of osmotic diuresis is to increase sodium concentration in the distal tubular fluid. This, in turn, increases the luminal negativity and hence transepithelial electrical gradient, a factor which stimulates net potassium secretion. As is evident from the data plotted in Figure 8-18, kaliuresis can be markedly enhanced if the elevation of tubular sodium concentration is induced by the presence of a poorly absorbable anion, such as sulfate.

In contrast, osmotic diuresis induced by hypertonic mannitol (a poorly absorbable non-electrolyte) in rats fed low-Na diet markedly reduced the contribution of the distal tubular potassium secretion to the total potassium excreted in urine, compared to hypertonic NaCl or Na_2SO_4 loading (Fig. 8-19). Also, it was found, but not shown here, that mannitol diuresis reduced proximal potassium reabsorption, a factor which contributed to the extent of urinary excretion of potassium.

That the diminished urinary excretion of potassium is not an inherent characteristic of the distal tubule is demonstrated by the plots shown in the lower left corner of Figure 8-18. These data are from rats fed low-Na, high-K diet and receiving an isotonic KCl solution mixed with hypertonic mannitol solution. The steep positive slope of the potassium-to-inulin TF/P ratios, including some values greater than unity, are indicative of the secretory capacity of the distal tubule for potassium. These results indicate further that sodium deprivation did not compromise the capacity of the distal tubule for potassium secretion.

Finally, maximal potassium secretion was observed when rats fed a high-K, low-Na diet received hypertonic Na_2SO_4 and isotonic KCl solutions along with dichlorophenamide, a diuretic agent. This diuretic is a potent carbonic anhydrase inhibitor, the effect is which is to interfere with sodium reabsorption in the proximal tubule, and hence induce natriuresis. The results, plotted in the upper corner of Figure 8-18, show a marked increase in net potassium secretion and urinary excretion (Fig. 8-19), which greatly exceeded those observed during the osmotic diuresis alone.

From these studies we may conclude that: (1) Neither the intratubular sodium concentration nor the filtered quantity of sodium entering the distal tubule was a rate-limiting factor if a one-to-one exchange were the mechanism of potassium secretion by the distal tubule. (2) The experimental dissociation of net sodium reabsorption and potassium secretion during osmotic diuresis and after injection of actinomycin D constitute strong evidence against a one-to-one Na-K exchange as the mechanism of potassium secretion. These findings, however, are consistent with an electrical coupling as the most likely mechanism of potassium secretion. (3) Inhibitory action of cardiac glycoside ouabain on both sodium reabsorption and potassium uptake at the peritubular membrane, mentioned earlier, is consistent with the view that active potassium reabsorption is in part responsible for the establishment of the transcellular potassium concentration gradient, a requirement for potassium secretion. (4) The intracellular concentration of potassium influences the net potassium secretion by the distal tubule and hence the extent of urinary excretion of this ion. Since intracellular concentration of potassium depends on the rate of potassium uptake at the peritubular membrane, a process mediated by Na-K stimulated ATPase, reduced cellular sodium concentration subsequent to sodium depletion could compromise potassium uptake and hence potassium secretion. (5) The extent of luminal negativity and therefore the magnitude of the transepithelial electrical gradient is a major determinant of net potassium secretion by the distal tubule.

These conclusions support the view that the electrical coupling between sodium and potassium, rather than a one-to-one Na-K exchange, is probably the major component of the mechanism mediating potassium secretion by the distal tubule. Recent studies by Burg and Stoner (1974), summarized in Table 8-2, suggest that since calculated potassium equilibrium potential from Nernst equation exceeded the measured transepithelial electrical potential, the observed high luminal potassium concentration cannot be accounted for by passive transport alone; at least part of the potassium secretion must be active.

To summarize, the data presented in Figures 8-17 to 8-19 suggest that the renal handling of potassium is a consequence of three sequential transport processes along the nephron: (a) net active reabsorption in the proximal tubule and the loop of Henle, (b) net secretion in the distal tubule primarily by passive electrical coupling and secondarily by active transport, and (c) net active reabsorption in the collecting tubule, with a potential for secretion.

From the foregoing discussion, it is evident that changes in potassium and sodium intake as well as alterations in blood levels of aldosterone profoundly influence net potassium secretion. Besides these, there are at least three other forcings which significantly modify potassium secretion by the distal tubule (Table 8-3). They are: (a) changes in plasma hydrogen ion concentration, (b) alteration in body water balance, and (c) selective action of some diuretics. Although renal mechanisms of hydrogen ion homeostasis and the action of diuretics are discussed in the ensuing chapters, the present discussion of renal handling of potassium would be incomplete without a brief mention of the effect of these forcings.

Plasma hydrogen ion concentration can be altered by fortuitous gain or loss of acid or alkali. Thus, both hyperventilation (respiratory in origin) and excess acid influx into the body (metabolic in origin) would lower the plasma hydrogen ion concentration, resulting in states of respiratory and metabolic alkalosis, respectively. The decrease in plasma hydrogen ion concentration causes hydrogen ions to be shifted from the cell into the plasma. To maintain electrical neutrality, there will be a concomitant increase in the cellular uptake of potassium. The resulting increase in the intracellular potassium concentration leads to an increase in the net secretion of this ion. Conversely, in acute respiratory and metabolic acidosis, conditions manifested by an increase in plasma hydrogen ion concentration, changes opposite to those mentioned above, will lead to a decrease in the cellular uptake of potassium and hence the net secretion of this ion.

In contrast, in chronic acidosis, there is an *increase* in net potassium secretion. The resulting condition, called *dissociated acidosis*, is characterized by excretion of alkaline urine despite acidosis (see Chapter 10).

It is apparent that, under the condition of acute hydrogen ion imbalance, potassium secretion is inversely related to hydrogen ion secretion. However, recent micropuncture studies, to be discussed later, have failed to show a clear-cut one-to-one exchange of potassium-hydrogen ions at the luminal membrane of the distal tubule.

Alteration in body water balance also influences potassium secretion by the distal tubule. Excessive loss of hypotonic fluid from the body, such as may occur in severe sweating, will lead to extracellular hypertonic dehydration (Chapters 1 and 3). This will induce a shift of water from the intracellular to the extracellular compartment, thereby increasing cellular concentration of potassium and hence net secretion of this ion. Conversely, excessive water intake results in extracellular hypotonic hydration. This will induce a shift of water from the extracellular to the intracellular compartment. The net effect is to reduce cellular concentration of potassium and hence net secretion of this ion.

Finally, chronic administration of some diuretics, such as chlorothiazide (a carbonic anhydrase inhibitor), furosemide and ethacrynic acid increases net potassium secretion. Although they differ in the site of action, they all interfere with sodium reabsorption, thereby increasing both tubular volume flow rate and sodium concentration. As mentioned earlier, both of these factors stimulate net potassium secretion. In contrast, mercurials and amiloride diuretics depress potassium secretion--the former by reducing the cellular uptake of potassium and the latter by decreasing the transepithelial electrical gradient.

PROBLEMS

8-1. What significant information has been obtained from the application of micropuncture, stop-flow microperfusion, and short-circuit current techniques to single nephrons and stop-flow experiments in whole kidney?

8-2. Briefly describe the extrarenal and intrarenal factors affecting iso-osmotic transport of sodium and water along the proximal tubule.

8-3. What experimental measurements do we need to decide whether an ion is transported actively or not?

8-4. Briefly explain the mechanisms whereby extracellular fluid expansion by intravenous mannitol and saline infusion induce natriuresis and diuresis.

8-5. How do changes in GFR modify tubular transport of sodium and water (a) in the proximal tubule and (b) in the loop of Henle?

8-6. State the currently accepted concept of K^+ secretion in the distal tubule and briefly outline the fundamental experiments which led to its development.

8-7. Micropuncture studies yielded the values of 10 and 0.5, respectively, for the tubular fluid-to-plasma concentration ratios of inulin and sodium at the end of the proximal tubule. If GFR was 120 ml/min and plasma sodium concentration was 140 mEq/L, calculate the fraction of filtered sodium reabsorbed along the proximal tubule.

8-8. In the table given below, indicate whether each forcing (during steady state) increases (+), decreases (-), or has no effect (0) on potassium secretion.

Forcings	Urinary Potassium Excretion
1. Respiratory acidosis	_____
2. Respiratory alkalosis	_____
3. Metabolic acidosis	_____
4. Metabolic alkalosis	_____
5. Sodium loading	_____
6. Sodium depletion	_____
7. Potassium loading	_____
8. Potassium depletion	_____
9. Water loading	_____
10. Administration of aldosterone	_____
11. Administration of spironolactone	_____
12. Administration of acetazolamide	_____
13. During mannitol or urea diuresis	_____

REFERENCES

1. Abodeely, D. A., and Lee, J. B.: Fuel of respiration of outer renal medulla. *Am. J. Physiol. 220*:1693-1700, 1971.

2. Arrizurieto-Muchnik, E. E., Lassiter, W. E., Lipham, E. M., and Gottschalk, C. W.: Micropuncture study of glomerulo-tubular balance in the rat kidney. *Nephron 6*:418-439, 1969.

3. Bank, N., and Aynedjian, H. S.: A micropuncture study of renal bicarbonate and chloride reabsorption in hypokalemic alkalosis. *Clin. Sci. 29*:159-170, 1965.

4. Bennett, C. M., Brenner, B. M., and Berliner, R. W.: Micropuncture study of nephron function in the Rhesus monkey. *J. Clin. Invest. 47*:203-216, 1968.

5. Bennett, C. M., Clapp, J. R., and Berliner, R. W.: Micropuncture study of the proximal and distal tubule in the dog. *Am. J. Physiol. 213*:1254-1262, 1967.

6. Berliner, R. W., and Bennett, C. M.: Concentration of urine in the mammalian kidney. *Am. J. Med. 42*:777-789, 1967.

7. Brenner, B. M., and Berliner, R. W.: Relationship between extracellular volume and fluid reabsorption by the rat nephron. *Am. J. Physiol. 217*:6-12, 1969.

8. Brenner, B. M., Falchuk, K. H., Keimowitz, R. I., and Berliner, R. W.: The relationship between peritubular capillary protein concentration and fluid reabsorption by the renal proximal tubule. *J. Clin. Invest. 48*:1519-1531, 1969.

9. Burg, M. B., and Stoner, L.: Sodium transport in the distal nephron. *Fed. Proc. 33*:31-36, 1974.

10. Clapp, R. J., and Robinson, R. R.: Distal sites of action of diuretic drugs in the dog nephron. *Am. J. Physiol. 215*:228-235, 1968.

11. Cohen, J. J., and Barac-Nieto, M.: Renal metabolism of substrate in relation to renal function. In: *Handbook of Physiology*, Section 8, *Renal Physiology*. Edited by J. Orloff and R. W. Berliner. Washington, D. C., American Physiological Society, 1973, pp. 909-1001.

12. Cortney, M. A.: Renal tubular transfer of water and electrolytes in adrenalectomized rats. *Am. J. Physiol. 216*:589-598, 1969.

13. Crabbe, J., and DeWeer, P.: Relevance of transport pool measurements in toad bladder tissue for the elucidation of the mechanism whereby hormones stimulate active sodium transport. *Arch. Ges. Physiol. 313*:197-221, 1969.

14. Curran, P. F., and MacIntosh, J. R.: A model system for biological water transport. *Nature 193*:347-348, 1962.

15. Daly, J. J., Roe, J. W., and Horrocks, P.: A comparison of sodium excretion following the infusion of saline into systemic and portal veins in the dog: evidence for a hepatic role in the control of sodium excretion. *Clin. Sci. 33*:481-487, 1967.

16. DeWardener, H. E.: The control of sodium excretion. In: *Handbook of Physiology*, Section 8, *Renal Physiology*. Edited by J. Orloff and R. W. Berliner. Washington, D. C., American Physiological Society, 1973, pp. 677-720.

17. DeWardener, H. E., Mills, I. H., Clapham, W. F., and Hayter, C. J.: Studies on the efferent mechanism of the sodium diuresis which follows the administration of intravenous saline in the dog. *Clin. Sci. 21*:249-258, 1961.

18. Diamond, J. M., and Bossert, W. H.: Standing gradient osmotic flow. A mechanism for coupling of water and solute transport in epithelia. *J. Gen. Physiol. 50*:2061-2083, 1967.

19. Dirks, J. H., Cirksena, W. J., and Berliner, R. W.: The effect of saline infusion on sodium reabsorption by the proximal tubule of the dog. *J. Clin. Invest. 44*:1160-1170, 1965.

20. Earley, L. E., and Daugharty, T. M.: Sodium metabolism. *New Eng. J. Med. 281*:72-86, 1969.

21. Earley, L. E., and Friedler, R. M.: The effects of combined renal vasodilation and pressor agents on renal hemodynamics and the tubular reabsorption of sodium. *J. Clin. Invest. 45*:542-551, 1966.

22. Earley, L. E., and Schrier, R. W.: Intrarenal control of sodium excretion by hemodynamic and physical factors. In: *Handbook of Physiology*, Section 8, *Renal Physiology*. Edited by J. Orloff and R. W. Berliner. Washington, D. C., American Physiological Society, 1973, pp. 721-762.

23. Edwards, B. R., Novakova, A., Sutton, R. A. L., and Dirks, J. H.: Effects of acute urea infusion on proximal tubular reabsorption in the dog kidney. *Am. J. Physiol. 224*:73-79, 1973.

24. Gertz, K. H.: Transtubuläre Natriumchloridflüsse und permeabilität für Nichtelektrolyte im proximalen und distalen Konvolut der Rattenniere. *Arch. Ges. Physiol.* *276*:336-356, 1963.

25. Giebisch, G.: Measurements of electrical potentials and ion fluxes on single renal tubules. *Circulation 21*:879-891, 1960.

26. Giebisch, G. : The contribution of measurements of electrical phenomena to our knowledge of renal electrolyte transport. *Prog. Cardiovas. Dis. 3*:463-482, 1961.

27. Giebisch, G.: Functional organization of proximal and distal tubular electrolyte transport. *Nephron 6*:260-281, 1969.

28. Giebisch, G.: Coupled ion and fluid transport in the kidney. *New Eng. J. Med. 287*:913-919, 1972.

29. Giebisch, G., and Malnic, G.: Some aspects of renal tubular hydrogen ion transport. *Proc. Intern. Congr. Nephrol. 4th Stockholm. 1*:181-194, 1970.

30. Giebisch, G., and Windhager, E. E.: Renal tubular transfer of sodium chloride and potassium. *Am. J. Med. 36*:643-669, 1964.

31. Giebisch, G., and Windhager, E. E.: Electrolyte transport across renal tubular membranes. In: *Handbook of Physiology*, Section 8, *Renal Physiology*. Edited by J. Orloff and R. W. Berliner. Washington, D. C., American Physiological Society, 1973, pp. 315-376.

32. Goldberg, M., McCurdy, D. K., Foltz, E. L., and Bluemle, L. W.: Effects of ethacrynic acid (a new saluretic agent) on renal diluting and concentrating mechanisms: evidence for site of action in the loop of Henle. *J. Clin. Invest. 43*:201-216, 1964.

33. Gottschalk, C. W.: Micropuncture studies of tubular function in the mammalian kidney. *Physiologist 4*:35-55, 1961.

34. Gottschalk, C. W.: Renal tubular function: lessons from micropuncture. *Harvey Lecture Ser. 58*:99-123, 1962-1963.

35. Gottschalk, C. W.: Osmotic concentration and dilution of the urine. *Am. J. Med. 36*:670-685, 1964.

36. Gottschalk, C. W., and Lassiter, W. E.: A review of micropuncture studies of salt and water reabsorption in the mammalian nephron. *Proc. Intern. Congr. Nephrol. 3rd Washington, D. C.,* 1966. Edited by Joseph S. Handler. New York: Karger, 1967, *Vol. 1*:357-373.

37. Gottschalk, C. W., and Lassiter, W. E.: Micropuncture methodology. In: *Handbook of Physiology*, Section 8, *Renal Physiology*. Edited by J. Oroloff and R. W. Berliner. Washington, D. C., American Physiological Society, 1973, pp. 129-143.

38. Howards, S. S., Davis, B. B., Knox, F. G., Dwight, F. S., and Berliner, R. W.: Depression of fractional sodium reabsorption by the proximal tubule of the dog without sodium diuresis. *J. Clin. Invest. 47*:1561-1572, 1968.

39. Jamison, R. L.: Micropuncture study of segments of thin loop of Henle in the rat. *Am. J. Physiol. 215*:236-242, 1968.

40. Jamison, R. L.: Micropuncture study of superficial and juxtamedullary nephrons in the rat. *Am. J. Physiol. 218*: 46-55, 1970.

41. Jamison, R. L., Bennett, C. M., and Berliner, R. W.: Countercurrent multiplication by the thin loops of Henle. *Am. J. Physiol. 212*:357-366, 1967.

42. Johnston, C. I., Davis, J. O., Howards, S. S., and Wright, F. S.: Cross-circulation experiments on the mechanism of the natriuresis during saline loading in the dog. *Circ. Res. 20*:1-10, 1967.

43. Katz, B., and Epstein, F. H.: The role of sodium-potassium-activated adenosine triphosphatase in the reabsorption of sodium by the kidney. *J. Clin. Invest. 46*:1999-2011, 1967.

44. Kill, F. Aukland, K., and Refsum, H. E.: Renal sodium transport and oxygen consumption. *Am. J. Physiol. 201*:511-516, 1961.

45. Koch, K. M., Aynedjian, H. S., and Bank, N.: Effect of acute hypertension on sodium reabsorption by the proximal tubule. *J. Clin. Invest. 47*:1696-1709, 1968.

46. Kokko, J. P.: Membrane characteristics governing salt and water transport in the loop of Henle. *Fed. Proc. 33*:25-30, 1974.

47. Koushanpour, E., Tarica, R. R., and Stevens, W. F.: Mathematical simulation of normal nephron function in rat and man. *J. Theor. Biol. 31*:177-214, 1971.

48. Krück, F.: Influence of humoral factors on renal tubular sodium handling. *Nephron 6*:205-216, 1969.

49. Landwehr, D. M., Klose, R. M., and Giebisch, G.: Renal tubular sodium and water reabsorption in the isotonic sodium chloride loaded rat. *Am. J. Physiol. 212*:1327-1333, 1967.

50. Landwehr, D. M., Schnermann, J., Klose, R. M., and Giebisch, G.: Effect of reduction in filtration rate on renal tubular sodium and water reabsorption. *Am. J. Physiol. 215*:687-695, 1968.

51. Lassiter, W. E., Mylle, M., and Gottschalk, C. W.: Net transtubular movement of water and urea in saline diuresis. *Am. J. Physiol. 206*:669-673, 1964.

52. Lassiter, W. E., Mylle, M., and Gottschalk, C. W.: Micropuncture study of urea transport in rat renal medulla. *Am. J. Physiol. 210*:965-970, 1966.

53. Lewy, J. E., and Windhager, E. E.: Peritubular control of proximal tubular fluid reabsorption in the rat kidney. *Am. J. Physiol. 214*:943-954, 1968.

54. Lockett, M. F.: Effects of saline loading on the perfused cat kidney. *J. Physiol. (Lond.) 187*:489-500, 1966.

55. Lowitz, H. D., Stumpe, K. O., and Ochwadt, B.: Micropuncture study of the action of angiotensin II on tubular sodium and water reabsorption in the rat. *Nephron 6*:173-187, 1969.

56. Malnic, G., and DeMello Aires, M.: Micropuncture study of chloride, bicarbonate and sulfate transfer in proximal tubules of rat kidney. *Am. J. Physiol. 218*:27-32, 1970.

57. Malnic, G., Klose, M., and Giebisch, G.: Micropuncture study of renal potassium excretion in the rat. *Am. J. Physiol. 206*:674-686, 1964.

58. Malnic, G., Klose, R. M., and Giebisch, G.: Micropuncture study of distal tubular potassium and sodium transport in the rat nephron. *Am. J. Physiol. 211*:529-547, 1966.

59. Malvin, R. L., Wilde, W. S., and Sullivan, L. P.: Localization of nephron transport by stop flow analysis. *Am. J. Physiol. 194*:135-142, 1958.

60. Marsh, D. J.: Solute and water flows in thin limbs of Henle's loop in the hamster kidney. *Am. J. Physiol. 218*:824-831, 1970.

61. McDonald, S. J., and DeWardener, H. E.: The relationship between the renal arterial perfusion pressure and the increased sodium excretion which occurs during an infusion of saline. *Nephron 2*:1-14, 1965.

62. Morgan T., and Berliner, R. W.: Permeability of the loop of Henle, vasa recta, and collecting duct to water, urea and sodium. *Am. J. Physiol. 215*:108-115, 1968.

63. Proverbio, F., Robinson, J. W. L., and Whittembury, G.:
    Sensitivities of Na-K ATPase and sodium extrusion mechanisms
    to ouabain and ethacrynic acid in the guinea pig cortex.
    Biochem. Biophys. Acta 211:327-335, 1970.

64. Rhodin, J.: Anatomy of kidney tubules. *Int. Rev. Cytol. 7*:
    485-534, 1958.

65. Richards, A. N., and Walker, A. M.: Methods of collecting fluid
    from known regions of the renal tubules of amphibia and of
    perfusing the lumen of a single tubule. *Am. J. Physiol. 118*:
    111-120, 1937.

66. Rodicio, J., Herrera-Acosta, J., Sellman, J. C., Rector, F. C.,
    Jr., and Seldin, D. W.: Studies on glomerulotubular balance
    during aortic constriction, ureteral obstruction and venous
    occlusion in hydropenic and saline-loaded rats. *Nephron 6*:
    437-456, 1969.

67. Schrier, R. W., McDonald, K. M., Marshall, R. A., and Lauler,
    D. P.: Absence of natriuretic response to acute hypotonic
    intravascular volume expansion in dogs. *Clin. Sci. 34*:57-72,
    1968.

68. Seely, J. F., and Boulpaep, E. L.: Electrical potentials across
    proximal and distal tubules of dog kidney. *Am. J. Physiol.
    221*:1084-1096, 1971.

69. Seely, J. F., and Dirks, J. H.: Micropuncture study of
    hypertonic mannitol diuresis in the proximal and distal tubule
    of the dog kidney. *J. Clin. Invest. 48*:2330-2340, 1969.

70. Selkurt, E. E., Womack, I., and Dailey, W. N.: Mechanism of
    natriuresis and diuresis during elevated renal arterial
    pressure. *Am. J. Physiol. 209*:95-99, 1965.

71. Shipp, J. C., Hanenson, I. B., Windhager, E. E., Schatzmann,
    H. J., Whittembury, G., Yoshimura, H., and Solomon, A. K.:
    Single proximal tubules of Necturus kidney. Methods for
    micropuncture and microperfusion. *Am. J. Physiol, 195*:
    563-569, 1958.

72. Skou, J. C.: The influence of some cations on adenosine
    triphosphatase from peripheral nerves. *Biochem. Biophys.
    Acta 23*:394-401, 1957.

73. Tanner, G. A., and Selkurt, E. E.: Kidney function in the
    squirrel monkey before and after hemorrhagic hypotension.
    Am. J. Physiol. 219:597-603, 1970.

74. Tobian, L., Coffee, K., and McCrea, P.: Evidence for a humoral factor of non-renal and non-adrenal origin which influences renal sodium excretion. *Trans. Assoc. Am. Physicians 80*: 200-206, 1967.

75. Ullrich, K. J., and Marsh, D. J.: Kidney, water and electrolyte metabolism. *Ann. Rev. Physiol. 25*:91-142, 1963.

76. Ussing, H. H.: The distinction by means of tracers between active transport and diffusion. *Acta Physiol. Scand. 19*: 43-56, 1949.

77. Ussing, H. H., and Zerahn, K.: Active transport of sodium as the source of electric current in the short-circuited isolated frog skin. *Acta Physiol. Scand. 23*:110-127, 1951.

78. Valtin, H.: *Renal Function: Mechanisms Preserving Fluid and Solute Balance in Health.* Little, Brown and Co., Boston, 1973.

79. Weinstein, S. W., and Klose, R. M.: Micropuncture studies on energy metabolism and sodium transport in the mammalian nephron. *Am. J. Physiol. 217*:498-504, 1969.

80. Whittembury, G., and Proverbio, F.: Two modes of Na extrusion in cells from guinea pig kidney cortex slices. *Arch. Ges. Physiol. 316*:1-25, 1970.

81. Wiederholt, M.: Effect of actinomycin-D on renal Na and K transport. *Proc. Ann. Meeting, Am. Soc. Nephrol., 2nd,* Washington, D. C., 1968.

82. Windhager, E. E.: *Micropuncture Techniques and Nephron Function.* Appleton-Century-Crofts, New York, 1968.

83. Windhager, E. E.: Some aspects of proximal tubular salt reabsorption. *Fed. Proc. 33*:21-24, 1974.

84. Windhager, E. E., Boulpaep, E. L., and Giebisch, G.: Electrophysiological studies on single nephrons. In: *Proc. Intern. Congr. Nephrol. 3rd, Washington, D. C.,* 1966. S. Karger, Basel, *Vol. 1*:35-47, 1967.

85. Windhager, E. E., Lewy, J. E., and Spitzer, A.: Intrarenal control of proximal tubular reabsorption of sodium and water. *Nephron 6*:247-259, 1969.

86. Wirz, H., Hargitay, B., and Kuhn, W.: Lokalisation des Konzentrierungsprozesses in der Niere durch direkte Kryoskopie. *Helv. Physiol. Pharmacol. Acta* 9:196-207, 1951.

87. Wirz, H., and Dirix, R.: Urinary concentration and dilution. In: *Handbook of Physiology*, Section 8, *Renal Physiology*. Edited by J. Orloff and R. W. Berliner. Washington, D. C., American Physiological Society, 1973, pp. 415-430.

Chapter 9

TUBULAR REABSORPTION AND SECRETION: CLASSIFICATION BASED ON OVERALL CLEARANCE MEASUREMENTS

In the preceding chapter, we analyzed the *sequential* processing of the filtrate and the mechanisms of tubular transport of major electrolytes and water along the various segments of the nephron. That analysis was largely based on successful application of micropuncture, microperfusion, and electrophysiological techniques at the level of a single nephron. Unfortunately, such techniques have been used to delineate the sequential processing of only a limited number of substances. To ascertain the renal handling of those solutes (mostly non-electrolytes) for which micropuncture data are scarce or as yet not available, we must resort to the standard overall clearance technique. Therefore, in this chapter, we shall expand on the materials presented in Chapter 6 and consider in more detail the *overall* (as opposed to sequential) processing of the major non-electrolyte constituents of the filtrate, using the standard clearance measurements. From such information we shall determine the net tubular transport of a substance by the kidney as well as classify the type of cellular transport process involved.

Insofar as the renal tubular processing of the filtrate is concerned, the solutes contained in the tubular fluid are transported by any one or a combination of three processes: bulk flow, simple passive diffusion, and carrier-mediated transport. The latter type of transport, however, is by and large the major mechanism for the net reabsorption or secretion of nearly all the important solutes present in the filtrate and plasma. It should be recalled from Chapter 4 that reabsorption and secretion refer to the *direction* of transport and not the underlying mechanisms. Thus, *reabsorption* refers to the transport of solutes from the tubular lumen into the peritubular capillary blood, while *secretion* refers to the transport of solutes from the peritubular capillary blood into the tubular lumen.

RENAL TITRATION CURVES:
CLASSIFICATION OF TUBULAR TRANSPORT

The capacity of the renal tubules for reabsorption and secretion varies depending on the type of solute being transported. To simplify this presentation, we may classify renal tubular transport into a *passive* process, which requires no expenditure of energy (e.g., urea transport) and an *active* process, which does require expenditure of energy (e.g., glucose and sodium transport). Note that the terms passive and active transport, as used here, imply that these processes represent the major contributing components in the overall transport of the given solute.

The renal handling of an actively transported solute may be further subdivided into two categories, depending on whether there is a maximum tubular transport capacity for that solute: (1) Those solutes for which there is a definite upper limit for unidirectional rate of transport, either reabsorptive or secretory in direction. Thus, as the quantity of solute delivered (filtered load) to the tubules for reabsorption is increased, the rate of reabsorption will increase only up to a certain maximal rate. Further increase in the filtered load presented to the tubules will not increase the rate of reabsorption. This limiting rate of reabsorption is called the *maximum tubular reabsorptive capacity* (Shannon et al., 1941, and Smith, 1955), and is designated by the symbol $\dot{T}m$. It denotes the maximum amount of a solute reabsorbed per minute, and its value varies with the substance involved. Similarly, there is also a *maximum tubular secretory capacity* which defines the limiting rate at which the tubules can secrete specific substances. Renal reabsorption of glucose and secretion of para-aminohippurate (PAH) are examples of actively transported solutes exhibiting tubular transport maximum. (2) Those solutes for which there is no definite upper limit for unidirectional rate of transport, and hence no $\dot{T}m$. Reabsorption of sodium along the nephron and secretion of potassium by the distal tubules are notable examples. Although sodium reabsorption is not a $\dot{T}m$-limited process, its net transepithelial reabsorption, as described in Chapter 8, is limited by the tubular flow rate, a factor influencing the cellular contact time which in part determines the rate of sodium diffusion from the tubular lumen into the renal tubule cell. Consequently, the reabsorption of sodium and like substances is called *gradient-time limited* transport.

Whether a substance is transported by a $\dot{T}m$-limited process or by a gradient-time limited process can be determined by simultaneous measurements of its filtered load and urinary excretion rate at varying plasma concentration. From these measurements, we can determine the net rate of reabsorption or secretion of the substance and whether or not it is transported by a $\dot{T}m$-limited process.

To illustrate the procedure, let us consider the renal transport of substance x with a permeability ratio of unity in a healthy subject. Using the techniques described in Chapter 6, we measure the renal clearance of substance x along with the clearance of inulin (C_{In}) as the concentration of x in the plasma ($[x]_p$), is progressively increased. Since inulin clearance is a measure of GFR, the filtered load of the substance for a given $[x]_p$ would be $C_{In} \cdot [x]_p$ or, more directly, GFR $\cdot [x]_p$. Assuming that in such an experiment GFR remains relatively constant, the filtered load of substance x should increase in direct proportion to the increasing plasma concentration of x. Since the urinary excretion rate of substance x (i.e., $\dot{V}_u \cdot [x]_u$), which can also be determined, is equal to the difference between the filtered load and the rate of tubular transport ($\dot{T}_x$) (see Equation 6-15), the value of the latter at a given plasma concentration would be:

$$\dot{T}_x = GFR \cdot [x]_p - \dot{V}_u \cdot [x]_u \qquad (9\text{-}1)$$

It should be recalled from Chapter 6 that if the substance x is reabsorbed, the sign of $\dot{T}_x$ would be positive, but if the substance x is secreted, the sign of $\dot{T}_x$ would be negative.

To determine whether the renal transport of x is by a $\dot{T}m$-limited process or not, we simply construct simultaneous plots of the filtered load (GFR $\cdot [x]_p$), the urinary excretion rate ($\dot{V}_u \cdot [x]_u$), and their calculated difference, i.e., the transport rate ($\dot{T}_x$), against the increasing plasma concentration of x ($[x]_p$). Such a combined plot, like those shown in Figures 9-1 and 9-2 (upper panels), is known as the *renal titration curves* for that substance; it determines the plasma concentration of the substance at which the "membrane carrier" is fully saturated (see discussion under *Glucose*, page 223).

Now if the substance x is transported by a $\dot{T}m$-limited process, we would expect the plot of $\dot{T}_x$ against $[x]_p$ to plateau at some value of $[x]_p$ and to remain constant thereafter. This is depicted by the theoretical reabsorption line parallel to the abscissa in Figure 9-1 (upper left graphs) for a substance transported by net reabsorption (e.g., glucose), and in Figure 9-2 (upper left graphs) for a substance transported by net secretion (e.g., PAH). Note that in both of these figures, the filtered load, the tubular transport, and the renal excretion rate are plotted against the filtered load and not the plasma concentration, as mentioned above. This is a more common way of plotting the titration curves. Note that plotting the filtered load against itself yields a 45 degree line through the origin, serving as a standard reference with which to compare the renal excretion rate.

On the other hand, if the renal transport of substance x is by a gradient-time limited process, such a plateau should not occur. This is depicted by the curvilinear line in Figure 9-1 (upper right graphs) for a substance transported by net reabsorption (e.g., sodium), and in Figure 9-2 (upper right graphs) for a substance transported by net secretion (e.g., potassium).

The lower graphs in Figures 9-1 and 9-2 depict the theoretical relationships between the fraction of the filtered load excreted by the kidneys ($\dot{V}_u \cdot [x]_u / GFR \cdot [x]_p$) as a function of the filtered load.

Note that this fraction is another expression of clearance ratio (see Chapter 6) and is obtained by dividing Equation 9-1 by the filtered load and rearranging terms:

$$\frac{\dot{V}_u \cdot [x]_u}{GFR \cdot [x]_p} = 1 \pm \frac{\dot{T}_x}{GFR \cdot [x]_p} \qquad (9-2)$$

In the case of a substance which is reabsorbed (Fig. 9-1) by $\dot{T}m$-limited process (e.g., glucose) the clearance ratio increases *sharply* and asymptotically toward the unity line. This is because when $\dot{T}_x = \dot{T}m$ (depicted by the vertical dashed line), the right-hand term in Equation 9-2 approaches zero as the filtered load is infinitely increased. In contrast, in the case of a substance not reabsorbed by $\dot{T}m$-limited process (e.g., sodium), the clearance ratio *gradually* approaches the unity line.

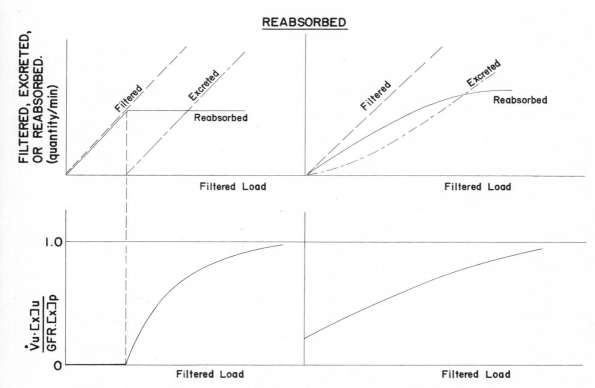

Figure 9-1. Theoretical relationships of renal titration curves (upper graphs) and clearance ratios (lower graphs) for a substance reabsorbed by $\dot{T}m$-limited process (e.g., glucose, left panel) and a substance reabsorbed by gradient-time limited process (e.g., sodium, right panel). [After Koch, A. (1960).]

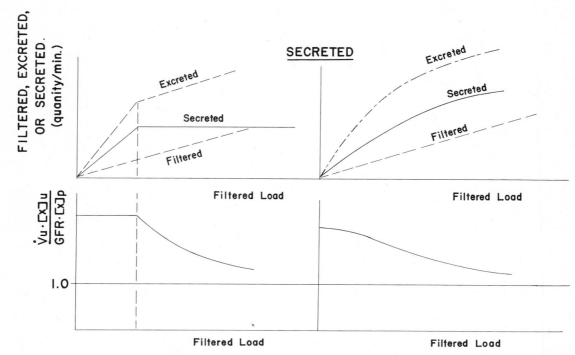

Figure 9-2. Theoretical relationships of renal titration curves (upper graphs) and clearance ratios (lower graphs) for a substance secreted by $\dot{T}m$-limited process (e.g., PAH, left panel) and a substance secreted by gradient-time limited process (e.g., potassium, right panel). [After Koch, A. (1960).]

In the case of a substance which is secreted (Fig. 9-2) by $\dot{T}m$-limited process (e.g., PAH), the clearance ratio begins at a value above unity (because $\dot{T}_x$ is positive in Equation 9-2) and sharply and asymptotically approaches the unity line. In contrast, in the case of a substance not secreted by a $\dot{T}m$-limited process (e.g., potassium), the clearance ratio gradually approaches the unity line.

Let us now inquire into the mechanisms and direction of net tubular transport of some important constituents of the filtrate as revealed from the application of the above concepts and titration studies. To facilitate presentation, we shall begin by considering those solutes which are transported by net reabsorption and then those which are transported by net secretion.

TUBULAR REABSORPTION

In this section we shall consider the renal transport of glucose, phosphate, sulfate, amino acids, organic anions, uric acid, and proteins, all of which with a few exceptions are reabsorbed by Tm-limited process. Because renal transport of glucose has been more extensively studied, its reabsorptive characteristics will be presented in more detail, so that it may serve as the prototype for the renal transport of the other substances mentioned above.

GLUCOSE

The classic clearance studies of Shannon and associates (1938, 1941) were the first in which the principles of titration curves were used to characterize the mechanism of renal transport of glucose in normal dogs. The conclusions and inferences drawn from these experiments have since become the framework for many of the subsequent studies designed to elucidate further the nature of the glucose transport system. Consequently, to facilitate understanding of these newer findings we shall begin by briefly enumerating the highlights of their conclusions.

1. Since at normal plasma glucose concentration the renal clearance of glucose was found to be zero, they concluded that all the filtered glucose must have been *reabsorbed*.

2. Because reabsorption was virtually complete, they reasoned that glucose must have been reabsorbed from the tubular fluid into the peritubular blood against a concentration gradient by an *active* process.

3. As the plasma concentration of glucose was progressively increased, they found that the tubular reabsorptive mechanisms became gradually *saturated*, so that glucose began to appear in the urine.

4. As the plasma glucose concentration was further increased, they observed that the transport mechanism became fully saturated, and the tubular reabsorption reached its *maximum limit* (Tm). Thereafter, Tm for glucose remained constant and unaffected by further increases in the plasma glucose concentration.

5. For a given animal, Tm for glucose was found to be stable during acute variations in the glomerular filtration rate, whether the changes were spontaneous or induced by obstruction of the abdominal aorta above the renal arteries or by hemorrhage.

On the basis of these findings, Shannon and co-workers suggested that the filtered glucose is reabsorbed by an *active, carrier-mediated* mechanism, the precise nature of which and the tubular site where glucose is reabsorbed remained to be determined. Micropuncture studies in rats (Walker et al., 1941; Frohnert et al., 1970) have subsequently shown that the tubular site where virtually all the filtered glucose is reabsorbed is the proximal tubule.

That glucose is in fact reabsorbed by a $\dot{T}m$-limited process was subsequently confirmed both in man (Smith et al., 1943) and in dog (Bradley et al., 1961). The human studies showed that in normal subjects $\dot{T}m$ for glucose was 375 ± 79.7 mg/min in 24 males and 303 ± 55.3 mg/min in 11 females tested. Both $\dot{T}m$ values are corrected to 1.73 m^2 body surface area. Furthermore, the dog studies showed that $\dot{T}m$ for glucose remained relatively constant in the face of modest changes in GFR, but was markedly decreased when GFR was greatly reduced (Coello and Bradley, 1964). This latter finding was attributed to a reduced overall function in those nephrons that are functioning and not to the existence of a glomerulotubular balance for glucose in any nephron.

CHARACTERISTICS OF GLUCOSE TITRATION CURVES. From the studies cited above as well as a number of others, a unifying picture of the general characteristics of renal transport of glucose has emerged. These are depicted in Figure 9-3, which illustrates the renal titration curves for glucose in man. To begin with, we see that as the plasma concentration of glucose ($[G]_p$) is gradually increased, the filtered load of glucose (GFR $\cdot$ $[G]_p$) increases linearly. Similarly, the tubular reabsorption of glucose ($\dot{T}_G$) (Equation 9-1) matches the filtered load and increases linearly with the plasma glucose concentration, so long as the latter remains below a value of 200 mg%. However, as the plasma concentration of glucose begins to exceed this value, a portion of the filtered glucose escapes tubular reabsorption and is therefore excreted in the urine (glucosuria). The plasma concentration at which glucose begins to appear in the urine (i.e., $[G]_p$ = 200 mg% in Fig. 9-3) is known as the *renal threshold concentration* for glucose. Note that this concentration is not synonymous with the plasma concentration that completely saturates the transport mechanism (i.e., $[G]_p$ = 400 mg% in Fig. 9-3). Note also that glucosuria occurs long before the transport mechanism is fully saturated. Two possible explanations for such a finding are discussed below.

As shown in Figure 9-3, the quantity of filtered glucose which escapes reabsorption, and hence is excreted in the urine, increases curvilinearly with the increasing plasma concentration until the latter exceeds a value of 400 mg%. Thereafter, the transport system becomes completely saturated and the quantity of filtered glucose reabsorbed will remain constant and independent of further increases in plasma glucose concentration. This constant reabsorption rate is called the *tubular reabsorption maximum* for glucose and is designated by the symbol $\dot{T}m_G$. At the maximal tubular reabsorption rate, the glucosuria will also become constant and a linear function of the plasma glucose concentration. Indeed, as the plasma glucose concentration exceeds 400 mg%, the slope of the excretion curve becomes parallel to the slope of the filtered curve.

As depicted in Figure 9-3, when the plasma glucose concentration varies between 200 and 400 mg%, both the amount of glucose reabsorbed or the amount excreted increase gradually, rather than abruptly, while

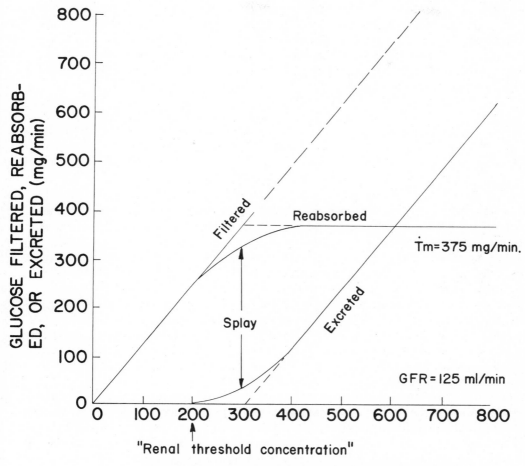

Figure 9-3. A typical titration curve for glucose in man. The heavy lines for reabsorption and excretion rates represent the actual experimental data, while the dashed lines represent the theoretical and extrapolated lines. [After Pitts, R. F. (1974).]

the filtered load increases linearly. The rounded regions of both the reabsorbed and excreted curves, which graphically relate $\dot{T}_G$ to the filtered load of glucose, are known as the *splay* of the titration curves. Of the various solutes which are reabsorbed by a $\dot{T}m$-limited process, glucose reabsorption shows a minimal degree of splay (Mudge, 1958).

The degree of splay in the glucose titration curves have been explained by two phenomena, which are not mutually exclusive: (1) the kinetics of tubular transport of glucose, and (2) the degree of morphological and functional heterogeneity of the nephron population within the kidney. Let us briefly examine each phenomenon and its significance as it affects renal glucose transport.

1. Kinetics of Glucose Transport. The kinetics of glucose transport has been suggested as a possible explanation for the degree of splay observed in its renal titration curves. This explanation can best be understood if we assume that the proximal tubular reabsorption of glucose involves the combination of the glucose molecule (G) with a membrane carrier (C) in a reversible reaction described by the following equilibrium equation:

$$K = \frac{[G] \cdot [C]}{[GC]} \tag{9-3}$$

where [G] is the concentration of glucose in the tubular fluid, [C] is the concentration of the free membrane carrier, [GC] is the concentration of the glucose-carrier complex at the surface of the luminal membrane, and K is the dissociation constant for the GC-complex.

As described in Chapter 7, the greater the affinity of glucose for the carrier molecule, the greater will be [GC], and hence the smaller the value of K. Conversely, the smaller the affinity of glucose for the carrier, the larger will be the product [G]·[C], and the larger the value of K. As long as [C] is large relative to [G], essentially all of the filtered glucose will be reabsorbed, and the clearance of glucose will be zero. However, as the plasma concentration of glucose and hence [G] in the proximal tubule increase, some glucose molecules will escape reacting with the free carrier molecules. Since the carrier has a finite affinity for glucose (that is, the value of K must be finite), a "supersaturating" concentration or one much higher than the renal threshold concentration of glucose is required to fully saturate the transport system. Consequently, glucose will appear in the urine long before the transport system is fully saturated or $\dot{T}m_G$ is reached.

2. Nephron Heterogeneity. A number of studies (Smith et al., 1943; Letteri and Wesson, 1965; Shankel et al., 1967) have shown that a considerable morphological and functional heterogeneity exists between the nephrons within the kidney. This heterogeneity is believed to be responsible for the marked difference between the glomerular and tubular functions of the active nephrons within the kidney, and has been suggested as a possible explanation for the observed splay in the glucose titration curves. Accordingly, some nephrons may have average filtration characteristics but subnormal tubular reabsorptive capacities. These nephrons will probably saturate more quickly and contribute to glucosuria at plasma glucose concentration considerably below the renal threshold level, hence before the overall $\dot{T}m$ for glucose is reached. The converse might also be true. Thus, there may be nephrons with subnormal filtration characteristics but with average tubular reabsorptive capacities. In short, this heterogeneity in the *glomerular-tubular* function of the active nephrons and their various morphological and functional

combinations could in part account for the incomplete reabsorption of glucose, and hence glucosuria, even at plasma glucose concentration considerably lower than the renal threshold for the whole kidney.

Clinically, the glucosuria seen in an otherwise healthy, young diabetic patient is due to an elevated plasma glucose concentration, since both GFR and $\dot{T}m$ for glucose are within normal limits. However, in elderly patients with long-standing diabetes, glucosuria may be absent despite the high plasma glucose concentration. This is due to a reduced GFR caused by deposition of mucopolysaccharide-protein complex in the glomerular capillary, a condition known as intercapillary glomerulosclerosis (Pitts, 1974).

A number of titration studies have shown that the renal transport of glucose exhibits a high degree of *structural specificity*. That is, glucose reabsorption is subject to competitive inhibition (see Chapter 7) when other sugars or substances of similar molecular structure are present in the filtrate. Thus, the sugar molecule having the highest affinity (low K_m) for the carrier molecule will tend to displace the sugar molecule with lower affinity (high K_m).

The most widely used substance for studying the structural specificity of glucose transport has been *phlorizin*, a phenolic glucoside. Lotspeich and Woronkow (1958) showed that intravenous infusion of small doses of phlorizin in dogs virtually blocked proximal reabsorption of glucose. This inhibition was found to be reversible when phlorizin infusion was stopped. These investigators suggested that the inhibitory effect of phlorizin on renal glucose reabsorption involves the competitive combination of phlorizin with the carrier of the glucose transport system in accordance with saturation kinetics. These results have been substantiated in the cat (Chan and Lotspeich, 1962) and in other mammalian species (Lotspeich, 1961).

On the basis of such studies, it is now accepted that the same glucose carrier system is used to transport other sugars, such as xylose, fructose, and galactose. However, glucose appears to have the highest affinity for the carrier, compared with these other sugars, so that when present it is preferentially reabsorbed. For an extensive theoretical treatment of renal glucose reabsorption, the reader is referred to excellent papers by Govaerts (1950) and Burgen (1956).

FACTORS AFFECTING $\dot{T}m$ FOR GLUCOSE. The concept of a stable $\dot{T}m$ for glucose and its independence of spontaneous or induced changes in the glomerular filtration rate, claimed by the earlier studies cited above, has been challenged by recent experiments. For example, Kruhoffer (1950) found in the rabbit a reversible reduction in the rate of glucose reabsorption despite the presence of a large glucose load when the GFR was reduced by dehydration or hemorrhage. He suggested that these changes were due to intermittency in the glomerular filtration rate in the single nephron, rather than to any change in the rate of glucose reabsorption by individual proximal convoluted tubules. More recently, Van Liew and co-workers (1967), using clearance techniques in the rat, observed a linear relationship between the rate of glucose reabsorption and the spontaneous reduction in the GFR. They suggested that this relationship may be an expression of the existence of glomerulotubular balance for glucose in a single nephron similar to that which exists for sodium or fluid reabsorption (see Chapter 8). Similar results have been obtained by Keyes and Swanson (1971) who examined $\dot{T}m_G$/GFR ratio in the dog, as an index of glomerulotubular function, during spontaneous or induced changes in GFR. From these studies, they suggested that the value of this ratio depends on (a) the number of functioning nephrons, and (b) the number of transport sites per nephron. The latter was assumed to vary directly (but not necessarily linearly) with the proximal tubular volume, a direct consequence of changes in the GFR. Accordingly, any factor that increases GFR would tend to increase the proximal tubular volume, thereby exposing more of the transport sites located on the luminal microvilli (brush border) to the tubular fluid and resulting in an increase in glucose reabsorption and hence $\dot{T}m_G$. Conversely, any factor which reduces the GFR should have the opposite effect. Thus, for a given GFR and within the physiological range, it is the combination of the number of functioning nephrons and the available transport sites that ultimately determine the maximum reabsorptive capacity of the kidney for glucose.

As was described in Chapter 8, any factor which tends to increase the GFR, such as expansion of the extracellular fluid volume (subsequent to intravenous fluid infusion, an experimental procedure used in all titration studies) will depress fluid reabsorption, while any factor which reduces GFR will enhance fluid reabsorption in the proximal tubule. Since this segment of the nephron is also the site of glucose reabsorption, it follows that any factor that alters fluid reabsorption here may secondarily induce parallel changes in glucose reabsorption. Hence, the experimentally determined $\dot{T}m$ for glucose may represent an "apparent" and not an absolute value for the tubular reabsorptive maximum, subject to body fluid homeostasis.

That alterations in sodium or fluid reabsorption in the proximal tubule, subsequent to spontaneous or induced changes in GFR, do indeed induce parallel changes in glucose reabsorption has been well documented in both rats and dogs. For example, Robson and co-workers (1968) found that the $\dot{T}m_G$/GFR ratio decreased in saline-loaded rats. This was due to an increase in GFR and a decrease in $\dot{T}m_G$ following saline diuresis. Since sodium reabsorption was also reduced subsequent to saline-loading (see also Chapter 8), they suggested that glucose reabsorption is in some manner coupled to sodium reabsorption in the proximal tubule.

In support of this concept, Kurtzman and associates (1972) found that in the dog glucose reabsorption is highly sensitive to changes in both GFR and sodium reabsorption. Furthermore, subsequent studies by these and other investigators have demonstrated that the effect of sodium reabsorption on solute reabsorption in the proximal tubule is not unique to glucose and represents a general phenomenon. Thus, alterations in sodium and water reabsorption in this nephron segment have a profound effect on reabsorption of other solutes besides glucose, such as phosphate (see discussion below) and bicarbonate (see Chapter 10).

In the case of glucose, the mechanism coupling its reabsorption to that of sodium has recently been clarified by direct micropuncture studies in the rat by Stolte and collaborators (1972). These investigators found that the net amount of glucose reabsorbed in the proximal tubule is directly influenced by the net amount of sodium and water reabsorbed by this nephron segment. Furthermore, they showed (a) that the rate of glucose reabsorption by the proximal tubule depends on both the concentration of glucose in the tubular fluid and the net rate of sodium and water reabsorption in this segment, and (b) that the glucose-sodium coupling mechanism accounted for a large fraction of the total amount of glucose reabsorbed by this nephron segment. On the basis of these findings, they suggested that the net transepithelial reabsorption of glucose involves at least two components: (1) a glucose-sodium coupling component, and (2) an active, carrier-mediated component with Tm-limited characteristics. However, as the concentration of glucose in the tubular fluid increases, the contribution of the active component to the total amount of glucose reabsorbed becomes negligible.

CELLULAR MECHANISM OF GLUCOSE TRANSPORT. The evidence presented thus far clearly suggests that the quantity of glucose normally filtered is almost completely reabsorbed in the proximal tubule by a two-component process. Although the underlying mechanisms for glucose transport by the first, or the glucose-sodium coupling component, is fairly well established (see Chapter 8), considerably less is known about the cellular mechanisms of glucose transport by the second, or the active transport component.

Our present concept of the cellular mechanism for active glucose transport across the proximal tubular cell is largely adapted from direct studies in the small intestine. In this tissue, glucose is actively reabsorbed from the lumen into the cells, where its concentration reaches a value higher than that in either the blood or the intestinal fluid (Crane, 1968). In an apparent contradiction to this concept, however, Krane and Crane (1959), using normal glucose concentration in the bathing medium, failed to show cellular accumulation of glucose by the kidney cortical slices. In contrast, in a later study, Kleinzeller and co-workers (1967), using a low concentration of D-glucose in the bathing medium, found significant cellular uptake of the sugar, with the intracellular concentration of D-glucose reaching a level higher than that in the extracellular fluid, thereby suggesting active transport of glucose at the luminal cell membrane. In a more recent study, Tune and Burg (1971), who measured glucose concentration simultaneously in the tubular fluid, cells, and the peritubular bath in isolated, perfused rabbit renal proximal tubules, have conclusively demonstrated that glucose is actively transported and that the site of the active transport is localized at the luminal cell membrane.

Although these and similar studies have contributed significantly to our understanding of the overall transepithelial transport of glucose in the kidney, they have not provided *direct* information on the cellular mechanism of the glucose transport system. Such information, however, has been obtained from recently developed techniques for isolation and biochemical characterization of the luminal cell membrane of the proximal tubule. An example is the recent comprehensive kinetic studies of the isolated luminal brush border of rabbit proximal tubule by Chesney and associates (1973). Using this preparation, these investigators have clearly demonstrated that the initial step in the glucose transport involves rapid interaction of glucose with the luminal cell membrane, a process which is both saturable and dependent upon the concentration of glucose and the membrane. Furthermore, this initial binding of glucose with the membrane is reversible and requires presence of calcium and magnesium and is inhibited competitively by phlorizin. Moreover, analysis of the relationship between the concentration of glucose and the binding of the sugar revealed the existence of two distinct receptor sites for the binding of glucose with the brush border membrane, one having a much greater binding affinity for glucose. Despite a number of differences in the kinetics characteristics of these two receptor sites, present evidence does not rule out the possibility that the two binding sites are mediated by a single membrane carrier protein whose affinity for binding is highly sensitive to the concentration of glucose.

On the basis of the various studies cited above, the following represents a tentative hypothesis for the probable steps involved in the cellular mechanisms of glucose transport across the mammalian proximal tubule cell. The first step in the transepithelial transport of glucose involves the active transport of the sugar from the tubular lumen into the proximal cell, across the brush border of the luminal cell membrane. Once inside the cell, because the intracellular concentration of glucose is higher than that in the peritubular fluid, glucose will be transported across the peritubular cell membrane down its concentration gradient by passive diffusion. However, because of the limited passive permeability of this membrane to glucose, transport across the peritubular cell membrane may also involve facilitated diffusion. Since solutes are reabsorbed iso-osmotically along the proximal tubule, the transepithelial reabsorption of glucose is accompanied by an osmotically equivalent quantity of water. In short, glucose is reabsorbed as an isotonic solution.

PHOSPHATE

Phosphate is the major constituent of the skeletal structures, which account for 80% of the total body stores of this substance. The remaining 20% occurs in the intracellular fluid and is associated with glycogen. Because of its prevalence in bone, the major function of phosphate concerns the metabolism of this tissue. However, phosphate also plays a vital role in carbohydrate metabolism and energy transformation and serves as an important blood buffer in the regulation of acid-base balance (see Chapter 10). Additionally, phosphate represents a significant constituent in a number of important compounds, such as phospholipids, phosphoproteins, nucleic acids, and nucleoproteins.

The daily requirement of phosphate is about 0.9 g for adults and somewhat higher for children (about 1.5 g) and pregnant women (about 2.5 g). The dietary phosphate is absorbed from the small intestine into the blood, where it exists in three fractions: (1) A lipid-phosphate fraction, with a concentration of about 8 mg%, (2) an ester-phosphate fraction, with a concentration of 1 mg%, and (3) a completely ionized inorganic fraction, with a concentration of 3 mg% (Hall, 1959). Since the plasma concentration of the inorganic phosphate fraction is the only one which is stabilized at 1.0 mM/L by renal reabsorption, the present discussion will be limited to this fraction.

CHARACTERISTICS OF PHOSPHATE TITRATION CURVES. Classic studies of Pitts and Alexander (1944) in normal and acidotic dogs and those of Lambert and associates (1947) and Anderson (1955) in man represent the earliest attempt to characterize the renal transport of phosphate by the application of titration techniques. Their findings, confirmed by subsequent studies in rat (Frick, 1968), dog (Agus et al., 1971), monkey (Vander and Cafruny, 1962), and man (Bijvoet, 1969) have generally established that the renal handling of phosphate is similar in many respects to that of glucose, but with two notable exceptions:

1. Since the $\dot{T}m$ for glucose reabsorption is set at such a high value (about 375 mg/min in man), it is normally never exceeded, indicating that the kidneys do not regulate the plasma concentration of glucose. In contrast, the $\dot{T}m$ for phosphate reabsorption is set at such a low value (0.1 mM/min in man) that a slight change in its plasma concentration produces marked changes in urinary excretion of phosphate. This implies that the kidneys do regulate the plasma concentration of phosphate.

2. As discussed earlier, the $\dot{T}m$ for glucose is relatively stable and is not influenced by ionic composition or hormone levels of the plasma. The $\dot{T}m$ for phosphate, however, is variable and is markedly influenced by the ionic composition of plasma and the circulating levels of parathyroid and adrenocortical hormones.

Figure 9-4 presents the renal titration curves for phosphate in the dog, which graphically illustrates the salient features of the renal transport of phosphate observed in this and other mammalian species, including man. As can be seen from this figure, the value of $\dot{T}m$ for phosphate in these studies averaged about 0.1 mM/min and was attained at a filtered load of about 0.125 mM/min. Furthermore, when GFR was altered by adjustment of dietary protein intake, a factor known to markedly influence GFR in dogs, $\dot{T}m$ was not affected.

Like glucose, the reabsorption of phosphate is virtually complete at normal plasma concentration. But, as the plasma concentration exceeds the renal threshold, the reabsorptive mechanism becomes saturated, resulting in urinary excretion of phosphate (phosphaturia).

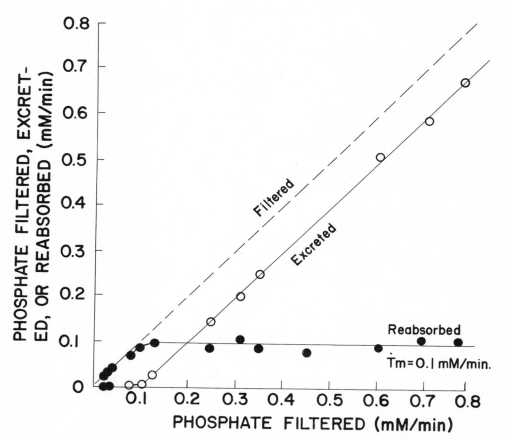

Figure 9-4. Renal reabsorption and excretion of phosphate as functions of the filtered load in the normal dog. [Redrawn from Pitts, R. F., and Alexander, R. S. (1944).]

Analogous to glucose, these findings suggest that the filtered phosphate is reabsorbed by an active, carrier-mediated process with Tm-limited characteristics. Likewise, the observed splay in the titration curves has been attributed to the kinetics of phosphate transport and the morphological and functional heterogeneity of the nephron population within the kidney, which have already been described.

A number of recent micropuncture studies in rats (Frick, 1968; Strickler et al., 1965), dogs (Agus et al., 1971), and monkeys (Vander and Cafruny, 1962) have established that, like glucose, the bulk of filtered phosphate is reabsorbed in the proximal tubule. However, in the rat, it has been shown that the loops of Henle and the distal and collecting tubules also have a limited capacity to reabsorb phosphate (Murayama et al., 1972). Furthermore, recollection micropuncture and whole kidney clearance studies by Puschett and associates (1972) have shown that the proximal reabsorption of phosphate, like glucose, is somehow coupled to that of sodium under a variety of experimental conditions, including the expansion of extracellular fluid volume, isotonic saline diuresis and aortic constriction.

FACTORS AFFECTING Ṫm FOR PHOSPHATE. A number of studies designed to elucidate the cellular mechanism of renal reabsorption of phosphate have revealed that several factors alter the Ṫm for phosphate and hence its renal transport. These findings are summarized in Figure 9-5.

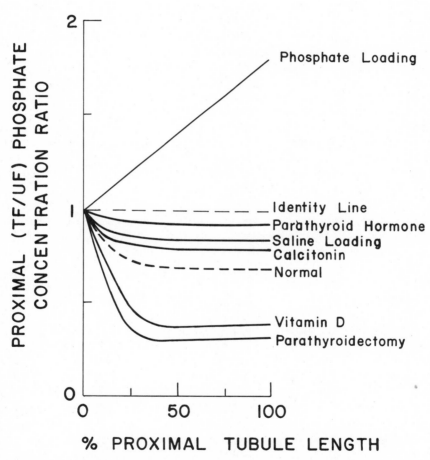

Figure 9-5. The proximal tubular fluid-to-ultrafiltrate (TF/UF) phosphate concentration ratios as functions of per cent of proximal tubule length under a variety of experimental conditions. The light dashed line is the identity line to which all the other lines should be compared. [Redrawn from Knox, F. G., Schneider, E. G., Willis, L. R., Strandhoy, J. W., and Ott, C. E. (1973).]

Pitts and Alexander (1944) showed that in the dog infusion of glucose sufficient to saturate the transport mechanism reduced the $\dot{T}m$, while infusion of phlorizin increased the $\dot{T}m$ for phosphate. From these observations they suggested that the cellular reabsorption of phosphate and glucose probably share a common mechanism.

By far the most important factors affecting renal reabsorption of phosphate are the circulating levels of the parathyroid and adrenocortical hormones. Prolonged administration of parathyroid hormone (PTH) markedly reduced $\dot{T}m$ for phosphate (Bijvoet, 1969), thereby depressing tubular reabsorption and increasing urinary excretion of phosphate. Micropuncture studies in the dog (Agus et al., 1971) have subsequently shown that the induced phosphaturia is due to the PTH-inhibition of phosphate reabsorption in both the proximal and distal tubules. Thus, administration of PTH increased the tubular fluid to ultrafiltrate (TF/UF) phosphate concentration ratio toward unity, while parathyroidectomy decreased this ratio considerably below unity compared to normal (Fig. 9-5).

A number of studies reviewed by Talmadge and Belanger (1968) have provided convincing evidence that the renal action of PTH is mediated by cyclic AMP. The probable mechanism of such an action was outlined briefly in Chapter 7. Accordingly, PTH present in the blood stimulates the adenylate cyclase located on the outer surface of the peritubular membrane, thereby increasing the intracellular production of cyclic AMP. The latter, by an as yet unknown mechanism, alters the permeability of the luminal cell membrane to phosphate, thereby decreasing its cellular uptake and reabsorption.

Like PTH, administration of excessive amount of adrenocortical hormone cortisone reduces the $\dot{T}m$ for phosphate, thereby promoting phosphaturia. This effect may represent the underlying mechanism for phosphaturia observed in patients with osteomalacia of hyperadrenocorticism (Pitts, 1974).

Since the discovery of thyrocalcitonin (TCT), the hypocalcemic-hypophosphatemic principle of the thyroid gland by Hirsch and co-workers (1964), its possible role in the renal transport of calcium and phosphate has been extensively studied. It has been found that TCT, besides stimulating the uptake of calcium and phosphate by the bone, thereby lowering the concentration of these ions in the blood, also stimulates urinary excretion of phosphate (increasing TF/UF ratio) in both normal and parathyroidectomized subjects (Singer et al., 1969). Since TCT causes hypocalcemia by the mechanism just mentioned, and because plasma concentration of calcium indirectly influences plasma phosphate concentration (normally concentrations of calcium and phosphate in the blood are reciprocally related), it has been suggested that the renal action of TCT may be a secondary phenomenon.

Another factor that influences renal reabsorption of phosphate is Vitamin D. Although its effect on urinary excretion of phosphate may reflect induces changes in the intestinal absorption of calcium and phosphate, parathyroid hormone, and bone metabolism, Vitamin D has been shown to have a direct stimulating effect on renal tubular reabsorption of phosphate. This effect is qualitatively similar to that of parathyroidectomy, that is, Vitamin D increases renal reabsorption of phosphate, as evidenced by a marked decrease in the proximal TF/UF phosphate concentration ratio shown in Figure 9-5 (Knox et al., 1973). It should be pointed out, however, that Vitamin D has a dual action: it stimulates the renal reabsorption of phosphate, while it simultaneously increases the plasma concentration of calcium. The latter effect, in turn, decreases the blood level of PTH, which in turn increases renal reabsorption of phosphate.

Both calcium and phosphate loading have been found to have a direct effect on renal tubular reabsorption of phosphate. Whereas hypercalcemia stimulates phosphate reabsorption, hyperphosphatemia depresses phosphate reabsorption. Indeed, consistent with the view that phosphate reabsorption is by an active, carrier-mediated process, the progressive increase in plasma phosphate concentration tends to saturate the transport mechanism and leads to phosphaturia. This has been confirmed by micropuncture studies by Strickler and associates (1965) who found a linear increase in the proximal TF/UF concentration ratio with hyperphosphatemia (Fig. 9-5).

Like glucose, tubular reabsorption of phosphate has been shown to be closely coupled to the reabsorption of sodium and water in the proximal tubule. Thus, any factor, such as saline loading, which depresses sodium reabsorption in this nephron segment will decrease phosphate reabsorption, as evidenced by an increase in TF/UF concentration ratio. The mechanisms underlying the phosphate-sodium coupling transport are presumably similar to those mentioned earlier for glucose. They are probably related to the factors that maintain glomerulotubular balance for sodium, which were described in Chapter 8.

Finally, studies in man have demonstrated a definite circadian rhythm for the urinary excretion of phosphate (Stanbury, 1958). Phosphate excretion was found to be minimal during the morning, becoming maximal during the afternoon and evening. No such study has been done in the dog or in any other mammalian species. In man, changes in the urinary excretion rate of phosphate were found to parallel those in plasma concentration. Furthermore, these changes followed parallel changes in the blood level of the parathyroid hormone. It has also been suggested that the normal variability of the $\dot{T}m$ for phosphate may be due to daily fluctuations in the rate of secretion of the parathyroid hormone (Aurbach and Potts, 1967). Despite these evidences, the exact nature of this circadian rhythm remains obscure.

SULFATE

Plasma concentration of inorganic sulfate is maintained within normal limits of 1.0 to 1.5 mM/L by a balance between the rate of its production from sulfur-containing amino acids and the rate of its excretion by the kidney. Renal titration studies in most mammalian species, including man (Mudge et al., 1973), similar to that depicted in Figure 9-6, have shown that the urinary excretion of sulfate is

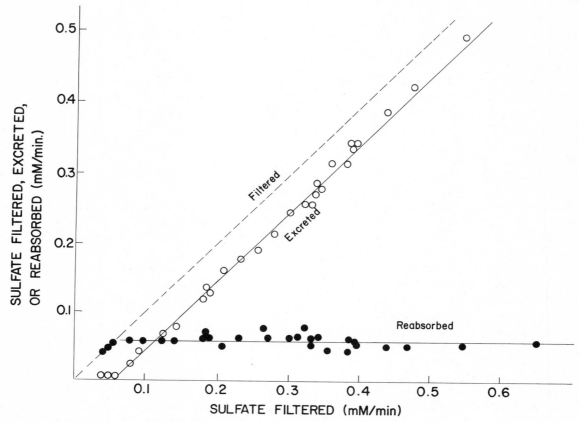

Figure 9-6. Renal reabsorption and excretion of sulfate as functions of the filtered load in the normal dog. [Redrawn from Lotspeich, W. D. (1947).]

normally far less than the filtered load, suggesting that the dominant mode of renal tubular transport of sulfate is by reabsorption.

These same studies have further shown that sulfate is reabsorbed by a $\dot{T}m$-limited process, exhibiting very little splay. Furthermore, they suggest that sulfate is absorbed by a mechanism similar to that of phosphate; that is, sulfate is reabsorbed by an active, carrier-mediated process.

Administration of glucose, phosphate, and amino acids, all of which are reabsorbed in the proximal tubule, has been found to inhibit sulfate reabsorption in this nephron segment. This finding suggests that the sulfate must also be reabsorbed in the proximal tubule, a conclusion which has been confirmed by stop-flow studies in the dog (Hierholzer et al., 1960).

The $\dot{T}m$ for sulfate, as measured by titration studies, was found to be of the same order of magnitude as that for phosphate. Like glucose, $\dot{T}m$ for sulfate was found to be sensitive to changes in GFR

(Berglund and Lotspeich, 1956). Furthermore, $\dot{T}m$ for sulfate could be depressed by infusion of glucose, sufficient to saturate the transport mechanism, and by infusion of hypertonic saline. As described in Chapter 8, the latter effect is due to the presence of an excessive amount of chloride, a readily reabsorbed anion, compared to the poorly reabsorbed sulfate anion. These studies suggest that sulfate is probably reabsorbed by the same cellular transport processes and carrier system that transports glucose and phosphate.

AMINO ACIDS

Plasma concentration of amino acids is maintained within normal limits of 2.5 to 3.5 mM/L by dynamic balance between the rate of dietary intake and its metabolic conversion as well as the rate of renal reabsorption of the quantity normally filtered. In addition, the kidneys participate in the transamination process (conversion of one amino acid to another) as well as the formation and excretion of ammonia to conserve major body electrolytes, such as sodium and potassium. This latter process constitutes an important mechanism in the renal regulation of acid-base balance and will be discussed in Chapter 10.

CHARACTERISTICS OF AMINO ACID TITRATION CURVES. As early as 1943, Pitts demonstrated that in the dog amino acids are reabsorbed by a $\dot{T}m$-limited process. In a subsequent study, when the effects of a number of amino acids on creatine (a compound structurally similar to glycine) reabsorption were compared, Pitts (1944) observed a competition for transport between structurally similar compounds. From these studies, Pitts concluded that there must be a single transport mechanism for the renal reabsorption of all amino acids. However, more recent evidence has clearly shown that there are at least three or more independent transport systems for the renal reabsorption of amino acids. For example, studies by Beyer and co-workers (1946, 1947) and Wright and associates (1947) have shown that some amino acids (e.g., lysine and arginine) are reabsorbed by a $\dot{T}m$-limited process, while others (e.g., histidine and methionine) are reabsorbed without exhibiting Tm-limited characteristics. Recent studies by Webber (1962, 1963) have confirmed earlier findings and have further demonstrated the existence of separate but sometimes overlapping pathways for the renal transport of neutral, basic, and acidic amino acids. Furthermore, stop-flow studies (Brown et al., 1961) have shown that most amino acids are reabsorbed in the proximal tubule. Also, reabsorption is active, since it occurs against a concentration gradient, as evidenced by a TF/P amino acid concentration ratio significantly below 1.0 in the proximal tubule.

Figures 9-7 and 9-8 illustrate the renal titration curves in the dog for two representative amino acids (glycine and lysine). These titration curves demonstrate many of the transport characteristics

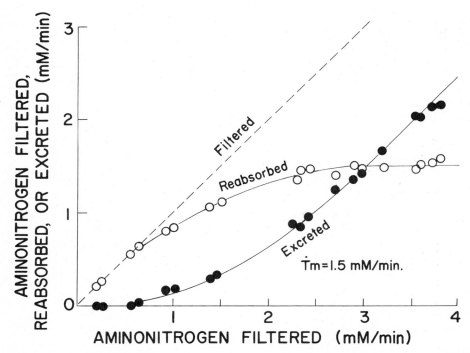

Figure 9-7. Reabsorption and excretion of aminonitrogen as functions of the filtered load in dogs in which glycine was infused to increase plasma concentration of aminonitrogen. [Redrawn from Pitts, R. F. (1943).]

common to most of the amino acids which have been studied. Note that the titration curves for glycine exhibit considerable splay, while that for lysine shows no splay. Also, the measured Tm for glycine is some 15-fold greater than that for lysine.

A number of studies have explored the possibility that factors other than the already mentioned glomerular-tubular balance may be responsible for the observed variations in the splay of the titration curves. A review of the available evidence (Young and Freedman, 1971) supports the concept that the *shape* of the titration curve is largely determined by the equilibrium constant of the transporting system. Thus, as the equilibration constant, K (Equation 9-3) approaches infinity (i.e., the Michaelis-Menten constant K_m approaches zero), the splay in the titration curve approaches zero. The low K_m value for glucose transport determined by micropuncture techniques and the high K_m value for amino acid transport obtained from studies of kidney cortex slices provide further corroborative evidence for this concept.

Several studies reviewed by Young and Freedman (1971) have clearly demonstrated that the renal transport of amino acids is influenced by

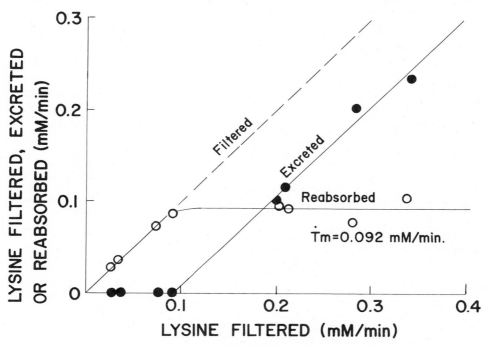

Figure 9-8. Reabsorption and excretion of lysine as functions of filtered load in the dog. [Redrawn from Wright, L. D., Russo, H. F., Skeggs, H. R., Patch, E. A., and Beyer, K. H. (1947).]

the presence of a number of substances, such as sodium and glucose, in the glomerular filtrate. For example, it has been shown that the uptake of amino acids by kidney cortex slices is diminished in a low-Na medium, and that the inhibition is complete in a Na-free medium. More direct evidence for the underlying mechanism has come from the study of the effect of sodium on amino acid transport in isolated proximal tubules and brush-border preparations. According to these studies, reabsorption of amino acids in the proximal tubule involves at least two sequential steps--namely, binding to the brush-border membrane and subsequent active transport into the cell. The binding step is found to be less sodium-dependent than the active transport step.

The influence of glucose on amino acid transport is best exemplified by Fanconi syndrome, a disease characterized by glucosuria associated with aminoaciduria. The underlying defect is believed to be due to a disruption of some common step in the reabsorptive pathway for glucose and amino acid. A number of clearance studies lend credence to the validity of this hypothesis. Thus, it has been found that intravenous infusion of glucose reduces renal reabsorption of amino acid. Similar inhibition is obtained by infusion of phlorizin, a competitive inhibitor of glucose transport, as well as some amino acids, such as lysine, glycine, and alanine. These findings are consistent with the above concept and further suggest that the competitive interaction between glucose and amino acid transport may be mediated via a Na-dependent ATPase system that provides energy for transport.

In summary, the available evidence indicates that amino acids are reabsorbed by an active, Na-dependent, carrier-mediated transport process in the proximal tubule similar to that described for glucose. But unlike the latter, there appear to be at least four separate transport systems for the reabsorption of the filtered amino acids: One mechanism transports the *neutral amino acids*, namely, alanine, valine, leucine, isoleucine, methionine, cysteine, serine, threonine, histidine, tyrosine, phenylalanine, and tryptophan. Another mechanism transports the *basic amino acids*, namely, cysteine, lysine, arginine, and ornithine. The third mechanism transports the *acidic amino acids*, namely, glutamic and aspartic acids. The fourth mechanism transports the *iminoglycine amino acids*, namely, glycine, proline, and hydroxyproline. Moreover, each transport mechanism is capable of reabsorbing more than one amino acid, but is influenced by competitive inhibition due to both structural and stereoisomeric configurations. Finally, because Tm for most amino acids studied is set very high, all the amino acids normally filtered are reabsorbed and none is excreted. Thus, like glucose, it appears that the kidney does not regulate the plasma concentration of amino acids.

ORGANIC ANIONS

The kidneys normally excrete a number of organic anions. The magnitude of their urinary excretion rate is markedly influenced by disturbances in body acid-base balance (Cooke et al., 1954; Grollman et al., 1961), being increased in *alkalosis* and decreased in *acidosis* (see Chapter 10 for definition of these terms). Cooke and associates (1954) have suggested that the organic aciduria represents a mechanism to regulate plasma chloride concentration in conditions of acid-base imbalance. Thus, in alkalosis the filtered chloride is reabsorbed while sodium is excreted in combination with organic anions. In contrast, in acidosis the filtered sodium is excreted in combination with chloride, instead of organic anions.

We shall now briefly describe the renal handling of some of the important organic anions found in the urine.

1. CITRATE. Citrate is the initial substrate of the tricarboxylic acid (TCA) cycle. It is both the source of energy for the kidney and the most abundant organic acid in the urine. Its urinary excretion helps to solubilize calcium, thereby reducing the possibility of calcium phosphate stone formation.

Because high concentration of citrate is toxic to the heart, conventional titration analysis of renal handling of citrate has not been made. However, within the limits of citrate concentration tolerated by the body, animal studies have shown that citrate titration curves exhibit considerable splay, suggesting that a $\dot{T}m$ for citrate reabsorption may actually exist. This conclusion is in part confirmed by studies of Grollman and co-workers (1961), who found that infusion of some intermediate components of the TCA cycle, such as oxaloacetate, succinate, fumarate, and malate block tubular reabsorption of citrate. In these studies, the citrate clearance became equal to GFR and never exceeded it, thus suggesting that these intermediate components of the TCA cycle competitively inhibit citrate reabsorption by the renal tubules.

2. α-KETOGLUTARATE. This substance is an important component of the TCA cycle and hence of the energy supply system of all the cells, including those of the renal tubules. Its plasma concentration is normally quite low, about 0.1 micromoles/ml, despite the fact that all the filtered α-ketoglutarate is reabsorbed. Its tubular reabsorption is active, since the cellular uptake from the tubular fluid occurs against the concentration gradient. Furthermore, tubular transport is $\dot{T}m$-limited, with the reabsorptive mechanism being saturated at a plasma concentration more than 20 times normal. The reabsorptive process exhibits relatively little splay. Because the renal threshold of α-ketoglutarate is considerably higher than its plasma concentration, the kidneys do not regulate the plasma concentration of this substance. The reabsorptive mechanism, therefore, serves to prevent the urinary loss of this important intermediary metabolite.

Besides being transported by the tubules, α-ketoglutarate is used by the renal tubule cells as a source of metabolic energy. It has been estimated that the kidneys use about 60% of the intravenously administered α-ketoglutarate, the remaining amount being used by the liver. This suggests that α-ketoglutarate is transported across both the luminal and peritubular renal cell membranes against the electrochemical gradient by a $\dot{T}m$-limited process (Sulamita and Pitts, 1964). Furthermore, these investigators observed that the $\dot{T}m$ for α-ketoglutarate is increased in acute respiratory and metabolic acidosis and is decreased in acute respiratory and metabolic alkalosis. These changes in the $\dot{T}m$ and the resulting effects on the tubular reabsorption of α-ketoglutarate were attributed to the induced changes in the intracellular pH of the renal tubule cells (see Chapter 10 for further discussion).

3. ACETOACETATE. Normally, all the filtered acetoacetate is reabsorbed actively by a $\dot{T}m$-limited process. However, in starvation and in uncontrolled diabetes mellitus, the urinary excretion rate rises in proportion to the increased plasma concentration.

4. β-HYDROXYBUTYRATE. This substance is also reabsorbed by an active, $\dot{T}m$-limited process. Its titration curves exhibit marked splay, with the renal threshold concentration being about 20 mg% in man.

5. LACTATE. Lactate is normally completely reabsorbed. Whether it is reabsorbed by a $\dot{T}m$-limited process is presently unresolved. However, in man when lactate plasma concentration exceeds the renal threshold concentration of about 60 mg%, its urinary excretion rate varies in proportion to increasing plasma concentration, suggesting a $\dot{T}m$-limited reabsorptive process (Pitts, 1974).

URIC ACID

In man the bulk of the excreted urinary nitrogen is in the form of urea and ammonia, with excretion of uric acid accounting for only 5% of the total. Despite this, there is a great deal of interest in the mechanism of renal transport of uric acid, the principal reason being the observed elevation of plasma uric acid concentration (hyperuricemia) in patients with gout. This is a metabolic disease characterized by painful inflammation of the joints accompanied by sodium urate deposition. The hyperuricemia is generally attributed to either an increase in the rate of uric acid synthesis, or a decrease in the rate of its renal excretion, or possibly a combination of the two (Wyngaarden, 1960).

Normally, the plasma concentration of uric acid is maintained between 4 to 6 mg% by a balance of three processes: (a) the rate of synthesis, (b) the rate of glomerular filtration, and (c) the rate of tubular transport (Gutman and Yü, 1961). A number of studies in most mammalian species, including man, have shown that the tubular transport of uric acid is bidirectional in the proximal tubule, with reabsorption and secretion occurring within the same tubular cell (Holmes et al., 1972). In the dog, however, stop-flow studies have shown that uric acid is only reabsorbed in the proximal tubule, but is both reabsorbed and secreted in the distal tubule.

Titration studies by Berliner and associates (1950) have shown that uric acid is reabsorbed actively by a $\dot{T}m$-limited process, with a maximum transport rate of about 15 mg/min per 1.73 m^2 body surface area in man. However, the maximum transport capacity normally is not exceeded, but can be saturated at plasma uric acid concentrations exceeding 15 to 20 mg%. Uric acid titration curves exhibit considerable splay, suggesting that the extent of splay, rather than the magnitude of $\dot{T}m$, may govern the urinary excretion rate of uric acid. Normally, more than 90% of the filtered uric acid is reabsorbed in the proximal tubule. Hence, tubular secretion must largely account for the bulk of uric acid excreted in the urine. In addition, because uric acid is lipid-insoluble, nonionic passive diffusion (see Chapter 10) plays no role in its tubular transport and, therefore, its urinary excretion. Consequently, changes in urinary pH which may occur in acid-base disturbances have no effect on its urinary excretion (Mudge et al., 1973).

Clinically, the hyperuricemia of gout may result from abnormal functioning of any one or a combination of those factors responsible for maintaining the plasma uric acid concentration at normal level. Thus, hyperuricemia may result from (a) an increase in the rate of synthesis of uric acid, (b) a reduction in the rate of glomerular filtration, and (c) an increase in the tubular reabsorption or a decrease in the tubular secretion. In man, the *pyrazinamide (PZA)* suppression test has been used extensively to localize the primary lesion causing hyperuricemia and to assess the relative effect of tubular secretion (Gutman et al., 1969). The premise for using this test has been that PZA (an antituberculosis drug) selectively blocks the tubular secretion of uric acid. Therefore, the quantity of uric acid excreted in the urine after PZA test must represent the quantity that escaped tubular reabsorption. Furthermore, the difference between the quantity of uric acid excreted before and after the PZA test represents the amount of uric acid that is secreted by the tubules. However, in a recent review of laboratory and clinical experiences with PZA, Holmes and associates (1972) have concluded that the inhibitory effect of this substance on tubular secretion is not as selective and complete as has been assumed. Therefore, further clinical use of PZA suppression test must be reevaluated.

PROTEINS

As mentioned in Chapter 5, the ultrafiltrate is virtually protein-free. However, stop-flow studies in dogs (Lathem et al., 1960) have shown that albumin, hemoglobin and other small molecular weight proteins are filtered at the glomerulus and are subsequently reabsorbed in the proximal tubule. Recent studies by Cortney and associates (1970), in which labelled proteins were injected into the rat proximal and distal tubules, have further revealed that the injected proteins are largely reabsorbed in the proximal tubule, but a smaller quantity is also reabsorbed in the distal tubule.

In man, about 0.5% of the total plasma albumin is filtered, yielding a filtrate albumin concentration of less than 30 mg%, compared to 4.0 g% in the plasma. Normally, virtually all the filtered albumin is reabsorbed in the proximal tubule by an active, T_m-limited process. In man, the T_m for albumin is estimated to be about 30 mg%, with the reabsorptive mechanism being saturated at a plasma concentration of about 6 to 7 g% (Pitts, 1974).

We conclude this section with Table 9-1, which summarizes the salient characteristics of the renal handling of the several important constituents of the filtrate which have already been discussed.

TABLE 9-1

Summary of Renal Transport of Some Important Constituents of the Filtrate

Substance	Mean Clearance in Physiological Conditions	Permeability Ratio	Tubular Reabsorption	Tubular Secretion
1. Magnesium	6 ml/min	50%	Proximal tubule; active.	Possible.
2. Calcium	1-3 ml/min	65%	Proximal tubule; active.	No.
3. Phosphate	3-10 ml/min	100%	Proximal tubule; active, Tm-limited; dependent on calcium.	Theoretically possible but never demonstrated.
4. Chloride	0.2-2 ml/min	100%	Proximal tubule; passive, follows sodium reabsorption; active in the ascending thick segment of the loop of Henle.	Unknown.
5. Sulfate	10 ml/min	50-100%	Both proximal and distal tubules; active with Tm being about the same as that for phosphate.	Unknown.
6. Amino Acids	Varies with nature of amino acid; but less than 5 ml/min.	Not known, probably 100%	Proximal tubule; Tm-limited.	Unknown.
7. Endogenous Creatinine	Grossly equal to glomerular clearance.	100%	Apparently none.	None or slight (dog).
8. Exogenous Creatinine	130% of glomerular clearance.	100%	Apparently none.	Certain (man).
9. Uric Acid	7-10 ml/min	Probably 100%	Both proximal and distal tubules; active, Tm-limited.	Occurs in distal tubule.

TABLE 9-1 (Cont.)

	Factors Increasing Clearance	Factors Decreasing Clearance	Organs Involved in Elimination from Body
1.	Increased blood magnesium; aldosterone.	Low blood magnesium.	Renal excretion 1/3; intestinal excretion 2/3.
2.	Blood calcium; Vitamin D; parathyroid hormone; presence of anions forming nonionizable salts of calcium, citrate, sulfate, etc.	Lowered blood calcium; thiazide diuretics.	Renal excretion 1/4; intestinal excretion 3/4.
3.	Diurnal variation, between noon and 8 PM; parathyroid hormone; acidosis; hypercalcemia.	Diurnal variation from midnight to midday; alkalosis; hypocalcemia; anterior pituitary growth hormone.	Renal excretion is predominant but not exclusive.
4.	Same as for sodium clearance; competition with bicarbonate; mercurial diuretics; saline diuretics.	Same as for sodium clearance; competition with bicarbonate; carbonic anhydrase inhibitors.	Renal excretion is almost exclusive in the absence of vomiting.
5.	Unknown.	Unknown.	Almost exclusively by kidney.
6.	Tubular competition between groups of amino acids.	Unknown.	Minimal physiological amino aciduria.
7.	Anything that increases glomerular filtration.	Anything that lowers glomerular filtration.	Exclusively by kidney.
8.	Anything that increases glomerular filtration.	Anything that lowers glomerular filtration.	Exclusively by kidney.
9.	Tubular inhibitors (e.g., probenecid) in high dose.	Tubular inhibitors (probenecid in low dose); and, above all, thiazide diuretics in normal therapeutic dose.	Exclusively by kidney; diminished in hyperuricemia.

TUBULAR SECRETION

With the exception of potassium (see Chapter 8) and hydrogen ions and ammonia (see Chapter 10), most of the substances which are normally secreted by the renal tubules are either weak acids or bases. These substances fall into one or more of the following classes: (1) They are not normal constituents of the plasma, such as drugs (e.g., penicillin and salicylate, a metabolic product of aspirin); (2) they are not metabolized by the body and are secreted virtually unchanged into the urine (e.g., p-aminohippurate, phenol red, and Diodrast-iodine, a radiopaque contrast material); and (3) they are slowly but incompletely metabolized (e.g., thiamine or Vitamin B_1).

Because p-aminohippurate has been widely used to measure the renal plasma flow (see Chapter 6) and is secreted by an active, $\dot{T}m$-limited process, its renal transport will be the only one described here. Its tubular transport, however, should serve as the prototype for the renal handling of the other substances secreted by the tubules.

P-AMINOPHIPPURATE

As mentioned in Chapter 6, p-aminohippurate (PAH), which is a weak organic acid, is secreted into the proximal tubule by a $\dot{T}m$-limited process. Its tubular transport exemplifies the renal handling of other similar substances, such as phenol red and Diodrast-iodine.

Although PAH is mostly secreted by the proximal tubule (Baines et al., 1968), some recent studies (Cho and Cafruny, 1970) have demonstrated that a smaller quantity of PAH is reabsorbed in this segment. Thus, there appears to be a *bidirectional* transport mechanism for PAH in the kidney. Although this small bidirectional transport of PAH does not appreciably influence the clearance of PAH, it certainly has a profound effect on the magnitude of $\dot{T}m$ for this substance.

Proximal secretion of PAH occurs by an active, carrier-mediated mechanism. The first step in its renal secretion consists of an uphill entry of PAH into the proximal cell across the peritubular membrane. The subsequent intracellular accumulation of PAH is believed to provide the driving force for its passive secretion across the luminal membrane and into the proximal lumen (Tune et al., 1969). Thus, the transepithelial transport of PAH appears to be active and occurring against a concentration gradient, since as mentioned in Chapter 8, there is no significant electrical potential gradient across the proximal cell membrane.

Figure 9-9 presents the renal titration curves for PAH in man. Note that like reabsorption of glucose, secretion of PAH and like substances involves active transport, characterized by a $\dot{T}m$-limited process. There is, however, considerable splay in the titration curves for the same reasons as those given for glucose reabsorption. In man, $\dot{T}m$ values for PAH, Diodrast-iodine, and phenol red average 80, 57, and 36 mg/min per 1.73 m^2 body surface area, respectively (Pitts, 1974).

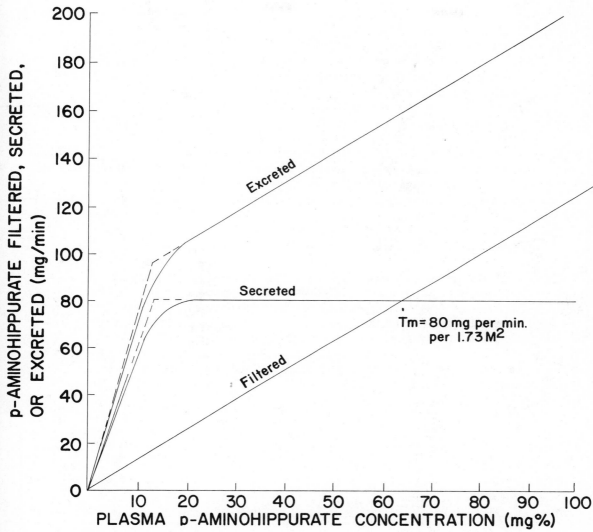

Figure 9-9. Secretion and excretion of p-aminohippurate as functions of plasma concentration in man. [Redrawn from Pitts, R. F. (1974).]

Intravenous infusion of PAH or Diodrast-iodine decreases tubular secretion of phenol red, suggesting that these substances are secreted by a common carrier system. However, it appears that PAH and Diodrast-iodine have greater affinity for the carrier, compared to phenol red, with competition for the carrier and eventual tubular secretion obeying the same kinetic laws that were outlined in Chapter 7.

PROBLEMS

9-1. Calculate the quantity of glucose filtered and the quantity
reabsorbed by the tubules under the following conditions:
  Plasma glucose concentration = 500 mg%
  Urinary excretion rate = 275 mg/min
  Inulin clearance = 130 ml/min
  Permeability ratio = 1.0

9-2. Calculate the quantity of Diodrast expressed as iodine, which
is filtered, and the quantity secreted by the tubules under the
following conditions:
  Plasma Diodrast-iodine concentration = 6 mg%
  Urinary excretion rate = 42 mg/min
  Inulin clearance = 130 ml/min
  Permeability ratio = 0.73

9-3. Complete Table 1 below by calculating the following:
  Quantity of glucose filtered, mg/min
  Quantity of glucose reabsorbed, mg/min
  Total quantity of glucose brought to the kidney, mg/min
  Plasma clearance of glucose, ml/min
  Extraction ratio for glucose
  (Assume GFR = 130 ml/min; RPF = 700 ml/min; and glucose
  permeability ratio = 1.0.)

Table 1

Plasma Glucose (mg%)	Urinary Excretion Rate (mg/min)	Glucose Filtered (mg/min)	Glucose Reabsorbed (mg/min)	Total Glucose Brought to Kidney (mg/min)	Plasma Glucose Clearance (ml/min)	Glucose Extraction Ratio
a. 50	0					
b. 100	0					
c. 288	0					
d. 500	275					
e. 700	535					
f. 1000	925					

9-4. Construct a graph with plasma glucose concentrations in mg% as
abscissa (0 to 1000 mg%) and the quantity of glucose filtered in
mg/min as ordinate (0 to 1500 mg/min). Plot the data from
Table 1.

9-5.   On the same graph plot the following data from Table 1 against
       plasma glucose concentration:
       a.   Glucose excreted, mg/min
       b.   Glucose reabsorbed, mg/min
       c.   Total glucose brought to kidney, mg/min

9-6.   At what plasma concentration does glucose first appear in the
       urine? _____

9-7.   What is the value of $\dot{T}m$ for glucose? _____

9-8.   Fill in the following table by reading the appropriate values
       from your graph:

                                        Plasma Glucose
                                   Concentration (mg%)
                              200   400   600   900

       a.   Glucose filtered, mg/min
       b.   Glucose reabsorbed, mg/min
       c.   Glucose excreted, mg/min
       d.   % of filtered glucose excreted
            (Note: calculated by dividing glucose excreted by
            glucose filtered and multiplying by 100.)

9-9.   How does the % of the filtered glucose which is excreted vary
       as the plasma glucose level increases? _____

9-10. If 100% of the filtered glucose were excreted, what would be
       the value for:
       a.   Glucose clearance? _____
       b.   Glucose extraction ratio? _____

9-11. Complete Table 2 given below by making the appropriate
       calculations. (Assume GFR = 130 ml/min; RPF = 700 ml/min;
       and PAH permeability ratio = 0.83.)

Table 2

Plasma PAH (mg%)	Urinary Excretion Rate (mg/min)	PAH Filtered (mg/min)	PAH Secreted by Tubules (mg/min)	Total PAH Brought to Kidney (mg/min)	Plasma PAH Clearance (ml/min)	PAH Extraction Ratio
a. 2	14					
b. 6	42					
c. 13	91					
d. 20	99.5					
e. 40	120.5					
f. 60	142.5					

9-12. Construct a graph similar to that for glucose and plot the
following ordinates against the plasma PAH concentration as
abscissa (ordinate range, 0 to 200 mg/min; abscissa range,
0 to 100 mg%):
a. PAH filtered, mg/min
b. PAH secreted by tubules, mg/min
c. PAH excreted in urine, mg/min
d. Total PAH brought to kidney, mg/min

9-13. At what plasma level does tubular secretion level off?

_____

9-14. What is the value of $\dot{T}m$ for PAH? _____

9-15. From your graph, fill in the following table:

	Plasma PAH Concentration (mg%)					
	4	8	15	30	50	70
a. PAH filtered, mg/min						
b. PAH secreted by tubules, mg/min						
c. PAH excreted in urine, mg/min						
d. $\dfrac{\text{PAH filtered}}{\text{PAH secreted by tubules}}$						

9-16. How does the ratio of filtered PAH to secreted PAH vary as the
plasma PAH level increases? _____

9-17. If the quantity of PAH secreted by the tubules became
insignificantly small compared to the quantity filtered,
what would be the value for:
a. PAH clearance? _____
b. PAH extraction ratio? _____

9-18. Construct a graph as follows:
a. As the left hand ordinate scale: Plasma clearance in
ml/min. Range 0 to 700 ml/min. Scale: 25 mm = 100 ml/min.
b. As the right hand ordinate scale: Extraction ratio.
Range 0 to 1.0. Scale: 25 mm = 0.14.
c. As the abscissae: Three separate scales, arranged one
below the other, representing plasma concentrations in mg%
as follows:
(1) Upper scale: Plasma Inulin Concentration.
Range: 0 to 500 mg%. Scale: 25 mm = 50 mg%.
(2) Middle scale: Plasma Glucose Concentration.
Range: 0 to 1000 mg%. Scale: 25 mm = 100 mg%.
(3) Lower scale: Plasma PAH Concentration.
Range: 0 to 100 mg%. Scale: 25 mm = 10 mg%.

9-19. On your graph plot the following clearances against the corresponding plasma concentrations:
a. Inulin clearance from Table 3, page 113.
b. Glucose clearance from Table 1, above.
c. PAH clearance from Table 2, above.

9-20. At an infinitely high plasma glucose level, which of the following would be true? (Check correct answer.)
a. Glucose clearance = glomerular filtration rate _____
b. Glucose clearance > glomerular filtration rate _____
c. Glucose clearance < glomerular filtration rate _____

9-21. At an infinitely high plasma PAH level, which of the following would hold? (Check correct answer.)
a. PAH clearance = glomerular filtration rate _____
b. PAH clearance > glomerular filtration rate _____
c. PAH clearance < glomerular filtration rate _____

9-22. Above what plasma PAH concentration does PAH clearance fall below the renal plasma flow? _____

REFERENCES

1. Agus, Z. S., Puschett, J. B., Senesky, D., and Goldberg, M.: Mode of action of cyclic adenosine 3',5'-monophosphate on renal tubular phosphate reabsorption in the dog. *J. Clin. Invest. 50*:617-626, 1971.

2. Anderson, J.: A method for estimating Tm for phosphate in man. *J. Physiol. (Lond.) 130*:268-277, 1955.

3. Aurbach, G. D., and Potts, J. T., Jr.: Parathyroid hormone. *Am. J. Med. 42*:1-8, 1967.

4. Baines, A. D., Gottschalk, C. W., and Lassiter, W. E.: Microinjection study of p-aminohippurate excretion by rat kidneys. *Am. J. Physiol. 214*:703-709, 1968.

5. Balagura, S., and Pitts, R. F.: Renal handling of α-ketoglutarate by the dog. *Am. J. Physiol. 207*:483-494, 1964.

6. Berglund, F., and Lotspeich, W. D.: Renal tubular reabsorption of inorganic sulfate in the dog, as affected by glomerular filtration rate and sodium chloride. *Am. J. Physiol. 185*:533-538, 1956.

7. Berliner, R. W., Hilton, J. G., Jr., Yü, T. F., and Kennedy, T. J., Jr.: The renal mechanism for urate excretion in man. *J. Clin. Invest. 29*:396-401, 1950.

8. Beyer, K. H., Wright, L. D., Russo, H. F., Skeggs, H. R., and Patch, E. A.: The renal clearance of essential amino acids: tryptophane, leucine, isoleucine and valine. *Am. J. Physiol. 146*:330-335, 1946.

9. Beyer, K. H., Wright, L. D., Skeggs, H. R., Russo, H. F., and Shaner, G. A.: Renal clearance of essential amino acids: their competition for reabsorption by the renal tubules. *Am. J. Physiol. 151*:202-210, 1947.

10. Bijvoet, O. L. M.: Relation of plasma phosphate concentration to renal tubular reabsorption of phosphate. *Clin. Sci. 37*: 23-36, 1969.

11. Bradley, S. E., Laragh, I. H., Wheeler, H. O., MacDowell, M., and Oliver, J.: Correlation of structure and function in the handling of glucose by nephrons of the canine kidney. *J. Clin. Invest. 40*:1113-1131, 1961.

12. Brown, J. L., Samiy, A. H., and Pitts, R. F.: Localization of aminonitrogen reabsorption in the nephron of the dog. *Am. J. Physiol. 200*:370-372, 1961.

13. Burgen, A. S. V.: A theoretical treatment of glucose reabsorption in the kidney. *Can. J. Biochem. Physiol. 34*: 466-474, 1956.

14. Chan, S. S., and Lotspeich, W. D.: Comparative effects of phlorizin and phloretin on glucose transport in the cat kidney. *Am. J. Physiol. 203*:975-979, 1962.

15. Chesney, R. W., Sacktor, B., and Rowen, R.: The binding of D-glucose to the isolated luminal membrane of the renal proximal tubule. *J. Biol. Chem. 218*:2182-2191, 1973.

16. Cho, K. C., and Cafruny, E. J.: Renal tubular reabsorption of p-aminohippuric acid (PAH) in the dog. *J. Pharmacol. Exp. Ther. 173*:1-12, 1970.

17. Coello, J. B., and Bradley, S. E.: Function of the nephron population during hemorrhagic hypotension in the dog with special reference to the effects of osmotic diuresis. *J. Clin. Invest. 43*:386-400, 1964.

18. Cohen, J. J., and Wittman, E.: Renal utilization and excretion

of α-ketoglutarate in dog: effect of alkalosis. *Am. J. Physiol. 204*:795-811, 1963.

19. Cooke, R. E., Segar, W. E., Reed, C., Etzweiler, D. D., Vita, M., Brusilow, S., and Darrow, D. C.: The role of potassium in the prevention of alkalosis. *Am. J. Med. 17*:180-195, 1954.

20. Cortney, M. A., Sawin, L. L., and Weiss, D. D.: Renal tubular protein absorption in the rat. *J. Clin. Invest. 49*:1-4, 1970.

21. Crane, R.: Absorption of sugars. In: *Handbook of Physiology*, Section 6, *Alimentary Canal*. Edited by C. F. Code. Washington, D. C., American Physiological Society, 1968, pp. 1323-1351.

22. Frick, A.: Reabsorption of inorganic phosphate in the rat. I. Saturation of transport mechanism. II. Suppression of fractional phosphate reabsorption due to expansion of extra-cellular fluid volume. *Arch. Ges. Physiol. 304*:351-364, 1968.

23. Frohnert, P., Höhmann, B., Zwiebel, R., and Baumann, K.: Free flow micropunture studies of glucose transport in the rat nephron. *Arch. Ges. Physiol. 315*:66-85, 1970.

24. Govaerts, P.: Interprétation physiologique des relations mathématique existant entre le taux du glucose sanguin et le débit urinaire de cette substance. *Acta Clin. Belg. 5*:1-13, 1950.

25. Grollman, A. P., Harrison, H. C., and Harrison, H. E.: The renal excretion of citrate. *J. Clin. Invest. 40*:1290-1296, 1961.

26. Gutman, A. B., and Yü, T. F.: A three-component system for regulation of renal excretion of uric acid in man. *Trans. Assoc. Am. Physicians 74*:353-365, 1961.

27. Gutman, A. B., Yü, T. F., and Berger, L.: Renal function in gout. III. Estimation of tubular secretion and reabsorption of uric acid by use of pyrazinamide. *Am. J. Med. 47*:575-592, 1969.

28. Hall, P. F.: *The Functions of the Endocrine Glands*. W. B. Saunders Co., Philadelphia, 1959.

29. Hierholzer, K., Cade, R., Gurd, R., Kessler, R. H., and Pitts, R. F.: Stop-flow analysis of renal reabsorption of sulfate in the dog. *Am. J. Physiol. 198*:833-837, 1960.

30. Hirsch, P. F., Voelkel, E. A., and Munson, P. L.: Thyrocalcitonin: Hypocalcemic hypophosphatemic principle of the thyroid gland. *Science 146*:412-413, 1964.

31. Holmes, E. W., Kelley, W. N., and Wyngaarden, J. B.: The kidney and uric acid excretion in man. *Kidney International 2*:115-118, 1972.

32. Keyes, J. L., and Swanson, R. E.: Dependence of glucose Tm on GFR and tubular volume in the dog kidney. *Am. J. Physiol. 221*: 1-7, 1971.

33. Kleinzeller, A., Kolinska, J., and Benes, I.: Transport of glucose and galactose in kidney cortex cells. *Biochem. J. 104*:843-851, 1967.

34. Knox, F. G., Schneider, E. G., Willis, L. R., Strandhoy, J. W., and Ott, C. E.: Site and control of phosphate reabsorption by the kidney. *Kidney International 3*:347-353, 1973.

35. Koch, A.: *The Kidney.* In: *Physiology and Biophysics*, edited by T. C. Ruch and H. D. Patton, 20th ed. W. B. Saunders Co., Philadelphia, 1973, pp. 844-872.

36. Krane, S., and Crane, R.: The accumulation of D-galactose against a concentration gradient by slices of rabbit kidney cortex. *J. Biol. Chem. 234*:211-216, 1959.

37. Kruhoffer, P.: *Studies on Water and Electrolyte Excretion and Glomerular Activity in the Mammalian Kidney.* Rosenkilde and Bagger, Copenhagen, 1950, pp. 76-85.

38. Kurtzman, N. A., White, M. G., Rogers, P. W., and Flynn, J. J., III,: Relationship of sodium reabsorption and glomerular filtration rate to renal glucose reabsorption. *J. Clin. Invest. 51*:127-133, 1972.

39. Lambert, P. P., Van Kessel, E., and Leplat, C.: Etude sur l'elimination des phosphates inorganiques chez l'homme. *Acta Med. Scand. 128*:386-410, 1947.

40. Lathem, W., Davis, B. B., Zweig, P. H., and Dew, R.: The demonstration and localization of renal tubular reabsorption of hemoglobin by stop flow analysis. *J. Clin. Invest. 39*: 840-845, 1960.

41. Letteri, J. M., and Wesson, L. G., Jr.: Glucose titration curves as an estimate of intrarenal distribution of glomerular filtrate in patients with congestive heart failure. *J. Lab. Med. 65*:387-405, 1965.

42. Lotspeich, W. D.: Renal tubular reabsorption of inorganic sulfate in the normal dog. *Am. J. Physiol. 151*:311-318, 1947.

43. Lotspeich, W. D.: Phlorizin and the cellular transport of glucose. *Harvey Lectures*, *Ser. 56*. Academic Press, New York, 1961, pp. 63-91.

44. Lotspeich, W. D., and Woronkow, S.: Some quantitative studies on phlorizin inhibition of glucose transport in the kidney. *Am. J. Physiol. 195*:331-336, 1958.

45. Mudge, G. H.: Clinical patterns of tubular dysfunction. *Am. J. Med. 24*:785-804, 1958.

46. Mudge, G. H., Berndt, W. O., and Valtin, H.: Tubular transport of urea, glucose, phosphate, uric acid, sulfate, and thiosulfate. In: *Handbook of Physiology*, Section 8, *Renal Physiology*. Edited by J. Orloff and R. W. Berliner. Washington, D. C., American Physiological Society, 1973, pp. 587-652.

47. Mudge, G. H., Cucchi, G., Platts, M., O'Connell, J. M. B., and Berndt, W. O.: Renal excretion of uric acid in the dog. *Am. J. Physiol. 215*:404-410, 1968.

48. Murayama, Y., Morel, F., and LeGrimellec, C.: Phosphate, calcium, and magnesium transfers in proximal tubules and loops of Henle, as measured by single nephron microperfusion experiments in the rat. *Arch. Ges. Physiol. 333*:1-16, 1972.

49. Pitts, R. F.: A renal reabsorptive mechanism in the dog common to glycine and creatine. *Am. J. Physiol. 140*:156-168, 1943.

50. Pitts, R. F.: A comparison of the renal reabsorptive processes for several amino acids. *Am. J. Physiol. 140*:535-547, 1944.

51. Pitts, R. F.: *Physiology of the Kidney and Body Fluids*. 3rd ed. Year Book Publishers, Inc., Chicago, 1974.

52. Pitts, R. F., and Alexander, R. S.: The renal absorptive mechanism for inorganic phosphate in normal and acidotic dogs. *Am. J. Physiol. 142*:648-662, 1944.

53. Puschett, J. B., Agus, Z. S., Senesky, D., and Goldberg, M.: Effects of saline loading and aortic obstruction on proximal phosphate transport. *Am. J. Physiol. 223*:851-857, 1972.

54. Robson, A. M., Srivastava, P. L., and Bricker, N. S.: The influence of saline loading on renal glucose reabsorption in the rat. *J. Clin. Invest. 47*:329-335, 1968.

55. Shankel, S. W., Robson, A. M., and Bricker, N. S.: On the mechanism of the splay in the glucose titration curve in advanced experimental renal disease in the rat. *J. Clin. Invest. 46*:164-172, 1967.

56. Shannon, J. A., Farber, S., and Troast, L.: The measurement of glucose Tm in the normal dog. *Am. J. Physiol. 133*:752-761, 1941.

57. Shannon, J. A., and Fisher, S.: The renal tubular reabsorption of glucose in the normal dog. *Am. J. Physiol. 122*:765-774, 1938.

58. Singer, F. R., Woodhouse, N. J. Y., Parkinson, D. K., and Joplin, G. F.: Some acute effects of administered porcine calcitonin in man. *Clin. Sci. 37*:181-190, 1969.

59. Smith, H. W.: *The Kidney, Structure and Function in Health and Disease.* Oxford University Press, New York, 1955.

60. Smith, H. W., Goldring, W., Chasis, H., Ranges, H. A., and Bradley, S. E.: The application of saturation methods to the study of glomerular and tubular function in the human kidney. *J. Mt. Sinai Hosp. N. Y. 10*:59-108, 1943.

61. Stanbury, S. W.: Some aspects of disordered renal tubular function. *Advan. Internal Med. 9*:231-282, 1958.

62. Stolte, H., Hare, D., and Boylan, J. W.: D-glucose and fluid reabsorption in proximal surface tubule of the rat kidney. *Arch. Ges. Physiol. 334*:193-206, 1972.

63. Strickler, J. C., Thompson, D. D., Klose, R. M., and Giebisch, G.: Micropuncture study of inorganic phosphate excretion in the rat. *J. Clin. Invest. 43*:1596-1607, 1965.

64. Sulamita, B., and Pitts, R. F.: Renal handling of α-ketoglutarate by the dog. *Am. J. Physiol. 207*:483-494, 1964.

65. Talmadge, R. V., and Belanger, L. F. (editors): *Parathyroid Hormone and Thyrocalcitonin (Calcitonin).* Excerpta Medica Foundation, New York, 1968.

66. Tune, B. M., and Burg, M. B.: Glucose transport by proximal renal tubules. *Am. J. Physiol. 221*:580-585, 1971.

67. Tune, B. M., Burg, M. B., and Patlak, C. S.: Characteristics of p-aminohippurate transport in proximal renal tubules. *Am. J. Physiol. 217*:1057-1063, 1969.

68. Vander, A. J., and Cafruny, E. J.: Stop flow analysis of renal function in the monkey. *Am. J. Physiol.* *202*:1105-1108, 1962.

69. Van Liew, J. B., Deetjen, P., and Boylan, J. W.: Glucose reabsorption in the rat kidney--dependence on glomerular filtration. *Arch. Ges. Physiol.* *295*:232-244, 1967.

70. Walker, A., Bott, P., Oliver, J., and MacDowell, M.: The collection and analysis of fluid from single nephrons of the mammalian kidney. *Am. J. Physiol.* *134*:580-595, 1941.

71. Webber, W. A.: Interactions of neutral and acidic amino acids in renal tubular transport. *Am. J. Physiol.* *202*:577-583, 1962.

72. Webber, W. A.: Characteristics of acidic amino acid transport in mammalian kidney. *Can. J. Biochem. Physiol.* *41*:131-137, 1963.

73. Wright, L. D., Russo, H. F., Skeggs, H. R., Patch, E. A., and Beyer, K. H.: The renal clearance of essential amino acids: arginine, histidine, lysine and methionine. *Am. J. Physiol.* *149*:130-134, 1947.

74. Wyngaarden, J. B.: On the dual pathogenesis of hyperuricemia in primary gout. *Arth. Rheum.* *3*:414-420, 1960.

75. Young, J. A., and Freedman, B. S.: Renal tubular transport of amino acids. *Clin. Chem.* *17*:245-266, 1971.

Chapter 10

RENAL REGULATION OF ACID-BASE BALANCE

In a healthy man, the arterial plasma concentration of hydrogen ions ($[H^+]_p$) expressed in pH units (pH = $-\log [H^+]$) is alkaline and ranges from 7.38 to 7.42, but may range from 7.0 to 7.8 in pathological states.

The alkalinity of blood is continuously threatened by endogenous influx of acids produced from the metabolism of the normal average diet. The acids produced are in two forms: (1) *Volatile acid* in the form of CO_2 produced (about 250 mM per kg of body weight) from the oxidative metabolism of the foodstuff, which upon hydration yields the weak carbonic acid (H_2CO_3):

$$CO_2 + H_2O \rightleftarrows H_2CO_3 \rightleftarrows H^+ + HCO_3^- \qquad (10\text{-}1)$$

The CO_2 thus produced is eliminated exclusively by the pulmonary system. (2) *Nonvolatile or fixed acid* produced from catabolism of the proteins in the diet. This yields an additional 1 mM of acid per kg of body weight in adults, and slightly higher amounts in infants and young children. For individuals on vegetarian diet, the nonvolatile component is mainly alkalis.

Besides the diet, the net influx of nonvolatile acid may increase in certain physiological and pathological conditions. Examples include lactic acid production in exercise and acetoacetic acid and β-hydroxybutyric acid production during uncontrolled diabetes mellitus.

If the nonvolatile acid is allowed to remain in the body, it clearly poses a serious threat to all normal life processes. Therefore, to prevent such a disaster, the nonvolatile acid must be neutralized and then excreted in suitable forms by the renal system.

It is clear that the normal alkalinity of the body fluids must be defended against the continuous daily influx of acid. This task of maintaining the blood pH within limits compatible with life is accomplished by the integrated actions of three important systems: (1) The *blood buffer system*, whose response is quick but can only make partial adjustment; (2) the *pulmonary system*, whose response is similarly quick but can make partial correction; and (3) the *renal system*, whose response is slow but completely corrects deviations in blood pH.

To better understand the mechanisms of renal regulation of blood pH, we shall begin this chapter with an overview of the functions of the blood buffers and the pulmonary system.

PHYSIOLOGICAL CHEMISTRY OF BLOOD BUFFERS

Regulation of normal blood pH involves both *passive* (or chemical) buffering, such as occurs in vitro, and *active* (or physiological) buffering, in which pulmonary and renal systems manipulate the plasma concentrations of the components of some passive blood buffers.

A *chemical buffer* consists of a mixture of a weak acid (or alkali) and its salt (Equation 10-1), and has the property of resisting changes in pH that would otherwise result from adding acid or alkali. This property may be defined quantitatively by plotting the amount of acid or alkali added against the pH. Such a plot yields a *sigmoidal* curve and is called the *titration curve* of the buffer.

Another way of defining this property is to apply the mass-action law to such a buffer mixture, yielding the well-known Henderson-Hasselbalch equilibrium equation:

$$pH = pK + \log \frac{[salt]}{[acid]} \qquad (10\text{-}2)$$

where [salt] and [acid] are the concentrations of salt and acid components of the buffer mixture, pH and pK are the negative logs of the [H^+] and the dissociation constant (K) of the weak acid, respectively. Accordingly, the strength of the buffer, i.e., its *buffering capacity*, depends on (a) the concentration of the buffer (the sum of the acid and salt concentrations) and (b) the nearness of the pH to the pK of the buffer. At equal salt and acid concentrations, the ratio term in Equation 10-2 becomes unity and its log equal to zero, in which case the pH becomes equal to the pK. At this pH, the buffering capacity is maximal, but because of the sigmoidal nature of the titration curve two thirds of this capacity is lost by moving the pH one unit to either side of the pK.

Whole blood is a *heterogeneous* mixture consisting of plasma and cell phases. Its major buffers are: inorganic phosphate, bicarbonate, and plasma proteins, all residing in the plasma phase, and the hemoglobin (Hb), residing in the red cell phase.

Insofar as *passive buffering* is concerned, the inorganic phosphate with a plasma concentration of 2 mM/L and a pK of 6.8 is

very poor. The bicarbonate buffer, however, with a plasma
concentration of 25 mM/L and a pK of 6.1, is a much stronger
passive buffer. In contrast, hemoglobin and plasma proteins are
by far the strongest passive buffers of the blood. These polyvalent
buffers provide a total concentration of some 50 mM/L (there are
normally 15.8 g% of Hb and 3.5 g% of plasma proteins in the blood)
and their pK's are so distributed as to yield a uniform maximal
buffering capacity over the full pathological pH range.

When it comes to *active buffering*, however, the important blood
buffers are inorganic phosphate and bicarbonate. The reason is that
selective renal excretion of the inorganic phosphate provides a means
of adjusting its plasma concentration by the renal system. The
bicarbonate buffer (Equation 10-1) is even more important, because
the concentration of its volatile acid component (CO_2) is manipulated
by the pulmonary system, while the concentration of its salt component
(HCO_3^-) is manipulated by the renal system.

Despite these differences in buffering capacity, all blood
buffers exist in equilibrium with the same plasma [H^+]. Therefore,
the ratio term in the Equation 10-2 for one buffer determines the
ratio term for all other buffers. This phenomenon is called the
isohydric principle and may be expressed as:

$$[H^+] = \frac{[HA]_1}{[A^-]_1} K_1 = \frac{[HA]_2}{[A^-]_2} K_2 \cdots \qquad (10-3)$$

where [HA] and [A^-] are the acid and salt concentrations of the
buffer pair, K is its dissociation constant, and subscripts 1 and 2
refer to the buffer species.

Because of the isohydric principle, a change in the buffering
capacity of the entire blood buffer system is reflected by a change
in the buffering capacity of one buffer pair. Hence, to understand
the response of the blood buffer system to acid-base disturbances, it
is sufficient to examine the behavior of only one of the blood buffer
pairs. For reasons mentioned earlier, of the four major blood buffers,
the *bicarbonate buffer* serves as the best candidate. Therefore,
disturbances in acid-base balance can be ascertained from studying
the behavior of the bicarbonate buffer and the regulation of its two
components by the pulmonary and renal systems.

CO_2 ABSORPTION CURVE OF TRUE PLASMA

The pulmonary and renal systems monitor the pCO_2 and [HCO_3^-] of
the true plasma, not the separated plasma. *True plasma* is plasma
which *includes* the buffering effect of the all-important Hb buffer.
Separated plasma is plasma which *excludes* such an effect. In the
province of acid-base regulation, the important differences between
the two types of plasma are in the behavior of their *CO_2 absorption*

curves. For true plasma, this curve is obtained as follows. Whole blood is exposed at 37°C to gas mixtures containing various known tensions of CO_2 and sufficiently high O_2 tension to completely saturate the hemoglobin with oxygen. After equilibration, the blood is centrifuged anaerobically and the total concentration of CO_2 in the plasma and the volume of CO_2 in the gas phase are determined. The latter is converted to pCO_2 and concentration units and is then subtracted from the total CO_2 in the plasma, to yield $[HCO_3^-]$ in the plasma. The plot of $[HCO_3^-]$ thus obtained at various CO_2 tensions against the pCO_2 of the gas mixture to which the blood was exposed yields the CO_2 absorption curve for the true plasma shown in Figure 10-1. In contrast, if we had separated the plasma first and then exposed it to various CO_2 tensions, we would get the other curve shown in Figure 10-1. Note that CO_2 absorption curve for the separated plasma is much flatter and does not go through the origin, because the buffering effect of Hb is now lacking. Note also that the steeper the CO_2 absorption curve, the more closely it follows the iso-pH line (see Fig. 10-4 and Equation 10-7), and hence the better is the buffering capacity.

It is clear that to faithfully describe the behavior of the whole blood buffers in acid-base disturbances from the bicarbonate buffer system, we must use the CO_2 absorption curve of the true plasma.

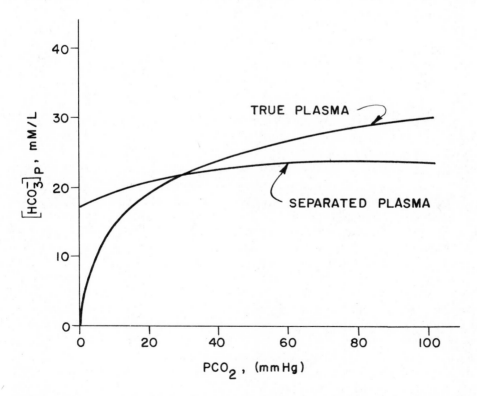

Figure 10-1. CO_2 absorption curve for true and separated plasma.

The necessity of dealing with the bicarbonate buffer system in true plasma has an important advantage, for the Henderson-Hasselbalch equation can be applied to the homogeneous plasma phase or the homogeneous red cell phase, but not to the heterogeneous whole blood. Applying the Henderson-Hasselbalch equation to the bicarbonate buffer of the true plasma yields:

$$pH = 6.1 + \log \frac{[HCO_3^-]_p}{[H_2CO_3]_p} \qquad (10\text{-}4)$$

where the subscript refers to the plasma. Since in the plasma the equilibrium for the formation of H_2CO_3 from CO_2 and H_2O (Equation 10-1) is far to the left, then the $[H_2CO_3]_p$ term in Equation 10-4 is proportional to the pCO_2 and is defined by Henry's law of gas solubility:

$$[H_2CO_3]_p = \alpha \ pCO_2 \qquad (10\text{-}5)$$

where α is the CO_2 solubility coefficient and has a value of 0.03 mM/L per mm Hg. Substituting Equation 10-5 into 10-4 yields:

$$pH = 6.1 + \log \frac{[HCO_3^-]_p}{0.03 \ pCO_2} \qquad (10\text{-}6)$$

Note that $[HCO_3^-]_p$ term is equal to the difference between the total CO_2 content of the plasma and that which is physically dissolved $(0.03 \ pCO_2)$.

Mathematically, as defined by Equation 10-6, and physiologically, pH is a dependent variable; its changes are determined by variations in pCO_2, which is the primary independent variable (direct input), and $[HCO_3^-]_p$, which is the secondary independent variable (indirect input). With this in mind, there are only three ways of graphically relating the three variables in this equation.

Figure 10-2 shows the plot of pH as a function of pCO_2. The data used to construct this and the other two plots (Figs. 10-3 and 10-4) are listed in Table 10-1. Note that as pCO_2 rises, the pH falls in clearly curvilinear fashion. Despite the fact that this plot represents the direct input-output relationship for the bicarbonate buffer system, it is not used.

Another way of relating these variables is by plotting $[HCO_3^-]_p$ as a function of pH. This plot, called the *bicarbonate-pH diagram*, was first introduced by Davenport (1958). As shown in Figure 10-3, it is linear, and the line is called the normal *buffer line*. The curvilinear line shown in this figure is called the *pCO2 = 40 mm Hg isobar*, meaning that the CO_2 tension is the same anywhere along the

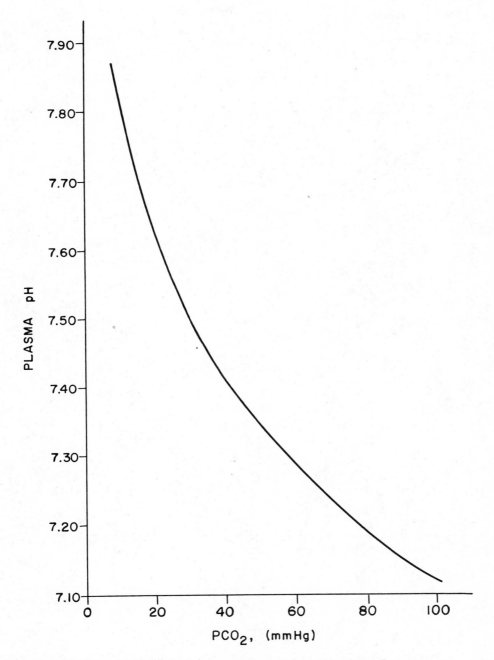

Figure 10-2. Relationship between plasma pH and pCO_2.

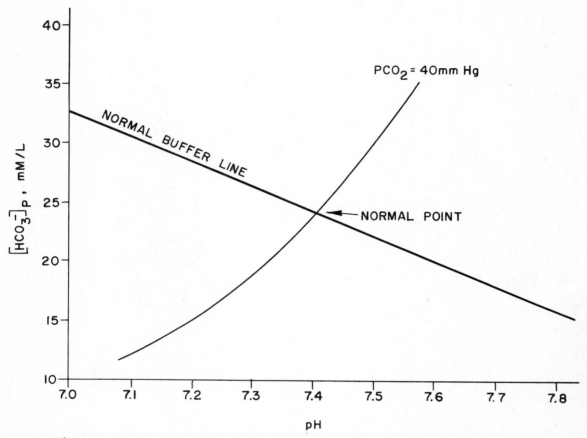

Figure 10-3. The bicarbonate-pH diagram of true plasma, with pCO_2 = 40 mm Hg isobar. [Redrawn from Davenport, H. W. (1958).]

curve. The data for plotting the pCO_2 isobar is obtained by first solving the Henderson-Hasselbalch equation for $[HCO_3^-]_p$:

$$[HCO_3^-]_p = 0.03 \ pCO_2 \times 10^{(pH - 6.1)} \qquad (10-7)$$

and then solving the equation for a given value of pCO_2 (such as pCO_2 = 40 mm Hg) and different values for pH ranging from 7.0 to 7.8. Note that for a pCO_2 < 40 mm Hg, the pCO_2 line will be shifted to the right, whereas for a pCO_2 > 40 mm Hg, it will be shifted to the left.

A third way of plotting these variables is to plot $[HCO_3^-]_p$ as a function of pCO_2. Such a plot, first introduced by Clark (1948)

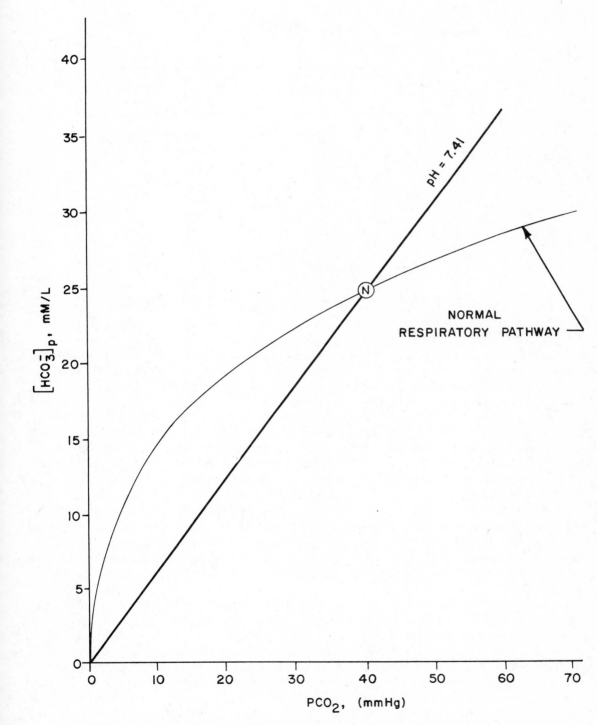

Figure 10-4. The bicarbonate-pCO$_2$ plot of true plasma, with radiating iso-pH = 7.41 line.

TABLE 10-1

Carbon Dioxide Absorption of Normal
Oxygenated True Plasma

pCO_2 (mm Hg)	$[HCO_3^-]_p$ (mM/L)	pH
10	15.2	7.82
20	19.4	7.62
30	22.0	7.50
40	24.0	7.41
50	25.6	7.36
60	26.9	7.29
70	28.0	7.24
80	28.9	7.19
90	29.8	7.15
100	30.4	7.12

[Data from Henderson, L. J. (1928).]

and refined later by Gray (1950, 1968) is called the *CO_2 absorption curve*. It is denoted as the "normal respiratory pathway" in Figure 10-4. The pH corresponding to any given pair of values for $[HCO_3^-]_p$ and pCO_2, as defined by Equation 10-6, is depicted by an *iso-pH line* radiating from the origin (Equation 10-7). Thus, the iso-pH = 7.41 line is defined by a line going from the origin through the normal point (N) defined here by $[HCO_3^-]_p$ = 25 mM/L and pCO_2 = 40 mm Hg. Note that when pH > 7.41, the iso-pH line will lie to the left, while for pH < 7.41 the iso-pH line will lie to the right of the normal iso-pH = 7.41 line.

The most striking feature of the CO_2 absorption plot is that it allows for complete visualization of the three variables of the plasma bicarbonate buffer system in one operation. Consequently, in this chapter we shall use this plot to discuss acid-base disturbances rather than the bicarbonate-pH diagram, although the latter is equally useful.

A closer examination of the CO_2 absorption curve reveals that as pCO_2 increases, such as may occur in hypoventilation, $[HCO_3^-]_p$ also increases, while the pH decreases. The blood reactions involved are shown in Figure 10-5. The rise in $[HCO_3^-]_p$ is due to neutralization of most of the added carbonic acid by the polyvalent proteinate, Pr^- (plasma protein and oxyhemoglobin), whose concentration decreases, but leaving the sum of the concentrations of bicarbonate and proteinate buffers unchanged. Furthermore, as the added CO_2 reduces the pH, the labile cations, B^+ (mainly Na^+ and K^+), formerly associated with the proteinate anions, are released to become associated with the bicarbonate ions. The fall in pH is buffered, however, because

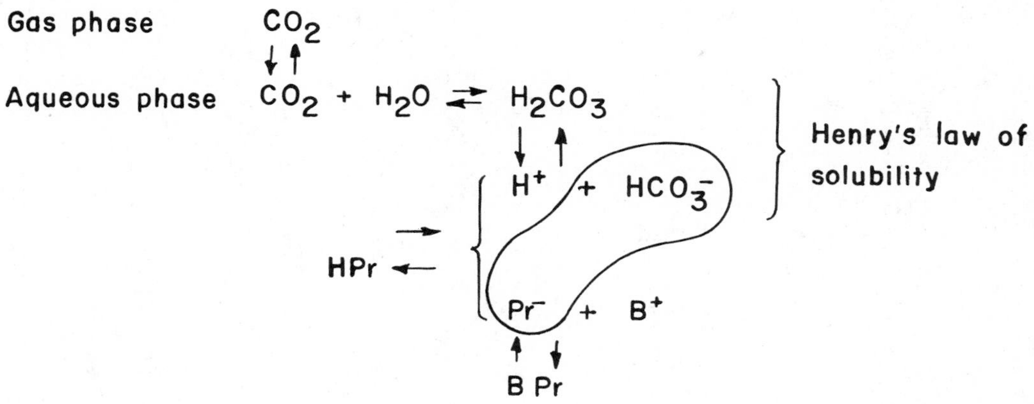

Figure 10-5. Reactions illustrating solubility of carbon dioxide in blood. [Redrawn from Muntwyler, E. (1968).]

the protein acids (HPr) that are formed ionize much less than the added carbonic acid. A precisely analogous but opposite sequence of reactions occurs in hyperventilation as the blood moves to the left of the normal point along the normal respiratory pathway.

STANDARD BICARBONATE CONTENT $\left([HCO_3^-]_{40}\right)$

Influx of fixed acids and alkalis into the blood causes disturbances in acid-base balance. How can this best be detected and measured? Obviously, determination of $[HCO_3^-]_p$ is not satisfactory because it is influenced as much by changes in pCO_2 as by influx of acid or alkali. The best way is to determine the level of the CO_2 absorption curve by measuring $[HCO_3^-]_p$ at some fixed, or standard, pCO_2. The standard pCO_2 usually used is 40 mm Hg, thereby eliminating the pulmonary compensation for acid-base disturbance. In practice, the whole blood sample is equilibrated at a pCO_2 of 40 mm Hg and a pO_2 of 150 mm Hg (to assure saturation of Hb with O_2) at a temperature of $37^{\circ}C$. The plasma bicarbonate, measured by subtracting dissolved CO_2 (= 0.03 pCO_2) from total CO_2 content, is called the *standard bicarbonate content* of true plasma (Astrup et al., 1960) and is symbolized as $[HCO_3^-]_{40}$. This is also a measure of the CO_2 content of the blood (Singer and Hastings, 1948) or of the body stores of alkali--or, as conventionally called, the *alkaline reserve* for neutralizing fixed acids. Thus, a decrease in $[HCO_3^-]_{40}$ indicates an increase in the influx of fixed acids, whereas an increase in $[HCO_3^-]_{40}$ indicates an increase in the influx of fixed alkali. These changes are reflected in downward and upward displacement of the CO_2 absorption curve, respectively. Just as the arterial pCO_2 is regulated by the pulmonary system, the $[HCO_3^-]_{40}$ is regulated by the renal system.

Clinically, the standard bicarbonate is not directly measured, but its deviation from normal, called *base excess* (BE) or *base deficit* (BD), is routinely approximated from measurement of arterial pCO_2 and pH and total hemoglobin (Hb). The validity of this estimation depends largely on the care with which the arterial blood is drawn and how quickly it is analyzed (Severinghaus et al., 1956a). The analyses of pCO_2 and pH are usually carried out on a blood gas analyzer, and of Hb on a co-oximeter. These values are then used to calculate, for example, base excess (or deficit) using the following equation (Siggaard-Andersen, 1964):

$$\text{Base Excess} = (1 - 0.0143 \text{ Hb}) \{ ([HCO_3^-]_p - $$

$$(9.5 + 1.63 \text{ Hb})(7.4 - pH_p)) - 24\} \qquad (10\text{-}8)$$

where 0.0143 is the number of milliliters of oxygen per gram of Hb in 100 ml of blood, Hb is the number of grams of hemoglobin in 100 ml of blood, (9.5 + 1.63 Hb) is the correction factor for absorption of CO_2 by Hb, and 7.4 and 24 are the assumed normal values for pH_p and $[HCO_3^-]_p$, which have already been defined. Note that the value of $[HCO_3^-]_p$ used in Equation 10-8 is calculated from pCO_2 and pH using the rearranged Henderson-Hasselbalch equation (Equation 10-7).

ELEMENTS OF ACID-BASE BALANCE

The regulation of acid-base balance involves two physiological regulators, the pulmonary and renal systems, which share one component in common--the blood buffer system (Fig. 10-6). The respiratory regulator controls arterial $pCO2$, as the direct input to this

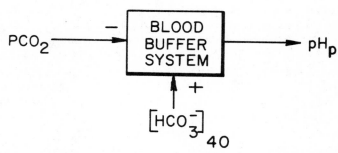

Figure 10-6. Scheme illustrating the elements of blood buffer system.

component, while the renal regulator controls $[HCO_3^-]_{40}$, as the indirect input to the same component. Before detailing the mechanisms whereby these two regulators stabilize the true plasma pH, the output of the blood buffer system, we need to understand some basic terminology, recommended at a recent symposium (Winters, 1966), which are used to describe acid-base disturbances.

Acidosis and *alkalosis* are *states* characterized by patterns of abnormalities in pCO_2, $[HCO_3^-]_p$, $[HCO_3^-]_{40}$, and pH_p. The first two are always disturbed, but the last two sometimes are and sometimes are not. It is, therefore, well to remember that *acidemia* (low "plasma" pH), such as may occur in hypercapnia (high pCO_2), and *alkalemia* (high "plasma" pH), such as may occur in hypocapnia (low pCO_2), refer only to one element in the patterns and are *not* synonymous with acidosis and alkalosis.

Every disturbance in acid-base balance has an *initial cause*, on the basis of which they are classified as *respiratory* or *metabolic*. Respiratory disturbances result from some initial forcing of the respiratory regulator that alters pCO_2, the direct input to the blood buffer system. Metabolic disturbances result from some initial forcing of the renal regulator (gain of fixed acid or alkali by the body) that alters $[HCO_3^-]_{40}$, the indirect input to the blood buffer system. Thus, the block diagram in Figure 10-6 neatly distinguishes the two classic causes of acid-base disturbances. In this block diagram, a minus sign near pCO_2 is a reminder that a step increase in this quantity causes a decrease in pH. Likewise, a plus sign near $[HCO_3^-]_{40}$ is a reminder that a step increase in this quantity causes an increase in pH. Further details of these relationships will be discussed later.

Disturbances in acid-base balance may be *uncompensated* (steady state error in pH) or *compensated* to various degrees (some or no steady state error in pH). The respiratory regulator compensates for metabolic disturbances, and the renal regulator compensates for respiratory disturbances. Each regulator will attempt to compensate for the effects of initial causes impinging on its own system, but because of proportional control,[*] a steady state error in pH will result. (It should be noted that this *within*-compensation, though it is tacitly recognized, is not called compensation.) The error in pH will then *elicit* a *second* compensation from the other regulator. Compensations for disturbances in acid-base balance refer *only* to this *cross-compensation* from the other regulator, and *not* to the within-regulator compensation.

Referring to Figure 10-4, uncompensated respiratory disturbances are portrayed by a displacement along the normal CO_2 absorption curve on the "normal respiratory pathway." Respiratory acidosis causes a displacement to the right, while respiratory alkalosis causes a displacement to the left, with no change in $[HCO_3^-]_{40}$. On the other hand, metabolic disturbances are portrayed by a shift in the CO_2 absorption curve, determined by a change in $[HCO_3^-]_{40}$. Thus, a fall

---

[*]See Appendix A for further details and definitions.

in $[HCO_3^-]_{40}$, as in metabolic acidosis, causes a downward shift, while a rise in $[HCO_3^-]_{40}$, as in metabolic alkalosis, causes an upward shift in the normal CO_2 absorption curve.

Let us now examine closely how pulmonary and renal regulators compensate for disturbances in acid-base balance.

AN OVERVIEW OF THE PULMONARY pH REGULATOR

Figure 10-7 shows an **orienting** functional diagram of the elements of the pulmonary pH regulator. For ease of presentation, it is divided into three components: the respiratory centers, the lungs and thorax, and the pulmonary gas exchanger. Briefly, the respiratory centers, located in the medulla oblongata and pons, monitor (designated by a small box on some arrows) at least six signals (shown by the arrows impinging on the left). As before, the plus or minus signs on any arrow indicate the directional effect of that forcing on the output of the appropriate box. The algebraic sum of these signals (neural integration) produces a net change in motor nerve impulses issued to the diaphragm and the thoracic muscles which control pulmonary ventilation ($\dot{V}_e$). As shown, the frequency of motor nerve impulses is a positive function of the sensitivity of the respiratory centers (K_c) to the given input signals. Likewise, the magnitude of pulmonary ventilation for a given motor nerve impulse is a negative function of the mechanical impedance (Z) of the lungs and thorax. Because ventilation is a cyclic process, the mechanical impedance is a function of airflow resistance (R), breathing frequency (f), and lung compliance (C):

$$Z = \sqrt{R^2 + \frac{1}{(\pi f C)^2}} \qquad (10\text{-}9)$$

The third component of the pulmonary pH regulator is the pulmonary gas exchanger. For clarity of presentation, it is divided into two phases: an O_2 exchanger and a CO_2 exchanger. The input to both exchangers is the ventilation equivalent ($\dot{V}_eE$), defined as the ratio of the pulmonary ventilation to the metabolic rate (MR). The outputs of the pulmonary gas exchanger are the partial pressures of O_2 and CO_2 in the arterial blood (P_aO_2 and P_aCO_2, respectively). The partial pressures of O_2 and CO_2 in the inspired air (P_iO_2 and P_iCO_2, respectively) represent the indirect inputs or properties of the exchanger. Note that for each component, the indirect input (property) determines its gain[*] (= output/input).

The other two systems shown in Figure 10-7, though not an integral part of the pulmonary pH regulator, are included for the sake of

---

[*]See Appendix A for further details and definitions.

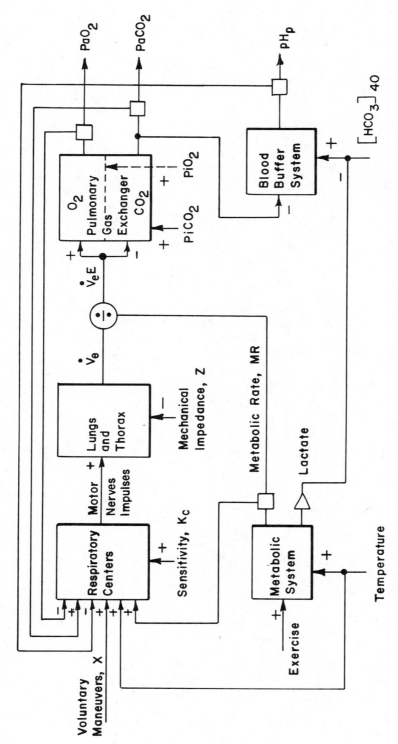

Figure 10-7. Scheme illustrating the components of the pulmonary pH regulator. [Modified and redrawn after Gray, J. S. (1968).]

completeness and subsequent integration of this regulator with the renal pH regulator.

The lower left-hand box represents the metabolic system (muscle, etc.) with metabolic rate (MR) and lactate as its outputs, and exercise as its input. The triangle on the arrow labelled lactate indicates that its production must exceed a critical *threshold level* before it can effectively alter $[HCO_3^-]_{40}$. The final element is the blood buffer system, shown by the box in the lower right-hand side, which we have already described.

FORCINGS AND RESPONSES OF THE PULMONARY pH REGULATOR

The steady state responses of the pulmonary pH regulator to some selected forcings are summarized in Table 10-2. Guided by the block diagram in Figure 10-7, verify the entries in this table by first considering the effect of each forcing at the level of the appropriate component and then follow the effect through the various feedback loops throughout the entire system. To illustrate, let us see how the pulmonary pH regulator cross-compensates for metabolic acidosis and alkalosis, the subject of present concern.

METABOLIC ACIDOSIS. Suppose a patient developed metabolic acidosis (as in diabetes mellitus or renal insufficiency) sufficient to lower his $[HCO_3^-]_{40}$ to 19 mM/L. If his ventilation remained unchanged, his arterial pCO_2 will remain constant, in which case the decrease in $[HCO_3^-]_{40}$ acting at the blood buffer system will lower the pH to 7.28. Consequently, as shown in Figure 10-8, the patient moves down the $pCO_2 = 40$ mm Hg iso-bar line to point A. But a fall in pH, acting through its feedback loop, stimulates ventilation, so that both $\dot{V}_e$ and $\dot{V}_eE$ rise. The increase in $\dot{V}_eE$ (induced by hyperventilation), acting at the exchanger, elevates P_aO_2 and lowers P_aCO_2. The latter effect causes the patient to move to the left of point A toward point B along a new CO_2 absorption curve, thereby raising the pH back toward the normal. This *induced respiratory alkalosis* constitutes the cross-compensation of the pulmonary pH regulator for metabolic acidosis.

How far left does the patient move along the new CO_2 absorption curve? Obviously not so far as complete pH compensation, for the lowered P_aCO_2, acting through its feedback loop, partially inhibits pH stimulation of ventilation. Thus, the patient's blood pattern settles down somewhere short of complete pH compensation, say at point B. Because the respiratory response to the metabolic acidosis is immediate, the patient's blood pattern does not follow the "dog-leg" pathway N→A→B, in separate steps. Actually, it follows the continuous pathway N→B shown on the "normal metabolic pathway."

METABOLIC ALKALOSIS. Exactly analogous, but opposite, changes occur if we induce a metabolic alkalosis sufficient to raise $[HCO_3^-]_{40}$

TABLE 10-2

Steady State Responses of the Pulmonary Regulator
to Some Selected Forcings

Disturbance Forcings	Maximum Ventilatory Gain (L/min)	Responses as Deviation from Normal				Arterial		
		MR	Motor Nerve Impulses	$\dot{V}_e$	$\dot{V}_eE$	pO_2	pCO_2	pH
Normal resting male	--	0.272	?	6.85	2.5	95	40	7.41
CO_2 inhalation – P_iCO_2↑	60	0	+	+	+	+	+	−
Altitude anoxia – P_iO_2↓	15	0	+	+	+	−	−	+
Metabolic acidosis – $[HCO_3^-]_{40}$↓	40	0	+	+	+	+	−	−
Metabolic alkalosis – $[HCO_3^-]_{40}$↑	−	0	−	−	−	−	+	+
Pulmonary impedance – Z↑	−	0	+	−	−	−	+	−
Respiratory depression – K_c↓	−	0	−	−	−	−	+	−
Voluntary hyperventilation – X↑	170	0	+	+	+	+	−	+
Fever – Temperature↑	20	+	+	++	+	+	−	+
Moderate exercise – MR↑	60	+	+	+	0	0	0	0
Severe exercise – MR↑, $[HCO_3^-]_{40}$↓	120	++	+++	+++	+	+	−	−

[Modified from Gray, J. S. (1968).]

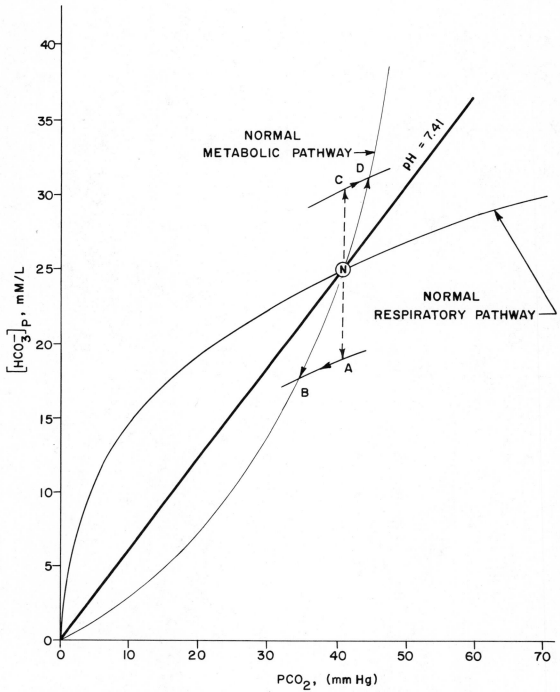

Figure 10-8. Scheme illustrating the pathways involved in pulmonary cross-compensation for metabolic disturbances.

to 30 mM/L (point C, Fig. 10-8). The patient hypoventilates (respiratory acidosis) and moves to the right of point C toward point D along a new CO_2 absorption curve, thereby lowering the pH toward normal. However, as before, the compensation is incomplete, and the patient's blood pattern settles down at point D. Again, the actual pathway that his blood follows is from point N to point D on the normal metabolic pathway, which represents the *partially cross-compensated* metabolic pathway.

It is clear that the pulmonary regulator provides an immediate, though incomplete, pH compensation in metabolic disturbances. The complete pH compensation is provided by adjustment of $[HCO_3^-]_{40}$ by the renal pH regulator, which is described next.

AN OVERVIEW OF THE RENAL pH REGULATOR

Disturbances in blood pH are prevented by continuous adjustment of the two inputs to the blood buffer system by the pulmonary and renal regulators. As described in the previous section, the pulmonary regulator manipulates pCO_2, which is one of the inputs determining pH (Fig. 10-6). The other input is the standard bicarbonate concentration ($[HCO_3^-]_{40}$), which is manipulated by the *renal pH regulator*. In this section we shall examine the operation of this regulator, component by component, as well as the intrarenal mechanisms mediating its response to acid-base disturbances.

THE STANDARD BICARBONATE POOL

Standard bicarbonate ($[HCO_3^-]_{40}$) was defined earlier as the bicarbonate concentration measured when blood is equilibrated *in vitro* with a pCO_2 of 40 mm Hg. Normally, its value is 25 mM/L.

Standard bicarbonate pool is determined by the influx or efflux of bicarbonate. Regardless of the route, two kinds of bicarbonate flux may be distinguished. *Controlled* fluxes consist of the *renal* excretion of acid or alkali, symbolized by $\dot{E}$. Acid excretion leads to accumulation of alkali, which will be neutralized by retained CO_2, producing an influx of bicarbonate into the body pool. Excretion of alkali leads to acid accumulation, which displaces CO_2 from bicarbonate, resulting in an efflux of bicarbonate from the body pool. The other kind of flux is a *fortuitous*, or accidental, flux, symbolized by $\dot{F}$, consisting of gains or losses of fixed acid or alkali by injection or via the GI tract or skin. The net bicarbonate flux ($\dot{HCO_3^-}$) is then the algebraic sum of these two fluxes, as illustrated in Figure 10-9.

The standard bicarbonate pool is the primary component in the renal pH regulator. Its functional *input* is the bicarbonate flux ($\dot{HCO_3^-}$), and its *output* is the standard bicarbonate content ($[HCO_3^-]_{40}$). An important *property* is time delay, emphasizing the slow renal adjustment of blood bicarbonate content. A second property is the

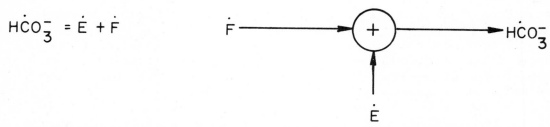

Figure 10-9. Factors determining the net flux of bicarbonate, $\dot{HCO_3}^-$, into the blood.

fluid volume of the whole pool, which converts an increment of $\dot{HCO_3}^-$ to a concentration, but we shall leave this as a constant and ignore it. But note that in the steady state of this pool (when $[HCO_3^-]_{40}$ is unchanging), the input ($\dot{HCO_3}^-$), which is the algebraic sum of $\dot{F}$ and $\dot{E}$, must be zero! For the first time in this book we have encountered a component whose steady state output can be determined only by following its changes *during a transient.* Its behavior is therefore governed by an *integral equation*,* but fortunately, it is easier to verbalize than symbolize it, as illustrated schematically in Figure 10-10.

If HCO_3^- influx exceeds HCO_3^- efflux during the transient, the steady state $[HCO_3^-]_{40}$ will have increased above its initial value, and vice versa. Note also that since $\dot{HCO_3}^-$ may be small compared to the large body pool, the transient tends to be long, even days or

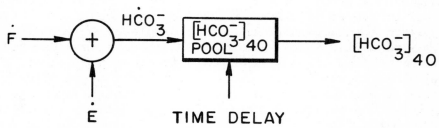

Figure 10-10. Schematic representation of factors determining standard bicarbonate concentration, $[HCO_3^-]_{40}$, in the blood.

---

*See Appendix A for further details and definitions.

weeks. In the block diagram, the property "time delay" is a reminder of this long transient and of the fact that we accumulate $H\dot{C}O_3^-$ over time to obtain the steady state output.

THE CELLULAR POOL

We have just described the body standard bicarbonate pool as though it were homogeneous. For most situations this simplified description is adequate, for the extracellular and intracellular compartments of the whole pool behave alike. In certain situations, however, the two compartments behave *oppositely*, so that the plasma $[HCO_3^-]_{40}$ may rise, while that of body cells falls, and vice versa. The result is a *dissociated* metabolic disturbance in acid-base balance; an intracellular acidosis and extracellular alkalosis, or vice versa, may occur *at the same time*.

The key element in this process appears to consist of opposite transfers of H^+ and K^+ ions across the cell membrane between the extra- and intracellular fluid compartments. If potassium salts are injected intravenously to produce a hyperkalemia, the K^+ ions enter body cells and H^+ ions leave them; this leaves an intracellular metabolic alkalosis and produces an extracellular metabolic acidosis. Conversely, if body K^+ is depleted to produce hypokalemia, K^+ ions leave body cells and H^+ ions enter them; this leaves an extracellular alkalosis and produces an intracellular acidosis (Fuller et al., 1955).

We shall represent this dissociated behavior by introducing another component, called the *cellular pool*. Its *input* is pH_p, normally 7.41. Its *output* is the pH of body cells (pH_c); although not easily measurable, it is lower than that of plasma and we assign to it an arbitrary normal value of 7.0. Its *property* is the plasma potassium concentration ($[K^+]_p$), normally about 5 mEq/L. For lack of precise information we relate these variables in the simplest possible form, as illustrated in Figure 10-11. So long as $[K^+]_p$ is normal, the

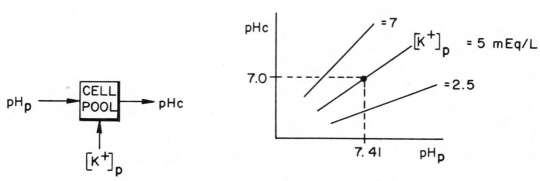

Figure 10-11. Schematic representation of factors affecting intracellular pH.

cellular and plasma pH simply rise and fall together. But, as noted in Chapter 8, a change in $[K^+]_p$ produces an inverse change in pH_p. Thus, an increase in $[K^+]_p$ will raise pH_c and lower pH_p, while a decrease in $[K^+]_p$ will produce the opposite effect. The possible mechanisms involved will be discussed later.

THE KIDNEYS

The kidneys have the ability to selectively excrete acid or alkali in the urine, measured not in terms of urine pH, but as mEq per day, which we have already symbolized as $\dot{E}$. To eliminate alkali, the kidneys excrete Na_2HPO_4 and $NaHCO_3$, both measured by titrating the urine with HCl back to pH 7.41. To eliminate acid, they excrete NaH_2PO_4 and synthesize NH_3 (largely from glutamine) for excretion as NH_4Cl; the acid phosphate is measured by back titration with NaOH, but the NH_4^+ is determined separately and added.

The average diet has a somewhat acid residue, so that $\dot{E}$ is normally about 50 mEq/day. In disturbances of acid-base balance, however, $\dot{E}$ may be as low as –300 or as high as +500 mEq/day.* The sign and magnitude of $\dot{E}$ appear to be determined by the pH within the renal tubular cells, which we can only assume behaves like pH_c of the cells in general. Again, for lack of precise data we assume a simple, negative, linear relationship for this behavior, as illustrated in Figure 10-12. Note that we have set the normal pH_c at 7.0 but specify a pH_c of 7.1 as the level at which the kidneys excrete a neutral urine ($\dot{E} = 0$). This allows the normal excretion of about 50 mEq of acid per day. The kidney property (K_k) determines the rate of acid or alkali

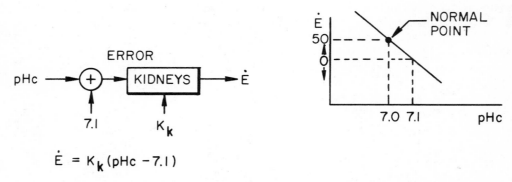

$$\dot{E} = K_k (pHc - 7.1)$$

Figure 10-12. Schematic representation of factors determining net renal acid excretion.

---

*Note: A negative $\dot{E}$ means excretion of alkali in urine.

excretion for a given pH error, and is thus the controller[*]
sensitivity. This property may be reduced by renal disease, as in
renal insufficiency, resulting in the accumulation of fixed acid,
to yield one kind of metabolic acidosis.

FORCINGS AND RESPONSES OF THE RENAL
pH REGULATOR

Synthesis of the foregoing components of the renal pH regulator
yields the block diagram shown in Figure 10-13. Note that one
component, the blood buffer system, is shared by both the pulmonary
and renal regulators, and that its output (pH_p) is a loop variable
for both regulators. In studying the renal regulator in isolation,
we can make pCO_2 an arbitrary constant, although we know it is a loop
variable in the pulmonary regulator (Fig. 10-7). Each regulator will
cross-compensate for the other. Just as the pulmonary regulator
cross-compensated for metabolic disturbances in acid-base balance,
we shall find that the renal regulator also cross-compensates for
respiratory disturbances in acid-base balance.

Excluding cross-compensation, all the disturbance forcings that
initially impinge on the renal regulator produce *metabolic* disturbances
in acid-base balance: (a) changes in fortuitous fluxes ($\dot{F}$) produce
either metabolic acidosis or alkalosis, (b) reductions in K_k produce a
metabolic acidosis, and (c) changes in $[K^+]_p$ produce *dissociated*
metabolic disturbances. Since these forcings are so important, let
us describe them more systematically:

A. CAUSES OF METABOLIC ALKALOSIS (ELEVATED $[HCO_3^-]_{40}$):
1. Gain of base from ingestion or injection of alkali, such as
alkaline salts for treatment of peptic ulcer.
2. Loss of acid from excessive vomiting of gastric HCl--if this
persists, K^+ ion depletion may result.

B. CAUSES OF METABOLIC ACIDOSIS (REDUCED $[HCO_3^-]_{40}$):
1. Gain of acid from ingestion of acid salts (NH_4Cl, for
example), or production of lactic acid in exercise, or of keto-acids
in fasting or uncontrolled diabetes mellitus, or loss of renal ability
to excrete acid (renal insufficiency).
2. Loss of base in alkaline body fluids, such as plasma lost
from burned skin surface, or severe diarrhea--if the latter persists,
K^+ ion depletion may be severe.

C. CAUSES OF DISSOCIATED METABOLIC DISTURBANCES:
1. Hyperkalemia from ingestion or injection of K^+ salts produces
extracellular acidosis and intracellular alkalosis.
2. Hypokalemia from K^+ ion loss (gastrointestinal fluids contain
higher $[K^+]$ than plasma), produces extracellular alkalosis and

---

[*]See Appendix A for further details and definitions.

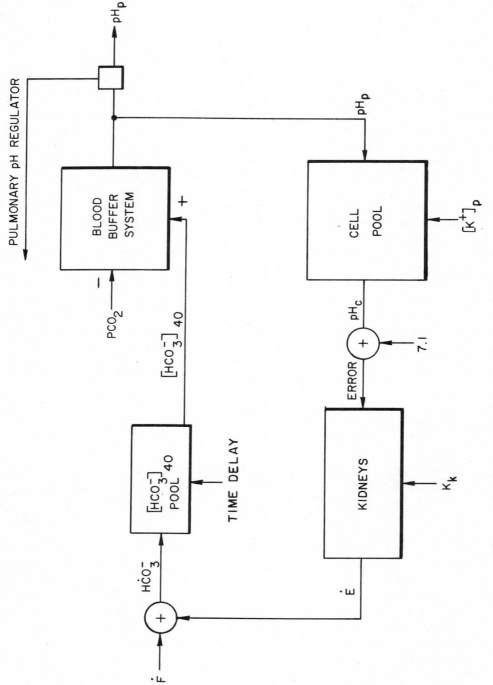

Figure 10-13. Synthesis of the renal pH regulator.

intracellular acidosis.

Still excluding cross-compensation, the renal regulator operates by *proportional* control, but with a new twist. A change in any of the three properties ($\dot{F}$, K_k, or $[K^+]_p$) will induce a *rate* of error development in pH; the error in pH will induce a compensatory *rate* of error correction. Since both are rates, the control is proportional and exhibits steady state error. The new twist is that with no control ($\dot{E}$ is not adjustable), the pH error will grow *endlessly*, with no steady state, but a fatal outcome.

Let us illustrate with the example of ingesting NH_4Cl to produce a metabolic acidosis; the NH_3 is converted to urea by the gut and liver, leaving an equivalent of HCl. One dose of NH_4Cl amounts to a *pulse* forcing, which will disturb the system, but since the forcing does not persist, the pH will *recover* to its original normal value. To examine the steady state response of NH_4Cl, we must use a *step* forcing, consisting of, say, 3 doses a day for as long as necessary to attain the steady state.

Guided by the block diagram, we start with a negative value for $\dot{F}$, the fortuitous influx of acid. The negative sign indicates that the fortuitous acid influx tends to reduce $[HCO_3^-]_p$ and hence $[HCO_3^-]_{40}$. This initiates a progressive fall in $[HCO_3^-]_{40}$, then pH_p, then pH_c. The latter initiates a progressive rise in renal excretion of acid, $+\dot{E}$, as a compensatory response. All these changes progress in magnitude until acid excretion matches acid ingestion; at this time the steady state is reached, though it may take a week or more. Now we find that $[HCO_3^-]_{40}$, pH_p, and pH_c are all low, as steady state errors, for it is the pH error that maintains the compensatory renal excretion.

Why did it take so long to reach the steady state? Not because of the kidney, for it responds promptly to changes in its own pH. The lag is due to the large $[HCO_3^-]_{40}$ pool, acting as a large alkaline reserve; the fortuitous influx of acid, even though continuous, was small compared to the size of the pool. What would have happened in the absence of control, i.e., with the feedback loop opened and $\dot{E}$ unadjustable? The persisting influx of acid would produce an endlessly falling $[HCO_3^-]_{40}$ and pH to zero, or death. Renal regulation is clearly a vital function.

Precisely analogous but opposite changes occur in metabolic alkalosis. To make sure you are getting the idea, trace through the block diagram in the same manner and analyze the renal response to such a disturbance.

Changes in $[K^+]_p$ produce *dissociated* metabolic acid-base disturbances. Guided by the block diagram, note that a rise in $[K^+]_p$, as by injection of K^+, will raise pH_c, lower acid excretion, or produce alkali excretion, thereby making $\dot{E}$ negative. Since $\dot{F}$, normally negative, is unchanged, their algebraic sum will be increasingly negative, causing $[HCO_3^-]_{40}$ and then pH_p to fall. In the steady state, there will be an extracellular metabolic acidosis, and an intracellular metabolic alkalosis.

RENAL CROSS-COMPENSATION

We have just seen that all the forcings that impinge *initially* on the renal regulator induce metabolic disturbances in acid-base balance, in spite of within-compensation by the renal regulator. As noted earlier, in the province of acid-base balance, this *within-compensation* is tacitly recognized, but is not called compensation; the latter term is reserved for what we here call *cross-compensation* between the two pH regulators. We learned that the pulmonary pH-regulator cross-compensates for metabolic disturbances arising in the renal pH-regulator. The abnormal pH_p induces a feedback adjustment of ventilation which corrects the pH_p, but only partially because of proportional control. This is called partial compensation (actually, partial cross-compensation). Furthermore, we saw that in metabolic disturbances, even with cross-compensation added to within-compensation, the correction of pH *was never complete*; there was only partial compensation. In fact, if the respiratory cross-compensation were somehow complete, disaster would result. The restoration of a normal pH would completely prevent renal within-compensation, and this would induce endlessly progressive and therefore fatal changes.

Let us now examine the reverse situation. All the forcings that impinge initially on the pulmonary regulator induce respiratory disturbances in acid-base balance, in spite of compensation *within* the pulmonary regulator. Again, this within-compensation is tacitly recognized, though it is not called compensation, but the cross-compensation provided by the renal regulator *is* called compensation. The abnormal pH_p induces a feedback adjustment of renal excretion which gradually corrects pH_p. Although the kidney *starts* the altered excretion immediately, it is *slow* in altering $[HCO_3^-]_{40}$ and pH_p. Accordingly, the respiratory disturbance may remain for some hours without detectable cross-compensation in the blood, though it is detectable in the urine. During this interval it is said to be uncompensated. Then, as time passes, the respiratory disturbance becomes partially compensated and eventually completely compensated, leaving *no steady state error*. The reason is that in response to pCO_2 forcing, the renal regulator operates by *integral* control. Let us see why.

Referring to the block diagram of the renal pH-regulator (Fig. 10-13), a respiratory disturbance consists of an abnormal pCO_2, elevated in acidosis, for example, with a low pH_p. The latter will lower pH_c, which will cause the kidneys to excrete extra acid ($\dot{E}$ becomes more positive). Since $\dot{F}$ is unaltered and normally negative, $\dot{HCO_3^-}$ becomes positive and $[HCO_3^-]_{40}$ begins to rise slowly, thereby slowly correcting pH_p. We might say the kidneys are inducing a *metabolic alkalosis* to counteract the *respiratory acidosis*. The key feature is that as long as pH_p is low, $[HCO_3^-]_{40}$ and pH_p will continue to rise, and this process cannot stop until pH_p is completely

corrected. At that time, $\dot{E}$ will have returned to normal and become
equal and opposite to $\dot{F}$. This is integral control, because the *rate*
of error correction is proportional to the *error*. Improvement must
continue as long as any error remains.

We found that complete respiratory cross-compensation for a
metabolic disturbance would be disastrous, but the reverse is not
true. Complete renal cross-compensation for a respiratory disturbance
has beneficial effects. Not only is the pH restored, but other errors
may undergo further correction. For example, restoration of pH in the
respiratory alkalosis that occurs during residence at high altitudes
removes the respiratory inhibition otherwise produced by alkalemia.
As a result, ventilation undergoes an additional compensatory increase,
further correcting the low pO_2. The pCO_2 will be further depressed,
but this alone (without alkalemia) is very well tolerated.

MECHANISMS OF RENAL pH REGULATION

Having just described the elements of renal regulation of
acid-base balance, we are now in a position to examine the mechanisms
involved in such a regulation.

As described in Chapter 4, the primary function of the kidney is
to *conserve* the major anions and cations of the body fluids, a
consequence of which is acid-base regulation. To maintain the total
quantities and concentrations of the major electrolytes within normal
limits, the kidneys must (a) stabilize the standard bicarbonate pool
by *obligatory* and *controlled* absorption of the filtered bicarbonate
and (b) excrete a daily load of 50 to 100 mEq of fixed (nonvolatile)
acids produced by metabolism. The fixed acids are excreted as
titratable acids and ammonium salts. The capacity of the kidneys
to perform these two functions is directly related to their ability
to stabilize the intra- and extracellular $[H^+]$ at normal levels. Let
us now examine the intrarenal mechanisms involved for each of these
functions.

1. OBLIGATORY BICARBONATE ABSORPTION IN THE PROXIMAL TUBULE

Normally 80 to 85% of the filtered bicarbonate is absorbed in
the proximal tubule. The key element of the absorption process is
the *exchange of hydrogen ions for sodium ions* across the luminal
border of the proximal cell membrane. As shown in Figure 10-14,
Na^+ moves across the luminal membrane down its electrochemical
gradient (depicted by the dashed arrow) into the cell. To maintain
electrical neutrality, H^+ is secreted actively (depicted by the circle
at the luminal membrane) from the cell into the tubular lumen
(Giebisch and Malnic, 1970). Once inside the tubule, H^+ combines
with the filtered HCO_3^- to form H_2CO_3. The carbonic acid thus formed

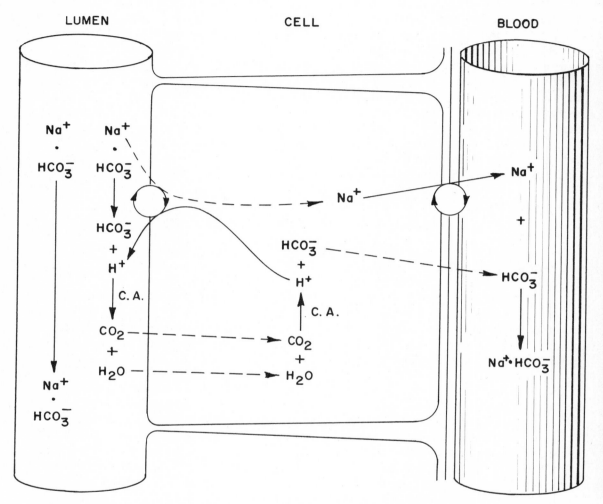

Figure 10-14. Scheme showing mechanism of obligatory bicarbonate absorption in the proximal tubule.

is readily dissociated into CO_2 and H_2O by the catalytic action of the enzyme *carbonic anhydrase* (CA), located in the tubular side of the luminal membrane (Rector et al., 1965). The presence of carbonic anhydrase at this site acts to reduce the steady-state concentration of carbonic acid that might otherwise limit H^+ secretion. The CO_2 thus formed in the lumen readily diffuses into the cell along its partial pressure gradient, and equilibrates with the CO_2 in the blood.

Because tubular H^+ is buffered by HCO_3^-, the entry of Na^+ into the cell must be electrically balanced by an anion. This is accomplished by either (a) passive diffusion of Cl^- down its electrochemical gradient, or (b) regeneration of HCO_3^- from cellular CO_2 and H_2O in the presence of carbonic anhydrase, with hydroxyl ion as its substrate (Maren, 1967). The result of either reaction leads to a net absorption of $NaHCO_3$ or $NaCl$ into the capillary blood. Note that Na^+ is absorbed by active process from the cell into the blood. This is depicted by the solid arrow and the circle on the peritubular side of the renal cell in Figure 10-14.

Similarly K^+ is absorbed as $KHCO_3$ or KCl into the capillary blood. However, it should be remembered (Chapter 8) that, in contrast to Na^+, the *transluminal* absorption of K^+ is *active* while *transcellular* transport is passive.

2. CONTROLLED BICARBONATE ABSORPTION IN THE DISTAL AND COLLECTING TUBULES

The remaining 10 to 15% of the filtered bicarbonate is absorbed mainly in the distal and collecting tubules by a mechanism which involves the *exchange of sodium ions for potassium or hydrogen ions*. The essence of this exchange mechanism, first proposed by Berliner and associates (1954), is illustrated in Figure 10-15. As shown, these authors postulated a "competitively shared" secretory pathway for hydrogen and potassium in exchange for sodium. This is depicted by the circle on the luminal side of the renal cell. Furthermore, they assumed that the intracellular $[H^+]$ and $[K^+]$ were the limiting factors in determining the competition between the net rate of active and passive secretion of H^+ and K^+, respectively, at the luminal pump in exchange for Na^+. As mentioned earlier, the intracellular $[H^+]$ and $[K^+]$ are in part determined by the plasma concentrations of these ions.

Except for the Na^+-H^+ and Na^+-K^+ exchange pump at the luminal border of the distal cell membrane, the reabsorptive pathways for bicarbonate are analogous to those described for the proximal tubule. Thus, as shown in Figure 10-15, the secreted H^+ ion combines with the filtered HCO_3^- to form H_2CO_3. The latter dissociates into CO_2 and H_2O. But unlike the proximal tubule, there is no luminal carbonic anhydrase involved in the dissociation reaction (Clapp et al., 1963). The CO_2 thus generated in the lumen diffuses into the cell and equilibrates with CO_2 in the blood. In the cell, the generated CO_2 is hydrated under the influence of carbonic anhydrase to yield HCO_3^- and H^+. The latter enters the secretory pathways, while the former is reabsorbed along with Na^+ into the blood. Also, as shown, the exchange of potassium for sodium leads to eventual reabsorption of 1 mole of $NaCl$ for every mole of $KHCO_3$ excreted. As mentioned in Chapter 8, the mechanism of Na^+-K^+ exchange on the peritubular side is by an active process and mediated by the Na^+-K^+ stimulated ATPase system (depicted by the circle in Fig. 10-15), while on the luminal side the Na^+-K^+ exchange occurs mainly by *electrical coupling* and is influenced by blood levels of aldosterone.

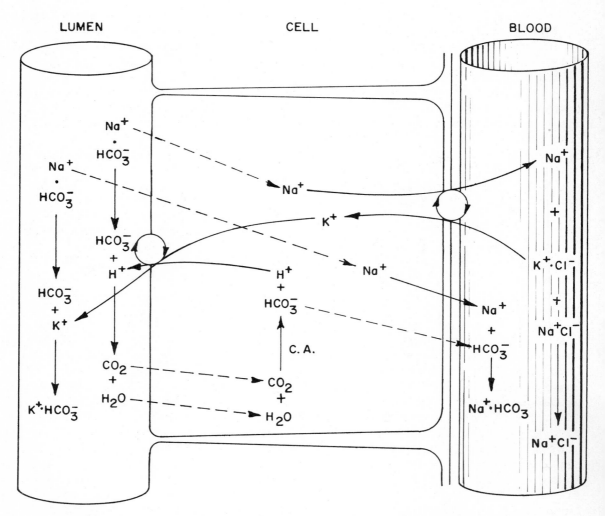

Figure 10-15. Scheme showing mechanism of controlled bicarbonate absorption in the distal and collecting tubules.

The Na^+-H^+ and K^+-H^+ ion exchange mechanisms are specialized to achieve different goals in the proximal and distal tubules. In the *proximal tubule*, a *large quantity* of hydrogen ions is exchanged for sodium or potassium ions against a low cell-to-lumen hydrogen ion concentration gradient. The net result is the absorption of nearly three fourths of the filtered $NaHCO_3$. In the *distal and collecting tubules*, a *small quantity* of hydrogen ions is exchanged for sodium ions against a high lumen-to-cell hydrogen ion concentration gradient. The net result is the absorption of the $NaHCO_3$, which escaped absorption in the proximal tubule.

Both obligatory and controlled bicarbonate absorption are influenced by at least five factors: (a) the "apparent" tubular reabsorptive capacity for bicarbonate, (b) the arterial pCO_2, (c) the plasma concentration of potassium, (d) the plasma concentration of chloride, and (e) the plasma levels of the adrenocortical hormones (glucocorticoids and mineralocorticoids). Let us examine the effects of each and their significance.

A. THE "APPARENT" TUBULAR REABSORPTIVE CAPACITY FOR BICARBONATE. Several earlier studies, using the previously described (Chapter 9) overall clearance methods and renal titration curves to characterize bicarbonate transport, demonstrated that the normal kidney handles bicarbonate transport as though there were a maximum tubular transport rate for this substance (Fig. 10-16). As shown, bicarbonate reabsorption increases linearly with increasing plasma concentration ($[HCO_3^-]_p$) until the latter reaches a value of about 25 mM/L, at which point the filtered load of the bicarbonate begins to exceed the tubular reabsorptive capacity. Thereafter, further increases in $[HCO_3^-]_p$ result in no further increase in tubular reabsorption, suggesting the existence of a tubular transport maximum ($\dot{T}m$) for bicarbonate.

Recent studies, however, have questioned the existence of a "true" $\dot{T}m$ for bicarbonate absorption. For example, Purkerson and associates (1969) found that in the rat the so-called maximum tubular transport capacity was highly sensitive to changes in GFR induced by expansion of the extracellular fluid volume, a procedure usually

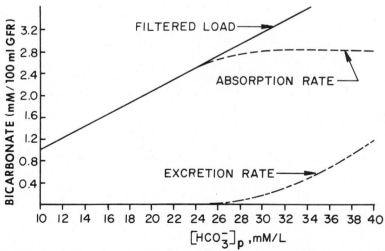

Figure 10-16. Renal reabsorption and excretion of bicarbonate as a function of the plasma concentration. [Redrawn from Pitts, R. F., Ayer, J. L., and Schiess, W. A. (1949).]

employed in $\dot{T}m$ determinations. Since expansion of extracellular volume is known to depress proximal sodium reabsorption and to reset the glomerular-tubular balance (Chapter 8), the possibility that the so-called "normal" patterns of titration curves for bicarbonate absorption (Fig. 10-16) may be an experimental artifact cannot be excluded. Similar conclusions have been reached by Slatopolsky and co-workers (1970) and Kurtzman (1970), who studied bicarbonate reabsorption in man and dog, respectively. Kurtzman (1970) found that expansion of the extracellular volume depressed bicarbonate reabsorption, and that this depression was related not to changes in GFR or $[HCO_3^-]_p$, but rather to the increase in the fractional sodium excretion. Although expansion of the extracellular volume decreased plasma potassium concentration, the depression of bicarbonate reabsorption was not related to the decrease in plasma potassium.

These findings strongly suggest that the net bicarbonate reabsorption is a function of GFR and hence of the degree of extracellular fluid (ECF) volume expansion: the reabsorption rate, and hence $\dot{T}m$, being high when ECF volume expansion is minimal, and low when ECF volume expansion is maximal, suggesting an *"apparent"* and not a *"true"* $\dot{T}m$ for renal transport of bicarbonate.

More recently, Bennett and associates (1975) have reinvestigated the renal titration curves for bicarbonate, and more specifically the effect of variations in GFR on its tubular reabsorption. In both hydropenic and ECF volume expanded dogs, they found a close functional relationship between the absolute rate of bicarbonate reabsorption and GFR at any plasma bicarbonate concentration. This tends to support the existence of an "apparent" but not a "true" $\dot{T}m$ for tubular reabsorption of bicarbonate. They have further suggested that the apparent reciprocal relationship between bicarbonate $\dot{T}m$ and ECF volume expansion observed previously and cited above might be due to an imperfect glomerular-tubular balance.

B. THE ARTERIAL pCO_2. A number of studies (Rector, 1973) have demonstrated that the apparent $\dot{T}m$ for the reabsorption of bicarbonate is very sensitive to changes in the arterial pCO_2. Thus, an increase in the arterial pCO_2 increases the apparent $\dot{T}m$ and, by the mechanisms depicted in Figure 10-14, increases the cellular regeneration of HCO_3^- and H^+. The resulting elevation of cellular $[H^+]$ increases the availability of H^+ for the Na^+-H^+ exchange process, thereby further increasing the cellular regeneration of HCO_3^- and its subsequent reabsorption into the blood. This relationship is illustrated in Figure 10-17. On the basis of these findings, Rector and associates (1960) have proposed that bicarbonate absorption may be mediated by two separate processes. One process has an apparent $\dot{T}m$ for HCO_3^- which is dependent on the arterial pCO_2 and independent of carbonic anhydrase activity. A second process is dependent on carbonic anhydrase and independent of the arterial pCO_2. Although these two processes can account for most of the bicarbonate reabsorbed by obligatory and controlled mechanisms, they lack direct experimental verification.

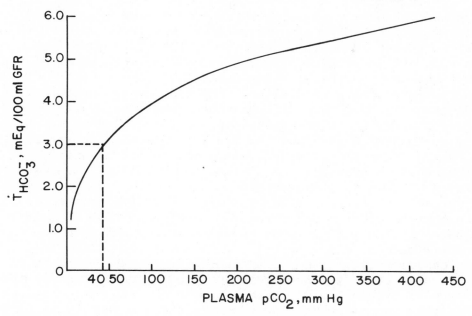

Figure 10-17. Relationship between net bicarbonate reabsorption, $\dot{T}_{HCO_3^-}$, and arterial pCO_2 in the dog. The curve approximates the experimental data obtained by Rector, F. C., Jr., Seldin, D. W., Roberts, A. D., Jr., and Smith, J. S. (1960).

The effect of arterial pCO_2 on net bicarbonate reabsorption represents the mechanism whereby the kidney cross-compensates for respiratory disturbances in acid-base balance. Thus, in *respiratory acidosis*, the rise in pCO_2 induces the kidneys, via the mechanism just described, to produce a metabolic alkalosis. Because of the integral control characterizing the renal cross-compensation, the kidneys will slowly increase $[HCO_3^-]_{40}$ by increasing HCO_3^- absorption as well as increasing acid excretion, thereby returning the blood back toward normal. Similarly, in *respiratory alkalosis*, the fall in pCO_2 decreases HCO_3^- absorption, thereby reducing $[HCO_3^-]_{40}$. Once again, because of the integral control, the kidneys slowly increase HCO_3^- excretion, thereby returning the blood pH back toward normal.

C. THE PLASMA CONCENTRATION OF POTASSIUM. A number of studies have shown that oral ingestion of potassium chloride (hyperkalemia) results in increased excretion of potassium bicarbonate in urine, and despite the development of the extracellular metabolic acidosis, the urine remains alkaline. This results in the so-called dissociated or "paradoxical" metabolic acid-base disturbance. Furthermore, it has been shown that administration of potassium salts produces a marked depression of HCO_3^- absorption, even when the filtered load of HCO_3^- is sufficient to saturate the reabsorptive mechanism (Fuller et al., 1955). This observed *inverse* relationship between the rate of HCO_3^- absorption and plasma potassium concentration (Fig. 10-18) is consistent with the view mentioned earlier that there appears to be a competition between K^+ and H^+ secretion by the distal tubule, and that the magnitude of ion secretion is related to the reciprocal of their concentrations in the renal tubular cells.

Changes in plasma potassium concentration, which produce dissociated metabolic acid-base disturbances, exert their effects on bicarbonate absorption in the distal and collecting tubules. As described in Chapter 8 and shown in Figure 10-15, hyperkalemia, induced by injection of potassium salt, produces three effects: (1) It enhances the transport of K^+ into the renal cells in exchange for cellular H^+ to maintain electrical neutrality. (2) This increased plasma hydrogen ion concentration is partly buffered by the plasma bicarbonate, resulting in the formation of H_2O and CO_2. The latter is eliminated by the lungs. Thus, hyperkalemia results in *extracellular metabolic acidosis*. (3) In the renal cells, the increased cellular potassium concentration favors the exchange of sodium with potassium; the latter is excreted as potassium bicarbonate. The increased filtered load of potassium and the associated anions (HCO_3^-) further augment renal excretion of $KHCO_3$. The result is the

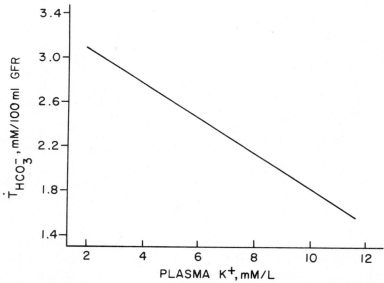

Figure 10-18. The relationship between net renal bicarbonate reabsorption, $\dot{T}_{HCO3}^-$, and plasma potassium concentration in the dog. The line approximates the experimental data obtained by Fuller, G. R., MacLeod, M. B., and Pitts, R. F. (1955).

formation of alkaline urine. In short, KCl loading results in *extracellular metabolic acidosis* accompanied by excretion of *alkaline urine*.

Of more clinical importance and interest is the reverse of the above condition, namely, *hypokalemic metabolic alkalosis*. The depletion of body stores of potassium due to diarrhea, vomiting, or hypersecretion of adrenal cortical hormones increases cellular hydrogen ion concentration at the expense of the plasma hydrogen ion concentration. The net result is the condition of *hypokalemic metabolic alkalosis* accompanied by excretion of acid urine.

In mild K^+ depletion, the contraction of the extracellular volume may be the underlying cause of alkalosis. Bicarbonate reabsorption can be decreased and hence alkalosis controlled by merely administering isotonic saline solution without supplementing K^+.

Recent micropuncture studies in rats, subjected to a variety of respiratory and metabolic acid-base disturbances, by Malnic and associates (1971, 1972) have further elucidated the roles of extracellular alkalosis and acidosis on K^+ and H^+ secretion by the distal tubules. These investigators found that the distal secretion of K^+ was *enhanced* in both respiratory and metabolic *alkalosis*, despite hypokalemia, while K^+ secretion was *depressed* in *acidosis*, despite hyperkalemia. Furthermore, the increase in K^+ secretion was associated with a rise in intratubular pH and hence a fall in intracellular pH. These findings in part confirm the K^+-H^+ competitive secretory concept and provide direct evidence that the intracellular H^+ ions determine the degree of K^+ secretion, while the intratubular bicarbonate load is the key factor determining the rate of H^+ secretion by the distal tubule.

D. THE PLASMA CONCENTRATION OF CHLORIDE. Like potassium, there is an inverse relationship between the plasma chloride concentration and the rate at which the filtered bicarbonate is reabsorbed. At present, the mechanism of this reciprocal relationship is not fully understood. One explanation may be the existence of the well-known *chloride-shift* in response to changes in HCO_3^- to maintain the electrical neutrality between the plasma and cell compartments. As a consequence of this reciprocal relationship, as plasma $[HCO_3^-]$ rises, $[Cl^-]$ in the plasma falls. This inverse relationship serves to maintain the sum of the plasma concentrations of bicarbonate and chloride approximately constant.

E. THE PLASMA LEVELS OF THE ADRENOCORTICAL HORMONES. The rate of bicarbonate reabsorption in the distal tubule is markedly influenced by changes in the secretion rate and blood levels of the adrenocortical hormones--glucocorticoids (cortisones) and mineralocorticoids (aldosterone). *Hypersecretion* of the adrenocortical hormones, as in Cushing's syndrome, and *hyperaldosteronism*, as in Conn's syndrome, both produce hypokalemia and hence dissociated extracellular *metabolic alkalosis*. The alkalosis is the result of the elevated plasma bicarbonate concentration caused by increased renal bicarbonate absorption (Fig. 10-18) and acid excretion. Conversely, *hyposecretion* of adrenocortical hormones or adrenal insufficiency, such as may occur in Addison's disease, results in hyperkalemia and hence extracellular *metabolic acidosis*, consequent to reduced renal bicarbonate absorption. In both these conditions, changes in bicarbonate absorption are secondary to hypo- and hyperkalemia produced by hyper- and hyposecretion of the adrenocortical hormones, respectively. The net effect is the development of a dissociated metabolic acid-base disturbance.

3. CONTROLLED EXCRETION OF TITRATABLE ACIDS AND AMMONIA

Absorption of Na^+ and K^+ along with HCO_3^- and Cl^- in the proximal tubule results in *no net gain* of H^+ by the tubular fluid. This is because the H^+ secreted is buffered mostly by the bicarbonate in the tubular fluid, thereby resulting in minimal acidification of urine by the end of this segment. The major sites of acidification of urine are the distal and collecting tubules. To understand the mechanism of acidification of urine by these segments, it should be recalled that in addition to HCO_3^- and Cl^-, the glomerular filtrate contains phosphate and sulfate, as well as organic acid anions.

Depletion of the standard bicarbonate pool results from the neutralization of strong acids, such as *sulfuric* and *phosphoric* acids, which are formed from the metabolism of dietary proteins and phospholipids. The neutralization of these acids results in the formation of CO_2, which is eliminated by the lungs, and the neutral salts (Na_2SO_4 and Na_2HPO_4), which are transported to the kidneys:

$$H_2SO_4 + 2NaHCO_3 \rightarrow Na_2SO_4 + 2H_2O + 2CO_2\uparrow \qquad (10-10)$$

$$H_3PO_4 + 2NaHCO_3 \rightarrow Na_2HPO_4 + 2H_2O + 2CO_2\uparrow \qquad (10-11)$$

The kidneys replenish the standard bicarbonate pool by excreting these neutral salts in two ways: (1) transformation into acid salts, by exchanging sodium ions with *ammonium ions*, and (2) conversion into free *titratable acids*, which can be excreted at the prevailing urinary pH. What determines by which method the kidney excretes the neutral salt is the difference between the pK_a of the salt and the hydrogen ion concentration of the tubular urine, or pH_u. The greater the ionization constant (K_a) for a given neutral salt, the smaller would be the pK_a. Thus, the larger the difference between pH_u and pK_a

$[(pH_u - pK_a)]$ the larger would be the quantity of the ionized neutral salt to be excreted. These salts are excreted exclusively as ammonium salts. Conversely, the smaller the ionization constant of the neutral salt, the larger would be the pK_a. Thus, the smaller the $(pH_u - pK_a)$, **the** smaller the quantity of the ionized neutral salts to be excreted. These salts can be excreted as titratable acids. For example, the sulfate salt, having a large ionization constant (low pK_a) is excreted as ammonium salt:

$$Na_2SO_4 + 2H_2CO_3 + 2NH_3 \rightarrow (NH_4)_2SO_4 + 2NaHCO_3 \qquad (10\text{-}12)$$

$$\text{(excreted)} \quad \text{(reabsorbed)}$$

while the phosphate salt, having a smaller ionization constant (high pK_a) is excreted as titratable acid:

$$Na_2HPO_4 + H_2CO_3 \rightarrow NaH_2PO_4 + NaHCO_3 \qquad (10\text{-}13)$$

$$\text{(excreted)} \quad \text{(reabsorbed)}$$

Therefore, the sum of the urinary excretion of titratable acid and ammonia is a measure of the total renal replacement of the standard bicarbonate pool.

Because chloride and sulfate anions are completely ionized at normal blood pH, they cannot be excreted as HCl or H_2SO_4. This is due to the fact that the presence of a small quantity of these acids in the urine, if not buffered, lowers the pH of tubular urine to a value of 1.0, which is far below the minimum pH of 4.5 generated by the distal tubular cells. Therefore, these anions must be excreted in combination with a substance which makes the tubular urine less acid. The kidney excretes chloride and sulfate anions in combination with ammonium ions (NH_4^+), which are readily produced by the distal and collecting tubular cells.

The normal kidney excretes almost twice as much acid combined with ammonia than it excretes titratable acid. However, as shown in Table 10-3, the diseased kidney excretes a lesser amount of acid combined with ammonia.

Let us now examine the mechanisms of formation of titratable acids and ammonium salts and their excretion in urine.

A. CONTROLLED EXCRETION OF TITRATABLE ACID. Formation and excretion of titratable acid is one process by which the kidney conserves Na^+ and replenishes the body bicarbonate pool and **thereby** **acidifies the urine.** The probable mechanism for this process is illustrated in Figure 10-19. The key element in the process is the

TABLE 10-3

Urinary Excretion of Acid in Man
in Health and Disease

Condition	mEq of Acid Excreted/Day	Ratio of Ammonia/Titratable Acid
1. Normal		
Acid combined with ammonia	30 - 50	
Titratable acid	10 - 30	1 - 2.5
2. Diabetic Ketosis		
Acid combined with ammonia	300 - 500	
Titratable acid	75 - 250	1 - 2.5
3. Chronic Renal Insufficiency		
Acid combined with ammonia	0.5 - 15	
Titratable acid	2.0 - 20	0.2 - 1.5

[From Pitts, R. F.: The renal regulation of acid base balance with special reference to the mechanism for acidifying the urine. I and II. *Science 102*:49-54, 81-85, July 20 and 27, 1945.]

quantity of filtered phosphate buffers. In the blood and hence the glomerular filtrate, the phosphate exists as both Na_2HPO_4 and NaH_2PO_4 with a concentration ratio ($[Na_2HPO_4]/[NaH_2PO_4]$) of 4:1. As shown, the exchange of hydrogen ions (produced from cellular hydration of CO_2) for sodium ions converts disodium phosphate (Na_2HPO_4) to monosodium phosphate (NaH_2PO_4), which is excreted as titratable acid in urine. This Na^+-H^+ exchange results in absorption of three of the nine Na^+ ions filtered, thereby altering the ($[Na_2HPO_4]/[NaH_2PO_4]$) ratio to 1:4 in the excreted urine. As a consequence of this exchange, sodium and bicarbonate are returned to the peritubular capillary blood, thereby replenishing the body stores of bicarbonate.

The rate of formation of titratable acid and its subsequent excretion are influenced by at least four factors: (1) the amount of buffer anions filtered and remaining in the tubular lumen; (2) the pK_a of these buffers; (3) the concentration of hydrogen ions in the tubular fluid; and (4) the plasma hydrogen ion concentration. Thus, the greater the filtered load of buffer anions and the closer their pK_a to pH_u, the greater is the quantity of the titratable acid excreted. Furthermore, the greater the hydrogen ion concentration in the blood (the lower the pH_p), as in acidosis, and hence that in the ultrafiltrate, the greater would be the rate of Na^+-H^+ exchange and ultimately the greater the reabsorption of $NaHCO_3$ into the blood.

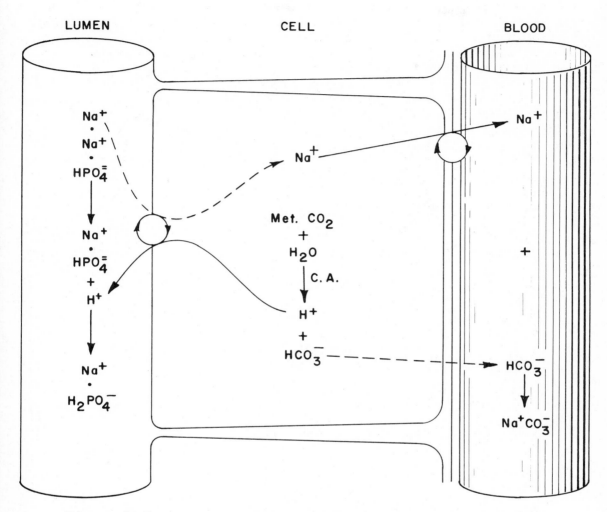

Figure 10-19. Scheme showing mechanism of controlled excretion of titratable acid in the distal and collecting tubules.

B. CONTROLLED EXCRETION OF AMMONIUM SALT. If the excretion of titratable acid were the only mechanism for renal acidification of urine, the magnitude of acid excretion would be limited by the amount of filtered phosphate buffers. That the kidney can excrete considerably more acid than can be accounted for by the amount of excreted titratable acid, even though the urinary pH normally would not fall below 4.5, is indicative that another process exists by which the kidney acidifies urine. This process is the formation of ammonia for the excretion of highly ionized neutral salts as ammonium salts, which in the process conserves sodium and replenishes the body bicarbonate pool. The mechanism of ammonia production and excretion of the ammonium salt is illustrated in Figure 10-20. As shown, the key element is the formation of ammonia within the renal cell mainly from glutamine extracted from the peritubular blood. The deamidation and deamination of each mole of glutamine, in the presence of the enzyme glutaminase, yields two moles of un-ionized ammonia (NH_3). In the tubular cells 99% of the ammonia thus produced exists as ammonium ions (NH_4^+), and only 1% as free NH_3. The un-ionized NH_3 is lipid-soluble and can diffuse freely across the renal cell membranes into the blood or lumen. In contrast, the ionized NH_4^+ is water-soluble and can diffuse much less readily from the cell into the lumen or peritubular blood. But as rapidly as one molecule

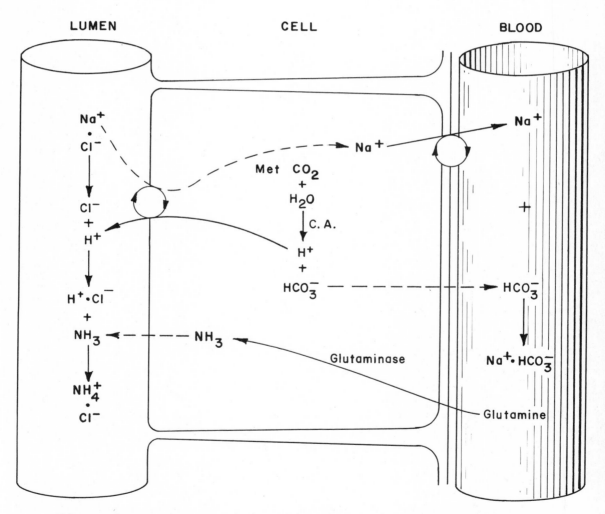

Figure 10-20. Scheme showing mechanism of controlled excretion of ammonium ions in the distal and collecting tubules.

of NH_3 diffuses out of the cell, it is immediately replaced by another molecule of NH_3 from dissociation of H^+ from NH_4^+:

$$NH_4^+ \rightarrow NH_3 + H^+ \qquad\qquad (10-14)$$

The H^+ ions thus produced become part of the cellular H^+ pool and therefore available for secretion into the lumen.

According to Brønstedt formulation, NH_4^+ is considered an acid because it yields an H^+ in alkaline solution, while NH_3 is considered a base because it accepts H^+ in acid solution. Therefore, as soon as the un-ionized NH_3 enters the lumen, it binds with H^+ and becomes *trapped* within the lumen as a relatively nondiffusible NH_4^+. In this manner, cellular ammonia is secreted into the lumen by passive *nonionic diffusion* without the expenditure of energy to maintain cell-to-urine pH gradient. This asymmetric diffusibility of NH_3 and NH_4^+ and the high pK of the NH_3/NH_4^+ buffer system (pK = 9.2) are, therefore, well-suited for Na^+-H^+ exchange with a minimum lowering of urinary pH.

The *nonionic diffusion* of ammonia just described exemplifies a common biological phenomenon in which the lipid-soluble component of a buffer pair (e.g., NH_3) can readily diffuse across the cell membrane, while its water-soluble component (e.g., NH_4^+) cannot. Such a process has potential clinical importance in promoting renal excretion of weak acids and bases. A notable example is its application in the treatment of phenobarbital poisoning (Valtin, 1973). The treatment involves intravenous infusion of mannitol and $NaHCO_3$ solutions. Infusion of the poorly absorbable mannitol will induce osmotic diuresis (Chapter 8), thereby reducing tubular reabsorption of phenobarbital. Infusion of $NaHCO_3$ will alkalinize the glomerular filtrate, thereby further reducing the passive reabsorption of the phenobarbital, a weak acid, by the nonionic diffusion process.

Although ammonia production and secretion are normally confined to the distal and collecting tubules, a number of recent studies (Pitts, 1973) have shown that in acidosis the proximal tubule can also produce and secrete ammonia. These same studies have further shown that the rate of ammonia secretion is influenced by at least three factors: (1) the degree of urinary acidity, (2) the degree of acidosis, and (3) the relative rates of flow of tubular fluid and peritubular capillary blood.

1. The effect of urinary pH on the net ammonia excretion ($\dot{E}_{NH_3}$) (production and secretion) is illustrated in Figure 10-21. As shown, during both normal acid-base state and metabolic acidosis, there is an inverse relationship between $\dot{E}_{NH_3}$ and pH_u. Thus, the lower the urinary pH (the more acid the urine), the greater is the net ammonia excretion.

2. Figure 10-21 also illustrates the effect of severity of acidosis on the rate of net ammonia excretion. It shows that for any given urinary pH, the rate of net ammonia excretion is higher during acidosis than during normal acid-base state. The increase in $\dot{E}_{NH_3}$

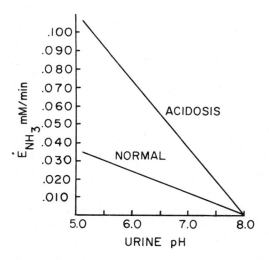

Figure 10-21. The relation between ammonia excretion, $\dot{E}_{NH_3}$ and urine pH in a single animal under conditions of normal acid-base balance and chronic acidosis. Urine pH was varied by intravenous infusion of $NaHCO_3$. [Redrawn from Pitts, R. F. (1948).]

during acidosis is most probably due to adaptive increase in renal production and secretion of ammonia and to a lesser extent to increased nonionic NH_3 diffusion and its luminal trapping. Thus, Lotspeich (1967) found that in NH_4Cl acidosis, a condition known to increase ammonia excretion, renal extraction of glutamine from peritubular blood was increased in rat, dog and man. Furthermore, in rat, he found a parallel adaptive increase in the synthesis of the enzyme glutaminase. The increase in ammonia excretion during NH_4Cl acidosis was found to be mediated by NH_4Cl-stimulation of DNA-dependent RNA synthesis by the kidney. Despite these and other extensive studies, the mechanism of adaptive increase in renal ammonia excretion in acidosis is at present not fully understood.

3. Besides urinary pH, the rate of diffusion of cellular NH_3 into the lumen is determined by the relative rates of flow of tubular fluid and peritubular blood. If the tubular fluid had the same pH as the blood, the peritubular blood, by virtue of its greater flow rate, would provide a favorable sink for diffusion of cellular NH_3. However, the slow tubular flow rate is more than offset by its lower pH, as compared to blood, for it makes it possible for 75% of the NH_3 produced within the renal cell to be diffused into the lumen and only 25% to be carried off by the blood. Of course, the situation can be reversed by any condition that causes the pH of the tubular fluid to approach or exceed the pH of the blood.

We conclude this section with a synthesis of the foregoing components of the intrarenal mechanisms of pH regulation, yielding the block diagram shown in Figure 10-22. Examination of this diagram reveals three important features of the renal pH regulator: (1) The intracellular $[H^+]$ is the main factor determining renal excretion of acid or alkali. (2) All variations in renal excretion of acid or alkali translate into variations in HCO_3^- ions entering renal blood. (3) Excretion of HCO_3^- may deplete body K^+.

Table 10-4 summarizes the responses of the renal pH regulator to some selected forcings already mentioned. It is clear that the *renal cell pH* is the key factor determining the renal excretion of acids or alkalis.

TABLE 10-4

Responses of the Renal pH Regulator to Some Selected Forcings

	Forcing	Condition	Plasma pH	Renal Cell pH	Urine
1.	NH_4Cl ingestion	Metabolic Acidosis	↓	↓	Aciduria
2.	CO_2 inhalation (acute)	Respiratory Acidosis	↓	↓	Aciduria
3.	K^+ depletion	Hypokalemic Alkalosis	↑	↓	Aciduria
4.	$NaHCO_3$ ingestion	Metabolic Alkalosis	↑	↑	Alkaluria
5.	Voluntary hyperventilation	Respiratory Alkalosis	↑	↑	Alkaluria
6.	K^+ injection	Hyperkalemic Acidosis	↓	↑	Alkaluria

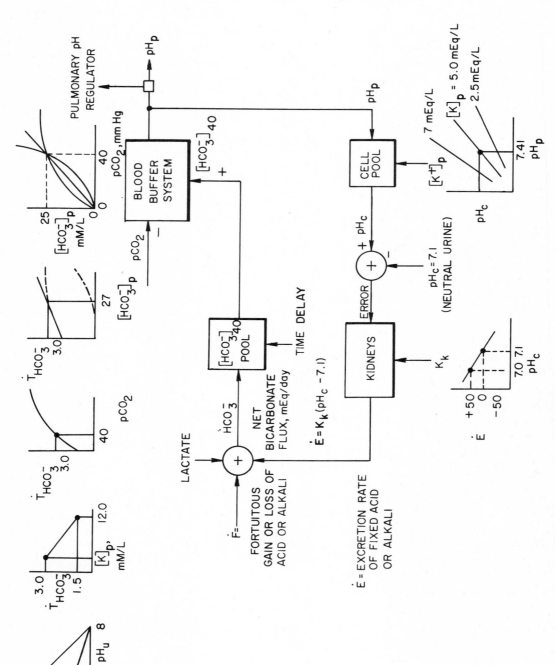

Figure 10-22. Synthesis of the renal pH regulator.

THE DUAL pH-REGULATOR: DISTURBANCES IN ACID-BASE BALANCE AND THEIR DIAGNOSES

From the foregoing analysis, it is clear that the ultimate regulation of acid-base balance entails coordinated, integrated function of the blood buffers and the pulmonary and the renal systems. Having studied the response characteristics of each system in isolation, we are now in a position to consider their combined response to acid-base disturbances, much the same way they operate in vivo in the body. For this purpose, we use the system's functional block diagram to analyze the mechanisms of within- and cross-compensation, and the $[HCO_3^-]_p$-pCO_2-pH plot to diagnose the disturbances in acid-base balance and as an aid in following the recovery and response to treatment.

Figure 10-23 presents the functional diagram of the dual pH-regulator. Note that the blood buffer system is shared by both the pulmonary and renal pH-regulators. To analyze the response of the dual pH-regulator to any acid-base disturbances, it is most helpful to proceed in two steps. First, analyze the within-compensation of the regulator to the forcing impinging on it. Then, if the forcing persists, proceed to analyze the cross-compensation from the other regulator. In such an analysis, you should recall that initial forcings for a *respiratory disturbance* in acid-base balance always impinge on the pulmonary system, which induces a within-compensated disturbance in pCO_2 and pH_p. If this disturbance persists, the renal pH-regulator cross-compensates by adjusting $[HCO_3^-]_{40}$, *slowly* but eventually completely. In contrast, the initial forcings for a *metabolic disturbance* in acid-base balance always impinge on the renal system, which induces a within-compensated disturbance in $[HCO_3^-]_{40}$ and hence pH_p. This disturbance induces *immediate* but *partial* cross-compensation from the pulmonary pH-regulator.

To diagnose disturbances in acid-base balance and to follow the recovery and response to treatment, we use the $[HCO_3^-]_p$-pCO_2-pH plot, similar to that shown in Figures 10-8 and 10-24. For this purpose, we need to elaborate further on some of the main features of such a plot germane to the present discussion.

The *normal respiratory pathway* is the familiar *in vitro* CO_2 absorption curve of true plasma. It identifies the blood response to changes in pCO_2 when $[HCO_3^-]_{40}$ is constant at 25 mM/L. Note that there is a whole family of CO_2 absorption curves, one for each level of $[HCO_3^-]_{40}$ other than 25 mM/L. In Figure 10-24, we have plotted two such curves, labelled high-gain and low-gain respiratory pathways. The data used to plot these, as well as the normal curve, are given in Table 10-5.

It should be apparent that at any moment a patient's blood pattern may lie on one of these curves. For each case, if we wish to know the value of $[HCO_3^-]_{40}$, we simply move along the patient's respiratory pathway to where the curve intersects with the iso-$pCO_2 = 40$ mm Hg line. Graphically, this procedure is

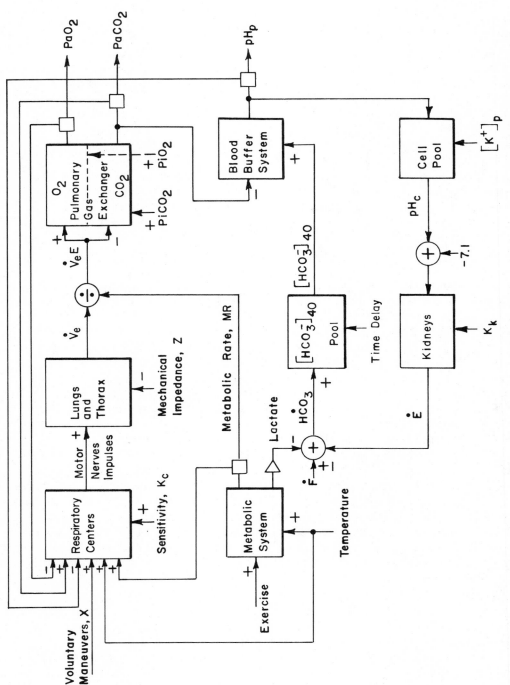

Figure 10-23. A functional block diagram of the dual pH-regulator.

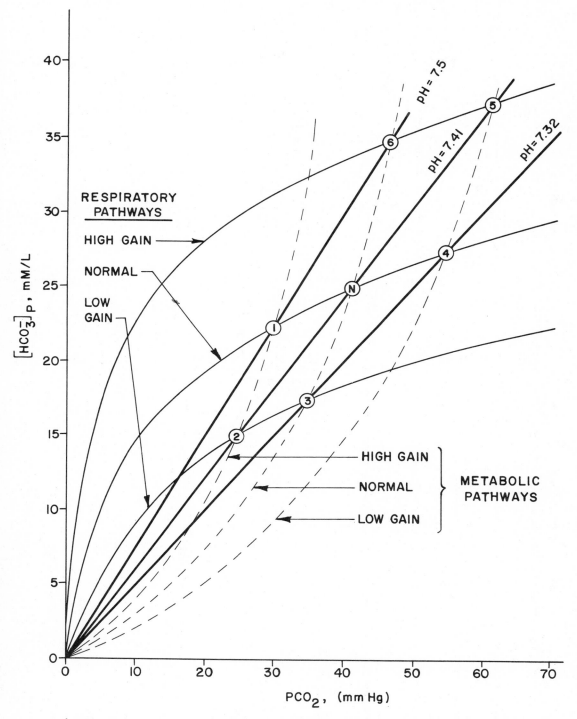

Figure 10-24. Respiratory and metabolic pathways drawn for data listed in Table 10-5. The three radiating iso-pH lines were obtained by drawing a straight line from the origin to these points: $pCO_2 = 48$ and $[HCO_3^-]_p = 37$; $pCO_2 = 59$ and $[HCO_3^-]_p = 37$; and $pCO_2 = 70$ and $[HCO_3^-]_p = 36$, respectively.

TABLE 10-5

Bicarbonate Concentration and pCO_2 Values for True Plasma Used to Plot Respiratory and Metabolic Pathways in Figure 11-24

Respiratory Pathways

pCO_2 (mm Hg)	Normal $[HCO_3^-]_{40}$	Low $[HCO_3^-]_{40}$	High $[HCO_3^-]_{40}$
	[HCO₃⁻]ₚ mM/L		
0	0	0	0
2.5	7.5	3.5	12.5
5.0	10.0	6.0	17.5
10.0	15.0	9.0	22.5
15.0	17.5	11.5	26.5
20.0	19.0	13.5	28.5
25.0	21.0	15.0	30.0
30.0	22.5	16.5	31.5
35.0	23.5	17.5	32.5
40.0	25.0	18.0	34.0
45.0	26.0	19.5	35.0
50.0	27.0	20.5	36.0
55.0	28.0	21.0	37.0
60.0	28.5	21.5	38.0
65.0	29.5	22.0	38.5
70.0	30.0	22.5	39.0

Metabolic Pathways

pCO_2 (mm Hg)	Normal gain	High gain	Low gain
	[HCO₃⁻]ₚ mM/L		
0	0	0	0
5.0	1.5	2.0	1.0
10.0	3.0	4.0	2.0
15.0	5.0	7.5	3.0
20.0	7.5	10.0	5.0
25.0	10.0	15.5	7.0
30.0	14.0	23.5	9.0
35.0	17.5	36.5	12.0
40.0	25.0		15.0
45.0	35.0		18.5
50.0			22.5
55.0			30.0
60.0			37.5

[Modified from Gray, J. S. (1968).]

analogous to exposing the patient's blood sample to pCO_2 = 40 mm Hg and determining its $[HCO_3^-]$. Moreover, if we wish to know what changes occur in the patient's blood pattern when the pulmonary regulator raises (hypoventilation) or lowers (hyperventilation) pCO_2 without renal cross-compensation (i.e., $[HCO_3^-]_{40}$ is constant), we simply move to the right (as for example from point N to point 4 in Figure 10-24) or to the left (from point N to point 1), respectively, along the patient's respiratory pathway.

The normal respiratory pathway, for which $[HCO_3^-]_{40}$ = 25 mM/L, represents the *completely uncompensated* (no renal cross-compensation) respiratory pathway. On the other hand, the radiating iso-pH = 7.41 line represents the *completely cross-compensated* respiratory pathway.

The other two curves, labelled high-gain and low-gain respiratory pathways, are followed during pulmonary cross-compensation for metabolic alkalosis and acidosis. The term "gain" here refers to the level of $[HCO_3^-]_{40}$: high-gain refers to elevated $[HCO_3^-]_{40}$, as in metabolic alkalosis, and low-gain refers to reduced $[HCO_3^-]_{40}$, as in metabolic acidosis. Thus, in metabolic acidosis, in which $[HCO_3^-]_{40}$ is reduced, the pulmonary cross-compensation causes the blood to move along a low-gain respiratory pathway toward the iso-pH = 7.41 line. As was shown in Figure 10-8, the combined effects of the metabolic acidosis and the induced respiratory alkalosis (partial pulmonary cross-compensation) are that the blood moves down along the curve labelled "normal metabolic pathway," such as that depicted by the curve connecting the normal point N to point 3 in Figure 10-24. Precisely analogous but opposite changes occur in metabolic alkalosis, so that the blood moves up along the normal metabolic pathway, such as that depicted by the curve connecting point N to point 6. Note that because changes in pH and pCO_2 have opposite effects on the respiratory center (Fig. 10-23) in both metabolic acidosis and alkalosis, there will only be a partial cross-compensation by the pulmonary regulator.

The *normal metabolic pathway* just described identifies the blood response to changes in $[HCO_3^-]_{40}$ when the gain for the pulmonary cross-compensation is constant. The term "gain" here refers to the state of pulmonary ventilation. Like the respiratory pathways, there is a whole family of metabolic pathways, depending on the *ventilatory state or gain* of the pulmonary cross-compensation. In Figure 10-24, we have plotted two such curves, labelled high-gain and low-gain metabolic pathways, respectively.

The curve labelled the high-gain (or hyperventilatory) metabolic pathway is followed during renal cross-compensation for respiratory alkalosis, which is initiated by some respiratory *stimulation* other than changes in pH or pCO_2. Examples include high altitude, anoxia, fever, and hysterical hyperventilation, all of which increase ventilation, yielding a lower pCO_2 for a given $[HCO_3^-]_{40}$. Thus, in chronic respiratory alkalosis, such as may occur during temporary residence at high altitudes (point 1, Fig. 10-24), the renal regulator will slowly but eventually completely cross-compensate for the alkalosis by inducing a *metabolic acidosis*, thereby returning the pH back toward normal. In Figure 10-24, this is depicted by moving the blood from point 1 to point 2, along the high-gain metabolic pathway.

The curve labelled the low-gain (or hypoventilatory) metabolic pathway is followed during renal cross-compensation for respiratory acidosis, which is initiated by some respiratory *inhibition* other than changes in pH or pCO_2. Examples include emphysema, asthma, chronic partial obstruction of airway, and depression of the respiratory centers, all of which reduce ventilation yielding a high pCO_2 for a given $[HCO_3^-]_{40}$. Thus, in chronic respiratory acidosis, such as may occur in pulmonary obstruction (point 4 in Fig. 10-24), the renal regulator will slowly but eventually completely cross-compensate for the acidosis by inducing a *metabolic alkalosis*, thereby returning the pH back toward normal. In Figure 10-24, this is depicted by moving the blood from point 4 to point 5, along the low-gain metabolic pathway. The only exception is the respiratory acidosis induced by *CO_2 inhalation*, which causes hyperventilation and hypercapnia. Although the pulmonary gain appears to be increased (hyperventilation), the renal cross-compensation follows the low-gain (hypoventilatory) pathway.

Thus, any patient's blood at any moment must lie on one of these families of metabolic pathways. If we wish to know the gain of the pulmonary cross-compensation, we simply note whether the patient's blood pattern lies to the left or to the right of the "normal metabolic pathway." Furthermore, if we wish to know what changes occur in the patient's blood pattern when the renal regulator raises or lowers $[HCO_3^-]_{40}$, we simply follow the normal metabolic pathway up or down, respectively. It should be remembered that in Figure 10-24, the radiating iso-pH line of 7.41 represents also the *completely cross-compensated* metabolic pathway, while the iso-pCO_2 = 40 mm Hg line represents no cross-compensation. Since respiratory cross-compensation for metabolic disturbances is immediate but only partial, the actual pathway followed is along neither the iso-pH = 7.41 line nor the iso-pCO_2 = 40 mm Hg line, but somewhere in between, namely the "normal metabolic pathway." Thus, the normal metabolic pathway represents *partially cross-compensated* metabolic pathway by the pulmonary regulator with a normal gain.

Using the functional diagram of the dual pH-regulator shown in Figure 10-23 and the respiratory and metabolic pathways shown in Figure 10-24, it is now easy to follow the development, compensation, recovery, or response to treatment in acid-base disturbances. To facilitate the use of the graph in Figure 10-24 in conjunction with the problems at the end of this chapter, the graph is divided into a number of areas demarcated by intersection of the various pathways, each defining a type of disturbance in acid-base balance. For any point plotted on this graph, such as those numbered 1 through 6, we can read off five pieces of information: $[HCO_3^-]_p$, pCO_2, pH, $[HCO_3^-]_{40}$, and the pulmonary gain. From this information, we can readily diagnose the disturbances in acid-base balance as acidosis or alkalosis, respiratory or metabolic or both, uncompensated, and partially or completely cross-compensated. Note that if both respiratory and metabolic acidosis (or alkalosis) are present, neither can or will be cross-compensated. Furthermore, since the graph in Figure 10-24 pertains only to plasma, it cannot at the same time display the cellular behavior in *dissociated* metabolic acid-base disturbances.

Now to help you discover for yourself the *simplicity* of diagnosing disturbances in acid-base balance and to master the materials presented, we end this chapter with a number of problems [taken in part from Gray (1968)]. To work out these problems, use the $[HCO_3^-]_p$-pCO_2-pH graph (Fig. 10-24) in conjunction with the block diagram of the dual pH-regulator. Remember that whenever the block diagram dictates a change in $[HCO_3^-]_{40}$, follow a metabolic pathway, and whenever it dictates a change in pCO_2, follow a respiratory pathway.

PROBLEMS

10-1. If a subject on the normal respiratory pathway has a pCO_2 of 40 mm Hg, (a) what is the pH? _____. (b) $[HCO_3^-]_p$? _____. (c) $[HCO_3^-]_{40}$? _____.

10-2. If he breathes CO_2 for 45 min to elevate his pCO_2 to 53.5 mm Hg, (a) what is the pH? _____. (b) $[HCO_3^-]_p$? _____. (c) $[HCO_3^-]_{40}$? _____. (d) Is this an acidemia, or alkalemia? _____. (e) Acidosis or alkalosis? _____. (f) Metabolic or respiratory? _____. (g) Compensated or uncompensated? _____. (h) A displacement on the normal respiratory pathway, or shift to a new one? _____.

10-3. If he voluntarily hyperventilates for 45 min to lower his pCO_2 to 29 mm Hg, (a) what is the pH? _____. (b) $[HCO_3^-]_p$? _____. (c) $[HCO_3^-]_{40}$? _____. (d) Is this an acidemia, or alkalemia? _____. (e) Acidosis or alkalosis? _____. (f) Metabolic or respiratory? _____. (g) Compensated or uncompensated? _____. (h) Displacement on the normal respiratory pathway, or shift to a new one? _____.

10-4. In the above examples, (a) do pH and pCO_2 vary together or oppositely? _____. (b) Do $[HCO_3^-]_p$ and pCO_2 vary together or oppositely? _____. (c) Can $[HCO_3^-]_p$ change without change in $[HCO_3^-]_{40}$? _____.

10-5.   (a) What is the $[HCO_3^-]_{40}$ for the higher curve? _____.
(b) The lower? _____.   (c) What kind of primary
disturbance would shift a person to one of these curves?
_____.   (d) Compensation for what kind of
disturbance would shift a person to one of these curves?
_____.

10-6.   A normal person develops a metabolic acidosis sufficient
to reduce his $[HCO_3^-]_{40}$ to 19 mM/L.   (a) If his respiratory
regulator made no cross-compensation, what pathways would
he follow? _____.   What would his pCO_2 be?
_____. $[HCO_3^-]_p$? _____.   pH? _____.
(b) If now his respiratory regulator is allowed to respond,
what pathway would he follow? _____.
What would his pCO_2 become? _____. $[HCO_3^-]_p$? _____.
pH? _____.   (c) Would he normally follow this "dog-leg"
pathway? _____.   Why? _____.
(d) What pathway will he actually follow? _____.

10-7.   A normal person develops a metabolic alkalosis sufficient
to raise his $[HCO_3^-]_{40}$ to 34 mM/L.   (a) If his respiratory
regulator made no cross-compensation, what pathway would
he follow? _____.   What would his pCO_2 be? _____.
$[HCO_3^-]_p$? _____.   pH? _____.   (b) If now his respiratory
regulator is allowed to respond, what pathway would he follow?
_____.   What would his pCO_2 become?
_____. $[HCO_3^-]_p$? _____.   pH? _____.   (c) Would he
normally follow this "dog-leg" pathway? _____.
Why? _____.   (d) What pathway will he
actually follow? _____.

10-8.   A normal person rides swiftly on a train from sea level to
an altitude which induces hyperventilation sufficient to
lower his pCO_2 to 29 mm Hg.   (a) What pathway did he follow?
_____.   (b) Identify the
disturbances in acid-base balance (i.e., respiratory or
metabolic, acidosis or alkalosis, uncompensated, partially
compensated, or fully compensated). _____.

10-9.   This person now remains at altitude for the next month.
(a) Does the initial cause persist? _____.
(b) Will compensation occur? _____.   (c) What regulator
will compensate? _____.   (d) Is it fast or slow? _____.
(e) Will the pH be corrected to normal? _____.   (f) What
input to the blood buffer system will be adjusted? _____.
(g) What pathway will be followed? _____.
(h) What will the steady state pH be? _____. $[HCO_3^-]_p$? _____.
$[HCO_3^-]_{40}$? _____. pCO_2? _____.   (i) Identify the
disturbance in acid-base balance. _____.   (j) Is he
hyperventilating more, or less, than when he arrived? _____.
(k) Is his pO_2 correction better, or worse, than when he
arrived? _____.

10-10.   This person now returns swiftly by train to sea level.
(a) Does this correct the initial cause? _____.
(b) What is his $[HCO_3^-]_{40}$? _____.   (c) Will his
hyperventilation disappear, or merely moderate?_____.
(d) What pathway did he follow? _____.   (e) What
is his pCO_2? _____.   pH? _____. $[HCO_3^-]_p$? _____.
(f) Identify this disturbance in acid-base balance.
_____.

10-11.   This person now remains at sea level for the next month.
(a) What will his $[HCO_3^-]_{40}$ do now? _____.
(b) What pathway will he follow? _____.
(c) What will his pH be? _____. $[HCO_3^-]_p$? _____.
pCO_2? _____.   (d) Was this fast or slow? _____.
(e) Have we gone full circle? _____.

10-12.   To make sure you are getting the idea, trace through in
the same four steps the case of a person who has a sudden,
persistent respiratory depression, which later on is
suddenly corrected.

10-13.   (a) In what disturbances of acid-base balance may the pH
be normal? _____.   (b) In what
disturbance may the pCO_2 be low? _____.
(c) In what disturbances may the $[HCO_3^-]_{40}$ be low? _____
_____.   (d) In what disturbances may the
renal excretion of acid be high? _____.
(e) Can you fully diagnose the type of disturbance from any
one of these? _____.

10-14.   Now that you have become familiar with the graph, it can be
simplified to three lines (Fig. 10-8), each running through
the normal point; the normal pH line, the normal respiratory
pathway, and the normal metabolic pathway.   For any point
plotted on such a graph you can tell whether pCO_2 is high or
low, pH is high or low, and $[HCO_3^-]_{40}$ is high or low.   From
this information you can diagnose any single disturbance and
any combination of disturbances in acid-base balance.

10-15.   Suppose a patient with a low $[HCO_3^-]_{40}$ was diagnosed as
having metabolic acidosis, when it was really a compensated
respiratory alkalosis; the patient was therefore given
$NaHCO_3$ by mouth.   (a) What pathway will be followed? _____
_____.   (b) What will happen to the pH?
_____.   (c) Does this help or hinder?
_____.

10-16.   Suppose a patient with a low pCO_2 was diagnosed as having
respiratory alkalosis, when it was really a metabolic acidosis;
the patient was therefore given CO_2 to breathe.   (a) What
pathway will be followed? _____.   (b) What will happen to
the pH? _____.   (c) Does this help or hinder? _____.

10-17.   The table below gives the blood gas findings for a normal
person and for eight patients with acid-base disturbances
(none breathing CO_2).

Patients	pCO_2 (mm Hg)	$[HCO_3^-]_p$ (mM/L)	$[HCO_3^-]_{40}$ (mM/L)	pH
Normal	40	25.0	25.0	7.41
1	45	35.0	33.0	7.50
2	60	37.5	33.0	7.41
3	54	27.5	25.0	7.32
4	47	20.0	18.5	7.25
5	35	17.5	18.5	7.32
6	25	15.0	18.5	7.41
7	29	22.0	25.0	7.50
8	33	32.0	33.0	7.60

Using the data in this table in conjunction with the plot
shown in Figure 10-24, answer the following questions:

(1)   Which patient has:
   a.   A fully compensated respiratory alkalosis? _____
   b.   A fully compensated respiratory acidosis? _____
   c.   A partially compensated metabolic alkalosis? _____
   d.   A partially compensated metabolic acidosis? _____
   e.   An uncompensated respiratory alkalosis? _____
   f.   An uncompensated respiratory acidosis? _____
   g.   A combined respiratory and metabolic acidosis? _____
   h.   A combined respiratory and metabolic alkalosis? _____
(2)   Which patient(s), if any, would you expect to be excreting
   acid _____ or alkali _____ in his urine, relative to
   normal?
(3)   If patients 1 and 5 in the table had a dissociated
   acid-base disturbance, which one would you expect to be
   excreting acid _____ or alkali _____ in his urine?
(4)   Which patient(s)'s blood pattern(s) lie(s) on a high
   gain _____ or low gain _____ metabolic pathway?
(5)   Which patient(s)'s blood pattern(s) lie(s) on a high
   gain _____ or low gain _____ respiratory pathway?
(6)   Which patient(s), if any, have acidemia _____ or
   alkalemia _____?
(7)   Which patient(s), if any, have elevated $[HCO_3^-]_{40}$? _____
(8)   Which patient(s), if any, have reduced $[HCO_3^-]_{40}$? _____
(9)   Starting with the normal point (N) in Figure 10-24 and
   using the numbers on this graph, indicate the *sequential
   changes* in blood pattern which occur in (1) sudden
   respiratory obstruction _____, (2) lasting a month _____,
   (3) sudden removal of the obstruction _____, and (4) a
   month later _____.

(10) Which patient(s), if any, would benefit if given NH_4Cl? _____

(11) Which patient(s), if any, would benefit if given $NaHCO_3$? _____

(12) Which patient(s), if any, represent a person in the apneic stage of asphyxia? _____

10-18. In the preceding problems, you were asked to diagnose disturbances in acid-base balance and to follow recovery and response to treatment using the now familiar $[HCO_3^-]_p$-pCO_2-pH diagram shown in Figure 10-24 in conjunction with the functional diagram shown in Figure 10-23. However, you will find that in many older writings in the literature and textbooks dealing with the subject of acid-base physiology, the $[HCO_3^-]_p$-pH diagram shown in Figure 10-23 is used instead. Therefore, you should attempt to answer the questions posed in the preceding problems using this diagram. The data needed to plot such a diagram are given below. It may prove to be a rewarding and eye-opening experience that you have learned about the simplicity of acid-base physiology the new way!

Data for Plotting True Plasma Buffer Curve

pH	$[HCO_3^-]_p$ (mM/L)
7.16	29.7
7.35	25.0
7.46	23.0
7.57	20.8

Data for Plotting pCO_2 = 40 mm Hg Isobar

pH	$[HCO_3^-]_p$ (mM/L)
7.00	9.6
7.05	10.7
7.10	12.0
7.15	13.5
7.20	15.1
7.25	17.0
7.30	19.0
7.35	21.3
7.40	24.0
7.45	27.0
7.50	30.0
7.55	33.8
7.60	37.6
7.65	42.6
7.70	47.8

REFERENCES

1. Astrup, P., Siggaard Andersen, O., Jørgensen, K., and Engel, K.: The acid-base metabolism--a new approach. *Lancet 1*:1035-1039, 1960.

2. Bennett, C. M., Springberg, P. D., and Falkinburg, N. R.: Glomerular-tubular balance for bicarbonate in the dog. *Am. J. Physiol. 228*:98-106, 1975.

3. Berliner, R. W., Kennedy, T. J., Jr., and Orloff, J.: Factors affecting the transport of potassium and hydrogen ions by the renal tubule. *Arch. Intern. Pharmacodyn. 97*:299-312, 1954.

4. Clapp, J. R., Watson, J. F., and Berliner, R. W.: Osmolality, bicarbonate concentration and water reabsorption in proximal tubule of the dog nephron. *Am. J. Physiol. 205*:273-280, 1963.

5. Clark, W. M.: *Topics in Physical Chemistry*. William & Wilkins Co., Baltimore, 1948.

6. Davenport, H. W.: *The ABC of Acid-Base Chemistry*. 4th ed. The University of Chicago Press, Chicago, 1958.

7. Fuller, G. R., MacLeod, M. B., and Pitts, R. F.: Influence of administration of potassium salts on the renal tubular reabsorption of bicarbonate. *Am. J. Physiol. 182*:111-118, 1955.

8. Giebisch, G., and Malnic, G.: Some aspects of renal tubular hydrogen ion transport. *Proc. Intern. Congr. Nephrol. 4th, Stockholm 1*:181-194, 1970.

9. Gray, J. S.: *Pulmonary Ventilation and Its Physiological Regulation*. Charles C Thomas, Publisher, Springfield, Ill. 1950.

10. Gray, J. S.: *Physiology Study Book*. Lecture notes in Physiology, Department of Physiology, Northwestern University Medical School, Chicago, 1968.

11. Henderson, L. J.: *Blood: A Study in General Physiology*. Yale University Press, New Haven, Connecticut, 1928.

12. Kurtzman, N. A.: Regulation of renal bicarbonate reabsorption by extracellular volume. *J. Clin. Invest. 49*:586-595, 1970.

13. Lotspeich, W. D.: Metabolic aspects of acid-base change. *Science 155*:1066-1075, 1967.

14. Malnic, G., De Mello Aires, M., and Giebisch, G.: Potassium transport across renal distal tubules during acid-base disturbances. *Am. J. Physiol. 221*:1192-1208, 1971.

15. Malnic, G., De Mello Aires, M., and Giebisch, G.: Micropuncture study of renal tubular hydrogen ion transport in the rat. *Am. J. Physiol. 222*:147-158, 1972.

16. Maren, T. H.: Carbonic anhydrase: chemistry, physiology and inhibition. *Physiol. Rev. 47*:595-781, 1967.

17. Muntwyler, E.: *Water and Electrolyte Metabolism and Acid-Base Balance*. The C. V. Mosby Co., St. Louis, 1968.

18. Pitts, R. F.: The renal regulation of acid base balance with special reference to the mechanism for acidifying the urine. I and II. *Science 102*:49-54, 81-85, July 20 and 27, 1945.

19. Pitts, R. F.: The renal excretion of acid. *Fed. Proc. 7*:418-426, 1948.

20. Pitts, R. F., Ayer, J. L., and Schiess, W. L.: The renal regulation of acid base balance in man: III. The reabsorption and excretion of bicarbonate. *J. Clin. Invest. 28*:35-44, 1949.

21. Pitts, R. F.: The role of ammonia production and excretion in regulation of acid-base balance. *New Engl. J. Med. 284*(1):32-38, 1971.

22. Pitts, R. F.: Production and excretion of ammonia in relation to acid-base regulation. In: *Handbook of Physiology*, Section 8, *Renal Physiology*. Edited by J. Orloff and R. W. Berliner. Washington, D. C., American Physiological Society, 1973, pp. 455-496.

23. Purkerson, M. L., Lubowitz, H., White, R. W., and Bricker, N. S.: On the influence of extracellular fluid volume expansion on bicarbonate reabsorption in the rat. *J. Clin. Invest. 48*:1754-1760, 1969.

24. Rector, F. C., Jr., Seldin, D. W., Roberts, A. D., Jr., and Smith, J. S.: The role of plasma CO_2 tension and carbonic anhydrase activity in the renal reabsorption of bicarbonate. *J. Clin. Invest. 39*:1706-1721, 1960.

25. Rector, F. C., Jr., Carter, N. W., and Seldin, D. W.: The mechanism of bicarbonate reabsorption in the proximal and distal tubules of the kidney. *J. Clin. Invest. 44*:278-290, 1965.

26. Rector, F. C., Jr.: Acidification of the urine. In: *Handbook of Physiology*, Section 8, *Renal Physiology*. Edited by J. Orloff and R. W. Berliner. Washington, D. C., American Physiological Society, 1973, pp. 431-454.

27. Severinghaus, J. W., Stupfel, M., and Bradley, A. F.: Accuracy of blood pH and pCO_2 determinations. *J. Appl. Physiol. 9*:189-196, 1956a.

28. Severinghaus, J. W., Stupfel, M., and Bradley, A. F.: Variations of serum carbonic acid pK' with pH and temperature. *J. Appl. Physiol. 9*:197-200, 1956b.

29. Siggaard-Anderson, O.: *The Acid-Base Status of the Blood*. 2nd ed. William & Wilkins Co., Baltimore, 1964.

30. Singer, R. B., and Hastings, A. B.: Improved clinical method for estimation of acid-base balance of human blood. *Medicine 27*:223-242, 1948.

31. Slatopolsky, E., Hoffsten, P., Purkerson, M., and Bricker, N. S.: On the influence of extracellular fluid volume expansion and of uremia on bicarbonate reabsorption in man. *J. Clin. Invest. 49*:988-998, 1970.

32. Valtin, H.: *Renal Function: Mechanisms Preserving Fluid and Solute Balance in Health*. Little, Brown & Co., Boston, 1973.

33. Winters, R. W.: Terminology of acid-base disorders. *Ann. N. Y. Acad. Sci. 133*:211-247, 1966.

Chapter 11

MECHANISM OF CONCENTRATION AND DILUTION OF URINE

In Chapter 8, while discussing the sequential processing of the filtrate along the loop of Henle, we alluded to the role of this nephron segment in concentrating and diluting the urine as deduced from the countercurrent multiplication principle. In this chapter, we shall elaborate on that summary and consider in more detail the principle of the countercurrent multiplication system and the evidence for its application to the kidney, the mechanism of concentration and dilution of urine deduced therefrom and its hormonal regulation, the measurement of the ability of the kidney to concentrate urine, and finally its modification in diuresis with special emphasis on the action of some selective diuretics and their potential therapeutic effects.

ANATOMY OF THE LOOP OF HENLE AND ITS BLOOD SUPPLY

The ability of the mammalian kidney to form a urine ranging in concentration from 1/6 isotonicity to 4 times isotonicity appears to be correlated with the length of the loop of Henle (Sperber, 1944). Thus, the longer the length of the loop of Henle (a condition related to the degree of inaccessibility of water, as in arid environment), the greater is the concentration of the excreted urine. This concentrating function of the loop of Henle presupposes that the fluid emerging from the loop and entering into the early distal tubule should be as hypertonic as ureteral urine. However, as we shall see shortly, micropuncture studies of fluid collected from the early distal tubule have shown clearly that this fluid is either hypotonic or isotonic with the plasma, but never hypertonic. Such findings imply that the site of the final concentration of urine must therefore be the collecting tubules. If so, then how does the sequential processing of the filtrate along the loop of Henle, as envisioned by the countercurrent multiplication hypothesis described in Chapter 8, contribute to the final concentration of urine emerging from the collecting tubules? To answer this question, we must first examine in greater detail the anatomical arrangement of the loop of Henle within the kidney and its blood supply.

As described in Chapter 8, the mammalian loop of Henle consists, sequentially, of a descending limb and an ascending limb. The descending limb consists of a short, thick segment, which is the late portion of the pars recta of the proximal tubule, followed by a long, thin segment. The ascending limb begins at the loop bend and consists of a short, thin segment, followed by a long, thick segment which is the early portion of the pars recta of the distal tubule. The extent of the development of the loop of Henle in a given nephron varies with the position of its renal corpuscle (Bowman's capsule and its associated glomerulus) within the cortex of the kidney. If the renal corpuscle of the nephron lies in the outer two thirds of the cortex (the so-called *cortical* nephron), the loop of Henle is relatively short. On the other hand, the *juxtamedullary* nephron (whose renal corpuscle lies in the inner third of the cortex, near the corticomedullary border) has a relatively long loop of Henle. The ratio of the cortical to the juxtamedullary nephrons is about 7 to 1 in man.

The physiological significance of this anatomical difference between these two types of nephrons and their population ratio may be considered as circumstantial evidence for their diverse roles in the renal regulation of water and electrolyte balance. Thus, the cortical nephrons are primarily concerned with the conservation of water and electrolytes, while the juxtamedullary nephrons play a major role in determining the ability of the kidney to concentrate and dilute urine, thereby adjusting the osmolality and volume of the excreted urine.

Figure 11-1 illustrates the salient structural features of the loop of Henle and its blood supply in the two types of nephrons. Of special interest here are the unique features of the blood supply to the juxtamedullary nephrons. Recent extensive anatomical studies (Fourman and Moffat, 1964) have shown that in the case of cortical nephrons the efferent arteriole breaks up to form the complex peritubular capillary network pervading the proximal and distal tubules. However, in the case of the juxtamedullary nephrons, the efferent arteriole gives rise to two distinct branches: One branch forms a similar capillary network surrounding the proximal and distal tubules, while a second branch proceeds directly into the medulla, where it forms a hairpin capillary loop, called the *vasa recta*, paralleling the loop of Henle. The vasa recta, thus formed, consists of a descending arterial limb and an ascending venous limb, joined together in the papillary region by a capillary plexus, depicted as a simple loop in Figure 11-1. As such, the vasa recta does not form a simple hairpin loop pervading the loop of Henle, but rather it consists of a descending and an ascending vascular bundle which are joined together at different medullary levels by a distinct capillary plexus. This anatomical arrangement of the vasa recta gives it the appearance of a distributed capillary bed with shunts between the descending and ascending limbs. As we shall learn later, this hairpin configuration of vasa recta with its associated shunts as well as its

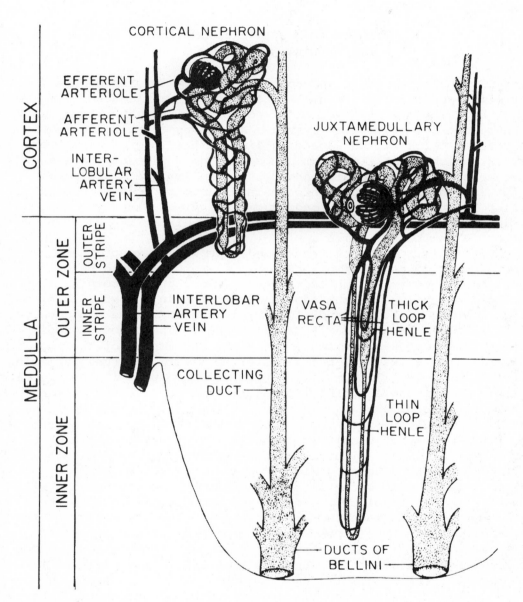

Figure 11-1. Comparison of gross structures and vascular supplies of cortical and juxtamedullary nephrons. [From PHYSIOLOGY OF THE KIDNEY AND BODY FLUIDS, 3rd ed., by R. F. Pitts. Copyright 1974, Year Book Medical Publishers, Inc., Chicago. Used by permission.]

slow blood flow rate profoundly influence the function of the loop of Henle in concentrating and diluting the urine.

Let us now see how these unique anatomical features of the loop of Henle and its associated blood supply contribute to concentration and dilution of urine as perceived by the countercurrent multiplication hypothesis described next.

PRINCIPLE OF COUNTERCURRENT MULTIPLICATION SYSTEM

In 1951, Hargitay and Kuhn proposed a theory for the mechanism of concentration and dilution of urine based on the premise that the loop of Henle, by virtue of its anatomical position within the kidney, acts as a countercurrent multiplier system. According to this theory, if the epithelial cells of the ascending limb of the loop of Henle were able to establish a small osmolar concentration difference between the fluid contents of the ascending and descending limbs at each level along the length of the loop, this small *transverse gradient* could be multiplied into a significant *longitudinal gradient* along the length of the loop by the *countercurrent* (opposite in direction) flow of tubular fluid in the two limbs.

Applying this concept to the kidney, one would expect that the isotonic fluid issuing from the proximal tubule should become progressively concentrated as it traverses along the descending limb of the loop, attaining maximum osmolality in the loop bend. Then, as the fluid travels up the ascending limb, it should become progressively hypotonic as it enters the early distal tubule. The osmotic gradient thus established between the two limbs along the length of the loop could result from either (1) net transfer of water from the descending limb to the ascending limb, or (2) net solute transport in the opposite direction. In either case, the initial transverse gradient at each level along the loop, which could be quite small, is multiplied into a significant gradient along the longitudinal medullary axis of the loop of Henle. The net result would be the development of a high osmolar concentration gradient along the medullary interstitium to which the collecting tubules would be exposed. The mechanism of formation of hypertonic urine is perceived to be the consequence of the osmotic equilibration of the collecting tubular fluid with the surrounding hypertonic medullary interstitium. The osmolality of the excreted urine would thus depend on the magnitude of the generated longitudinal gradient, which in turn is governed by (a) the magnitude of the initial transverse gradient (the so-called "single effect"); (b) the length of the loop of Henle; (c) the solute and water permeability of the epithelia of the descending and ascending limbs; and (d) the flow rate in the loop of Henle, the collecting tubule and the vasa recta, as well as interactions between these structures.

To better visualize the operation of the countercurrent multiplication system, let us consider the model shown in Figure 11-2. Initially, at time zero (upper left corner) the descending

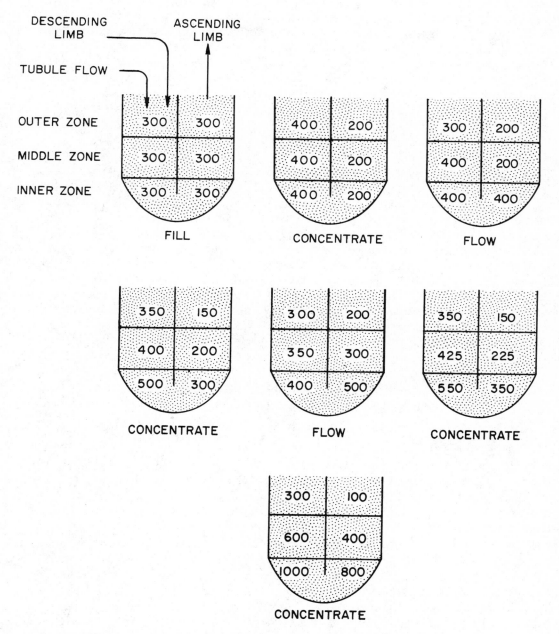

Figure 11-2. A model depicting the operation of the countercurrent multiplication in the loop of Henle.

and ascending limbs are shown to be filled with fluid containing 150 mM/L of sodium chloride, for a total osmolality of 300 mOsm/L, which is iso-osmotic with the plasma. Three representative medullary cells capable of active solute transport (mainly sodium chloride) from the ascending to descending limbs are considered. They are designated outer, middle, and inner zones. The first step in the operation of the countercurrent multiplication is the establishment of the transverse gradient. This is accomplished by the active transport of enough sodium chloride from the ascending limb to the descending limb to create a maximum transverse gradient of about 200 mOsm/L. The next step involves the *flow* of the contents of the cell in the outer zone out of the ascending limb into the distal tubule, while an equal volume of fluid having a concentration of 300 mOsm/L enters from the proximal tubule into the descending limb. The subsequent steps are the repeat of the previous ones. That is, each *flow* step is followed by a *concentrate* step until the final steady state concentrate condition shown at the bottom of Figure 11-2 is reached.

From this model, it is evident that the magnitude of the longitudinal gradient depends on (a) the magnitude of the initial transverse gradient, (b) the length of the loop of Henle, and (c) the tubular flow rate. Thus, in the steady state, the mechanism of urine concentration depends on the operation of two processes: (1) The countercurrent multiplication of the concentration between the two limbs of the loop of Henle, which establishes an osmolar concentration gradient within the medullary interstitium from cortex to the tip of the papilla. (2) The osmotic equilibration of the adjacent collecting tubular fluid with the surrounding hypertonic medullary interstitium. As we shall see later, the medullary vasa recta complements the operation of both processes and enhances their efficiency by removing water in excess of solutes so as to preserve the hypertonicity generated within the medullary interstitium.

EXPERIMENTAL EVIDENCE FOR EXISTENCE OF COUNTERCURRENT MULTIPLICATION SYSTEM IN THE LOOP OF HENLE

The original experimental verification of the countercurrent multiplication hypothesis was provided by Wirz and colleagues (1951). These investigators found that when *in situ* frozen sections of kidney of hydropenic (thirsty) rats were thawed under microscope, the cortical tissue fluid melted at the same temperature as the arterial blood. This implied that the fluids in the proximal and distal tubules, which are located in the cortex, were iso-osmotic with the blood. However, the fluid contained in the tissues from the outer and inner medulla melted at progressively lower and lower temperatures, compared with the arterial blood, indicating that the fluids in the medullary structures, namely, the loop of Henle, collecting tubule, and vasa recta, became increasingly hyperosmotic relative to the blood. Figure 11-3 presents graphically a summary of their findings. It shows that as we proceed from the cortex toward the papilla, in the longitudinal direction (in the figure from left to right across the kidney), the tissue fluid becomes progressively hyperosmotic, while in a given transverse level (in the figure along the vertical direction within a zone) the fluid osmolality remains the same. Subsequent micropuncture studies (Gottschalk and Mylle, 1959) discussed below, however, showed that the fluid collected from the early distal tubule was hypo-osmotic and became iso-osmotic by the middle of the convoluted segment. Although these micropuncture data do not invalidate the concept of increasing longitudinal gradient, they demonstrate that the

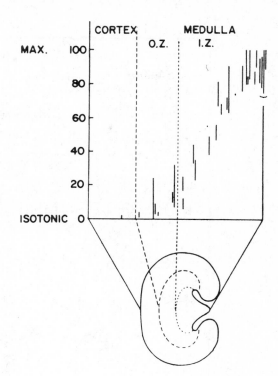

Figure 11-3. Osmolality of tissue slices from the cortex, the outer zone (O.Z.) and the inner zone (I.Z.) of the medulla of the kidney of hydropenic rat. Ordinate scale is the measured tonicity expressed as percentage of maximum. [From Wirz, H., Hargitay, B., and Kuhn, W. (1951).]

tubular fluids at a given transverse level do not have exactly the same osmolality. The earlier observations of Wirz and associates (1951) have recently been confirmed (Bray, 1960).

Gottschalk and Mylle (1959) were the first to make a systematic micropuncture study of the various segments of the nephron in both rat and hamster, thereby providing the most impressive evidence in support of the countercurrent multiplication in the loop of Henle and its role in concentration and dilution of urine. They found that in rats the fluids collected from the proximal tubule remained iso-osmotic (fluid-to-plasma or F/P osmolality ratios equal to unity), regardless of whether the ureteral urine was hypo- or hyperosmotic. Furthermore, they observed that in hydropenic rats forming highly concentrated urine, the fluid collected from the early distal convoluted tubule was consistently hypo-osmotic (F/P osmolality ratios less than unity), and became iso-osmotic in the second half of the distal convolution, but never hyperosmotic. These findings, which are summarized in Figures 11-4 and 11-5 clearly demonstrate that the formation of hyperosmotic urine is a consequence of the collecting tubular function, thus providing strong experimental evidence in support of the countercurrent multiplication theory.

As mentioned earlier, the observed hypotonicity of the fluid entering the early distal convoluted tubule can be the result of either two processes: (a) hyperosmotic reabsorption of solute from the ascending limb, or (b) secretion of water into this segment. If the first process--namely, solute reabsorption in excess of water--is the mechanism, then the only solute present in sufficient quantity in this segment is sodium chloride.

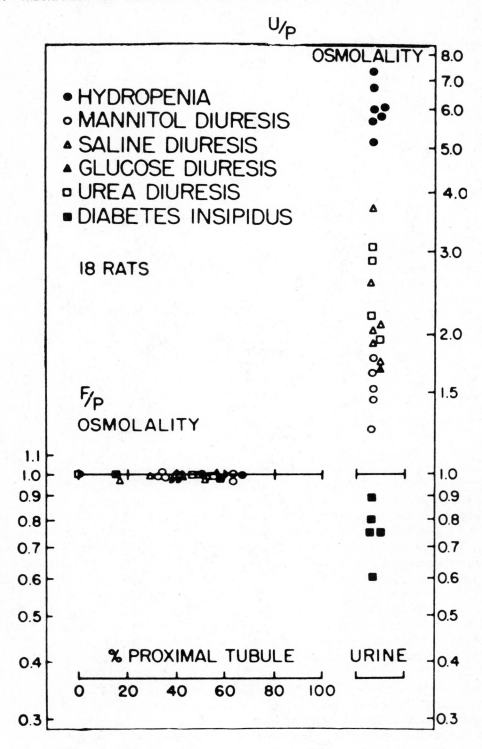

Figure 11-4. Comparison of fluid-to-plasma (F/P) osmolality ratios of fluid collected from the proximal convoluted tubule with the urine-to-plasma (U/P) osmolality ratios in rats under different diuretic states. [From Gottschalk, C. W., and Mylle, M. (1959).]

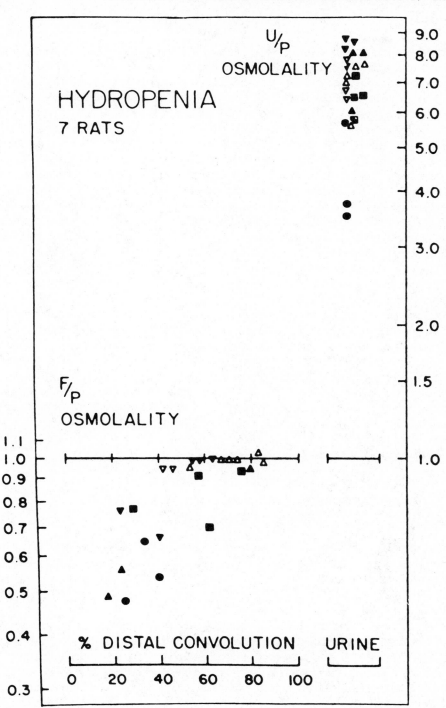

Figure 11-5. Comparison of fluid-to-plasma (F/P) osmolality ratios of fluid collected from distal convoluted tubule with the urine-to-plasma (U/P) osmolality ratios during hydropenia. Different symbols refer to different rats. [From Gottschalk, C. W., and Mylle, M. (1959).]

To differentiate between these two processes, Gottschalk and Mylle (1959) induced osmotic diuresis by infusion of either a nonabsorbable solute, such as mannitol, or sodium chloride, and determined the F/P osmolality ratios in the fluid collected from the early distal tubule. As shown in Figure 11-6, when diuresis was induced by intravenous infusion of 25% solution of mannitol, urine flow increased up to 80 times that of the hydropenic state, and the F/P osmolality ratios in the early distal convoluted tubule were low but not less than 0.6. Similar results were obtained during glucose diuresis, a solute not known to be reabsorbed in the loop of Henle. However, when diuresis was induced by intravenous infusion of 5% sodium chloride solution, urine flow rate increased to the same level as with mannitol and glucose, but the F/P osmolality ratios in the early distal convoluted tubule were as low as 0.3. During both sodium chloride diuresis and mannitol or glucose diuresis, the fluid collected from the second half of the distal convoluted tubule was iso-osmotic with the plasma.

The increase in the degree of hypotonicity of the early distal fluid during sodium chloride diuresis, compared with mannitol or glucose diuresis, was taken as a strong evidence that this observed hypotonicity is due to hyperosmotic reabsorption of sodium chloride from the ascending limb of the loop of Henle and not secretion of water. Thus, they suggested that it is this hyperosmotic solute reabsorption that is responsible for the development of the transverse gradient, which when multiplied leads to the establishment of a significant longitudinal osmolality gradient in the surrounding medullary interstitium.

A PROPOSED MODEL FOR THE OPERATION OF THE COUNTERCURRENT MULTIPLICATION SYSTEM IN THE LOOP OF HENLE

On the basis of these micropuncture studies and other evidence cited above, Gottschalk and Mylle (1959) proposed the first working model for the countercurrent multiplication hypothesis as it applies to the kidney. The salient features of their model are depicted in Figure 11-7.

This model envisions that sodium ions, by an active mechanism analogous to that described for the proximal tubule (see Chapter 8), and chloride ions, as a consequence of electrochemical gradient established by sodium movement, are reabsorbed from the relatively water-impermeable ascending limb of the loop of Henle into the surrounding medullary interstitium until a limiting gradient of 200 mOsm/kg of water has been established between the medullary interstitium and the fluid in the ascending limb. This *single effect* of osmolar concentration gradient is then multiplied as the fluid in the descending limb comes into osmotic equilibrium with the surrounding hypertonic medullary interstitium by diffusion of water out of and sodium chloride into the descending limb. The overall effect would be that an increasing osmolar concentration gradient is established in the longitudinal direction within the

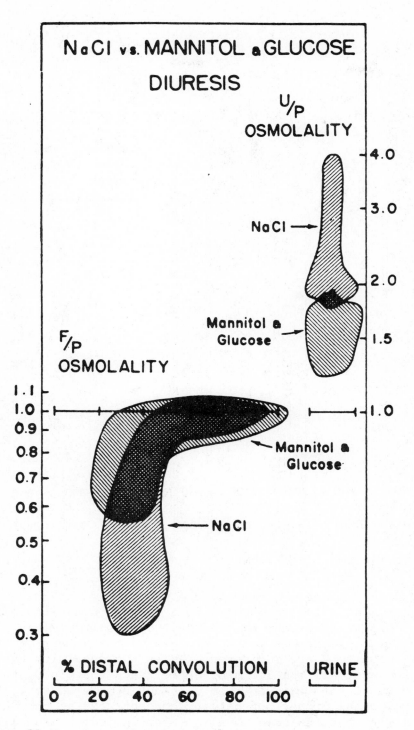

Figure 11-6. Comparison of fluid-to-plasma (F/P) osmolality ratios of fluid collected from the distal convoluted tubule and urine-to-plasma (U/P) osmolality ratios during hypertonic sodium chloride diuresis with those during hypertonic mannitol and glucose diureses. [From Gottschalk, C. W., and Mylle, M. (1959).]

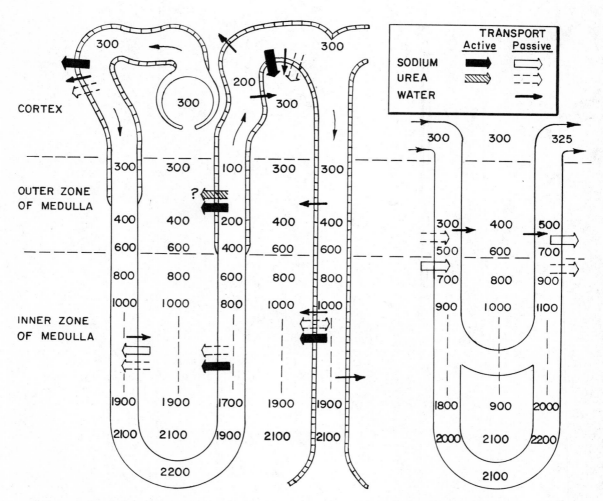

Figure 11-7. Diagram depicting the proposed countercurrent multiplication system in a nephron with a long loop and in the vasa recta. The numbers represent hypothetical osmolality values. No quantitative significance is to be attached to the number of arrows, and only net movements are indicated. As is the case with the vascular loops, not all the loops of Henle reach the tip of the papilla, and hence the fluid in them does not become as concentrated as that of the final urine, but only as concentrated as the medullary interstitial fluid at the same level. [Redrawn from Gottschalk, C. W., and Mylle, M. (1959).]

interstitium, extending from the corticomedullary border to the tip of the papilla, as was found by Wirz and associates (1951). The osmolality of the urine issuing from the collecting tubule was assumed to be the consequence of passive osmotic equilibration of the fluid in this nephron segment (mainly by reabsorption of water in excess of solute) with the surrounding hypertonic medullary interstitium. Thus, in this manner, the fluid in the collecting tubule becomes progressively hypertonic as the filtrate traverses along this nephron segment from the corticomedullary border to the tip of the papilla. Furthermore, consistent with the micropuncture studies summarized in Figure 11-4, they suggested that in the presence of ADH, the epithelium of the collecting tubule is maximally water-permeable, thereby further enhancing the osmotic equilibration of the fluid in the collecting tubule with the surrounding hypertonic medullary interstitium. Moreover, they postulated that the degree to which the urine in the collecting tubule is concentrated depends on the relative rates of filtrate flow along the loop of Henle and the collecting tubule. As described in Chapter 8, a slow rate of filtrate flow tends to increase the tubular transit time, thereby prolonging the contact time between the luminal fluid and the tubular epithelium. This would favor a maximum attainment of osmotic equilibration of tubular fluid with the surrounding hypertonic medullary interstitium and hence a greater concentration of urine. The effect of flow rate on urine concentration is further enhanced by the presence of ADH. Under the influence of this hormone, there is a greater osmotic flow of water out of the collecting tubule into the hypertonic medullary interstitium, thus reducing the filtrate volume and its flow rate, which further augment the osmolar concentration of the fluid in the collecting tubule and hence the osmolality of the excreted urine.

As illustrated in Figure 11-7 and envisioned by this model, the vasa recta plays an important role in the maintenance of the longitudinal hypertonicity of the medullary interstitium with which the collecting tubular fluid comes into osmotic equilibrium. Furthermore, renal handling of urea within the medulla contributes significantly to the efficiency of the urinary concentration by the loop of Henle. Because of their importance, the roles of both vasa recta and urea in the operation of the countercurrent multiplication will be discussed later in separate sections of this chapter.

A number of micropuncture studies have substantiated the basic elements of the above model. While collecting fluids from the loop of Henle near the papilla, Ullrich and Jarausch (1956) found that the hypertonicity of the medullary tissues previously observed by Wirz and associates (1951) was due largely to increased concentration of sodium chloride and urea in this region. In a later study, Jamison and colleagues (1967), using partial nephrectomy and tissue excision techniques to expose the medullary structures, found that the fluid collected from the medullary portion of the ascending limb was significantly hypo-osmotic relative to that of the adjacent descending limb, with a mean difference in osmolality of about 117 mOsm/kg of water (Fig. 11-8). A lower concentration of sodium chloride in the

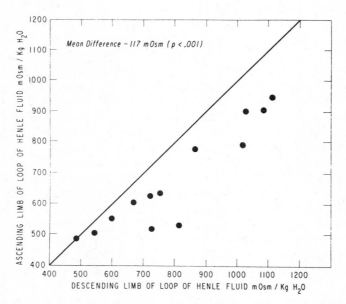

Figure 11-8. Comparison of osmolalities of fluids from ascending limbs and adjacent descending limbs of the loop of Henle. [From Jamison, R. L., Bennett, C. M., and Berliner, R. W. (1967).]

ascending limb fluid accounted for nearly 90% of this difference. These results corroborate those of Gottschalk and Mylle (1959) and strongly suggest that active reabsorption of sodium chloride from the ascending limb, rather than water secretion into this segment, is the step which leads to the development of the *initial transverse gradient* (the so-called "single effect") necessary for the development of the *longitudinal medullary interstitial gradient* by the loop of Henle, with which the collecting tubule equilibrates.

As predicted by the countercurrent hypothesis, Gottschalk (1961) found that in hydropenic rats, in which plasma ADH concentration is high, fluid collected from the loop of Henle and the vasa recta near the tip of the papilla are essentially in osmotic equilibrium with urine collected from the adjacent collecting tubule. This is illustrated in Figure 11-9, which also shows that in animals with diabetes insipidus the collecting tubule urine was hypo-osmotic relative to the fluid collected from the adjacent loop of Henle and vasa recta. However, the hypertonicity of the latter fluids was much less compared to that of the hydropenic rats. Furthermore, a comparison of the osmolality of the fluid in the distal tubule between intact hydropenic rats and rats with diabetes insipidus during sodium chloride diuresis showed a marked reduction in the F/P ratios in this segment, with eventual decrease in U/P osmolality ratios. These results, reproduced in Figure 11-10, provide unequivocal evidence for the effect of ADH on the water permeability of the epithelia of the distal convoluted and collecting tubules and

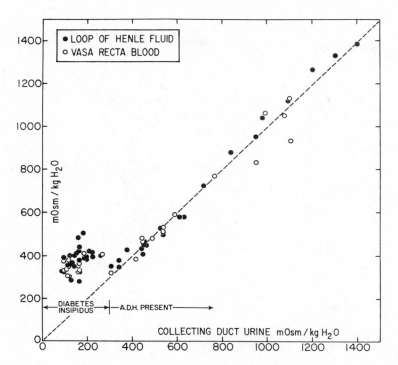

Figure 11-9. Relation between the osmolality of collecting
tubule urine and fluids from loops of Henle and vasa recta blood
in various normal desert rodents and in hamsters with experimental
diabetes insipidus. Some of the values obtained in the presence
of antidiuretic hormone (ADH) are from hamsters with diabetes
insipidus following the administration of exogenous ADH. [From
Gottschalk, C. W. (1961).]

the role of this hormone in concentration and dilution of urine. The
intracellular mechanism mediating the action of ADH in these nephron
segments will be discussed later in this chapter.

PRESENT CONCEPT OF THE COUNTERCURRENT
MULTIPLICATION SYSTEM BASED ON RECENT
DIRECT MICROPERFUSION STUDIES ALONG THE
LOOP OF HENLE AND COLLECTING TUBULE

The main premise of the model proposed by Gottschalk and Mylle
(1959) and depicted in Figure 11-7 is threefold: (1) The transverse
gradient (the so-called "single effect") between the ascending and
descending limbs of the loop of Henle is developed by active
hyperosmotic reabsorption of sodium along the entire length (both
thin and thick segments) of the water-impermeable ascending limb;
(2) the fluid in the descending limb becomes iso-osmotic with the
surrounding hypertonic medullary interstitium by both osmotic

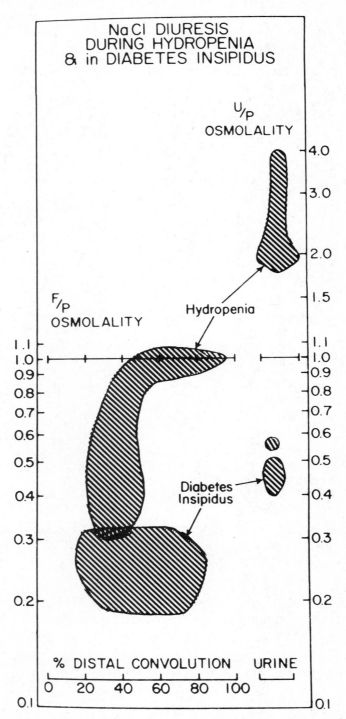

Figure 11-10. Comparison of fluid-to-plasma (F/P) osmolality ratios of fluid collected from distal convoluted tubule and urine-to-plasma (U/P) osmolality ratios during sodium chloride diuresis in normal hydropenic rats and in rats with experimental diabetes insipidus. [From Gottschalk, C. W. (1961).]

abstraction of water from and diffusive entry of sodium chloride into the descending limb; and (3) the osmolality of the excreted urine is the consequence of osmotic equilibration of the collecting tubule with the surrounding hypertonic medullary interstitium primarily by water reabsorption, a process enhanced by ADH.

Although the overall pattern of concentration and dilution of urine, as envisioned by this model, has been largely confirmed by subsequent micropuncture studies, its underlying assumptions, however, could not be tested until very recently. As described in Chapter 8, recent advances in microperfusion technique of isolated segments of rabbit renal tubules have made it possible to delineate more precisely (a) the nature of the solute pump in the ascending limb of the loop of Henle, which is responsible for the development of the initial transverse gradient, and (b) the mechanism of osmotic equilibration of the fluid in the descending limb and collecting tubule with the surrounding hypertonic medullary interstitium. These experiments have made it possible to test the assumptions of the above model, and more specifically to answer the following *five* questions: (1) What is the precise mechanism by which the transverse gradient (the "single effect") is established? More specifically, is it the active reabsorption of sodium or not? (2) Is the transverse gradient developed along the entire length of the ascending limb (including both thin and thick segments), or is it only confined to the thick segment? (3) Is the epithelia of the ascending limb impermeable to the osmotic flow of water? This is a fundamental prerequisite for the development of hypotonicity in this loop segment, and hence the transverse gradient. (4) Is the osmotic equilibration of the descending limb with the surrounding hypertonic medullary interstitium accomplished primarily by osmotic reabsorption of water and secondarily by solute entry, or do both processes operate about equally? And (5) is the osmolality of the excreted urine a consequence of osmotic equilibration of the collecting tubular fluid with the surrounding hypertonic medullary interstitium, primarily by water reabsorption or solute retention, or both?

The following represents a summary of the most important of these studies which have led to a revision and refinement of the above countercurrent multiplication model. To facilitate presentation and to be consistent with the sequence of events in the operation of the countercurrent multiplication process, we shall discuss this evidence under the headings of ascending and descending limbs of the loop of Henle and the collecting tubule.

ASCENDING LIMB OF THE LOOP OF HENLE

Micropuncture studies of Gottschalk and Mylle (1959) in rat, cited earlier, revealed that fluids collected from the early distal convoluted tubule had tubular fluid-to-plasma osmolality ratios of less than unity (Fig. 11-5), thus suggesting hyperosmotic reabsorption of sodium chloride along this nephron segment. On the basis of these and other studies (Fig. 11-6), they proposed that as the filtrate traverses from the papilla toward the cortex along the ascending limb it becomes progressively hypo-osmotic relative to the surrounding medullary interstitium. This hypotonicity was attributed to (a) hyperosmotic reabsorption of sodium chloride, by active sodium and passive chloride transport, along the entire length of the ascending limb, and (b) relative impermeability of the ascending limb epithelia to osmotic flow of water. Recent studies discussed below, however, have questioned the validity of the first assumption but have confirmed the accuracy of the second.

As described in Chapter 8, Burg and Stoner (1974) and Kokko (1974), perfusing isolated segments of rabbit renal tubules, found that in contrast to all other segments of the nephron examined, the transepithelial electrical gradient across the thick segments of the ascending limb of the loop of Henle was *positive* (see Table 8-2) with respect to the bath (the peritubular interstitial fluid). Substitution of sodium-free perfusate, choline chloride, for sodium chloride enhanced this electrical positivity, while substitution of a chloride-free perfusate abolished it. Furthermore, using the criteria described in Chapter 8, these investigators demonstrated that the reabsorption of sodium chloride in the thick segment of the ascending limb is accomplished by active chloride transport, which induces positive diffusion of sodium out of the lumen. In a related study, Burg and associates (1973) showed that furosemide, ethacrynic acid, and mercurial diuretics, when present in the lumen of the thick ascending limb, induce diuresis by inhibiting active chloride transport. However, placing the diuretic agents in the bath (the peritubular fluid) had no effect.

That the ascending limb epithelia (both thin and thick segments) are relatively impermeable to the osmotic flow of water is now well established. Using microperfusion techniques, Morgan and Berliner (1968) found that the descending limb epithelia were more than twice as permeable to the osmotic flow of water as the ascending limb epithelia. Furthermore, the water permeability of the epithelia of either limb was unaffected by addition of ADH to the perfusion solution. These findings have recently been confirmed (Kokko, 1974).

To summarize, the studies cited above have provided unequivocal evidence that the transverse gradient (the so-called "single effect") is not generated by active sodium and passive chloride reabsorption along the entire length of the ascending limb, as suggested by Gottschalk and Mylle (1959). Rather, it is developed as a consequence of active chloride and passive sodium reabsorption, a process confined only to the thick segment of the water-impermeable ascending limb of the loop of Henle.

DESCENDING LIMB OF THE LOOP OF HENLE

The question of the mechanism of the osmotic equilibration of the descending limb of the loop of Henle with the surrounding hypertonic medullary interstitium has now been largely resolved. It should be recalled that in their model, Gottschalk and Mylle (1959) suggested that the osmotic equilibration was accomplished by both diffusion of water out of and sodium chloride into the descending limb, since the epithelial membranes were permeable to both solutes and water. However, subsequent studies, discussed below, have shown that this osmotic equilibration is largely accomplished by osmotic reabsorption of water with secondary diffusive entry of solutes, mainly urea and sodium chloride.

Lassiter and associates (1961) observed that in the hamster the tubular fluid-to-plasma concentration ratios for inulin in the thin limbs of the loop of Henle near the papilla averaged about 11, while the tubular fluid-to-plasma osmolality ratios averaged only about 2.8. Since inulin is neither reabsorbed nor secreted throughout the nephron, its tubular fluid-to-plasma concentration ratio is usually taken as a measure of water reabsorption along the nephron. Thus, the higher tubular fluid-to-plasma concentration ratio for inulin compared to that for osmolality in the same region of the loop of Henle strongly suggests that osmotic equilibration is accomplished largely by preferential reabsorption of water rather than the diffusive entry of solutes.

That the progressive increase in the hypertonicity of the fluids in the descending limb, as required by the countercurrent multiplication hypothesis, is largely due to reabsorption of water into the hypertonic medullary interstitium has been confirmed by Kokko (1970) and more recently by Jamison (1974). Using isolated, perfused rabbit descending limb, Kokko (1970) found that this segment of the nephron is highly permeable to water but is relatively impermeable to solutes. Furthermore, the water permeability of the descending limb was found to be much greater than that of the proximal tubule. Jamison (1974) observed that osmotic reabsorption of water accounted for about 65% of the osmotic equilibration of the descending limb fluid with the surrounding hypertonic medullary interstitium, while diffusive entry of urea and sodium chloride accounted for 25% and 10%, respectively. These findings have attributed a somewhat greater role to solute entry than that predicted by the passive countercurrent multiplication model of inner medulla (discussed below) proposed by Kokko and Rector (1972). In that model, water reabsorption accounted for 96%, while solute entry (mainly urea) accounted for only 4% of the osmotic equilibration of the descending limb fluid with the surrounding hypertonic medullary interstitium.

PASSIVE COUNTERCURRENT MULTIPLICATION IN INNER MEDULLA. Using the technique of perfusing the isolated segments of rabbit renal tubules developed by Burg and associates (1966), Kokko (1970, 1972) examined the permeability properties of the epithelia of the thin segments of rabbit loop of Henle. He found that the thin descending limb had a high osmotic water permeability, but was relatively impermeable to sodium chloride and urea. In contrast, the thin ascending limb had a zero osmotic water permeability, but was very permeable to sodium chloride and only moderately permeable to urea. The thick ascending limb, as mentioned earlier, was relatively impermeable to osmotic flow of water and passive sodium chloride and urea transport. In addition, Morgan and Berliner (1968) found that the distal tubule and the cortical and outer medullary segments of the collecting tubule were impermeable to urea, both in the presence and absence of ADH, but showed enhanced permeability to water in the presence of ADH. This differential permeability to water and urea was suggested as an explanation for the high luminal and interstitial urea concentration observed in the cortical and outer medullary regions, a condition created by osmotic water abstraction secondary to hyperosmotic sodium chloride reabsorption from the thick ascending limb of the loop of Henle. In the inner medulla, however, they found that the presence of ADH enhanced not only the water permeability of the collecting tubule, but also its permeability to urea, an effect unique to this segment. This would favor urea accumulation within the inner medulla, thereby promoting its diffusive entry, along its concentration gradient, into the thin segments of both ascending and descending limbs of the loop of Henle, as well as the adjacent vasa recta.

On the basis of these findings, Kokko and Rector (1972) proposed a strictly passive countercurrent multiplication for the concentrating mechanism in the inner medulla. The essential steps involved in the development of concentration gradient within the inner medulla by this model, as depicted in Figure 11-11, are: (1) Hyperosmotic reabsorption of sodium chloride from the water-impermeable thick ascending limb induces osmotic reabsorption of water from the distal tubule and outer medullary and cortical collecting tubular segments; (2) this water abstraction, along with active reabsorption of sodium chloride accompanied by osmotic reabsorption of water in these tubular segments, raises luminal concentration of urea to very high levels; (3) upon reaching the inner medulla, the high urea concentration favors its passive diffusion from the collecting tubule into the surrounding medullary interstitium; (4) the resulting accumulation of urea in the inner medullary interstitium promotes passive diffusion of urea into the descending and ascending limbs of the loop of Henle, and eventually into the outer medullary and cortical tubular segments; (5) this *recycling* of urea from the inner medullary collecting tubule through the loop of Henle to the outer medullary and cortical tubular segments induces further osmotic abstraction of water from the adjacent descending thin limb and inner medullary collecting tubule; (6) water abstraction from the descending thin limb raises its luminal concentration of sodium chloride, thereby promoting passive diffusion of sodium chloride out of the ascending thin limb into the interstitium, as the filtrate traverses along this segment toward the outer medulla; (7) the resulting accumulation of sodium chloride within the inner medulla raises medullary interstitial osmolar concentration, thereby promoting further osmotic reabsorption of water from the adjacent collecting tubule, thus increasing the concentration of the non-absorbable solutes (X_S), and hence the concentration of the excreted urine; (8) the vasa recta serves as a passive vehicle for removal of excess water and solutes reabsorbed from the loop of Henle and the collecting tubule, thereby preserving the medullary longitudinal osmolar concentration gradient.

The validity of this model has recently been tested by Jamison and his associates (1973, 1974) in rats with hereditary hypothalamic

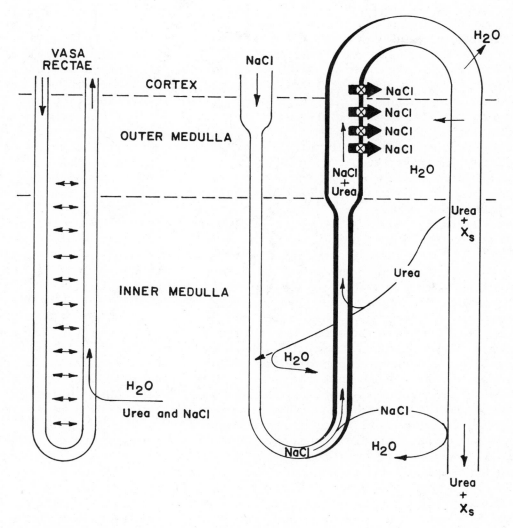

Figure 11-11. Diagram depicting the countercurrent multiplication system without active transport in the inner medulla. Thick lines on the ascending limb indicate water-impermeability, and X_S designates a non-absorbable solute. [Redrawn from Kokko, J. P., and Rector, F. C., Jr. (1972).]

diabetes insipidus (Brattleboro strain). In these rats, the tip of the papilla protrudes beyond the main body of the kidney, thereby making it accessible for direct micropuncture. Using this preparation, these investigators determined the flow and composition of fluids collected from the end of the thin descending limb (the loop bend) and adjacent collecting tubule during water diuresis and after ADH-induced antidiuresis and compared them with those collected from similar regions in normal rats. The mean osmolality in the fluid collected from the end of the collecting tubule near the papilla was 230 $\pm$ 26 in water diuresis and 667 $\pm$ 94 in ADH-induced antidiuresis in the

Brattleboro rats, compared to 1216 ± 118 mOsm/kg of water in the normal rats.

The contribution of water abstraction from and solute addition to the descending limb as a means of osmotic equilibration of its content with the surrounding hypertonic medullary interstitium was determined in both the Brattleboro and normal rats. Jamison and his associates found that in the Brattleboro rats, solute addition accounted for 33% of the increased osmolality of the fluid along the descending limb during water diuresis and 40% during antidiuresis. However, in the normal hydropenic rats, solute addition accounted for 35% of the increased osmolality along the descending limb.

An important finding of their study was that the quantity of urea remaining at the end of the descending thin limb (the loop bend) was equivalent to more than 300% of the quantity filtered at the glomerulus in the Brattleboro rats during ADH-induced antidiuresis, compared to over 600% in the normal antidiuretic rats. Assuming that there was no secretion of urea into the proximal tubule of the juxtamedullary nephron, any quantity of urea exceeding 100% of that filtered at the glomerulus must have been added to the tubular fluid as it traversed along the descending limb. They estimated that the net addition of urea into the descending limb accounted for 86 to 92% of the total increase in urea concentration along this segment of the nephron. These findings, additionally, lend credence to the earlier observations and suggestions of Lassiter and associates (1964) and of Kokko and Rector (1972) that there is a recycling of urea through the loop of Henle, a phenomenon that plays a significant role in the concentration of urine by the countercurrent multiplication mechanism, which will be discussed later in this chapter.

To summarize, studies reported by Jamison (1974) indicate that water abstraction accounts for 60 to 67% of the increased osmolality of the descending limb fluid and solute entry for 33 to 40% of the total. Moreover, the added solute is not exclusively urea; sodium chloride contributes the major fraction. Although these findings generally support the passive countercurrent multiplication model of Kokko and Rector (1972), they do not support its prediction that water abstraction accounts for 96% of the increased osmolality of the descending limb fluid, while solute entry (primarily urea) accounts for the remaining 4%.

COLLECTING TUBULE

Recent meticulous anatomical studies of the kidney (Oliver, 1968) have revealed that the collecting tubule differs from the nephron in its origin and in its morphological structure. The mammalian collecting tubule develops from the ureteral bud, which in turn is derived from the *metanephric duct*. In contrast, the nephron, which consists of the proximal tubule, the loop of Henle and the distal tubule, is derived from the *mesonephros* via the nephrogenic vesicle. In the course of development and growth, the mature collecting tubule, unlike the nephron, does not become a separate unit, but instead forms a series of paired tubes, giving it a tree-like appearance, which begins in the cortex and terminates in the papilla. In the human kidney, an average of 11 distal tubules empty into the beginning of a collecting tubule. Thereafter, the collecting tubules fuse (two into one) a total of eight to nine times, eventually forming the duct of Bellini. It is estimated that each duct of Bellini collects fluid from some 3000 to 6000 nephrons. Because of this complex arrangement, the term *collecting tubule system* has been suggested for this portion of the renal tubule (Jamison, 1974).

The role of the collecting tubule in concentration and dilution of urine is ultimately related to its anatomical layout within the cortex and medulla of the kidney, as well as the selective effect of ADH on the permeability of its epithelia to water and urea (Grantham and Burg, 1966; Morgan and Berliner, 1968; Bowman and Foulkes, 1970).

Until recently, it was assumed that in the absence of ADH the entire collecting tubule was impermeable to osmotic flow of water (Gottschalk and Mylle, 1959). However, recent *in vitro* perfusion studies have shown that in the absence of ADH only the cortical and outer medullary segments of the collecting tubule are impermeable to osmotic flow of water, while the terminal portion is both permeable to water and can reabsorb solute, mainly sodium and urea (Jamison, 1974).

The ability of the terminal portion of the collecting tubule to reabsorb both water and solutes (urea and sodium with its associated anion) suggests that the collecting tubule not only plays an important role in concentrating urine, as required by the countercurrent multiplication hypothesis, but also participates in the dilution of urine. These findings indicate that the collecting tubule plays a more important role in the regulation of water and electrolyte balance than has previously been realized.

Figure 11-12 incorporates the various experimental evidence presented in this section and depicts the salient features of the present concept of the operation of the countercurrent multiplication system in the loop of Henle and the subsequent concentration of urine in the adjacent collecting tubule.

As shown, the countercurrent multiplication process is initiated in the outer medulla. Here, hyperosmotic, active reabsorption of chloride accompanied by passive transport of sodium out of the water-impermeable thick segment of the ascending limb increases the osmolar concentration of the surrounding medullary interstitium. This exposes the fluids in the adjacent descending limb and collecting tubule in this region to an hypertonic environment, to which they adjust by osmotic loss of water (in the case of the collecting tubule) as well as entry of solutes (in the case of the descending limb). The result is an increase in the concentration of sodium chloride in the descending limb and an increase in the concentration of urea in the collecting tubule. The latter effect results from (a) osmotic abstraction of water as a consequence of hyperosmotic reabsorption of sodium chloride from the thick ascending limb, and (b) osmotic reabsorption of water accompanying active sodium and passive chloride

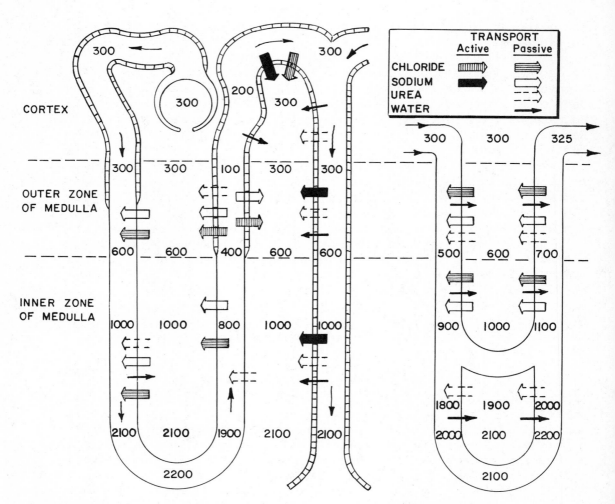

Figure 11-12. Diagram depicting the operation of the countercurrent multiplication system based on recent evidence discussed in the text. As in Figure 11-7, the numbers represent hypothetical osmolality values. Also, no quantitative significance is to be attached to the number of arrows, and only net movements are indicated.

reabsorption from the distal tubule and the cortical and outer medullary segments of the collecting tubule.

In the inner medulla, in the absence of active solute reabsorption from the water-impermeable thin ascending limb, the generated outer medullary interstitial gradient is not only maintained but is also enhanced by two processes: (a) passive reabsorption of sodium chloride and (b) recycling of urea. Osmotic abstraction of water from the outer medullary descending limb increases the concentration of sodium chloride in the filtrate reaching the inner medullary segment. As this filtrate traverses the thin ascending limb, the high luminal sodium chloride concentration favors its passive diffusion along the concentration gradient out of the ascending limb into the surrounding inner medullary interstitium. This increases the surrounding interstitial osmolar concentration while at the same time dilutes the fluid in the water-impermeable thin ascending limb. The inner medullary interstitial osmolar concentration is further increased by the recirculation of urea from the adjacent collecting tubule through the surrounding interstitium into the loop of Henle. The net result of the increase in the inner medullary interstitial osmolar concentration is further osmotic abstraction of water, not only from the thin descending limb, but also from the adjacent collecting tubule. The latter process is greatly enhanced in the presence of ADH.

To summarize, in the steady state, the operation of the various processes mentioned above lead to the development of a steep longitudinal gradient within the medulla, increasing from the cortex to the tip of the papilla, to which the fluids in the adjacent descending limb and collecting tubules are exposed and will equilibrate. The efficiency of this operation is enhanced by vasa recta, which, as we shall learn shortly, removes excess water and solutes reabsorbed from the loop of Henle and collecting tubule, thereby preserving the longitudinal gradient established in the medulla.

ROLE OF UREA IN THE COUNTERCURRENT MULTIPLICATION SYSTEM

Results of several micropuncture studies have suggested that renal transport of urea not only increases the ability of the kidney to concentrate urine, but also enhances the ability of the kidney to concentrate urine with non-urea solutes. To understand how these diverse functions are accomplished, let us examine the sequential processing of urea along the various nephron segments.

Micropuncture studies in hamsters (Lassiter et al., 1961), rats (Ullrich et al., 1963), and dogs (Clapp, 1965) have shown that the tubular fluid-to-plasma concentration ratio for urea ($[TF/P]_u$) was about one half that for inulin by the time the filtrate had reached the end of the proximal convoluted tubule, suggesting that about 50% of the filtered urea is reabsorbed along this nephron segment. Moreover, the urea-to-inulin $[TF/P]$ approached a value of unity by the time filtrate had entered the early distal convoluted tubule, suggesting that somehow an amount of urea equal to that reabsorbed in the proximal tubule was added to the tubular fluid as the filtrate traversed the loop of Henle. Since the fluid collected from the loop bend had a urea-to-inulin $[TF/P]$ considerably higher than unity, this urea must have been added to the tubular fluid along the descending limb of the loop of Henle. Furthermore, they found that $[TF/P]$ for inulin increased from a value of 3.0 at the end of the proximal tubule to a value of 6.9, by the time the filtrate had reached the early distal convoluted tubule, suggesting a net reabsorption of water along the loop of Henle. In short, as the filtrate traverses the loop of Henle, osmotic reabsorption of water from and passive diffusive entry of urea into the descending limb increases urea concentration along this loop segment.

In a recent study, Lassiter and associates (1966) provided direct evidence for the accumulation of urea in the loop of Henle and its participation in the countercurrent multiplication process. They found a $[TF/P]_u$ of about 17 in the fluid collected from the loop bend, compared to a value of 1.5 in the late proximal tubule fluid. This finding suggested that as the filtrate travels down the descending limb of the loop of Henle, urea is added to this nephron segment. Furthermore, by the time filtrate reaches the middle of the collecting tubule, the urea load is reduced by about 35%. This decrease in urea load in the late portion of the collecting tubule implies that urea is reabsorbed from this segment, presumably by passive diffusion, into the medullary interstitium, an idea first suggested by Berliner and associates (1958) and confirmed by recent micropuncture studies (Wirz and Dirix, 1973).

The results of the various experiments cited above are summarized in Table 11-1 for the rat, and their extrapolations to the human kidney are given in Table 11-2. These data show that normally in man about 50% of the filtered urea is reabsorbed along the nephron, while the remainder is excreted into the urine. Furthermore, comparing the percentage of filtered urea remaining in the fluid collected from different segments of the nephron in Tables 11-1 and 11-2 reveals that urea concentrations in the fluids collected from the loop bend and the early distal convoluted tubules are much higher than can be accounted for by the urea which had escaped proximal reabsorption, suggesting that urea is effectively recirculated within the renal medulla. This *recirculation of urea* involves its reabsorption from the distal and collecting tubules and its subsequent diffusion into the descending and ascending limbs of the loop of Henle (Fig. 11-13). Moreover, as mentioned earlier (see also Chapter 8), this recirculation of urea serves to establish a steep longitudinal medullary interstitial gradient by concentrating not only urea but also non-urea solutes, such as sodium chloride. This is made evident by comparing the percentage of total osmolality of fluid in different nephron segments due to the various solutes listed in Tables 11-1 and 11-2.

The extent of urea recycling appears to be correlated with the length of the loop of Henle within the medulla. The longer the length of the loop, the greater is the recycling of urea and its subsequent accumulation within the medulla, and hence the greater is the final osmolality of the excreted urine. The recycling of urea is further augmented by the selective action of ADH on the water and urea permeability of the distal and collecting tubules. ADH enhances the urea permeability of only the medullary segment of the collecting tubule, while at the same time it increases the water permeability of all segments of both the distal and collecting tubules (Bowman and Foulkes, 1970). As shown in Figure 11-13, both of these factors contribute to the high osmolality of the excreted urine in antidiuresis.

As mentioned in Chapter 8, in antidiuresis, although the molar concentrations of the fluid collected from the loop of Henle and the urine are approximately equal, the relative amounts of sodium and urea

TABLE 11-1

Relative Flow Rates and Concentrations of Water, Sodium, Urea, and Potassium in Different Nephron Segments of Rat Kidney

Nephron Segments	Percentage Remaining*				Percentage of Total Osmolality		
	Water	Sodium	Urea	Potassium	Sodium	Urea	Potassium
Glomerulus	100.0	100.0	100.0	100.0	46.5	2.3	1.5
End of Proximal Tubules	23.0	23.0	44.7	16.4	46.5	4.4	1.0
Loop of Henle (Bend)	17.0	47.1	605.3	86.9	33.3	20.8	1.9
Early Distal Tubules	17.0	9.5	133.0	3.7	35.6	24.4	0.4
End of Distal Tubules	6.0	2.9	77.1	26.7	23.3	30.0	6.7
End of Collecting Tubules	0.24	0.1	26.3	11.9	4.3	55.0	15.7

*For the method of calculation see Chapter 8.
[From Koushanpour, E., Tarica, R. R., and Stevens, W. F. (1971).]

TABLE 11-2

Relative Flow Rates and Concentrations of Water, Sodium, Urea,
and Potassium in Different Nephron Segments of Human Kidney

Nephron Segments	Percentage Remaining*				Percentage of Total Osmolality		
	Water	Sodium	Urea	Potassium	Sodium	Urea	Potassium
Glomerulus	100.0	100.0	100.0	100.0	46.5	1.6	1.6
End of Proximal Tubule	20.0	20.0	50.0	16.0	46.5	4.0	1.3
Loop of Henle (Bend)	16.0	33.3	576.0	57.6	33.3	20.0	2.0
Early Distal Tubules	16.0	9.4	165.0	3.8	37.0	22.5	0.5
End of Distal Tubules	4.8	3.3	76.8	27.0	28.6	22.9	8.1
End of Collecting Tubules	0.8	0.7	48.0	9.6	14.4	33.3	6.6

*For the method of calculation see Chapter 8.
[From Koushanpour, E., Tarica, R. R., and Stevens, W. F. (1971).]

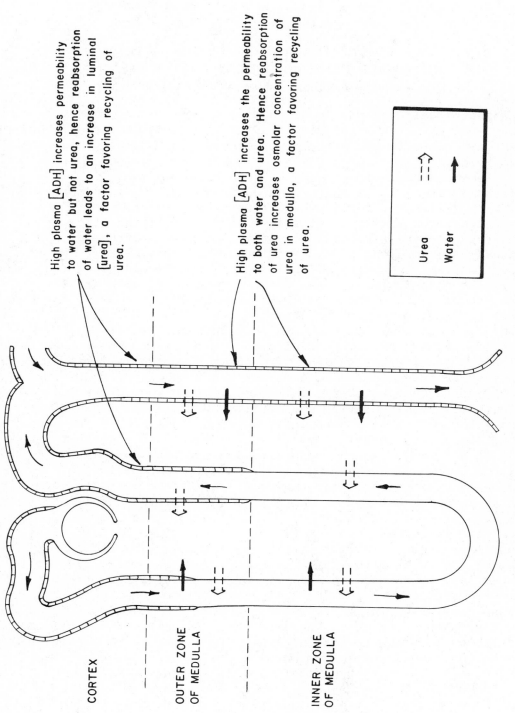

Figure 11-13. A schematic diagram depicting the recirculation of urea within the renal medulla.

in these two samples are inversely related: sodium is high and urea is low in the loop bend, whereas the opposite is true for the urine. However, this inverse relationship is abolished following sodium loading, a procedure known to reduce active sodium reabsorption in both distal and collecting tubules (Giebisch et al., 1964).

ROLE OF VASA RECTA IN THE COUNTERCURRENT MULTIPLICATION SYSTEM: THE COUNTERCURRENT DIFFUSION EXCHANGER

The anatomical arrangement of the medullary blood vessels described earlier not only provides the vehicle for delivery of the important nutrients to the medullary tissues, but also provides a means of removing the water and solutes which have entered the interstitial regions from the various tubular structures. As we shall learn shortly, it is the efficiency of this latter function, acting as a passive countercurrent diffusion exchanger, that can markedly enhance or limit the effectiveness of the performance of the countercurrent multiplication system in the loop of Henle, and consequently the concentration and dilution of urine.

The transient operation of the countercurrent multiplication system in the loop of Henle leads to accumulation of both sodium chloride and water in the medullary interstitium. Obviously, for the countercurrent system to be effective, neither sodium chloride nor water can accumulate in the medulla without a limit. In the steady state, once the longitudinal gradient is established, both sodium chloride and water must be removed by the medullary blood flow as fast as they are reabsorbed from the ascending (for sodium chloride) and descending (for water) limbs of the loop of Henle. Since the fluid leaving the ascending limb of the loop of Henle is *hypotonic* compared to that entering the descending limb of the loop, the blood leaving the medulla must be more hypertonic than that entering it. To maintain the medullary longitudinal gradient established by the countercurrent multiplication in the loop of Henle, the major problem is to prevent the excessive loss of fluid containing large amounts of osmotically active solutes. This is the function of the vasa recta. A possible explanation for this function is as follows.

In the presence of active reabsorption of chloride and passive movement of sodium from the thick segment of the ascending limb of the loop of Henle, the descending limb of the vasa recta behaves similarly to that of the loop of Henle--that is, sodium chloride enters (by passive diffusion) and water leaves (by osmosis). However, because blood flows faster in the vasa recta (see Fig. 6-5) than the tubular fluid flows in the loop of Henle (Table 11-1), the blood in the descending vasa recta approaches the interstitial osmolality at a level slightly below that in the descending limb of the loop of Henle. Consequently, as the blood enters the ascending vasa recta, it would have a slightly higher osmolality than the surrounding medullary interstitium (Fig. 11-12). This higher osmolality will result in a net diffusion of sodium chloride out of and water into the ascending limb of the vasa recta. However, because of the same difference in the rates of blood and tubular fluid flows mentioned above, the discrepancy in reaching the osmotic equilibrium with the surrounding medullary interstitium would persist. The net result is that the blood leaving the medulla would have a slightly higher osmolality than that entering it. This diffusion of sodium chloride out of the ascending limb of the vasa recta and its subsequent entry into the descending limb of the vasa recta, via the medullary interstitium, and the osmotic flow of water in the opposite direction is the basis for referring to the vasa recta as the *passive countercurrent diffusion exchanger*.

From the above analysis, it follows that the more nearly the osmolality of the blood leaving the medulla (via the ascending limb of the vasa recta) approaches that entering it (via the descending limb of vasa recta), the less sodium chloride will be lost from the medulla, and hence the greater would be the magnitude of the medullary longitudinal gradient. One factor that contributes to this unequal osmolality is the rate of medullary blood flow. The higher the medullary blood flow, the less time available for osmotic equilibration. Hence, the greater would be the rate of solute washout from the medulla, thereby reducing the medullary longitudinal gradient, which eventually lowers the osmolality of the excreted urine. Let us see why.

As described in Chapter 6 (see Fig. 6-5), Thornburn and associates (1963) showed that the blood flow in the inner medulla, which contains the vasa recta, is very slow compared to the blood flow in the cortical region. This slow medullary blood flow rate appears to be well suited for the passive countercurrent exchanger function of the vasa recta. Thus, dehydration or administration of small doses of ADH, either of which decreases the medullary blood flow, leads to accumulation of urea and sodium chloride in the medulla, thereby increasing the longitudinal gradient and hence the concentration of urine. On the other hand, administration of large doses of vasoactive drugs, including ADH, produces diuresis, the mechanism of which is at present poorly understood (Lever, 1965). In contrast, water and osmotic diuresis and diabetes insipidus, all of which tend to increase the medullary blood flow, promote solute washout from the medullary interstitium, thereby reducing the longitudinal gradient and hence the concentration of urine. In short, an increase in blood flow in the medullary blood vessels will tend to decrease urine concentration, whereas a decrease in the blood flow will have the opposite effect.

Another factor modifying the medullary blood flow consists of changes in the systemic arterial pressure. While cortical blood flow obeys autoregulation, a phenomenon described in Chapter 5, the medullary blood flow does not. In fact, experimental evidence has shown that the medullary blood flow varies directly with changes in the systemic arterial blood pressure (Thurau, 1964). Perfusion of the kidney with arterial pressure of up to 250 mm Hg, though it did not alter the GFR because of autoregulation, produced a significant decrease in urine osmolality. This was due to a marked increase in the medullary blood flow which varied with the perfusion pressure and thus did not obey the autoregulatory mechanism. In osmotic diuresis, although the medullary blood flow is increased, the increase in GFR (due to intravascular volume expansion) further reduces the medullary osmotic gradient (see Chapter 8), thereby yielding a more dilute urine. On the basis of these findings, it has been suggested (Thurau, 1964) that this asymmetric effect of the arterial blood pressure on the cortical and medullary blood flows represents a means by which the mammalian kidney is capable of changing the urinary concentration in response to variation of the blood pressure without affecting the glomerular filtration rate.

Finally, the macula densa-renin-angiotensin feedback system, which was described in Chapter 5, also plays an important role in adjusting the medullary blood flow. Its function is to prevent the dissipation of the normal transverse gradient, thus assuring the development of the normal medullary longitudinal gradient necessary for the production of a hypertonic urine. The significance of this mechanism in the overall renal regulation of water and electrolyte balance will be described in Chapter 12.

MEASUREMENT OF THE CONCENTRATING AND DILUTING ABILITY OF THE KIDNEY

From the foregoing discussion, it is clear that the ability of the kidney to concentrate and dilute urine depends on the functions of the loop of Henle and the distal and collecting tubules. We learned that the fluid emerging from the proximal tubule remains iso-osmotic, regardless of the osmolality of the excreted urine. However, as the filtrate traverses the descending limb, it becomes hyperosmotic as a consequence of the countercurrent multiplication process following the hyperosmotic reabsorption of sodium chloride from the water-impermeable ascending limb of the loop of Henle. The reabsorption of sodium chloride, without the osmotic accompaniment of water, in the ascending limb leaves behind an amount of water free of solute, thereby making the fluid remaining in the tubule hypotonic. For this reason, this water, which is not reabsorbed, is referred to as the "*solute-free*" water, and the ascending limb is known as the *diluting segment*.

As was pointed out earlier, the degree of hypotonicity of the fluid in the ascending limb determines the magnitude of the transverse gradient, a factor which in turn governs the magnitude of the longitudinal gradient developed in the medullary interstitium. It is the latter osmolar concentration gradient that eventually determines the degree of concentration of fluid emerging from the collecting tubule and hence the osmolality of the excreted urine. The latter is a consequence of the ability of the collecting tubule to reabsorb water in excess of solute, a process greatly enhanced by ADH, and thereby to adjust its osmolality to that of the surrounding hypertonic medullary interstitium. For this reason, the collecting tubule is referred to as the *concentrating segment*.

Thus, in the final analysis, the ability of the kidney to concentrate and dilute urine depends on the functions of the ascending limb of the loop of Henle and the collecting tubule. The former determines the volume of "solute-free" water excreted in the urine, whereas the latter determines the quantity of the osmotically active solutes or the *osmolar concentration* of the excreted urine. For this reason, it is of great clinical importance and potential diagnostic value to determine the relative amounts of water and osmotically active solutes that are not reabsorbed (and are therefore excreted in the urine).

Although in animal studies, it is possible to assess the functions of the ascending limb and collecting tubule directly, techniques for such a direct observation in man are not yet available. Therefore, in clinical practice, a qualitative estimate of the functions of these tubular segments and hence of the concentrating and diluting ability of the kidney is obtained by measuring the osmolar concentration of urine relative to that of plasma as well as the volume of excreted urine, using the standard clearance technique described in Chapter 6. The rationale for applying this method to determining the concentrating and diluting ability of the kidney is as follows.

Micropuncture studies cited earlier have shown that most of the filtrate is reabsorbed iso-osmotically along the proximal and distal tubules, while the remaining small fraction is reabsorbed in the loop of Henle and the collecting tubule, where its osmolality undergoes considerable modification. Thus, any deviation in the osmolality of the excreted urine from isotonicity must reflect relative reabsorptive changes in water and solutes along these tubular segments. Hence, excretion of a concentrated urine implies net reabsorption of water in excess of solute, whereas excretion of a dilute urine implies just the opposite. Accordingly, to obtain a qualitative estimate of the concentrating and diluting ability of the kidney, one need simply measure the renal clearance of the osmotically active solutes present in the blood and compare it with the renal clearance of solute-free water. Let us now examine the operational definitions of these clearances and their physiological meanings (Wesson, 1969).

Osmolar clearance, symbolized by C_{Osm}, may be defined as the volume of plasma which contains the same quantity of the osmotically active solutes excreted in 1 minute in urine. It is calculated by dividing the total amount of the osmotically active solutes excreted in the urine per minute (the product of urine osmolality (U_{Osm}) and urine volume (V)), by the plasma osmolality (P_{Osm}):

$$C_{Osm}(ml/min) = \frac{U_{Osm}(mOsm/L) \cdot V(ml/min)}{P_{Osm}(mOsm/L)} \tag{11-1}$$

Because both U_{Osm} and P_{Osm} are measured by cryoscopical method--that is, by freezing-point depression--their values include the contribution of both electrolytes and non-electrolytes. In a fasting but otherwise normal individual, osmolar clearance varies between 2 to 3 ml/min, and is relatively independent of urine flow.

Solute-free water clearance is defined as the difference between the volume of urine excreted per minute (V) and the osmolar clearance

(C_{Osm}) calculated from Equation 11-1:

Solute-free water clearance (ml/min) = V(ml/min) - C_{Osm}(ml/min)

$$(11-2)$$

If the urine is neither concentrated nor dilute, that is, if it is iso-osmotic with the plasma ($U_{Osm} = P_{Osm}$), it follows from the definition of the osmolar clearance (Equation 11-1) that $V = C_{Osm}$ in Equation 11-2, and the solute-free water clearance would be zero. However, if the urine is concentrated, that is, if U_{Osm} is much greater than P_{Osm}, and V is very small, as would be the case during dehydration, C_{Osm} would be greater than V, and their difference would be *negative*. This negative solute-free water clearance is designated by the symbol $T^C_{H_2O}$, and it means that there is a net reabsorption of water. That is why the excreted urine is *hypertonic*. The superscript "c" in the symbol $T^C_{H_2O}$ signifies that the net reabsorption of water occurs in the concentrating segment of the nephron, namely, the collecting tubule. On the other hand, if the urine is dilute, that is, if U_{Osm} is much smaller than P_{Osm}, and V is relatively large, as would be the case during water ingestion or diuresis, C_{Osm} would be less than V, and their difference would be *positive*. This *positive* solute-free water clearance is designated by the symbol C_{H_2O}, and it means that water is not reabsorbed and hence is excreted in the urine. That is why the urine is *hypotonic*. In short, a negative solute-free water clearance means net reabsorption of water in excess of solutes and hence excretion of an hypertonic urine. In contrast, a positive solute-free water clearance means net excretion of water in excess of solutes and hence formation of an hypotonic urine. Thus, $T^C_{H_2O}$ is equal to $-(C_{H_2O})$.

To further illustrate the physiological meanings of osmolar clearance as well as the negative and positive solute-free water clearances, let us consider the following two cases:

1. In a normal man, restriction of fluid intake results in elaboration of a urine some 4 to 5 times more concentrated than the plasma. In such a circumstance, urine flow may reach a value as low as 0.5 ml/min. Assuming a plasma osmolality of 300 mOsm/L, U_{Osm} would have a value of 5 x 300 mOsm/L = 1,500 mOsm/L, and the osmolar clearance would be:

$$C_{Osm}(ml/min) = \frac{1,500 (mOsm/L) \times 0.5 (ml/min)}{300 (mOsm/L)} = 2.5 \text{ ml/min} \qquad (11-3)$$

Because urine is hypertonic, there must have been a net reabsorption of water, and hence a negative solute-free water clearance ($T^C_{H_2O}$):

$$T^C_{H_2O}(ml/min) = V - C_{Osm} = 0.5(ml/min) - 2.5(ml/min)$$

$$= -2.0 \; ml/min \qquad (11-4)$$

This negative solute-free water clearance means that the osmotically active solutes which were present in 2.5 ml of blood (C_{Osm} = 2.5 ml/min) were excreted in 0.5 ml of hypertonic urine, resulting in a net reabsorption of 2.0 ml of solute-free water back into the blood. In this manner, the kidneys have conserved water to dilute the body fluids, thereby decreasing the plasma osmolality toward normal.

    2. In contrast, ingestion of a liter or more of water by a normally hydrated man will increase urine flow to as much as 20 ml/min, while at the same time it may decrease urine osmolality to 0.1 that of the plasma. Again, assuming a plasma osmolality of 300 mOsm/L, U_{Osm} = 0.1 x 300 mOsm/L = 30 mOsm/L, and

$$C_{Osm}(ml/min) = \frac{30(mOsm/L) \; x \; 20(ml/min)}{300(mOsm/L)} = 2.0 \; ml/min \qquad (11-5)$$

    Because urine is hypotonic, there must have been relatively less water reabsorption, and hence a positive solute-free water clearance (C_{H_2O}):

$$C_{H_2O}(ml/min) = V - C_{Osm} = 20(ml/min) - 2.0(ml/min)$$

$$= 18.0 \; ml/min \qquad (11-6)$$

This positive solute-free water clearance means that the osmotically active solutes which were present in 2.0 ml of blood (C_{Osm} = 2.0 ml/min) were excreted in 20 ml of hypotonic urine, resulting in a net loss of 18.0 ml of solute-free water from the body. In this manner, the kidneys have excreted water to concentrate the body fluids, thereby increasing the plasma osmolality toward normal.

    Thus, by manipulating the reabsorption of water and osmotically active solutes, the kidneys adjust the volume and osmolality of the body fluids. The outcome of this adjustment is reflected in the volume and osmolality of the excreted urine as measured by osmolar and solute-free water clearances. However, as pointed out in Chapter 1, the kidneys appear to be more effective in protecting the body against dilution than concentration. The kidneys cannot replace the excessive fluid lost from the body, and therefore must be aided by direct fluid replacement.

HORMONAL REGULATION OF CONCENTRATION AND DILUTION OF URINE

In the preceding sections, we stated that in the mammalian kidney the final volume and osmolality of the excreted urine ultimately depend on the extent of osmotic equilibration of the fluids in the collecting tubules with the surrounding hypertonic medullary interstitium. Briefly, there are three factors that contribute to this osmotic equilibration: (1) Osmotic reabsorption of water from the distal and collecting tubules, a process greatly enhanced in the presence of the *antidiuretic hormone* (ADH); (2) passive reabsorption of urea from the same tubular segments, as well as *ADH-enhanced* passive urea reabsorption from the inner medullary collecting tubule, which initiates the recycling of urea within the renal medulla; and (3) active reabsorption of the sodium, which had escaped reabsorption in the proximal tubule and the loop of Henle, along with its associated anion from the same tubular segments, a process profoundly influenced by the circulating level of another hormone, namely, the adrenocortical hormone *aldosterone* (see also Chapter 8). It therefore follows that any factor that influences the plasma concentration of ADH and aldosterone must exert a marked effect on the final volume and osmolality of the excreted urine.

To better understand the roles of these two hormones in the concentration and dilution of urine, and hence in the regulation of the final volume and osmolality of the excreted urine, it is necessary to closely examine the sites and mechanisms of their cellular actions as well as the factors governing their effects on the target tissues. To facilitate this presentation and subsequent discussion, we shall include a brief survey of the biosynthesis, secretion, and metabolism of each hormone and the factors affecting them.

MECHANISM OF ACTION OF ANTIDIURETIC HORMONE (ADH)

BIOSYNTHESIS, SECRETION, AND METABOLISM. It has been established that injection of crude extracts of the posterior lobe of the pituitary gland (neurohypophysis) into mammals produces three distinct physiological responses: (1) It causes uterine contraction, an action referred to as the *oxytocic* effect; (2) it raises the systemic arterial blood pressure, an action referred to as the *vasopressor* effect; and (3) it decreases the volume of excreted urine, an action referred to as the *antidiuretic* effect (Kamm et al., 1928). Subsequent purification and separation of the crude extracts led to the successful isolation and synthesis of three chemically distinct hormones, each exhibiting the oxytocic, vasopressor, and antidiuretic effects to varying degrees (Du Vigneaud, 1956). Structurally, all three hormones are nonapeptides with molecular weights of slightly over 1000 and comprising a cyclic unit, formed by a disulfide-bridged pentapeptide and a tripeptide side chain unit. The three hormones are named oxytocin, [8-arginine]-vasopressin, and [8-lysine]-vasopressin.

Of these, [8-arginine]-vasopressin (AVP), which has an arginine
residue in the 8 position in the side chain, is the most prevalent
form of the posterior pituitary hormone found in mammals. It has
been isolated as the natural hormone in man, dog, rat, rabbit, and
sheep. In contrast, [8-lysine]-vasopressin (LVP), in which a lysine
residue replaces the arginine residue in the 8 position in the side
chain, has been isolated only from the hog pituitary. Although all
three hormones cause antidiuresis, the antidiuretic effects of AVP
and LVP are some 100 times that of oxytocin. For this reason, the
two *vasopressins* are customarily referred to as the *antidiuretic
hormones* or ADH.

It is generally accepted that vasopressins are primarily
synthesized in the *supraoptic* nucleus, whereas oxytocin is synthesized
in the *paraventricular* nucleus of the hypothalamus. The synthesized
hormones are then carried by *neurosecretory granules* through the
hypothalamo-hypophyseal nerve tracts into the neurohypophysis, where
they are stored for subsequent release into the circulation (Sachs,
1967). Recent studies have confirmed this concept and have further
clarified the role of the neurosecretory granules in the biosynthesis
and transport of the neurohypophyseal hormones. According to these
new findings, the neurosecretory granules contain a group of small
molecular weight proteins, called *neurophysin*, which bind oxytocin
and vasopressins. As such, neurophysin serves as both "precursor"
and "carrier" of the neurohypophyseal hormones, thereby providing a
vehicle for their transport from the hypothalamus to the posterior
lobe of the pituitary gland, where they are stored. Subsequent to
proper stimulation, the appropriate hormone is then separated from
the neurophysin protein and is released as a free polypeptide into
the circulation (Wuu et al., 1971).

The plasma concentration of ADH, based on bioassay of pressor
activity of pure [8-arginine]-vasopressin (400 pressor units per mg)
is about 5 microunits (μU), or 5×10^{-5} μg per ml plasma, in normal
subjects (Share, 1967). The plasma concentration of the hormone is
maintained by a dynamic balance between the rates of its biosynthesis
and secretion into the circulation, and the rate of its removal from
the blood. Although the rates of biosynthesis and secretion of
vasopressins are at present not well understood, they appear to be
largely dependent on the blood volume and its osmolality, with the
latter being the major stimulus (see Chapter 12 for further details).
However, there is little disagreement about the rates and major routes
of removal of ADH from the circulation. Results of numerous clearance
studies have shown that ADH is removed from the blood by three major
routes: (1) hepatic clearance and metabolic inactivation by the
liver; (2) renal clearance and excretion in the urine; and (3)
utilization by the renal tubular target tissues (Lauson, 1967).
Furthermore, clearance studies in dogs and rats have shown that only
half of the injected ADH reaches the kidney, while the other half is
cleared and inactivated by the liver. Of the amount of ADH that
reaches the kidney, approximately half is excreted in the urine.
Since ADH does not appreciably bind to plasma proteins, it is
therefore filtered at the glomerulus and is subsequently reabsorbed.
Hence, its renal clearance and urinary excretion represent that

fraction of the filtered hormone which has escaped tubular reabsorption. The circulatory half-life of injected ADH averaged about 6.5 min in these studies.

SITES AND MODES OF CELLULAR ACTION. The classic experiments of Verney (1947) were the first to define the nature of the ADH-releasing stimulus, the target organ, and its response characteristics. Verney found that intracarotid injection of hypertonic saline or sucrose solution reduced previously established water diuresis in conscious dogs. Moreover, a sustained 2% increase in the osmolality of blood was sufficient to produce a 90% reduction in maximal water diuresis. This response was completely abolished following removal of the posterior lobe of the pituitary gland. In a later study, Jewell and Verney (1957) showed that oliguria (a marked reduction of urine volume) resulted whenever the hypertonic solution reached the supraoptic nucleus. On the basis of these findings, Verney and associates postulated that the cells of the supraoptic nucleus act as the "osmoreceptors" responding to alterations in the osmotic pressure or osmolality of the blood perfusing them. Since these cells were known to produce ADH, they postulated further that the release of this hormone increased the osmotic reabsorption of water by the kidney, a factor accounting for the inhibition of water diuresis and concentration of the excreted urine. Although subsequent studies confirmed the above mechanism for the release of ADH and its overall renal action (Share, 1967; see also Chapter 12), localization of ADH-responsive target tissues within the nephron and the mode of its cellular action had to await the application of micropuncture and microperfusion techniques to the kidney tubules.

Micropuncture and microperfusion studies of the distal and collecting tubules, cited earlier, have clearly established that (a) the distal and collecting tubules are the only ADH-responsive target tissues within the kidney, and (b) ADH not only increases the osmotic water permeability of these tubular segments, but it also enhances the passive urea permeability of the inner medullary collecting tubule. Furthermore, it has been shown (Morel et al., 1965) that ADH causes an increase in the osmotic water permeability of the luminal membrane of the renal cells in these tubular segments, but has no effect on the water permeability of the peritubular membrane. However, to have any effect on the permeability of the luminal membrane, ADH must be added to the surface of the peritubular membrane, which is the blood side of the distal and collecting tubules. Thus, the antidiuretic effect of ADH is obtained only when the hormone reaches the distally located nephron segments by way of the blood vessels. Consequently, the ADH which is filtered at the glomerulus is exposed to the luminal side of the tubular cell, and therefore, insofar as water reabsorption is concerned, it has no physiological effect.

In summary, ADH-enhanced osmotic reabsorption of water in the distally located nephron segments appears to be a consequence of some as yet unknown intracellular biochemical processes which are presumed to be initiated by the exposure of the surface of the peritubular membrane to ADH. Exactly how the presence of ADH at the peritubular surface initiates these complex cellular processes, and how these processes in turn bring about alterations in the osmotic water permeability of the luminal surface, have been the subject of considerable investigations.

Our present knowledge of the mechanism of cellular action of ADH has largely been derived from an extension of studies in anuran membrane (toad urinary bladder) to mammalian renal tubules (Orloff and Handler, 1964, 1967). In toad bladder, it has been found that when ADH is added to the fluid in contact with the *serosal* (peritubular or blood) side, it causes an increase in both diffusional and osmotic reabsorption of water from the *mucosal* (luminal or urinary) side of the epithelial membrane. However, placing the ADH in the fluid bathing the mucosal side produces no effect, suggesting that ADH cannot enter the cell. In contrast, osmotic transfer of water from the mucosal side to the serosal side was increased when cyclic AMP was placed in the fluid bathing either the serosal or mucosal side, suggesting that cyclic AMP can enter the cell. From these studies, the following general inferences have been made: (1) The barrier for the osmotic reabsorption of water lies within the mucosal side of the epithelial membrane; (2) ADH, acting on the serosal side, somehow causes an increase in the osmotic water permeability of the mucosal side; and (3) since cyclic AMP mimics the action of ADH, its cellular concentration somehow might mediate the ADH-enhanced water reabsorption. This latter inference is based on the postulated role of the newly discovered cyclic AMP (Sutherland et al., 1968) as the "second messenger," mediating the hormone-stimulated biological response of a variety of target tissues (see Fig. 7-9).

In a series of elegant experiments, Grantham and associates (1969, 1971) have extended these observations to the mammalian nephron, thereby providing the most direct experimental evidence for the site of action and the cellular mechanism of ADH-enhanced water reabsorption. Using isolated fragments of rabbit cortical collecting tubule, they found that, in the absence of ADH, when the peritubular surface of the tubular segment was exposed to hypo-, iso-, and hyperosmotic solutions, the tubular cells behaved like an osmometer: shrinking in hyperosmotic and swelling in hypo-osmotic solutions. However, no such response was observed when the luminal surface of the tubular segments was exposed to the same solutions. In contrast, when ADH was added to the fluid bathing the peritubular surface, the previously unresponsive luminal surface became "active" and once again the tubular cells behaved like an osmometer. However, no osmometer-like effect was observed when ADH was added to the fluid bathing the luminal surface. In contrast, when cyclic AMP was added to the fluid bathing either the peritubular or luminal surfaces, the tubular cells once again behaved as an osmometer. Electron microscopic examination of both ADH-stimulated and cyclic AMP-stimulated tubular fragments revealed an increase in the size of the existing aqueous channels (intercellular space with tight junction; see Fig. 8-11) within the tubular cells, an observation which in part accounted for the altered osmotic water permeability. From these findings, analogous to those for the anuran membrane, the following general conclusions were drawn: (1) The luminal membrane of the tubular cell constitutes the barrier for the osmotic reabsorption of water; (2) ADH-stimulation of the peritubular membrane of the tubular cell somehow increases the water permeability of the luminal membrane; and (3) since cyclic AMP mimics the action of ADH but, unlike the latter, it can enter the renal cells, ADH-enhanced water reabsorption is somehow mediated by the intracellular production of cyclic AMP which, in an unknown manner, alters the water permeability of the luminal membrane.

The mystery of the intracellular processes initiated by ADH-stimulation has now been partly resolved by additional experiments. The results of these experiments have led to the formulation of the hypothesis shown in Figure 11-14, depicting the cellular action of ADH. From the functional point of view, we may divide the various biochemical reactions involved into two sequential steps: (1) An ADH-dependent formation of cyclic AMP (cyclic **AMP** breakdown within the cell is independent of the hormone); and (2) cyclic AMP-dependent phosphorylation of the proteins in the luminal membrane, thereby bringing about altered water permeability (dephosphorylation of the luminal membrane is independent of the hormone). Let us now consider the details of these two steps, starting with the interaction of ADH with the peritubular membrane.

Experiments with the isolated perfused collecting tubules, cited above, have shown that ADH induces osmotic reabsorption of water from these epithelia only when the hormone is present in the fluid bathing the peritubular membrane. From this, it has been inferred that the *receptor for ADH* must be located on the outer surface of the peritubular membrane of the tubular cell. Moreover, since cyclic AMP has been found to mimic the cellular action of ADH, it is postulated that the stereospecific binding of ADH with the receptor somehow activates enzymatic production of cyclic AMP. It has been shown (Sutherland et al., 1968) that the enzyme *adenylate cyclase*, located in the inner surface of the cell mambrane, catalyzes the formation of *cyclic AMP* from *adenosine triphosphate (ATP)*. The latter is supplied by cellular breakdown of *glycogen*, a reaction stimulated by both ADH and cyclic AMP (Fig. 11-14).

The concentration of cyclic AMP thus formed within the cell is regulated by a cytoplasmic enzyme called *cyclic AMP-phosphodiesterase*. This enzyme which is not influenced by ADH converts cyclic AMP into 5'-AMP, an inactive degradation product. Therefore, cyclic AMP-phosphodiesterase plays an important role in the cellular metabolism of cyclic AMP and the extent to which it mediates ADH-induced water reabsorption. Inhibition of this enzyme by reagents such as theophylline, aminophylline, or chlorpropamide can potentiate the effect of ADH or exogenous cyclic AMP on osmotic water reabsorption (Berndt et al., 1970).

The precise mechanism whereby the intracellular formation of cyclic AMP induces altered water permeability of the luminal membrane is presently not well understood. However, on the basis of several

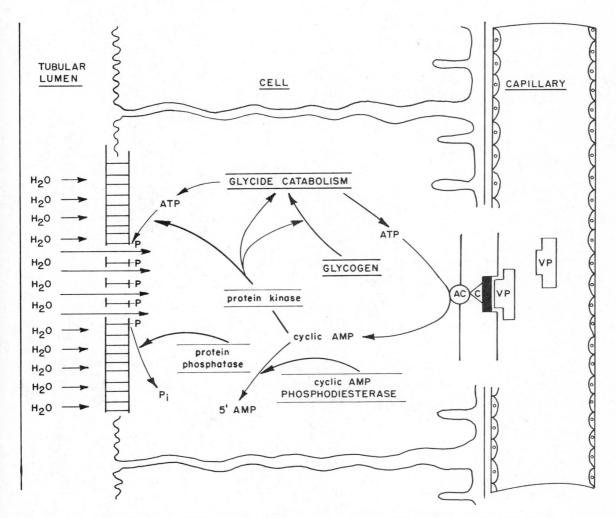

Figure 11-14. Scheme depicting the proposed mechanism of cellular action of ADH. VP designates a molecule of vasopressin or ADH, and the triangle designated C represents the hypothetical coupler which connects the membrane-bound receptor (dark rectangle) to the catalytic site of the adenylate cyclase (AC). [Modified from Dousa, T. P. (1973).]

in vitro microperfusion as well as isolated cell experiments, the following picture has emerged. Intracellular formation of cyclic AMP stimulates an intracellular enzyme called *protein kinase*, which catalyzes the transfer of gamma-phosphate of ATP to serine or threonine residues of the *protein phosphatase*. The latter is located on the inner surface of the luminal membrane of the renal cell. Thus, cyclic AMP, by activating protein kinase, may bring about *phosphorylation* of the luminal membrane, the postulated consequence of which is the alteration of the structure of the luminal membrane, and thereby an increase in its osmotic water permeability.

The scheme depicted in Figure 11-14 represents a mixture of both experimentally verified and postulated steps which may be involved in the cellular action of ADH. As such, it has served a useful purpose not only in synthesizing the various experimental and theoretical information, but also in guiding future research. Thus, it has helped to elucidate the nature of pathogenesis of *nephrogenic diabetes insipidus*. This is a disease characterized by polyuria and a decrease or loss of the ability of the kidney to increase the osmolality of urine in response to exogenous ADH. Although the exact mechanism underlying its pathogenesis is at present not well understood, results of a number of experiments suggest that the defect may be due to a decrease in ADH-stimulated cyclic AMP formation within the renal cell (Dousa, 1974).

In summary, the overall effect of renal action of ADH is to modify the net reabsorption of water in the distal and collecting tubules, yielding a concentrated urine. Consistent with the ideas developed in the previous section, we may consider the volume of urine excreted per minute (V) as the algebraic sum of osmolar and solute-free water clearances:

$$V = C_{Osm} + C_{H_2O} \tag{11-7}$$

In the presence of ADH, there is a net increase in the water permeability of the luminal cell membrane, allowing the water to follow the osmotic gradient established across the membrane. The consequence of this water reabsorption is an increase in C_{Osm} and a decrease in C_{H_2O} (actually an increase in negative solute-free water clearance, $T^C_{H_2O}$), yielding a concentrated urine, having osmolality about the same as that found in the renal papilla. However, in the absence of ADH, reduced water reabsorption in these distally located nephron segments increases C_{H_2O} and hence C_{Osm} leading to the excretion of a dilute urine with osmolality very much less than that of papillary urine. In both cases, however, the fluid collected from the loop bend is hyperosmotic, although that collected in the presence of ADH has three to four times higher osmolality than that obtained in the absence of ADH.

MECHANISM OF ACTION OF ALDOSTERONE

PRODUCTION AND SITE OF ACTION. The modern history of the renal action of aldosterone began in the late 1940's, when Roemmelt and associates (1949) found that in adrenalectomized dogs only 2 to 2.5% of the total filtered sodium escaped tubular reabsorption, a deficiency that was corrected by administration of the crude extracts of the adrenal gland. Subsequent purification and isolation of the crude extracts identified the sodium-retaining substance as an

18-aldehyde derivative of corticosterone and hence it was named *aldosterone* (Simpson and Tait, 1955).

Aldosterone is synthesized from cholesterol in the *zona glomerulosa* of the adrenal cortex. Its biosynthesis is regulated by several factors, of which dietary intake of sodium is the most prominent. In normal subjects whose sodium intake varies between 50 and 200 mEq/day, 50 to 250 µg of aldosterone is produced per day, of which about 10% is excreted in urine (Knochel and Whale, 1973). Clearance studies have shown that the renal clearance of aldosterone is about 14% of that of inulin, suggesting that about 86% of the filtered aldosterone is reabsorbed by the renal tubules (Siegenthaler et al., 1964).

In normal subjects kept in supine position for 3 consecutive days and given a daily dose of 10 mEq sodium/100 mEq potassium, plasma concentration of aldosterone showed a distinct diurnal rhythm. It varied from 55 ± 7 ng/100 ml plasma at 8 a.m. to 33 ± 5 ng/100 ml plasma at 11 p.m. (Williams et al., 1972). Although the physiological significance of this diurnal variation in plasma concentration is at present not known, it is believed to be mediated by variations in the secretion of the anterior pituitary adrenocorticotrophic hormone, ACTH.

The sites of renal action of aldosterone have been localized by both stop-flow and micropuncture experiments. Stop-flow studies (Vander et al., 1958) have shown that administration of aldosterone to adrenalectomized dogs lowers the high sodium concentration found in the fluids emerging from the distally located nephron segments. This suggested that the renal action of aldosterone is confined to the distal and collecting tubules, a conclusion which was subsequently confirmed by free-flow micropuncture studies (Hierholzer et al., 1965). They found that in adrenalectomized rats the high $[TF/P]_{Na}$ in the distal tubules was reduced after administration of aldosterone. However, no difference in the $[TF/P]_{Na}$ in the proximal tubule was noted between the normal and adrenalectomized animals, a finding which was has also been confirmed in dogs (Wright et al., 1969). Other kinds of evidence, however, have implicated the action of aldosterone in the proximal tubule. Thus, when tritiated aldosterone was injected into the rats it appeared in both the proximal and distal tubules. Moreover, actinomycin D (see discussion below for mechanism) inhibited a portion of proximal tubular sodium reabsorption in adrenalectomized rats treated with aldosterone (Mulrow and Forman, 1972). Despite this, the proximal tubular action of aldosterone remains controversial and has yet to be verified by free-flow micropuncture experiments. Thus, from available evidence we may conclude that the renal action of aldosterone is confined to the distal and collecting tubules, where it enhances the reabsorption of about 2% of the filtered sodium. As described in Chapter 8, the resulting reduction in the luminal concentration of sodium increases the luminal negativity, a factor which by electrical coupling enhances secretion of either potassium or hydrogen ions in exchange for sodium. Hence, potassium or hydrogen ion secretion is secondary to the primary action of aldosterone on sodium transport.

To summarize, reabsorption of sodium in the distal and collecting tubules occurs as a consequence of *two* mechanisms: One mechanism consists of *aldosterone-independent* active reabsorption of most of the sodium, by a process analogous to that described for the proximal tubule (see Chapter 8). The second mechanism consists of *aldosterone-dependent* active reabsorption of a small fraction of the remaining sodium (about 2% of the filtered load). When considered in a short-term situation, the quantity of sodium reabsorbed by the second mechanism is very small. However, the long-term loss of this amount of sodium from the body consequent to aldosterone deficiency is indeed very serious and detrimental to life.

FACTORS REGULATING BIOSYNTHESIS. A number of studies (see reviews by Müller, 1971; Williams and Dluhy, 1972) have shown that the biosynthesis of aldosterone from cholesterol is influenced by three major factors, each acting on different sites along the biosynthetic pathway shown in Figure 11-15. This scheme assumes that there is only one type of aldosterone-producing cell and that there is only one biosynthetic pathway for aldosterone. To facilitate presentation, we have divided this pathway into three stages: (1) The conversion of cholesterol into pregnenolone, designated as the *early pathway*; (2) the conversion of pregnenolone into corticosterone, designated as the *middle pathway*; and (3) the conversion of cortico- sterone into aldosterone, designated as the *late pathway*. On the basis of this division, the various stimuli influencing aldosterone biosynthesis may be classified into those which affect the early, middle, or late pathway.

Results of extensive studies in both animals and man have shown that stimuli that influence the early pathway are all of *acute* nature, while those that act on the late pathway are all of *chronic* nature. Included in the first category are the renin-angiotensin system, acute changes in sodium and potassium intake, and blood levels of ACTH. Of these, the first two are the most important, while ACTH plays only a minor role in aldosterone biosynthesis. The second category includes chronic sodium and potassium loading and/or depletion, and their combinations. It should be remembered that increased production of aldosterone caused by acute stimuli is a consequence of increased activity in both the early and late pathways. The increase in the activity of the late pathway is due to a secondary increase in corticosterone production consequent to increased activity in the early pathway. Thus, acute infusion of renin or angiotensin stimulates the early pathway, and hence increases the production of aldosterone. Similarly, acute infusion or oral ingestion of potassium as well as chronic potassium loading enhances aldosterone production, while chronic potassium depletion or sodium loading inhibits its production. The potassium effect on aldosterone production has been shown to be independent of the renin-angiotensin system. Let us now consider in more detail the effect of each of these stimuli on aldosterone biosynthesis.

A. Renin-Angiotensin System. As mentioned in Chapter 5, renin is an enzyme produced by the *granular cells* of the juxtaglomerular

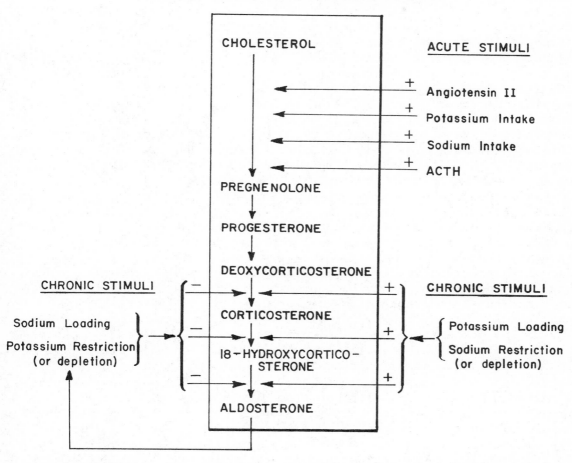

Figure 11-15. Scheme summarizing the sites of action of acute and chronic stimuli on the biosynthesis of aldosterone. A plus sign (+) above the arrows indicates stimulation, and a minus sign (-) indicates inhibition. [Modified from Müller, J. (1971).]

apparatus in response to (a) changes in renal blood flow (a direct consequence of alterations in blood volume) and (b) changes in the osmolality or sodium load in the distal tubular fluid passing by the *macula densa cells*. For the present, we will focus only on the changes in blood volume and their effects upon renin production, and hence aldosterone biosynthesis.

Briefly, a decrease in the circulating blood volume leads to a reduction in the renal blood flow. This is monitored by the granular cells of the juxtaglomerular apparatus, causing an increase in renin production by these cells. This renin acts on its circulating substrate, angiotensinogen (found chiefly in the alpha-2-globulin fraction of plasma) to split off the decapeptide angiotensin I, which is biologically inactive. However, upon passing through the lung, which is rich in converting enzyme, angiotensin I is converted into the biologically active octapeptide angiotensin II. This substance has at least three known effects: (1) It is a potent vasoconstrictor; (2) it has a direct effect on sodium transport by the kidney; and (3) it stimulates the zona glomerulosa cells to secrete aldosterone (Vander, 1967). The latter effect enhances plasma levels of aldosterone, which in turn increases sodium reabsorption, accompanied by osmotic reabsorption of water, from the distal and collecting tubules. This would lead to an increase in the circulating blood volume, thereby closing the negative feedback loop. Most of the animal studies have shown that renin-angiotensin levels and aldosterone secretion change in parallel fashion following alterations in blood volume and/or sodium intake. Further details of this feedback loop as well as that initiated by the macula densa cells will be discussed in Chapter 12.

B. Changes in Sodium-Potassium Balance. The second category of stimuli affecting aldosterone biosynthesis consists of acute changes in dietary intake of sodium and potassium as well as chronic loading and/or restriction of these ions. The former influences the early pathway, whereas the latter acts on the late pathway.

Like angiotensin II, acute alterations of sodium and potassium intake stimulate the early pathway, thereby increasing the conversion of cholesterol to pregnenolone and eventually the secretion of aldosterone. In contrast, chronic loading and/or restriction of sodium and potassium alter aldosterone secretion by directly modifying the activity of the late pathway. Thus, either chronic potassium loading or sodium restriction causes an increase in aldosterone production, whereas sodium loading or potassium restriction produces a marked decrease in aldosterone production. An additional effect of these chronic stimuli is that by modifying the activity of the late pathway, they modulate the rate of response or the "sensitivity" of the aldosterone secretion to various acute stimuli. Furthermore, as depicted in Figure 11-15, restriction of sodium intake and potassium loading have an *additive stimulatory* effect on aldosterone production. In contrast, restriction of potassium intake and sodium loading have an *additive inhibitory* effect on the rate of biosynthesis of aldosterone. However, if severely sodium-depleted subjects are also potassium-restricted, aldosterone secretion is found to decrease to subnormal levels, suggesting the predominant effect of potassium (Williams and Dluhy, 1972). In short, in normal man, it is the dynamic interrelationship between sodium and potassium balance that ultimately determines the effect of these ions on aldosterone secretion and their potentiating effect in response to various acute stimuli.

C. Role of ACTH. As depicted in Figure 11-15, ACTH enhances aldosterone production by stimulating the early biosynthetic pathway. Its stimulatory effect is enhanced when the zona glomerulosa is sensitized by the action of chronic stimuli on the late biosynthetic pathway. Under normal conditions, ACTH plays a minor role in the biosynthesis of aldosterone, except for mediating its diurnal secretion.

D. Other Factors. Since changes in aldosterone secretion are often associated with parallel changes in water and electrolyte balance and hence edema formation, factors controlling its biosynthesis have received considerable attention in clinical medicine. Of particular interest are the factors controlling aldosterone secretion in *anephric man* and the consequences of the *loss of sodium-retaining effect* of aldosterone after prolonged administration.

In anephric man, in which the renin-angiotensin system is absent, it has been found that the increase in plasma aldosterone concentration that normally occurs upon assuming upright posture is abolished. It should be remembered that, in a normal subject, assuming upright posture decreases central venous volume and hence the circulating blood volume (due to pooling of the blood in the lower extremities by gravity) and thereby stimulates aldosterone production by the renin-angiotensin mechanism described above. Numerous studies in man and animals, referred to above, have shown a direct effect of alteration in potassium balance as well as plasma potassium levels on aldosterone secretion. Moreover, it has been found that aldosterone secretion in anephric man increases in response to stressful stimuli, a possible consequence of parallel changes in ACTH. On the basis of this evidence, it has been suggested that in anephric man, the most important factor controlling aldosterone secretion is potassium balance, with ACTH playing a secondary role. Another factor controlling aldosterone secretion in anephric man is the prolonged administration of anticoagulant *heparin*, which is required for hemodialysis therapy. Prolonged administration of this substance produces hypoaldosteronism, the mechanism of which is at present not known (Williams and Dluhy, 1972).

The other condition of clinical interest is the *loss of sodium-retaining effect* of aldosterone following prolonged administration. When aldosterone is administered for several days to normal subjects, the kidney escapes from the sodium-retaining, but not the potassium-losing effect of the hormone (August et al., 1958). The onset of the escape is related to the amount of dietary sodium intake. Although the mechanism of this escape phenomenon is at present not known, it is believed to be responsible for the absence of edema in patients with primary aldosteronism. The failure of the escape mechanism is thought to contribute to the edematous states in patients with congestive heart failure, liver cirrhosis with ascites, and nephrosis.

In summary, it is evident that under normal condition of dietary salt intake, the basal rate of aldosterone secretion is controlled by the additive effect of the renin-angiotensin system and the plasma level of potassium. This is complemented by an additional effect of dietary sodium and potassium intake which potentiate aldosterone secretion in response to acute stimuli. In short, changes in dietary intake of sodium and potassium, by virtue of the effect of these ions on the late biosynthetic pathway, sensitize (potentiate) the zona glomerulosa to acute stimuli which act on the early biosynthetic pathway. Thus, with identical plasma levels of angiotensin II, aldosterone production is found to be greater in sodium-restricted than in sodium-loaded subjects. However, potassium restriction has an adverse effect on angiotensin II-stimulated aldosterone secretion. As depicted in Figure 11-15, there exists a negative feedback loop between potassium restriction (or depletion) and aldosterone secretion. Since potassium loss from the body via the kidney is itself a consequence of increased aldosterone secretion, stimulation of aldosterone by angiotensin II is *self-limited* by the potassium loss it causes.

MODES OF CELLULAR ACTION. Our present understanding of the mechanism of action of aldosterone and its effect on sodium transport in the mammalian kidney has largely been derived from extensive studies of sodium transport in isolated toad urinary bladder. Results of numerous studies (Sharp and Leaf, 1966), employing both short-circuit and isotope dilution techniques (see Chapter 8), have revealed the following general characteristics for sodium transport across isolated toad urinary bladder. The *direction* of net transbladder sodium transport is from the *mucosal* (urinary) side to the *serosal* (blood) side of the bladder. Sodium is transported across the mucosal barrier by *passive diffusion* down its electrochemical gradient. Once inside the epithelial cells, the accumulated sodium is then *actively* transported by the membrane-bound Na^+-K^+ activated ATPase pump across the serosal barrier against its electrochemical gradient. This active transport is "electrogenic"; it occurs without obligatory coupled movement of an anion in the same direction or a cation in the opposite direction. The extrusion of sodium out of the cell leads to the separation of charges (sodium ions), which gives rise to the measured electrical potential gradient. The effect of aldosterone on sodium transport was first demonstrated in the isolated toad bladder (Crabbé, 1961). When 3×10^{-10} M of aldosterone (an amount considerably less than plasma aldosterone concentration, which is about 10^{-8} M) was added to the fluid bathing the serosal surface, it caused an increase in the short-circuit current, which is equivalent to an increase in active sodium transport, after a *latent period* of 45 to 90 minutes. This increase in active sodium transport was independent of the concentration of aldosterone in the bathing fluid. The response also occurred after the withdrawal of the hormone from the bathing fluid during the latent period. Subsequent studies (Sharp and Leaf, 1966) showed that this latent period was not due to slow accumulation of the hormone in the tissue, since maximal tissue hormone concentration could be achieved only 30 minutes after the hormone exposure. Nevertheless, one to four hours were required before a detectable change in the active sodium transport could be measured.

Similar results have been obtained in the intact mammalian kidney (Sharp and Leaf, 1966). When aldosterone is injected into the renal artery of dogs and rats, a latent period of 45 to 120 minutes elapses before antinatriuresis is detected. In the rat, the peak of aldosterone effect on sodium transport after a single injection occurred when the hormone was virtually absent from the circulation.

In both the isolated toad urinary bladder and the intact mammalian kidney, the antinatriuretic effect of aldosterone is inhibited by actinomycin D, puromycin, and cycloheximide, which are all well-known inhibitors of protein synthesis. In the mammalian kidney, however, these inhibitors failed to block the kaliuretic effect of aldosterone. This finding indicates that the aldosterone induced renal reabsorption of sodium and secretion of potassium may occur by two separate pathways (see Chapter 8).

Exactly how aldosterone stimulates sodium transport has been the subject of intensive investigation. Several types of studies, using toad urinary bladder and adrenalectomized rat kidney, have led to the formulation of a currently accepted hypothesis depicting the cellular action of aldosterone and the mechanism of its stimulation of sodium transport.

The observed latent period before the onset of aldosterone effect led Crabbé (1961) to suggest that stimulation of sodium transport by aldosterone involves intracellular synthesis of an active intermediate substance. Since then, in a series of intricate experiments, Edelman and his associates (Edelman and Fimognari, 1968; Feldman et al., 1972) have identified the nature of this active intermediate substance and have consequently proposed the *induction theory* of aldosterone action. According to this theory, as depicted in Figure 11-16, aldosterone present in the blood crosses the serosal (peritubular) membrane by chemical diffusion and enters the cytoplasm of the epithelial cell, where it stereospecifically binds noncovalently with an *aldosterone-receptor* protein. Studies of the time course of uptake of tritiated aldosterone by the four conventional cell fractions (nucleus, cytosol, mitochondria, and microsomes) have identified cytosol as the fraction containing the initial cytoplasmic aldosterone-receptor protein. This cytoplasmic binding is characterized by a latent period of 30 to 45 minutes, exclusive of the time required for the onset of the hormone effect. The cytoplasmic aldosterone-receptor complex is then *translocated* into the nucleus, where it binds noncovalently with the acceptor sites on the *nuclear chromatin*. The formation of this complex somehow activates deoxyribonucleic acid (DNA)-dependent synthesis of ribonucleic acid (RNA). This is called *gene transcription*, meaning that the information in the DNA is "transcribed" into RNA. The RNA, thus synthesized, is called the messenger RNA (mRNA), because it leaves the nucleus and enters the cytoplasm where it induces *de novo* synthesis of protein. This step is called *translation*, meaning that the nucleotide of mRNA is "translated" into the amino acid sequence of the synthesized protein. The *aldosterone-induced-protein* (AIP) thus synthesized, through a series of poorly understood reactions, mediates the increase in the transepithelial sodium transport.

Support for the induction theory have come from a number of experiments (Feldman et al., 1972). It has been shown that actinomycin D and cycloheximide inhibit aldosterone-induced sodium transport by inhibiting the DNA-dependent RNA synthesis of AIP. *Actinomycin* inhibits transcription by binding to the guanosine residue of DNA, while *cycloheximide* inhibits translation. In the

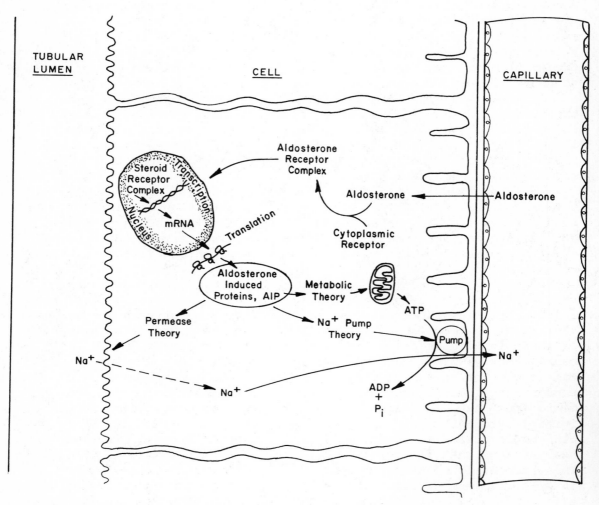

Figure 11-16. Scheme depicting the proposed mechanism of cellular steps involved in aldosterone-stimulated sodium transport. [Modified from Feldman, D., Funder, J. W., and Edelman, I. S. (1972).]

rat, inhibition of DNA-dependent synthesis of RNA by actinomycin D abolished the antinatriuretic effect of aldosterone but not its kaliuretic effect. Recent studies (Lifschitz et al., 1973) have confirmed these findings in the dog and have shown further that actinomycin D failed to abolish the aldosterone-enhanced hydrogen ion secretion. These findings suggest that the effect of aldosterone on potassium and hydrogen ion secretion is independent of DNA-dependent RNA synthesis. Furthermore, the effect of aldosterone of increasing both the hydrogen and potassium secretion appears to occur by a pathway different from that involved in the transport of sodium and may involve a common biochemical pathway for hydrogen and potassium (see Chapters 8 and 10).

Spironolactone, a competitive aldosterone antagonist, inhibits binding of aldosterone to both cytosol and nuclear receptor proteins. However, it has no effect on the uptake of tritiated aldosterone by the other two cell fractions or the plasma concentration of the hormone (Edelman, 1972). This is in contrast to inhibition of aldosterone effect by actinomycin D (inhibits transcription) and *ouabain* (inhibits Na^+-K^+ activated ATPase), which do not displace the hormone from the receptor sites.

The underlying assumption of the induction hypothesis of the cellular mechanism of aldosterone-stimulated sodium transport is the DNA-dependent synthesis of RNA, which in turn induces the synthesis of a new protein, the AIP. The only direct experimental proof for the synthesis of this protein, which may be a permease, a membrane component, or a carrier molecule, is the recent report of Benjamin and Singer (1974). Using electrophysiological and biochemical techniques, they demonstrated aldosterone-induced synthesis of a low-molecular-weight protein (about 12,000) in isolated toad urinary bladder. The synthesized protein had a high specificity for aldosterone, as revealed by the inhibitory effects of actinomycin D and spironolactone.

How does AIP increase sodium transport? Based on the accepted model of transepithelial sodium transport described earlier (see also Chapter 8, Fig. 8-7) and as depicted in Figure 11-16, three theories have been advanced to explain the action of AIP: (1) The sodium pump theory--AIP increases the activity of Na^+-K^+ activated ATPase pump at the serosal (peritubular) membrane, and hence increases sodium tra port; (2) the permease theory--AIP facilitates the entry of sodium across the mucosal (luminal) membrane, thereby providing more sodium for the pump to work on; and (3) the metabolic theory--AIP stimulates mitochondrial synthesis of ATP, hence raising cellular ATP/ADP ratio. Let us consider the consequence of each theory and its supporting evidence.

The sodium pump theory, advanced by Goodman and associates (1969), is based on the finding that aldosterone potentiated the effect of vasopressin on sodium transport under anaerobic conditions in the isolated toad urinary bladder. This finding implicates aldosterone as activating the membrane-bound Na^+-K^+ ATPase pump, and hence increasing sodium transport. However, direct experimental proof from assaying the Na^+-K^+ ATPase activity in response to aldosterone is lacking. Time course studies of single injection of aldosterone have shown that its effect on sodium transport peaks at 3 to 4 hours and disappears after 6 hours. In contrast, multiple injection of the hormone is required to detect its effect on Na^+-K^+ ATPase activity, which begins 6 hours after hormone expression and peaks at 24 to 36 hours (Feldman et al., 1972). Moreover, the response is not specific to aldosterone, and is seen after administration of *corticosterone* and *dexamethasone*, a steroid with predominant glucocorticoid activity and no effect on sodium transport. Both nonspecificity and delayed increase in the Na^+-K^+ ATPase activity may be due to noncovalent binding of aldosterone with glucocorticoids receptors within the cytoplasm.

The permease theory, advanced by Sharp and Leaf (1966) is based on the concept that AIP increases the passive influx of sodium across the luminal membrane, thereby indirectly increasing the active extrusion of sodium across the peritubular membrane. If AIP acts on the rate-limiting membrane at the urinary surface, there should be an increase in the intracellular sodium concentration. Alternatively, if AIP acts on the rate-limiting membrane at the blood surface, there should be a decrease in the intracellular concentration of sodium. Measurement of intracellular sodium concentration of epithelial cells isolated from the toad urinary bladder have shown that both aldosterone and vasopressin increased intracellular sodium concentration (Handler et al., 1972). Since vasopressin increases the permeability of the luminal membrane, aldosterone must have produced similar effect with respect to sodium. Similar increase in intracellular sodium concentration was obtained after exposure of the cells to ouabain. In contrast, *amiloride*, a diuretic agent which inhibits sodium transport to the same extent as ouabain, decreased intracellular sodium concentration, suggesting that amiloride inhibited the passive influx of sodium across the luminal membrane. These results, however, are in variance with those of Lipton and Edelman (1971) who, using similar preparations, found no detectable change in the intracellular sodium concentration. They suggested that AIP has a bipolar effect; it enhances simultaneously plasma sodium influx at the luminal membrane and active sodium efflux at the peritubular membrane.

Further support for the permease theory comes from direct measurement of transepithelial electrical resistance. If AIP acts on the sodium influx step, it should reduce transepithelial electrical resistance (see Fig. 8-7). However, if AIP acts on the sodium efflux step, there should be no change in resistance. Electrophysiological measurements have shown that aldosterone caused a small decrease in transepithelial electrical resistance in toad urinary bladder (Civan and Hoffman, 1971).

The metabolic theory, advanced by Edelman and Fimognari (1968), is based on the concept that AIP stimulates oxidative metabolism, thereby increasing the rate of supply of high energy intermediates which would act as a pacemaker for the sodium transport system. Therefore, the increase in sodium influx at the luminal membrane is secondary to enhanced active sodium efflux at the peritubular membrane. This hypothesis was prompted by the striking dependence of aldosterone-stimulated sodium transport on the presence of exogenous oxidative substrates of tricarboxylic acid cycle in isolated toad urinary bladder preparation.

Experimental evidence supporting the metabolic theory comes from several types of studies in isolated toad urinary bladder preparation (Feldman et al., 1972): (1) In bladders depleted of oxidative substrates the normal aldosterone-stimulated increase in sodium transport does not occur. However, addition of substrate to aldosterone-treated bladders causes an immediate increase in sodium transport (no latent period). This suggests that synthesis of AIP may occur in the absence of oxidative substrates, but that energy metabolism is required for the expression of its effects. (2) The aldosterone effect is maintained by any substrate that leads to the formation of pyruvate or oxaloacetate, as well as glucose. (3) Several inhibitors of oxidative phosphorylation in mitochondria (such as rotenone and amobarbital) inhibit the aldosterone-induced effect in toad bladder, but do not block its response to vasopressin or amphotericin B. In the absence of aldosterone, amphotericin B increases net transbladder sodium transport, presumably by increasing the rate of sodium influx at the mucosal barrier. The results obtained with the inhibitors imply that the mitochondrial nicotinamide adenine dinucleotide dehydrogenase (NADH) pathway is specifically involved in the mediation of aldosterone-induced increase in sodium transport. (4) Renal citrate synthase activity decreases after adrenalectomy. It increases after administration of physiological concentrations of aldosterone with a time-course paralleling the urinary sodium-potassium response to the hormone. Furthermore, stimulation of citrate synthase could be blocked by spironolactone at concentrations that inhibit urinary electrolyte changes. In contrast, glucocorticoids had no inhibitory effect on renal citrate synthase activity.

At present, available evidence favors both the permease and metabolic theories as possible modes of cellular action of aldosterone on sodium transport. However, there are many unresolved questions about the nature of action of AIP. There is as yet no direct experimental verification of the role of AIP on the observed increase in the net transport of sodium in aldosterone-sensitive tissues. Moreover, the stoichiometric relationship, if any, between the synthesis of AIP and net sodium transport is yet to be demonstrated.

We conclude this section by summarizing the net operation of the countercurrent multiplier system and the effects of ADH and aldosterone on this operation. As illustrated schematically in Figure 11-17, the input to the countercurrent multiplier system is the *transverse osmolality gradient* ($\Delta[Os]_T$), established at the corticomedullary border between the descending (DL) and ascending (AL)

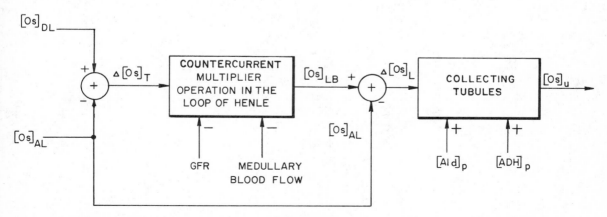

Figure 11-17. Schematic representation of net operation of the countercurrent multiplier system.

limbs of the loop of Henle. The output of the countercurrent multiplier system, to which the adjacent collecting tubule equilibrates, is the magnitude of the *longitudinal osmolality gradient* ($\Delta[Os]_L$). This is the difference between the osmolality of the fluid in the loop bend ($[Os]_{LB}$) and $[Os]_{AL}$. The magnitude of this gradient depends on both GFR and the medullary blood flow. Thus, an increase in either GFR or the medullary blood flow leads to a decrease in the time required for osmotic equilibration between the tubular fluid and the medullary interstitium (indicated by a negative sign next to appropriate arrows). This results in a decrease in $\Delta[Os]_L$, and hence an increase in solute washout into the urine. The osmolality of urine issuing from the collecting tubule depends not only on the osmolality of the fluid leaving the loop of Henle, but also on the rate of water and sodium reabsorption and the effects of ADH and aldosterone on the tubular processes involved. As shown, an increase in the plasma levels of both hormones leads to formation of an hyperosmotic urine (indicated by a positive sign next to appropriate arrows), whereas a decrease in their plasma levels produces the opposite effects.

PHYSIOLOGY OF DIURESIS: DIURETICS, AND THEIR ACTIONS

DIURESIS AND ITS CLASSIFICATION

Diuresis is defined as an increase in urine volume flow (V), usually in excess of 2 ml/min. This increase in urine flow could result from interference with two normal tubular functions: (1) Reduced osmotic reabsorption of water, leading to increased solute-free water clearance (C_{H_2O}) and hence *water diuresis*; and (2) reduced solute reabsorption, primarily sodium ions with associated anions, leading to increased osmolar clearance (C_{Osm}) and hence *solute* or *osmotic diuresis*. In both cases, there is an increase in urine volume flow which is the basis for diuresis. Therefore, we may classify diuretic states as either water or osmotic diuresis. Let us now briefly examine the conditions which produce these diuretic states.

1. WATER DIURESIS. Normally, water diuresis results from excessive fluid intake. The resulting hemodilution reduces the blood concentration of ADH, and hence diminishes its effectiveness in promoting osmotic reabsorption of water in the distally located nephron segments.

Clinically, there are two pathological conditions which alter the normal effect of ADH, and hence lead to water diuresis. One is *diabetes insipidus*, a condition characterized by subnormal synthesis and release of ADH, caused by some hypothalamic lesions. The second is *nephrogenic diabetes insipidus*, a condition characterized by the loss of the responsiveness of the distal tubular epithelium to ADH.

2. OSMOTIC DIURESIS. As discussed in Chapter 8, any freely filterable, water soluble, non-absorbable, or poorly absorbable solute increases urine flow by retarding osmotic reabsorption of water and hence sodium reabsorption in selective segments of the nephron. Such a substance is called an *osmotic diuretic* and the ensuing diuresis is called *osmotic diuresis*. In this type of diuresis, there is a parallel increase in both *osmolar* and *solute-free water* clearances.

Osmotic diuresis may also be induced by intravenous infusion of any solution which tends to increase blood volume and systemic arterial blood pressure, and hence GFR and medullary blood flow. As pointed out in Chapter 8, intravenous infusion of a large quantity of *isotonic saline* inhibits sodium reabsorption in the proximal tubule in both rat (Landwehr et al., 1967) and dog (Dirks et al., 1965), leading to increased urinary excretion of sodium and water. This natriuresis, resulting from reduced tubular reabsorption of sodium, occurs even in the presence of aldosterone and reduced GFR (De Wardener et al., 1961). That the inhibition of the proximal sodium reabsorption may be a consequence of potentiation of a *natriuretic hormone* during isotonic saline infusion has been inferred from cross-circulation experiments (Johnston et al., 1967). Thus, cross-circulation of blood from a saline-loaded donor dog to a normal recipient dog produced significant natriuresis, even when sodium load was decreased by aortic constriction above the renal arteries. Despite extensive research, the existence of such a hormone lacks direct endocrinological proof at present.

The most widely used osmotic diuretic agent is *mannitol*, a non-absorbable solute which is freely permeable at the glomerulus and is neither reabsorbed nor secreted. *Urea*, which is freely filtered but is partially reabsorbed by flow-dependent passive diffusion along the nephron, is a close second. Intravenous infusion of these solutes has a dual effect: (a) They cause an expansion of the extracellular volume which, through its cardiovascular effect, leads to an increase in GFR and medullary blood flow. Both of these factors contribute to enhanced natriuresis. (b) Presence of these solutes in the tubular filtrate will obligate water, retarding its osmotic reabsorption, a factor markedly limiting diffusive entry of sodium across the luminal membrane into the renal tubule cell. The result is a reduction in the transtubular sodium transport, a factor contributing to enhanced natriuresis.

Recent recollection micropuncture studies in dogs (Seely and Dirks, 1969) have shown that the major inhibitory effect of mannitol on sodium reabsorption occurs along the ascending limb (the diluting segment) of the loop of Henle, with a somewhat lesser inhibition of sodium reabsorption in the proximal tubule. Thus, during mannitol diuresis, the proximal inhibition of sodium reabsorption, though comparatively small, results in an increased delivery of filtrate to the distally located nephron segments. In the loop of Henle, the resulting increased tubular flow rate decreases sodium reabsorption in the ascending limb, thereby reducing the *transverse gradient* and hence the medullary longitudinal osmolar gradient. The latter effect reduces the extent of osmotic equilibration of the fluid in the collecting tubule with the surrounding medullary interstitium, a factor accounting for enhanced natriuresis during mannitol diuresis. Another factor contributing to this natriuresis is the increased medullary blood flow during the mannitol diuresis. Thus, the increase in both the medullary blood flow and the tubular flow rates contribute to solute washout from the medulla, thereby reducing the medullary concentration gradient, which leads to excretion of a relatively dilute urine.

Figure 11-4 shows the comparative diuretic effects of some commonly used osmotic diuretic agents. It is evident that the final osmolality of the excreted urine depends on several factors: (a) Whether the osmotically active solute present in the ultrafiltrate is reabsorbed or not. Thus, infusion of mannitol, which is not reabsorbed, causes excretion of a more dilute urine than infusion of sodium chloride, which is reabsorbed throughout the nephron. (b) The extent to which an osmotically active solute is reabsorbed determines the degree of induced osmotic diuresis. Thus, infusion of glucose, which is reabsorbed by a Tm-limited process only in the proximal tubule, results in a greater diuresis (and hence a more dilute urine) than urea infusion. The latter is reabsorbed to varying degrees throughout the nephron. (c) Whether the osmotically active solute infused dissociates in solution or not (and hence the number of particles in solution) is another determinant of the degree of induced diuresis. Thus, infusion of sodium sulfate (Na_2SO_4) results in a greater diuresis (and hence a more dilute urine) than NaCl infusion. This is because Na_2SO_4 yields *three* osmotically active particles in solution, whereas NaCl yields only *two*. Moreover, sulfate ion is a poorly absorbable solute compared to chloride ion. (d) Whether the subject is in a state of water imbalance or not. Thus, infusion of any osmotic diuretic agent causes a greater diuresis in a well-hydrated subject (positive water balance) than in a hydropenic subject (negative water balance). (e) Whether ADH or aldosterone levels in the blood are within normal limits or not, and whether the subject is receiving exogenous doses of these hormones. Thus, infusion of any osmotic diuretic agent to a patient with diabetes insipidus causes excretion of a more dilute urine (greater diuresis) compared to a normal individual.

DIURETICS AND THEIR CLASSIFICATION

Diuretics are a group of pharmacological agents that cause an increase in urine volume flow. However, the major purpose of diuretic therapy is not to increase urine volume flow, but rather to rid the body of excess sodium and water, to reduce the extracellular volume, and hence to eliminate edema and associated hypertension.

The commonly used diuretics may be classified in terms of (a) chemical structures, (b) sites of action along the nephron, or (c) whether they interfere with solute (primarily NaCl) or water reabsorption along the nephron. Most of the commonly used diuretics exert their effects primarily by interfering with sodium chloride reabsorption along one or more segments of the nephron. Their effects on water reabsorption occur secondarily, due to the osmotic

effect of unreabsorbed sodium and its associated anions.
Consequently, most of the diuretics may be classified as osmotic
diuretics, which, with few exceptions, cause a parallel increase in
both osmolar and solute-free water clearances. Therefore, from a
functional point of view, we will classify the various diuretic drugs
as osmotic diuretics according to their sites of action along the
nephron.

METHODS USED TO ASSESS SITES OF ACTION OF DIURETICS

Our present knowledge of the sites and the mechanisms of action
of the commonly used diuretics has been derived from the application
of clearance, stop-flow, micropuncture, and microperfusion techniques
to the study of renal function.

As described in Chapter 6, measurement of renal clearance of a
substance provides a means of assessing the integral function of the
whole kidney. Application of this technique to assess renal effects
of diuretics has yielded three kinds of information: (1) The
magnitude of diuretic-induced natriuresis, expressed as the fraction
of filtered sodium excreted ($U_{Na} \cdot V/GFR \cdot P_{Na}$); (2) diuretic-induced
changes in urinary electrolyte composition; and (3) evaluation of
diuretic-induced changes in concentrating and diluting mechanisms
from changes in solute-free water clearance (C_{H_2O}). Of these, the
latter information has provided considerable insight into the possible
sites of diuretic action. Thus, it has been shown that any diuretic
agent that interferes with sodium chloride reabsorption in the
proximal tubule will tend to increase C_{H_2O}, whereas any diuretic
agent that interferes with sodium chloride reabsorption in the distal
tubule will tend to reduce C_{H_2O} (Seldin et al., 1966).

Stop-flow technique, as described previously in Chapter 8,
though a useful tool, has several shortcomings. Nevertheless,
its application has provided "gross" segmental localization
of the diuretic effects on tubular transport along the nephron.

By far the most direct information about the sites and mechanisms
of diuretic action has come from those studies in which micropuncture
and microperfusion techniques were employed. Without going into
specifics of these techniques (see Chapter 8 for details), we shall
now describe the sites and modes of action of some commonly used
diuretics along the nephron (Fig. 11-18) as revealed by these studies.

SITES AND MODES OF ACTION OF SPECIFIC DIURETICS ALONG THE NEPHRON

1. PROXIMAL TUBULE. In the proximal tubule, the filtered
sodium is reabsorbed as NaCl and as NaHCO$_3$. As described in Chapter
10, in both cases the transtubular reabsorption of sodium results
from its passive entry into and its active extrusion out of the
tubule cell (Fig. 10-14). Reabsorption of filtered chloride ion

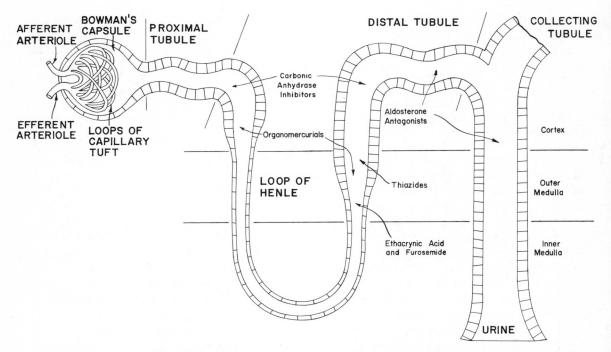

Figure 11-18. Scheme showing the sites of action of the commonly used diuretics along the nephron.

occurs passively along the electrochemical gradient established by sodium movement. However, as illustrated in Figure 10-14, reabsorption of filtered HCO_3^- ion occurs by a more complicated mechanism. It involves *carbonic anhydrase* catalysis of cellular hydration of CO_2 and the subsequent cellular generation of H^+ and HCO_3^- ions. The H^+ ion thus generated is exchanged for Na^+ ion at the luminal cell membrane (a process promoting CO_2 formation and its cellular entry) while the generated HCO_3^- ion is reabsorbed by passive diffusion into the blood. Thus, the key to HCO_3^- ion reabsorption is the carbonic anhydrase-catalyzed generation of H^+ ion. Accordingly, diuretic agents that exert their effects in the proximal tubule may be classified as those which directly interfere with sodium reabsorption and those which indirectly interfere with sodium reabsorption by inhibiting carbonic anhydrase-catalyzed H^+ ion generation and its exchange for Na^+ ion. The latter has become the most popular type of diuretic for inhibiting sodium reabsorption in the proximal tubule and hence inducing natriuresis.

Carbonic Anhydrase Inhibitors. *Acetazolamide* (Diamox) is the sulfonamide most frequently used to inhibit carbonic anhydrase activity. For a detailed discussion of the chemistry and pharmacology of this **class** of drugs, the interested reader is referred to an excellent review by Maren (1967).

The major effect of acetazolamide is the inhibition of Na^+-H^+

exchange at the luminal membrane of the proximal tubule (Fig. 11-18), where the major fraction of sodium bicarbonate is reabsorbed. This drug inhibits the intracellular hydration of CO_2, a primary source of cellular H^+ ion. Consequently, it inhibits sodium bicarbonate reabsorption, thereby increasing its urinary excretion and making the urine alkaline. Similarly, it inhibits sodium bicarbonate reabsorption in the distal tubule, a factor contributing to increased luminal negativity and enhanced potassium secretion (see Chapters 8 and 10 for details).

Acute administration of acetazolamide leads to production of an alkaline urine due to marked increase in urinary excretion of sodium, potassium, and bicarbonate (Table 11-3). Additionally, it causes 10 to 30% reduction in GFR and inconsistent changes in RPF. Thus, the hemodynamic effect of the drug must be taken into consideration when evaluating its renal effect.

Chronic administration of acetazolamide leads to the development of mild to moderate *hyperchloremic*, *metabolic acidosis*, and eventually results in the loss of diuretic effectiveness and the return of urinary electrolyte composition to pre-drug pattern. This latter response is called the *refractory state* and its mechanism is not known.

Another potent carbonic anhydrase inhibitor is *chlorothiazide* (Diuril), a heterocyclic sulfonamide. It is an orally effective diuretic which is widely used in clinical treatment of edema and associated hypertension.

Acute administration of this drug to both dog and man (Beyer, 1958) leads to marked increase in urinary excretion of sodium, potassium, chloride, and bicarbonate (Table 11-3). However, in contrast to acetazolamide, chronic administration of chlorothiazide leads to development of *hypochloremic*, *hypokalemic, metabolic alkalosis*. Moreover, the chloriuretic potency of this drug is impaired by neither metabolic alkalosis (in contrast to organomercurials) nor metabolic acidosis (in contrast to acetazolamide). In addition, administration of chlorothiazide to dogs (Earley et al., 1961) and man (Au and Raisz, 1960) has no significant effect on the urinary concentrating mechanism. These findings suggest that besides inhibiting carbonic anhydrase activity, chlorothiazide must also interfere with chloride reabsorption in the early distal convoluted tubule, where urine is hypotonic. The molecular mechanism mediating this effect is, however, not known.

2. LOOP OF HENLE. As described previously in Chapter 8, the major site of sodium chloride reabsorption in the loop of Henle is the ascending limb (the diluting segment). Thus, any agent that interferes with sodium chloride reabsorption in this nephron segment will tend to reduce the transverse gradient, which through the operation of the countercurrent multiplication mechanism will eventually lead to excretion of a dilute urine. For this reason, the diuretics which inhibit sodium chloride reabsorption in the ascending limb are by far the most potent natriuretics (Table 11-3), since they inhibit the renal concentrating and diluting mechanism. There are three diuretics that fall into this category: organomercurials, ethacrynic acid, and furosemide.

TABLE 11-3

Changes in Urinary Composition and Relative Natriuretic Potency
of Some Commonly Used Diuretics

Diuretics	Sites of Action	Effects on Excretion				% Maximal Fraction of Filtered Sodium Excreted
		Sodium	Potassium	Chloride	Bicarbonate	
Ethacrynic Acid	AL	+	+	+	0	25
Furosemide	AL	+	+	+	0	25
Organomercurials	AL, DT	+	-*	+	0	20
Chlorothiazide	PT, DT	+	+	+	+*	8
Aminophylline	Not known	+	+	+	+	5
Acetazolamide	PT, DT	+	+	+*	+	5
Spironolactone	DT	+	-	+*	+	3
Triamterene	DT	+	-	+*	+	3

(*) means that the effect is not consistently seen, (+) means increase, (-) means decrease, and (0) means no change.

PT = proximal tubule; DT = distal tubule; AL = ascending limb of the loop of Henle.
[Modified from Goldberg, M. (1971).]

A. Organomercurials. Until the recent development of orally effective diuretic agents, such as ethacrynic acid and furosemide, organomercurials had been the most widely used natriuretic agents. Intramuscular injection of organomercurials stimulates natriuresis and chloriuresis and inhibits kaliuresis (Table 11-3). Their chronic administration leads to development of *hypochloremic, metabolic alkalosis*, with eventual loss of diuretic effectiveness. This refractory state, however, can be reversed by administration of agents that raise plasma chloride levels and acidify the body fluids (Levy et al., 1958).

Despite widespread usage of the organomercurials in the past four decades, the mechanism of their diuretic effects remains mysterious, but their sites of action have recently been defined.

Early clearance and stop-flow studies implicated both the proximal and distal tubules as the major sites of action of organomercurials. However, subsequent micropuncture studies (Dirks et al., 1966) have revealed that the organomercurials have no effect on sodium reabsorption in the accessible portions of the proximal tubule in hydropenic dogs with or without fluid replacement. This suggested a more distal site of action, which was later confirmed by Clapp and Robinson (1968), who found that in dogs organomercurials increased the [TF/P] osmolality in the distal tubule.

More recent micropuncture studies in the dog (Evanson et al., 1972), however, have revealed that the primary site of action of organomercurials is the inhibition of sodium reabsorption in the loop of Henle (presumably the ascending limb), with no detectable inhibition of sodium reabsorption in the proximal tubule. The same studies also showed that this drug inhibited potassium secretion in the distal tubule, even after potassium loading, a procedure which should enhance potassium secretion. Although this latter finding implies that organomercurials may somehow inhibit the membrane bound Na^+-K^+ activated ATPase activity in the distal tubule, the issue is far from being settled at present.

Exactly how organomercurials inhibit sodium reabsorption in the ascending limb and distal tubule (Fig. 11-18) remains a controversial issue. However, it is believed that the ionization of mercury is an intermediate step, a process greatly enhanced when plasma hydrogen ion concentration is increased (acid pH). Thus, acidosis promotes diuretic effectiveness of organomercurials, whereas alkalosis inhibits it. This may perhaps be the reason why the metabolic alkalosis that develops in chronic administration of this drug leads to the loss of its diuretic effectiveness.

Clinically, organomercurials are commonly used to rid the body of edema arising from cardiac malfunction (e.g., congestive heart failure). They have also been used to eliminate edema in patients with liver cirrhosis. However, they should not be used in edematous patients with renal disease.

B. Ethacrynic Acid and Furosemide. Although ethacrynic acid (a derivative of phenoxyacetic acid) and furosemide (a sulfamylbenzene derivative of anthranilic acid) are chemically dissimilar, they produce similar diuretic effects in the kidney. Numerous micropuncture studies in rats (Duarte et al., 1971; Morgan et al., 1970), dogs

(Bennett et al., 1967; Clapp and Robinson, 1968; Dirks and Seely, 1970) and monkeys (Bennett et al., 1968) have clearly shown that the major site of renal action of both of these diuretic drugs is the ascending limb of the loop of Henle (Fig. 11-18). Both drugs inhibit sodium chloride reabsorption in the ascending limb, thereby increasing the concentration of these ions in the tubular fluid and eventually their urinary excretion (Table 11-3). The resulting increase in the osmolality of the ascending limb fluid reduces the transverse gradient, which through the operation of the countercurrent multiplication mechanism would lead to a reduction in the medullary longitudinal osmolar concentration gradient and hence production of a dilute urine. Additionally, both diuretics produce marked kaliuresis (Table 11-3), presumably by stimulating potassium secretion in the distal tubule. The mechanism mediating this effect is not known.

3. DISTAL AND COLLECTING TUBULES. In the distal and collecting tubules, reabsorption of sodium occurs by two separate mechanisms; one is aldosterone-dependent and the other is not. Thus, inhibition of sodium reabsorption in these distally located nephron segments may be accomplished by two types of diuretics; those that interfere with the action of aldosterone and those that do not. Spironolactone is an example of the first category, while triamterene and amiloride are examples of the second category. The feature common to all three is that they inhibit potassium secretion and indirectly induce natriuresis.

A. Spironolactone. This is a steroid which is a competitive antagonist of the renal action of aldosterone. It binds with cytoplasmic receptors of aldosterone, and thereby interferes with aldosterone-stimulated sodium reabsorption in the distal and collecting tubules (Fig. 11-18). The inhibitory effect of spironolactone can be reversed, however, by raising the blood level of aldosterone. Therefore, spironolactone can be used as an effective diuretic in normal subjects but not in adrenalectomized patients.

B. Triamterene and Amiloride. These are two drugs which have recently been developed and are orally effective antikaliuretics. They operate independently of aldosterone and hence can be used as effective diuretics in adrenalectomized patients.

THE XANTHINE DIURETICS

This class of drugs is among the oldest of the modern diuretics. They include caffeine, theobromine, and theophylline. Of these, theophylline is the one most frequently used.

As mentioned earlier, theophylline inhibits phosphodiesterase. This leads to intracellular accumulation of cyclic AMP. Thus, the diuretic effect of theophylline may be related to the inhibition of sodium reabsorption by cyclic AMP, an idea confirmed by the recent observation that dibutyryl cyclic AMP (an analogue that readily enters the cell) inhibits sodium reabsorption in the proximal tubule (Agus et al., 1971). The modes and sites of action of caffeine and theobromine are not known.

Since xanthine diuretics affect a variety of organ systems, including the cardiovascular system, the mechanism of their renal action remains obscure. At present, they are not used as standard diuretics in clinical medicine.

SUMMARY

Diuresis may be induced either by interference with sodium chloride reabsorption (osmotic diuresis) or by interference with water reabsorption (water diuresis). Most of the clinically used diuretic drugs exert their effects by interfering with sodium chloride reabsorption. Hence, they all behave as osmotic diuretics. Of these, the most potent are the carbonic anhydrase inhibitors, such as acetazolamide, which have their effects on sodium bicarbonate reabsorption in the proximal tubule. Furosemide, ethacrynic acid, and organomercurials, though they may have an inhibitory effect on proximal sodium reabsorption, exert their effects primarily in the ascending limb of the loop of Henle. Antikiuretic agents inhibit sodium-potassium exchange in the distal and collecting tubules either by antagonizing the action of aldosterone (e.g., spironolactone) or by a mechanism unrelated to aldosterone (e.g., triamterene and amiloride).

PROBLEMS

11-1.   There are two types of nephrons within the human kidney.
(a) Name them and give their relative population ratio;
(b) briefly outline the similarities and differences in their blood supply; and (c) briefly describe the functional contribution of each to the regulation of volume and composition of body fluids.

11-2.   Briefly outline the main features of the countercurrent multiplication principle as it applies to the kidney.

11-3.   Discuss the various types of experimental evidence that have been marshalled to support the operation of the countercurrent multiplication system within the kidney.

11-4.   Briefly describe the role of urea recirculation within the renal medulla in concentration and dilution of urine, and indicate how this role is affected by ADH.

11-5.   What is the role of the blood supply in the vasa recta in concentration and dilution of urine?

11-6.   How do the expansion of the extracellular fluid volume and hypertension affect countercurrent multiplication process in the loop of Henle? Do you expect the final urine to be more concentrated or dilute relative to normal?

11-7.   Define osmolar and solute-free water clearances and briefly describe their potential clinical use in assessing the ability of the kidney to concentrate urine.

11-8.   Indicate the sites of action of ADH and aldosterone within the nephron and briefly outline the cellular mechanisms mediating their effects.

11-9.   What are the physiological differences between diabetes insipidus and nephrogenic diabetes insipidus? Could you distinguish between the two types of diabetes by administration of ADH, and why?

11-10. List the major factors that influence aldosterone biosynthesis in the zona glomerulosa of the adrenal cortex and their proposed sites of action along the biosynthetic pathway.

11-11. What is meant by aldosterone escape phenomenon? Does it have any clinical significance?

11-12. What factors regulate aldosterone biosynthesis and secretion rate in anephric man?

11-13. What is the mechanism by which postural changes affect aldosterone biosynthesis and secretion rate?

11-14. Define diuresis and diuretics and briefly classify the major types of diuretic agents and the factors governing their use in research and clinical practice.

11-15. Of the various commonly used diuretics, which ones are the most potent and why?

11-16. Why is Na_2SO_4 solution a more effective osmotic diuretic than NaCl solution?

REFERENCES

1. Agus, Z. S., Puschett, J. B., Senesky, D., and Goldberg, M.: Mode of action of parathyroid hormone and cyclic adenosine 3',5'monophosphate on renal tubular phosphate reabsorption in the dog. *J. Clin. Invest.* 50:617-626, 1971.

2. Au, W. Y. W., and Raisz, L. G.: Studies on the renal concentrating mechanism. V. Effect of diuretic agents. *J. Clin. Invest.* *39*:1302-1311, 1960.

3. August, J. T., Nelson, D. H., and Thorn, G. W.: Response of normal subjects to large amounts of aldosterone. *J. Clin. Invest.* *37*:1549-1555, 1958.

4. Benjamin, W. B., and Singer, I.: Aldosterone-induced protein in toad urinary bladder. *Science 186*:269-272, 1974.

5. Bennett, C. M., Clapp, J. R., and Berliner, R. W.: Micropuncture study of the proximal and distal tubule of the dog. *Am. J. Physiol.* *213*:1254-1262, 1967.

6. Bennett, C. M., Brenner, B. M., and Berliner, R. W.: Micropuncture study of nephron function in the Rhesus monkey. *J. Clin. Invest.* *47*:203-216, 1968.

7. Berliner, R. W., Levinsky, N. G., Davidson, D. G., and Eden, M.: Dilution and concentration of the urine and the action of antidiuretic hormone. *Am. J. Med.* *24*:730-743, 1958.

8. Berndt, W. O., Miller, M., Kettyle, W. M., and Valtin, H.: Potentiation of the antidiuretic effect of vasopressin by chlorpropamide. *Endocrinology 86*:1028-1032, 1970.

9. Beyer, K. H.: The mechanism of action of chlorothiazide. *Ann. N.Y. Acad. Sci.* *71*:363-379, 1958.

10. Bowman, F. J., and Foulkes, E. C.: Antidiuretic hormone and urea permeability of collecting ducts. *Am. J. Physiol.* *218*: 231-233, 1970.

11. Bray, G. A.: Freezing point depression of rat kidney slices during water diuresis and antidiuresis. *Am. J. Physiol.* *199*: 915-918, 1960.

12. Burg, M. B., Grantham, J. J., Abramow, M., and Orloff, J.: Preparation and study of fragments of single rabbit nephrons. *Am. J. Physiol.* *210*:1293-1298, 1966.

13. Burg, M. B., Stoner, L., Cardinal, J., and Green, N.: Furosemide effect on isolated perfused tubules. *Am. J. Physiol.* *225*:119-124, 1973.

14. Burg, M. B., and Stoner, L.: Sodium transport in the distal nephron. *Fed. Proc.* *33*:31-36, 1974.

15. Civan, M. M., and Hoffman, R. E.: Effect of aldosterone on electrical resistance of toad bladder. *Am. J. Physiol.* *220*:324-328, 1971.

16. Clapp, J. R.: Urea reabsorption by the proximal tubule of the dog. *Proc. Soc. Exp. Biol. Med. 120*:521-523, 1965.

17. Clapp, J. R., and Robinson, R. R.: Distal sites of action of diuretic drugs in the nephron. *Am. J. Physiol. 215*:225-235, 1968.

18. Crabbé, J.: Stimulation of active sodium transport by the isolated toad bladder with aldosterone in vitro. *J. Clin. Invest. 40*:2103-2110, 1961.

19. De Wardener, H. E., Mills, I. H., Clapham, W. F., and Hayter, C. J.: Studies on the efferent mechanism of the sodium diuresis which follows the administration of intravenous saline in the dog. *Clin. Sci. 21*:249-258, 1961.

20. Dirks, J. H., Cirksena, W. J., and Berliner, R. W.: The effect of saline infusion on sodium reabsorption by the proximal tubule of the dog. *J. Clin. Invest. 44*:1160-1170, 1965.

21. Dirks, J. H., Cirksena, W. J., and Berliner, R. W.: Micropuncture study of the effect of various diuretics on sodium reabsorption by the proximal tubule of the dog. *J. Clin. Invest. 45*:1875-1885, 1966.

22. Dirks, J. H., and Seely, J. F.: Effect of saline infusion and furosemide on the dog distal nephron. *Am. J. Physiol. 219*:114-121, 1970.

23. Dousa, T. P.: Role of cyclic AMP in the action of antidiuretic hormone on kidney. *Life Sciences 13*:1033-1040, 1973.

24. Dousa, T. P.: Cellular action of antidiuretic hormone in nephrogenic diabetes insipidus. *Mayo Clin. Proc. 49*:188-199, 1974.

25. Duarte, C. G., Chomety, F., and Giebisch, G.: Effect of amiloride, ouabain, and furosemide on distal tubular function in the rat. *Am. J. Physiol. 221*:632-639, 1971.

26. Du Vigneaud, V.: Trail of sulfur research: From insulin to oxytocin. *Science 123*:967-974, 1956.

27. Earley, L. E., Kahn, M., and Orloff, J.: The effects of infusions of chlorothiazide on urinary dilution and concentration in the dog. *J. Clin. Invest. 40*:857-866, 1961.

28. Edelman, I. S., and Fimognari, G. M.: On the biochemical mechanism of action of aldosterone. *Recent Progr. Hormone Res. 24*:1-44, 1968.

29. Edelman, I. S.: The initiation mechanism in the action of aldosterone on sodium transport. *J. Steroid Biochem.* *3*:167-172, 1972.

30. Evanson, R. L., Lockhart, E. A., and Dirks, J. H.: Effect of mercurial diuretics on tubular sodium and potassium transport in the dog. *Am. J. Physiol.* *222*:282-289, 1972.

31. Feldman, D., Funder, J. W., and Edelman, I. S.: Subcellular mechanisms in the action of adrenal steroids. *Am. J. Med.* *53*:545-560, 1972.

32. Fourman, J., and Moffat, D. B.: Observations on the fine blood vessels of the kidney. *Proc. Symp. Zool. Soc. Lond.* *11*:57-71, 1964.

33. Giebisch, G., Klose, R. M., and Windhager, E. E.: Micropuncture study of hypertonic NaCl loading in the rat. *Am. J. Physiol.* *206*:687-693, 1964.

34. Goldberg, M.: Renal tubular sites of action of diuretics. In: *Renal Pharmacology.* Edited by J. W. Fisher and E. J. Cafruny. Appleton-Century-Crofts, New York, 1971, pp. 99-119.

35. Goodman, D. D., Allen, J. E., and Rasmussen, H.: On the mechanism of action of aldosterone. *Proc. Nat. Acad. Sci. USA* *64*:330-337, 1969.

36. Gottschalk, C. W., and Mylle, M.: Micropuncture study of the mammalian urinary concentrating mechanism: evidence for the countercurrent hypothesis. *Am. J. Physiol.* *196*:927-936, 1959.

37. Gottschalk, C. W.: Micropuncture studies of tubular function in the mammalian kidney. *Physiologist* *4*:35-55, 1961.

38. Grantham, J. J., and Burg, M. B.: Effect of vasopressin and cyclic AMP on permeability of isolated collecting tubules. *Am. J. Physiol.* *211*:255-259, 1966.

39. Grantham, J. J., Ganote, C. F., Burg, M. B., and Orloff, J.: Paths of transtubular water flow in isolated renal collecting tubules. *J. Cell Biol.* *41*:562-576, 1969.

40. Grantham, J. J.: Mode of water transport in mammalian renal collecting tubules. *Fed. Proc.* *30*:14-21, 1971.

41. Handler, J. S., Preston, A. S., and Orloff, J.: Effect of aldosterone on the sodium content and energy metabolism of epithelial cells of the toad urinary bladder. *J. Steroid Biochem.* *3*:137-141, 1972.

42. Hargitay, B., and Kuhn, W.: Das Multiplikations-prinzipals Grundlage der Harnkonzentrierung in der Niere. *Z. Elektrochem.* *55*:539-558, 1951.

43. Hierholzer, K., Wiederholt, W., Holzgreve, H., Giebisch, G., Klose, R. M., and Windhager, E. E.: Micropuncture study of renal transtubular concentration gradients of sodium and potassium in adrenalectomized rats. *Arch. Ges. Physiol.* *285*:193-210, 1965.

44. Jamison, R. L., Bennett, C. M., and Berliner, R. W.: Countercurrent multiplication by the thin loops of Henle. *Am. J. Physiol. 212*:357-366, 1967.

45. Jamison, R. L., Buerkert, J., and Lacy, F.: Micropuncture study of Henle's thin loop in Brattleboro rats. *Am. J. Physiol. 224*:180-185, 1973.

46. Jamison, R. L.: Recent advances in the physiology of Henle's loop and collecting tubule system. *Circ. Res. 34(Suppl. I)*: 91-100, 1974.

47. Jewell, P. A., and Verney, E. B.: An experimental attempt to determine the site of the neurohypophyseal osmoreceptors in the dog. *Phil. Trans. B240*:197-324, 1957.

48. Johnston, C. I., Davis, J. O., Howards, S. S., and Wright, F. S.: Cross-circulation experiments on the mechanism of the natriuresis during saline loading in the dog. *Circ. Res. 20*: 1-10, 1967.

49. Kamm, O., Aldrich, T. B., Grote, I. W., Rowe, L. W., and Bugbee, E. P.: The active principles of the posterior lobe of the pituitary gland. I. The demonstration of the presence of two active principles. II. The separation of the two principles and their concentration in the form of potent solid preparations. *J. Am. Chem. Soc. 50*:573-601, 1928.

50. Knochel, J. P., and Whale, M. G.: The role of aldosterone in renal physiology. *Arch. Internal Med. 131*:876-884, 1973.

51. Kokko, J. P.: Sodium chloride and water transport in the descending limb of Henle. *J. Clin. Invest. 49*:1838-1846, 1970.

52. Kokko, J. P.: Urea transport in the proximal tubule and the descending limb of Henle. *J. Clin. Invest. 51*:1999-2008, 1972.

53. Kokko, J. P., and Rector, F. C., Jr.: Countercurrent multiplication system without active transport in inner medulla. *Kidney International 2*:214-223, 1972.

54. Kokko, J. P.: Membrane characteristics governing salt and water transport in the loop of Henle. *Fed. Proc. 33*:25-30, 1974.

55. Koushanpour, E., Tarica, R. R., and Stevens, W. F.: Mathematical simulation of normal nephron function in rat and man. *J. Theor. Biol. 31*:177-214, 1971.

56. Landwehr, D. M., Klose, R. M., and Giebisch, G.: Renal tubular sodium and water in the isotonic sodium chloride loaded rat. *Am. J. Physiol. 212*:1327-1333, 1967.

57. Lassiter, W. E., Gottschalk, C. W., and Mylle, M.: Micropuncture study of net transtubular movement of water and urea in nondiuretic mammalian kidney. *Am. J. Physiol. 200*:1139-1147, 1961.

58. Lassiter, W. E., Mylle, M., and Gottschalk, C. W.: Net transtubular movement of water and urea in saline diuresis. *Am. J. Physiol. 206*:669-673, 1964.

59. Lassiter, W. E., Mylle, M., and Gottschalk, C. W.: Micropuncture study of urea transport in rat renal medulla. *Am. J. Physiol. 210*:965-970, 1966.

60. Lauson, H. D.: Metabolism of antidiuretic hormones. *Am. J. Med. 42*:713-744, 1967.

61. Lever, A. F.: The vasa recta and countercurrent multiplication. *Acta Med. Scand. Suppl. 434*:1-43, 1965.

62. Levy, R. I., Weiner, I. M., and Mudge, G. H.: The effects of acid-base balance on diuresis produced by organic and inorganic mercurials. *J. Clin. Invest. 37*:1016-1023, 1958.

63. Lifschitz, M. D., Schrier, R. W., and Edelman, I. S.: Effect of actinomycin D on aldosterone-mediated changes in electrolyte excretion. *Am. J. Physiol. 224*:376-380, 1973.

64. Lipton, P., and Edelman, I. S.: Effects of aldosterone and vasopressin on electrolytes of toad bladder epithelial cells. *Am. J. Physiol. 221*:733-741, 1971.

65. Maren, T. H.: Carbonic anhydrase: chemistry, physiology and inhibition. *Physiol. Rev. 47*:597-781, 1967.

66. Morel, F., Mylle, M., and Gottschalk, C. W.: Tracer microinjection studies of effect of ADH on renal tubular diffusion of water. *Am. J. Physiol. 209*:179-187, 1965.

67. Morgan, T., and Berliner, R. W.: Permeability of loop of Henle, vasa recta and collecting duct to water, urea and sodium. *Am. J. Physiol. 215*:108-115, 1968.

68. Morgan, T., Tadokoro, M., Martin, D., and Berliner, R. W.: Effect of furosemide on Na^+ and K^+ transport studied by microperfusion of the rat nephron. *Am. J. Physiol. 218*:292-297, 1970.

69. Müller, J.: *Regulation of Aldosterone Biosynthesis*. Springer-Verlag, New York, 1971.

70. Mulrow, P. J., and Forman, B. H.: The tissue effects of mineralocorticoids. *Am. J. Med. 53*:561-572, 1972.

71. Oliver, J.: *Nephrons and Kidneys*. Harper & Row, New York, 1968.

72. Orloff, J., and Handler, J. S.: The cellular mode of action of antidiuretic hormone. *Am. J. Med. 36*:686-697, 1964.

73. Orloff, J., and Handler, J. S.: The role of adenosine 3',5'-phosphate in the action of antidiuretic hormone. *Am. J. Med. 42*:757-768, 1967.

74. Pitts, R. F.: *Physiology of Kidney and Body Fluids*. 3rd ed. Year Book Publisher, Chicago, 1974.

75. Roemmelt, J. C., Sartorius, O. W., and Pitts, R. F.: Excretion and reabsorption of sodium and water in the adrenalectomized dogs. *Am. J. Physiol. 159*:124-136, 1949.

76. Sachs, H.: Biosynthesis and release of vasopressin. *Am. J. Med. 42*:687-700, 1967.

77. Seely, J. F., and Dirks, J. H.: Micropuncture study of hypertonic mannitol diuresis in the proximal and distal tubule of the dog kidney. *J. Clin. Invest. 48*:2330-2339, 1969.

78. Seldin, D. W., Eknoyan, G., Suki, W. W., and Rector, F. C., Jr.: Localization of diuretic action from the pattern of water and electrolyte excretion. *Ann. N.Y. Acad. Sci. 139*:328-343, 1966.

79. Share, L.: Vasopressin, its bioassay and the physiological control of its release. *Am. J. Med. 42*:701-712, 1967.

80. Sharp, G. W. G., and Leaf, A.: Mechanism of action of aldosterone. *Physiol. Rev. 46*:593-633, 1966.

81. Siegenthaler, W. E., Peterson, R. E., and Frimpter, G. W.: The renal clearance of aldosterone and its major metabolites. In: *Aldosterone, A Symposium*. Edited by E. E. Baulier and P. Robel. F. A. Davis Company, Philadelphia, 1964, pp. 51-72.

82. Simpson, S. A., and Tait, J. F.: Recent progress in methods of isolation, chemistry and physiology of aldosterone. *Recent Progr. Hormone Res. 11*:183-210, 1955.

83. Sperber, I.: Studies on the mammalian kidney. *Zool. Bidrag Uppsala 22*:249-432, 1944.

84. Sutherland, E. W., Robison, G. A., and Butcher, R. W.: Some aspects of the biological role of adenosine 3',5'-monophosphate (cyclic AMP). *Circulation 37*:279-306, 1968.

85. Thornburn, G. D., Kopald, H. H., Herd, J. A., Hollenberg, M., O'Morchae, C. C. C., and Barger, A. C.: Intrarenal distribution of nutrient blood flow determined with Krypton[85] in the unanesthetized dog. *Circ. Res. 13*:290-307, 1963.

86. Thurau, K.: Renal hemodynamics. *Am. J. Med. 36*:698-719, 1964.

87. Ullrich, K. J., and Jarausch, K. H.: Untersuchungen zum Problem der Harnkonzentrierung und Harnverdünnung: über die Verteilung der Elektrolyte. Harnstoff, Aminosäuren und exogenem Kreatinin in Rinde und Mark der Hundeniere bei verschiedenen Diuresezuständen. *Arch. Ges. Physiol. 262*:537-550, 1956.

88. Ullrich, K. J., Schmidt-Nielsen, B., O'Dell, R., Pehling, G., Gottschalk, C. W., Lassiter, W. E., and Mylle, M.: Micropuncture study of composition of the proximal and distal tubular fluid in rat kidney. *Am. J. Physiol. 204*:527-531, 1963.

89. Vander, A. J., Malvin, R. L., Wilde, W. S., Lapides, J., Sullivan, L. P., and McMurray, V. M.: Effects of adrenalectomy and aldosterone on proximal and distal tubular sodium reabsorption. *Proc. Soc. Exp. Biol. Med. 99*:323-325, 1958.

90. Vander, A. J.: Control of renin release. *Physiol. Rev. 47*:359-382, 1967.

91. Verney, E. B.: The antidiuretic hormone and the factors which determine its release. *Proc. Roy. Soc. B 135*:25-106, 1947.

92. Wesson, L. G., Jr.: *Physiology of the Human Kidney*. Grune & Stratton, New York, 1969.

93. Williams, G. H., Cain, J. P., Dluhy, R. G., and Underwood, R. H.: Studies of the control of plasma aldosterone concentration in normal man. I. Response to posture, acute and chronic volume depletion, and sodium loading. *J. Clin. Invest. 51*:1731-1742, 1972.

94. Williams, G. H., and Dluhy, R. G.: Aldosterone biosynthesis: interrelationship of regulatory factors. *Am. J. Med. 53*: 595-605, 1972.

95. Wirz, H., Hargitay, B., and Kuhn, W.: Lokalisation des Konzentrierungsprozesses in der Niere durch direkte Kryoskopie. *Helv. Physiol. Pharmacol. Acta 9*:196-207, 1951.

96. Wirz, H., and Dirix, R.: Urinary concentration and dilution. In: *Handbook of Physiology*, Section 8, *Renal Physiology*. Edited by J. Orloff and R. W. Berliner. Washington, D. C., American Physiological Society, 1973, pp. 415-430.

97. Wright, F. S., Knox, F. G., Howards, S. S., and Berliner, R. W.: Reduced sodium reabsorption by the proximal tubule of DOCA-escaped dogs. *Am. J. Physiol. 216*:869-875, 1969.

98. Wuu, T. C., Crumm, S., and Saffran, M.: Amino acid sequence of porcine neurophysin-I. *J. Biol. Chem. 246*:6043-6063, 1971.

Chapter 12

RENAL REGULATION OF EXTRACELLULAR VOLUME AND OSMOLALITY

Although each complex mammalian physiological system is developed to do a specific task, several of them are organized to perform one or more integrated functions. Of these functions, none is more essential to a normal life than that of *stabilizing* and maintaining a constant *internal environment* despite a wide variety of disturbances. A failure to achieve this stability or *homeostasis*, resulting from a breakdown in the various regulatory processes involved, poses a definite threat to life.

In a multicellular organism, such as man, several elaborate and specialized organ systems have the common task of minimizing or eliminating such a threat. In Chapter 1, we presented the salient, organizational features of these organ systems and collectively called them the *renal-body fluid regulating system*. As was depicted in Figure 1-1, this system is composed of metabolic, gastrointestinal, cardio-vascular, pulmonary, cutaneous and renal subsystems. Although basic knowledge of the function of each of these subsystems is necessary, it was pointed out that only through an understanding of the interaction among them can one hope to gain an insight into the complex regulatory mechanisms involved in the body fluid homeostasis.

In the preceding chapters, we presented a systematic *analysis* of the components of body fluids, the various aspects of renal function, and their roles in the overall regulation of the constancy of the internal environment in the face of a wide variety of disturbances. Briefly, we learned that the distribution of water and solutes within the various body fluid compartments, in the steady state of normality, depends on the adjustment of rates of fluid influx into and out of the body. We pointed out that of these, only the rate of renal efflux is subject to internal regulation in response to body needs in the face of external perturbations. The renal adjustment of fluid efflux was seen to be a function of the factors governing the formation of the glomerular filtrate and its subsequent sequential modification by tubular reabsorptive and secretory processes. Hence, in the final analysis, regulation of renal effluxes is ultimately determined by those factors--both renal and extrarenal in origin--that regulate GFR and renal transport rates. Furthermore, since the volume and composition of the renal efflux reflect renal adjustment of these parameters in the blood compartment, which is in dynamic equilibrium with the other body fluid compartments, the regulation of renal efflux is the key to the ultimate regulation of the volume and composition of body fluids.

As mentioned in the preceding chapters, renal regulation of volume and osmolality of body fluids is influenced by the functional state of gastrointestinal, cardiovascular, pulmonary, and neuroendocrine systems. Of these, the gastrointestinal system influences primarily the rate of normal delivery of water and solutes into the body, and hence indirectly influences kidney function. On the other hand, the cardiovascular, pulmonary and neuroendocrine systems exert a direct influence on the intra- and extrarenal mechanisms responsible for the maintenance of body fluid homeostasis.

In this chapter, we shall attempt to *synthesize* the materials presented in the preceding chapters by considering the functional characteristics, and more importantly, the pertinent input-output relationships of these subsystems, using the already familiar *functional* or *control diagram*.

MAJOR COMPONENTS OF THE RENAL-BODY FLUID REGULATING SYSTEM

Figure 12-1 presents schematically a simplified functional diagram of the renal-body fluid regulating system. To get a "feel" for what this diagram represents and to facilitate subsequent discussion, let us examine briefly the salient features of each subsystem and identify its functional role in the overall operation of the system.

For the purpose of this presentation, we may divide the renal-body fluid regulating system into four separate but interacting subsystems:

1. The *gastrointestinal (G.I.) system*, which provides the most important route of fluid entry into, and a normal route of fluid loss out of, the body. Thus, fluid intake is the only input to this system, while fluid loss (normally as feces) and fluid absorption represent the two important outputs. Not shown is fluid lost through fistulae (e.g., gastric), which represents an abnormal but important output for the system. In pathological conditions such as vomiting and diarrhea, excessive fluid lost from the G.I. system may pose a serious threat to water and electrolyte balance. Because different kinds and amounts of solutes may be lost in each of these conditions, in adults reduction in the extracellular fluid volume (dehydration) usually leads to secondary and acute changes in acid-base balance (see Chapter 10). Therefore, alteration in the fluid intake and excessive fluid loss in disease are two of the ways by which the operation of the renal-body fluid regulating system can be disturbed.

2. The *cardiovascular system*, composed of a circulatory apparatus and a tissue exchanger, which are not shown in the

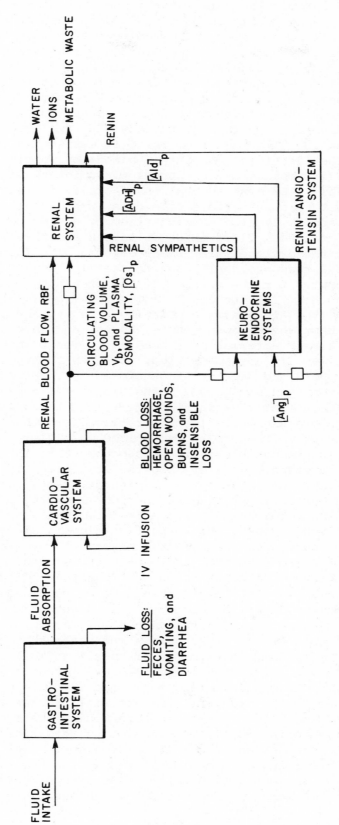

Figure 12-1. A simplified functional diagram of the major components of the renal-body fluid regulating system.

functional diagram. The *circulatory apparatus* consists of a double heart, which mechanically pumps the blood containing fluid and nutrients absorbed by the G.I. system to the various tissues and organs of the body, including the neuroendocrine and renal systems. The *tissue exchanger* consists of the thin-walled capillaries, which supply all tissues. Water, electrolytes, and nutrients move in both directions across the capillary walls as a result of regional hydrostatic pressure gradients and electrochemical forces. In the functional diagram, two inputs are shown for the cardiovascular system: the fluid absorbed from the G.I. system and intravenous infusion. The latter is, of course, a mode of forcing fluid into the body in circumstances when normal fluid intake via the G.I. system is not possible. Because absorption of orally ingested fluid is associated with a considerable time delay, the renal response to such a volume expansion is also characterized by a time delay. In contrast, intravenous fluid infusion causes a rather immediate expansion of the extracellular fluid volume, with little or no time delay in renal response. Although the cardiovascular system has multiple outputs, for the purpose of the present discussion we have shown only three: (a) the renal blood flow (RBF), (b) the circulating blood volume (V_b) and plasma osmolality ($[Os]_p$), and (c) the blood loss, as in hemorrhage, open wounds, burns, and insensible loss. Hemorrhage, either arterial or venous, involves a loss of both plasma and blood cells. If not controlled, it leads to hypotension, circulatory shock and death. As mentioned in Chapter 3, fluids discharged from open wounds and burns are lost from the interstitial space. Since the interstitial fluid is similar to plasma, except for the amount of proteins, its loss is reflected in the intravascular volume, a factor which must be recognized when fluid replacement is indicated. The insensible fluid loss occurs through the pulmonary and cutaneous subsystems. However, because it ultimately comes from the blood, it is included here for completeness. Note that the second output serves as an input to both the renal and the neuroendocrine systems. A *small box* on any arrow indicates that the signals being conveyed are *monitored* by the respective organ systems.

3. The *neuroendocrine systems* consist of three major components: the autonomic nervous system, the hypothalamus-pituitary system, and the adrenal gland. As depicted in the functional diagram, two inputs impinge on this system: one is the circulatory blood volume and plasma osmolality, and the second is the output of the renin-angiotensin system, namely, angiotensin II ($[Ang]_p$). Once again, the small box on both of the input arrows indicates that the neuroendocrine system monitors the circulating blood volume, the plasma osmolality and the blood level of angiotensin II. As we shall learn shortly, changes in V_b are monitored by peripheral *stretch receptors* in both the high-pressure arterial and low-pressure venous sides of the circulation, which in turn modify the sympathetic outflow to the kidney and indirectly the rate of synthesis and release of antidiuretic hormone, and hence its plasma concentration ($[ADH]_p$). In contrast, changes in $[Os]_p$ are monitored by the hypothalamic *osmoreceptors*, thereby altering the rates of synthesis and release of ADH and hence its plasma concentration. Changes in the plasma level

of angiotensin II produce a direct effect on the rate of synthesis of aldosterone by the zona glomerulosa of the adrenal cortex and its release into the circulation, and consequently its plasma concentration ($[Ald]_p$). Thus, as shown, the three output signals emerging from the neuroendocrine systems are: the sympathetic outflow to the kidney, $[ADH]_p$, and $[Ald]_p$.

4. The *renal system* represents the final and the most important component of the renal-body fluid regulating system. As we learned, the renal system indirectly maintains the constancy of the internal environment by directly monitoring the volume and osmolality of the circulating blood, thereby stabilizing the volume and osmolality of the extracellular fluid compartment. The kidney does this by carefully adjusting the rate of elimination of water, ions, and metabolic wastes. As shown, the output signals from the neuroendocrine systems modulate the renal function, and thereby the rate of excretion of water and ions.

As depicted in Figure 12-1, the renal system represents the primary regulatory organ whose function is directly modified by two other systems, namely, the cardiovascular and neuroendocrine systems. These two systems represent the *extrarenal* components of the renal-body fluid regulating system. Let us now examine in detail the functional organization and operational characteristics of the intra- and extrarenal components of the renal-body fluid regulating system, beginning with a review of the renal components.

A. THE RENAL COMPONENT

Figure 12-2 presents a functional diagram of the renal regulator developed on the basis of the materials presented in the preceding chapters. Note that in this and subsequent diagrams, a *plus sign* next to an input arrow impinging on a box means that the forcing increases the output signal, whereas a *minus sign* implies just the opposite.

The upper portion of Figure 12-2 depicts the four major components of the *renal regulator*: The glomerular ultrafilter, the proximal tubule, the loop of Henle and the distal and collecting tubules. To get a "feel" for the operation of the renal regulator as it pertains to the present discussion, let us analyze it component by component, beginning with the glomerular ultrafilter component in the upper left corner.

Consistent with what we have learned earlier (Chapter 5) the rate of glomerular filtration (GFR) is proportional to the effective glomerular filtration pressure (ΔP_f), with the ultrafilter permeability (k_g) as the limiting proportionality constant. The magnitude of ΔP_f is determined by the algebraic sum (depicted by a circle with a plus sign inside) of the glomerular capillary pressure (P_g) and the glomerular capillary protein oncotic pressure (π_g). The magnitude of P_g is a function of the systemic arterial pressure (P_{AS}) and the resistance of the renal vascular bed, shown in the lower portion of the diagram. The resistance of the renal vascular bed is a positive function of the renal sympathetic activity. The magnitude of π_g is a function of plasma protein oncotic pressure (π_p) (not shown), which in turn is dependent upon the rate of protein intake or

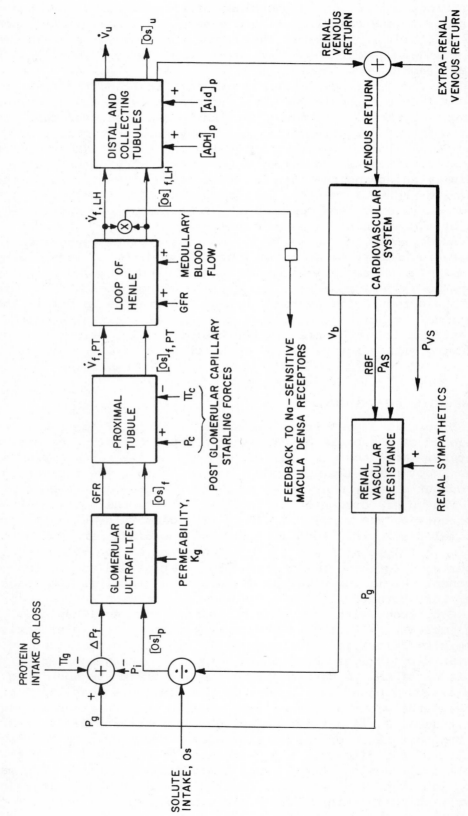

Figure 12-2. A functional diagram of the renal regulator.

loss. The osmolality of the filtrate ($[Os]_f$), emerging from the glomerular ultrafilter, is equal to the osmolality of the protein-free fraction of plasma ($[Os]_p$). The latter is determined by the intake of the osmotically active solute (O_s) and the circulating blood volume (V_b). This relationship is depicted in the diagram by a circle with a division sign inside.

The functional diagram reveals that an important determinant of both $[Os]_p$ and π_p is the *volume of circulating blood*, whose magnitude is determined by the *cardiac output*, which in turn depends on the *venous return*. The latter, as shown in the lower right-hand corner, is determined by the algebraic sum of the renal and extrarenal venous returns. The magnitude of the former depends on the algenraic sum of the tubular processing of the filtrate by all the functioning nephrons. The magnitude of the latter depends on *three* major factors: (1) the rate of oral intake of water, (2) the rate of extrarenal loss of water and solutes, such as insensible loss, respiration, sweat, and stool, and (3) fortuitous gain or loss of water and solutes, such as intravenous infusion, hemorrhage, vomiting, diarrhea, gastric fistula, plasma loss through burned skin, and open wounds.

In the *proximal tubule* (PT), depicted by the second box in the upper portion of the diagram, approximately two thirds of the filtered water and solutes is reabsorbed iso-osmotically, yielding a filtrate tubular volume flow of $\dot{V}_{f,PT}$ and a filtrate osmolality of $[Os]_{f,PT}$ at the end of this segment. As shown, the reabsorption of the filtrate along this nephron segment depends mainly on the transepithelial transport of sodium, with reabsorption rate being influenced by changes in GFR and in postglomerular capillary pressure (P_C), and protein oncotic pressure (π_C), the so-called Starling forces. Thus, as described in Chapter 8, an increase in GFR, as by intravenous fluid infusion, increases the velocity of filtrate flow and reduces the time required to establish the sodium diffusion gradient across the luminal membrane, thereby decreasing the net transepithelial sodium and hence filtrate reabsorption. Likewise, an increase in P_g, beside causing an increase in ΔP_f and hence GFR, also induces further hemodynamic changes in the postglomerular capillaries (the peritubular capillary network), which leads to a reduction of filtrate reabsorption in the proximal tubule. The rise in P_g is transmitted to the peritubular capillary network, where it induces a proportional rise in the capillary hydrostatic pressure (P_C). Since the transcapillary movement of the filtrate from the peritubular interstitium to the blood depends largely on the hydrostatic pressure gradient (see Chapter 8), the rise in P_C opposes such a gradient. Hence, an increase in either GFR or P_g, or both, tends to reduce filtrate reabsorption in the proximal tubule, resulting in a net urinary excretion of solute (primarily sodium) and water. Conversely, an increase in π_C, induced by high protein intake, selective increase in efferent arteriolar resistance, or excessive loss of water (hemoconcentration) increases filtrate reabsorption in this nephron segment.

In the *loop of Henle* (LH), depicted by the third box in the upper portion of the diagram, the filtrate volume and its osmolality undergo considerable modification, consistent with the operation of the countercurrent multiplication process described earlier (Chapters 8 and 11). As shown, the volume ($\dot{V}_{f,LH}$) and osmolality ($[Os]_{f,LH}$) of the filtrate emerging from the ascending limb are influenced by changes in GFR and the renal medullary blood flow.

An increase in GFR reduces the net reabsorption of sodium chloride from the ascending limb by a mechanism analogous to that described for the proximal tubule, thereby increasing the sodium load ($\dot{V}_{f,LH} \cdot [Na]_{f,LH}$) emerging from this nephron segment. This is depicted by the circle with the multiplication sign inside. Likewise, an increase in the medullary blood flow causes solute washout from the medullary interstitium by the mechanism described in Chapter 11, and hence reduces the longitudinal gradient in the medullary interstitium. The consequence of this reduced gradient is a decrease in solute (sodium chloride and urea) concentration along the descending limb, and hence in the fluid entering the ascending limb. Thus, an increase in the medullary blood flow causes an increase in $[Os]_{f,LH}$, secondary to a decrease in the longitudinal gradient in the medullary interstitium. As shown, changes in the sodium concentration or sodium load (depicted by a circle with a multiplication sign inside) of the fluid emerging from the loop of Henle by way of the ascending limb are monitored (depicted by a small box on the arrow) by the sodium-sensitive tubular receptors at the macula densa. These receptors constitute the afferent limb of a negative feedback mechanism believed by some (Thurau et al., 1967) to play an important role in the regulation of GFR. The pros and cons of this concept, as well as the physiological role of the macula densa receptors in the renal regulation of the extracellular volume and osmolality, will be discussed later in this chapter.

In the *distal and collecting tubules*, depicted by the last box in the upper portion of the diagram, the filtrate undergoes its final change in volume and osmolality. The final volume ($\dot{V}_u$) and osmolality ($[Os]_u$) of the excreted urine are the result of two simultaneous processes: (1) the exposure of the tubular fluid traversing along this nephron segment to the surrounding medullary interstitium, having a steep osmolar concentration gradient along its longitudinal axis, and (2) the exposure of the peritubular side of the tubular cell membrane to the circulating levels of aldosterone and antidiuretic hormone. As described in Chapter 11, the steeper the longitudinal osmolality gradient in the medullary interstitium, the smaller would be the volume and the greater would be the osmolality of the excreted urine. An increase in the blood level of either aldosterone or ADH would also yield the same result. A factor which limits the final volume and osmolality of the excreted urine is the limited adaptive reabsorptive capacity of the distal and collecting tubules. Thus, an increase in the volume of filtrate entering these nephron segments would overwhelm their reabsorptive capacity, leading to increased renal excretion of solute and water.

Note that the renal processing of the filtrate at each tubular segment returns to the blood nearly all the filtered solutes and water. This is depicted by the arrow emerging from the distal tubule and labelled "renal venous return." Thus, in this manner, the renal regulator stabilizes directly the blood volume and its osmolality, and indirectly those of the extravascular and intracellular fluid compartments.

B. THE EXTRARENAL COMPONENTS

As depicted in Figure 12-1, the renal regulation of blood volume and osmolality is influenced by the normal functioning of three major organ systems: the gastrointestinal, cardiovascular, and neuroendocrine systems. The effects of alterations in the G.I. function in health and disease on body fluid homeostasis are mediated via the induced changes in the volume and osmolality of the circulating blood. The influence of the G.I. system on renal function is indirect and for the sake of simplicity we shall not discuss its function to any extent. Therefore, in the present discussion and hereafter, we shall refer to the cardiovascular and neuroendocrine systems as the extrarenal components of the renal-body fluid regulating system. Let us now examine the role of each separately.

1. THE CARDIOVASCULAR SYSTEM. As depicted in the lower portion of Figure 12-2, the cardiovascular system supplies a relatively constant fraction of cardiac output, as renal blood flow (RBF), to the kidney for processing. As discussed in Chapter 5, the constancy of the renal blood flow, for a given systemic arterial pressure (P_{AS}) is determined by the intrarenal vascular resistance, which in part is influenced by the activity of renal sympathetic nerves. The magnitude of RBF is in part determined by the cardiac output, which in turn depends on the venous return to the heart. The latter, in turn, is in part determined by the renal venous return whose volume and osmolality are subject to renal regulation.

In terms of body fluid homeostasis, the cardiovascular system provides continuous information about two parameters of the circulating blood: *volume* and *osmolality*. Changes in blood volume are translated into changes in systemic arterial (P_{AS}) and venous (P_{VS}) pressures. Changes in P_{AS} are continuously monitored by the *stretch receptors* located in the high-pressure vascular bed (carotid sinus and aortic arch baroreceptors) and in the kidney (afferent arteriolar baroreceptors). Changes in P_{VS} are monitored by the *stretch receptors* in the low-pressure vascular bed (left and right atria). The afferent information arising from these receptors is then monitored by the appropriate components of the neuroendocrine system, leading to alterations in the blood levels of aldosterone and ADH. Changes in blood osmolality ($[Os]_p$) are likewise monitored by the neuroendocrine system, which also lead to alteration of blood levels of these hormones.

2. THE NEUROENDOCRINE SYSTEMS. As mentioned earlier, the neuroendocrine systems consist of three major components: the autonomic nervous system, the hypothalamus-pituitary system, and the adrenal gland. The input to these systems consists of changes in P_{AS}, P_{VS}, and $[Os]_p$, as well as changes in $[Ang]_p$. As depicted in Figure 12-1, the changes in these parameters will induce changes

in the sympathetic outflow to the kidney and blood levels of aldosterone and ADH, leading to alterations in renal excretion of sodium and water, and hence in the volume and osmolality of the blood.

The foregoing analysis reveals two important operational features of the renal-body fluid regulating system. (1) The *renal system* plays a central role in maintaining the constancy of the internal environment, a direct consequence of stabilizing the volume and composition of the blood. (2) The function of the renal regulator is partly modified by the *cardiovascular* and *neuroendocrine* systems.

As we proceed in this section, it is important to bear in mind these essential features, as outlined above, which will be fully described below. Because they occupy the central theme of this chapter, we might restate them briefly. The kidneys stabilize the volume and composition of the blood, and hence indirectly the extracellular fluid. Changes in volume and composition of the blood initiate compensatory responses from the cardiovascular and neuroendocrine systems, which in turn modify renal function.

With this brief outline of the functions of the major components of the renal-body fluid regulating system, we are now ready to consider in detail, and as revealed by recent studies, the various factors involved in the regulation of volume and osmolality of the blood and hence indirectly that of the extracellular fluids.

REGULATION OF OSMOLALITY VERSUS VOLUME

Since the osmolality of the blood and hence of the extracellular fluid is in part determined by its volume, it is of special interest to inquire into the nature of interplay of the regulatory mechanisms involved in stabilizing the osmolality and volume of the extracellular fluid. In general, as long as the quantity of the osmotically active solutes in the extracellular fluid remains unaltered, any change in its volume due to fortuitous loss or gain of fluid is regulated by adjustment of renal efflux of osmotically active solutes. On the other hand, if there is a loss of osmotically active solutes, which is the case in most instances of fluid disturbance, restoration of the osmolality of the extracellular fluid volume depends on the readjustment of its volume. This is accomplished by adjustment of renal efflux of water.

The question of whether the regulation of volume precedes regulation of osmolality, or vice versa, has been the subject of intensive investigation. However, the issue, which is of considerable academic and clinical interest, continues to be controversial and has not been resolved. The bulk of the available experimental evidence (see reviews by Gauer et al., 1970; Share and Claybaugh, 1972) appears to favor the concept that changes in blood volume initially induce a change in aldosterone-stimulated renal reabsorption of sodium. The resulting change in plasma osmolality will induce a secondary change in the blood volume via ADH-stimulated renal reabsorption of water. Therefore, it seems reasonable to state that the renal regulation of volume and osmolality of the blood, and hence the extracellular fluid, are ultimately determined by the dynamic interplay of those renal and extrarenal factors which modify the normal rates of synthesis and release of ADH and aldosterone and their cellular action in the distal and collecting tubular epithelia.

Since ADH is primarily concerned with renal reabsorption of water, its regulation will affect primarily the plasma osmolality and secondarily the blood volume. On the other hand, because aldosterone is primarily concerned with renal reabsorption of sodium as isotonic solution, its regulation will affect primarily the blood volume and secondarily the plasma osmolality. Consequently, to facilitate presentation, we shall discuss the factors regulating the plasma levels of ADH (and hence osmolality) and aldosterone (and therefore volume) separately.

REGULATION OF PLASMA OSMOLALITY: CONTROL OF WATER EXCRETION

Regulation of plasma osmolality largely depends on the dynamic balance between the rates of influx and efflux of water into and out of the body. Of these fluxes, only the rate of renal efflux is subject to internal regulation.

Regulation of renal excretion of water is ultimately determined by the factors which influence the rates of synthesis and release of ADH into the blood and its cellular action in the distal and collecting tubular epithelia. There are two physiological stimuli for the synthesis and release of ADH: First, the *plasma osmolality*, which acts via the *osmoreceptors* located in or near the hypothalamus. Second, the *blood volume*, which, through induced changes in the systemic arterial (P_{AS}) and venous (P_{VS}) pressures, acts via the *stretch* or *volume receptors* located in the carotid sinus, aortic arch and left atrium. Let us now consider the response characteristics of these receptors and their relative contribution to the rates of synthesis and release of ADH and hence the renal excretion of water.

A. OSMORECEPTORS

HYPOTHALAMIC OSMORECEPTORS. As mentioned in Chapter 11, as early as 1947, Verney, in a series of now classic experiments, demonstrated that a sustained 5-minute infusion of an hypertonic solution of saline or sucrose (but not urea, which enters the cells) into the arterial blood supply of the hypothalamus of dogs reduced a pre-established water diuresis. The changes in renal response were brought about by as little as 1 to 2% change in the osmolality of the perfusing arterial blood. On the basis of these findings, Verney proposed that there must be receptor cells in or near the hypothalamus sensitive to changes in the effective osmotic pressure of the extracellular fluid bathing them. He called these cells the *"osmoreceptors."* Subsequent studies (Jewell and Verney, 1957; Jewell, 1963) located these osmoreceptors in the vicinity of the supraoptic nucleus of the hypothalamus.

According to the osmoreceptor concept developed by Verney and his associates, an increase in the osmolality of the blood supplying the osmoreceptor cells leads to an increase in the cellular uptake of osmotically active solutes accompanied by osmotic entry of water. This would result in the swelling of the osmoreceptor cells, which would in turn stimulate the receptor endings to increase their neural discharge. The increase in the frequencies of impulses arising from the osmoreceptor cells will eventually lead to an increase in the synthesis of ADH by the hypothalamus-pituitary system and its release into the blood. The resulting increase in $[ADH]_p$ will then cause an increase in osmotic reabsorption of water from the distal and collecting tubules, thereby reducing C_{H_2O}. Although the details of how the increase in the osmolality of the extracellular fluid, to which the osmoreceptors are exposed, leads to an increase in neural discharge and eventual increase in synthesis and release of ADH remain entirely speculative, **considerable** evidence supports the osmoreceptor concept. Without being exhaustive, we shall cite two recent relevant studies as examples. For a more detailed review of evidence supporting the osmoreceptor theory, the interested reader is referred to the references cited by these two reports and a recent review by Share and Claybaugh (1972).

The most direct evidence supporting the osmoreceptor concept comes from recent studies of Johnson and associates (1970). They found that in conscious sheep, a decrease in the plasma osmolality of 1.2% produced a 2 to 1 microunits/ml reduction in $[ADH]_p$, a change sufficient to bring about a detectable water diuresis. A further support for the osmoreceptor concept comes from recent electrophysiological studies of Durham and Novin (1970). They recorded slow potential changes from the region of the supraoptic nucleus in response to infusion of hypertonic solution into the rabbit carotid artery. From their observations, they concluded that the supraoptic nucleus contains osmoreceptors which respond to rapid changes in osmolality of the circulating body fluids.

In summary, as depicted in Figure 12-3, changes in plasma osmolality ($[Os]_p$) are monitored by the osmoreceptors in the supraoptic nucleus of the hypothalamus, which in turn regulate the synthesis and release of ADH into the blood. The resulting change in the plasma concentration of ADH will in turn modulate the rate of osmolar reabsorption of water from the distal and collecting tubules. Thus, an increase in $[Os]_p$ leads to an increase in ADH release and hence in $[ADH]_p$, with eventual decrease in solute-free water clearance (C_{H_2O}) and hence antidiuresis. Conversely, a decrease in $[Os]_p$ will produce the opposite effects: decrease in $[ADH]_p$, increase in C_{H_2O} and water diuresis. In the diagram, the *negative sign* next to the arrow labelled $[ADH]_p$ indicates that ADH normally *decreases* C_{H_2O} by increasing osmotic reabsorption of water in the distally located nephron segments.

Of clinical interest is the marked water diuresis (in excess of 2.5 liters/day) seen in patients with diabetes insipidus. This could result from lesion(s) in or near the supraoptic nucleus of the hypothalamus-pituitary system, leading to a marked decrease in synthesis and release of ADH and hence an increase in C_{H_2O}. The

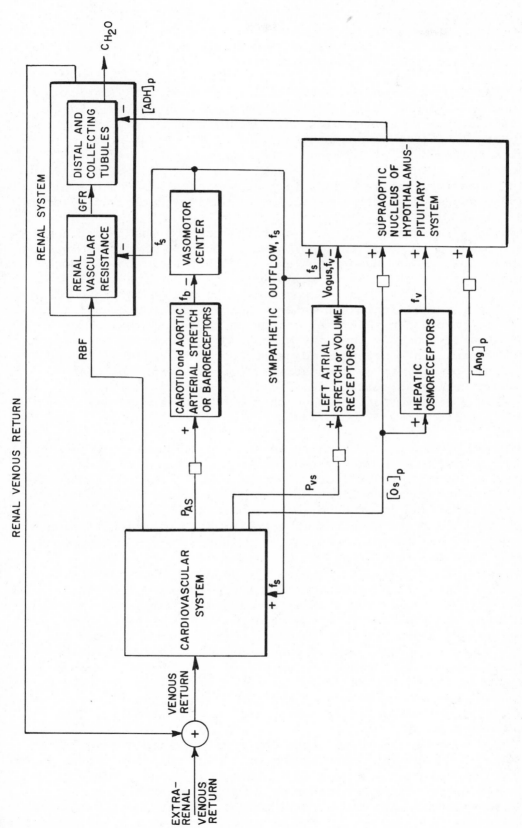

Figure 12-3. A functional diagram of the extrarenal regulation of ADH release and renal excretion of water.

insatiable urge of these patients to drink water (polydipsia) has been considered secondary to a primary polyuria (marked excretion of hypotonic urine) and dehydration resulting from the disruption of synthesis and release of ADH mechanism.

THIRST CENTER. Numerous studies in conscious rats (Stricker, 1969) and goats (Anderson, 1971) have provided convincing evidence that, in addition to osmoregulation, hypothalamus plays an important role in regulation of water drinking in thirst. The thirst sensitive center is believed to be located in the anterolateral region of the hypothalamus. Stimulation of this region in rats and goats elicits drinking behavior, while lesions in this area abolish the normal drinking response to water deprivation or administration of hypertonic saline.

Available evidence indicates that the role of the thirst center in water balance is equal in importance to that of the ADH-releasing supraoptic nucleus of the hypothalamus. Both centers appear to be activated by the same afferent stimuli--namely, changes in plasma osmolality and blood volume. However, the thirst center responds by controlling the oral influx of water, whereas the ADH-releasing center responds by regulating the renal efflux of water. In this manner, through dynamic, coordinated, integrated dual actions of these centers, there is a continuous adjustment of total body water and hence of the osmolality of the extracellular fluid in the face of various disturbing stimuli. To preserve the simplicity of presentation, we have not included the thirst center and its input-output signals in Figure 12-3.

HEPATIC OSMORECEPTORS. There is growing evidence that the liver plays an important role in osmoregulation, presumably by monitoring the osmotic pressure of the portal venous blood. The existence of hepatic osmoreceptors was first postulated by Haberich (1968) after observing that infusion of hypertonic saline solution into the portal vein of conscious rats resulted in antidiuresis, whereas infusion of water resulted in diuresis. As depicted in Figure 12-3, Haberich suggested that the renal response was mediated via a reflex modification of ADH-releasing system by the hepatic branch of the vagus nerve (f_v). Further support for the existence of hepatic osmoreceptors has come from studies of Niijima (1969), who recorded the frequency of impulses from the hepatic branch of vagus nerve of isolated guinea pig livers perfused with hypertonic solutions of saline, glucose, sucrose, and mannose. He found that the frequency of afferent impulses increased in direct proportion to the increase in the osmolality of the perfusion fluid. However, in contrast to the hypothalamic osmoreceptors, a minimum of 6% increase in the osmolality of the perfusing fluid was required to stimulate the portal osmoreceptors.

Recent evidence indicates that the hepatic receptors are more sensitive to changes in concentration of sodium chloride in the portal vein blood than those of osmolality. Thus, Passo and associates (1973) have reported that infusion of hypertonic saline, but not hypertonic sucrose, into the hepatic portal vein of anesthetized cats for 90 minutes produced a significant natriuresis 30 minutes after the onset of infusion. However, infusion of both hypertonic saline and sucrose solutions into the femoral vein failed to alter the urinary excretion of sodium. Furthermore, they showed that bilateral vagotomy abolished the response to portal vein infusion. From these results, they concluded that, at least in the cat, liver contains specific receptors which monitor sodium chloride concentration in the portal vein and which via the vagus nerve can reflexly alter the urinary excretion of sodium. Further support for the existence of hepatic sodium receptors comes from a recent study by Andrews and Orbach (1974), who found an increase in the frequency of afferent impulses recorded from the hepatic branch of the vagus nerve of the isolated rabbit livers perfused with hypertonic saline solution.

Despite these evidences the question of whether the hepatic receptors are sensitive to sodium chloride concentration or osmolality of the portal vein blood is at present not fully resolved. Furthermore, the extent and relative contribution of the portal osmoreceptors to the overall regulation of water balance remains to be explored.

B. STRETCH OR VOLUME RECEPTORS

As depicted in Figure 12-3, there are *two* groups of stretch or volume receptors whose activities influence the rate of synthesis and release of ADH. The first group is located in the *left atrium*, where they monitor the volume of blood returning to the left ventricle. Because of their anatomical location, the left atrial receptors have also been called the low-pressure venous vascular bed receptors. The second group is found in two locations. One set is located in the *carotid sinus*, which is a dilatation of the internal carotid artery at the point where common carotid artery divides into the external and internal carotid arteries. Another set is located in the *aortic arch*, just proximal to the exit of the aorta from the left ventricle. Because of their anatomical locations, the carotid sinus and aortic arch receptors have also been called the high-pressure arterial vascular bed baroreceptors. That these two groups of receptors represent the afferent limb of a reflex mechanism for the control of ADH release is now well established.

1. LEFT ATRIAL STRETCH RECEPTORS. Henry and associates (1956) were the first to demonstrate the role of the left atrial stretch-sensitive volume receptors in the reflex regulation of ADH release. They showed that inflation of a small rubber balloon inserted into the left atrial appendage of an anesthetized dog produced an increase in urine flow after a latent period of 5 to 10 minutes. The reflex nature of the renal response was subsequently established by Henry and Pearce (1956), who showed that cooling the vagus nerve abolished the urinary response to left atrial balloon distention. Since the increase in urine flow in these studies was due largely to an increase in water excretion, they suggested that the renal response was a consequence of a reflex inhibition of ADH release by left atrial balloon distention. Although these conclusions were based largely

on indirect evidence, subsequent studies generally have supported their validity and have further delineated the nature of the reflex pathway and its response characteristics. The following represents a summary of some of the more important studies which have provided the experimental evidence for the left atrial receptor component of the reflex regulation of ADH release.

Baisset and Montastruc (1957) provided the first direct evidence that the increase in the left atrial pressure by balloon inflation produced a decrease in the antidiuretic activity of the plasma. This was subsequently confirmed by Shu'ayb and associates (1965), who observed an increase in urine flow and a decrease in plasma concentration of ADH in anesthetized dogs following an increase in left atrial pressure by balloon inflation. Moreover, they showed that both renal and hormonal effects could be abolished by vagotomy, thereby confirming the reflex nature of both responses. In a similar study, Arndt and associates (1963) observed hemodynamic changes, in addition to hormonal and renal responses, in anesthetized dogs following an increase in left atrial pressure by balloon inflation. They found that the increase in both osmolar and solute-free water clearances were accompanied by an increase in clearances of inulin and PAH, despite a reduction in cardiac output and arterial blood pressure. That the hemodynamic changes were in part responsible for the renal and hormonal responses have further been verified in unanesthetized dogs (Lydtin and Hamilton, 1964). These authors found that increasing the left atrial pressure by tightening a pursestring suture around the mitral valve caused an increase in arterial blood pressure, renal blood flow, urine flow, and urinary sodium excretion.

Although the studies cited above provide substantial support for the existence of a left atrial stretch receptor reflex regulating ADH release, they do not rule out the contributing effects of accompanying hemodynamic changes. The latter could have resulted from large increases in left atrial pressure which were used in the above studies. Moreover, the methods used to determine plasma ADH activity were variable and unsatisfactory. To resolve the issue and to determine whether the left atrial stretch reflex is normally of physiological significance, Johnson and associates (1969) reexamined the problem by determining the renal and hormonal response to much smaller increases in the left atrial pressure. They found that small increases in the left atrial transmural pressure (P_{LA}) up to 7 cm of water produced by balloon inflation in anesthetized dogs produced a linear decrease in the peripheral arterial plasma concentration of ADH. The latter was determined by bioassay in the ethanol-anesthetized rat after extraction and concentration of the hormone. The decrease in $[ADH]_p$ was associated with a significant increase in urine flow and a decrease in urine-to-plasma (U/P) osmolality ratio and a negative solute-free water clearance ($T^C_{H_2O}$). The left atrial distention-induced renal and hormonal responses were not affected by concomitant changes in plasma osmolality or intravenous infusion of ADH. From these findings, they concluded that the left atrial stretch-sensitive volume receptors play a major role in the regulation of plasma ADH level, a concept which is now well established (Share and Claybaugh, 1972).

Considerable evidence (Gauer and Henry, 1963; Gauer et al., 1970) have generally established that the vagal afferents enter the *vasomotor center* in the medulla oblongata with secondary connection to the supraoptic region of the hypothalamus, which controls the rate of synthesis and release of ADH. The impulses in the vagal afferents have an inhibitory effect on the hypothalamus and hence on ADH release. Since the vasomotor center (which, as described below, is the site of neural control of the cardiovascular system) also receives afferent inhibitory impulses from the carotid sinus and aortic arch baroreceptors, it has been suggested (Share and Claybaugh, 1972) that the vagal afferents may in part determine the extent of information transmitted by the arterial baroreceptors. Thus, the influence of the baroreceptor afferents on the vasomotor center becomes dominant only when the impulse activity in vagal afferents is reduced.

To summarize, as depicted in Figure 12-3, an increase in the blood volume leads to an increase in the systemic venous pressure (P_{VS}) and eventually the left atrial pressure (P_{LA}), which is monitored (indicated by a small box on the arrow) by the left atrial stretch receptors. Stimulation of these receptors leads to an increase in the frequency of impulses in the vagal afferents (f_v) to the hypothalamic centers. Apparently, the vagal impulses arriving in these regions inhibit the synthesis and release of the ADH by the supraoptic nucleus of the hypothalamus, thereby reducing the plasma concentration of ADH. The decrease in $[ADH]_p$ leads to a decreased osmotic reabsorption of water from the distal and collecting tubules, and hence to an increase in solute-free water clearance (C_{H_2O}) and diuresis.

There are a number of other stimuli besides direct changes in blood volume that bring about reflex changes in $[ADH]_p$ and C_{H_2O}. The most important of these are changes in the ambient temperature and body posture. Recent experiments in human subjects (Segar and Moore, 1968) have shown that these stimuli bring about a redistribution of blood in the low-pressure intrathoracic vessels, which is monitored by the left atrial volume receptors, thereby causing reflex variations in $[ADH]_p$ and C_{H_2O}. Thus, exposure to *cold* or *heat* caused a marked *decrease* or *increase* in $[ADH]_p$, respectively, without any accompanying change in $[Na^+]_p$, $[Cl^-]_p$, or total solute concentrations. Since there was no change in plasma osmolality, changes in $[ADH]_p$ could not be mediated via the hypothalamic osmoreceptors. These changes, however, may be explained on the basis of redistribution of blood volume. It is well known that cooling causes peripheral vasoconstriction, which leads to an increase in the central blood volume. The resulting increase in the venous return will eventually cause an increase in the left atrial pressure and the intrathoracic "volume receptor" activity, which in turn causes inhibition of the hypothalamic centers. However, during exposure to heat, marked peripheral vasodilation results in a decrease in the central blood volume, leading to a decrease in the activity of volume receptors and an eventual increase in ADH release. In short, exposure to cold causes diuresis, whereas exposure to heat results in antidiuresis.

Postural changes lead to a redistribution of central blood volume and hence alter the activity of volume receptors. Thus, in *recumbent* position, the increase in central blood volume leads to an increase in left atrial pressure and inhibition of ADH release. In a *sitting* position, the left atrial pressure decreased somewhat, leading to eventual increase in ADH release. Upon *standing*, the left atrial pressure falls markedly, resulting in a lesser inhibition of the hypothalamus and an eventual increase in ADH release. Thus, assuming an upright position results in antidiuresis, whereas a recumbent position leads to diuresis. During sleep, the production of a concentrated urine is for the most part due to a reduction of blood pressure, which more than offsets the effect of reduced ADH release. Other agents that stimulate ADH release are: emotion, exercise, anesthesia, and nicotine. The agents inhibiting ADH release include alcohol, caffeine, and CO_2 inhalation.

In a subsequent study, Moore (1971) found that the diluting and concentrating ability of the intact human kidney, as indicated by the U/P osmolality ratio, was a *sigmoidal* function of plasma ADH concentration. As shown in Figure 12-4, when $[ADH]_p = 0.7$ μU/ml, the kidney neither dilutes nor concentrates (U/P = 1.0), allowing the kidney to excrete about 18 liters of water per day. When $[ADH]_p$ increases from 0.7 to 4.0 μU/ml, the U/P osmolality ratio increases linearly. However, an increase in $[ADH]_p$ above this level has no effect on the concentrating ability of the kidney. The significance of this sigmoidal relationship is that the maximal renal water conservation could be achieved by the release of moderate amounts of ADH. This allows for a normal kidney function in spite of moderate daily bodily activity, fluctuations in body and ambient temperatures, fortuitous fluid intake or loss, and postural changes.

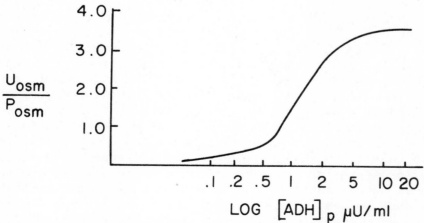

Figure 12-4. Relationship between U_{osm}/P_{osm} and the logarithm of plasma ADH concentration in man. The curve approximates the data of Moore (1971), which were fitted by the equation: $Y = 0.11 + 1.35x - 0.12x^2$.

2. CAROTID SINUS AND AORTIC ARCH BARORECEPTORS. As depicted in Figure 12-3, a number of studies (Heymans and Neil, 1958; Korner, 1971) have established that changes in the systemic arterial pressure (P_{AS}) are monitored (indicated by small box on the arrow) by the *stretch-sensitive* receptors located in the carotid sinus and aortic arch. Thus, an increase in P_{AS} stimulates these receptors, resulting in an increased frequency of impulses travelling in the baroreceptor component of the Hering nerve (for the carotid sinus) and the depressor nerve component of the vagosympathetic trunk (for the aortic arch). It has been found that the mean and the pulse pressure components of the blood pressure interact non-additively, so that at higher mean pressures the superimposed pulse pressure is a less effective stimulus in eliciting response from these receptors (Koushanpour and McGee, 1969). The afferent impulse arising from these baroreceptor nerves (f_b) will then enter the vasomotor center, where they inhibit the sympathetic nuclei (both the cardioaccelerator and vasoconstrictor centers) and by reciprocal inhibition stimulate the parasympathetic nuclei (the cardioinhibitor center). The result would be a net decrease in the frequency of sympathetic outflow (f_s) to (a) the kidneys, (b) the heart and blood vessels (indicated by the box labelled "cardiovascular system"), and (c) the hypothalamus-pituitary system. The decrease in sympathetic outflow to the cardiovascular system will lead to bradycardia and reduced vasoconstriction, the combined effects of which are to restore P_{AS} toward normal and hence close the negative feedback loop. Note that, as depicted here, the vasomotor center constitutes the site where the negative feedback occurs. Conversely, a decrease in P_{AS} results in a decreased f_b and hence less inhibition of the vasomotor center. This would lead to a net increase in sympathetic outflow, which by the same mechanism leads to restoration of blood pressure toward normal. In short, changes in P_{AS}, brought about by, for example, changes in *blood volume*, will induce appropriate compensatory responses from the baroreceptor reflex system.

That the baroreceptors do indeed play a significant role in the regulation of blood volume is now well established. Perlmutt (1963) observed that bilateral occlusion of common carotid arteries (a maneuver which reduces the blood pressure at the carotid sinus) for 5 minutes in vagotomized (left atrial and aortic arch receptors eliminated), hydrated dogs reduced solute-free water clearance after a latent period of 5 to 15 minutes. Share and Levy (1962) showed that bilateral occlusion of common carotid arteries in vagotomized dogs resulted in an increase in plasma concentration of ADH. This effect was blocked by carotid sinus denervation. In a subsequent study, Share (1965) showed that if the systemic arterial blood pressure was maintained at a constant level, bilateral occlusion of common carotid arteries increased $[ADH]_p$ even in dogs with intact vagi. Subsequently, Share (1967) showed that the rise in $[ADH]_p$ which normally occurs after bilateral common carotid occlusion could be prevented by simultaneous inflation of a balloon in the left atrium. Furthermore, when the carotid sinuses of an anesthetized, vagotomized dog were perfused at normal mean and pulse pressure, no rise in $[ADH]_p$ occurred following hemorrhages of up to 50% of the blood volume. In another study, Share and Levy (1966) showed that variations in arterial pulse pressure at the carotid sinus influence ADH release. Thus, they observed an increase in $[ADH]_p$ when flow through the carotid sinuses of the dog was changed from pulsatile to nonpulsatile. The effectiveness of nonpulsatile flow as a stimulus to baroreceptors is now well established (Koushanpour and McGee, 1969).

These studies indicate that a decrease in P_{AS}, acting through the carotid sinus baroreceptor mechanisms, brings about a reflex increase in $[ADH]_p$. The latter effect will eventually lead to a reduction in C_{H_2O} and antidiuresis. The opposite result, namely, water diuresis, follows an increase in P_{AS}. Essentially similar results have been obtained for the aortic arch baroreceptors (Share and Claybaugh, 1972).

At present, the information about the neural pathways mediating the sympathetic inhibition of ADH release is meager. For simplicity of presentation, we have depicted it as a single pathway in the block diagram. Finally, as shown, sympathetic outflow to the kidneys modifies the renal vascular resistance and hence GFR. Thus, an increase in sympathetic outflow should lead to a decrease in C_{H_2O}. This is in part substantiated by the studies of Karim and associates (1971), who found a decrease in renal sympathetic activity with left atrial balloon inflation.

Thus, it appears that changes in P_{AS} and P_{VS} resulting from a deliberate or sudden change or shift in blood volume induce a dual effect upon the renal system: (a) alteration of the sympathetic outflow to the kidneys and (b) modification of the rates of synthesis and release of ADH by the hypothalamus-pituitary system. Their integrative effects at the hypothalamus-pituitary and renal systems would induce a coordinated corrective response in the renal system.

A number of studies (Gauer et al., 1970) have attempted to determine the relative potency and contribution of the low-pressure and high-pressure vascular bed stretch receptors in the reflex regulation of ADH release. It now appears that the left atrial receptors are more sensitive to small changes in blood volume than the carotid sinus and aortic arch receptors. That is, the left atrial receptors constitute the first line of defense against nonhypotensive changes in blood volume. Thus, as long as blood loss does not exceed 10% of the blood volume, the hemorrhage is nonhypotensive and does not activate the high-pressure vascular bed receptors. The renal response is essentially mediated through the left atrial stretch receptors. However, when hemorrhage is hypotensive--that is, when it exceeds 10% of the blood volume--the reduced P_{AS} activates the arterial baroreceptor reflex, thereby initiating compensatory adjustment of renal response by the mechanism described above and depicted in Figure 12-3.

C. INTERACTIONS BETWEEN OSMOTIC AND VOLUME STIMULI

Having delineated the functional characteristics of the elements of the ADH-releasing system, we are now ready to inquire into the question of interaction between them and to assess their relative roles in the regulation of water balance and hence the plasma osmolality. This problem has recently been studied by Zehr and associates (1969) and Johnson and co-workers (1970) in conscious sheep. Zehr and his associates (1969) found that in water deprivation, the reduced blood volume lowers the left atrial pressure, thereby reflexly decreasing the vagal inhibition of ADH release from the hypothalamus-pituitary system. Concurrently, the increased plasma osmolality stimulates the osmoreceptors to stimulate ADH release. Thus, in water deprivation both osmotic and volume elements act together to stimulate ADH release and hence to increase renal conservation of water. In contrast, iso-osmotic or hypo-osmotic expansion of the extracellular fluid volume in either the normally hydrated or dehydrated sheep resulted in a reduction of ADH release regardless of the direction of changes in plasma osmolality. From these findings they concluded that the left atrial stretch receptors play a major role in ADH release, a conclusion not warranted in view of the subsequent findings of Johnson and co-workers (1970). These investigators, using similar preparations, compared in conscious sheep the effects of iso-osmotic changes in blood volume and iso-volemic changes in plasma osmolality separately, and combinations of the volume and osmolality stimuli. When applied separately, iso-osmotic changes in blood volume or iso-volemic changes in plasma osmolality elicited appropriate, expected responses from the volume and osmotic receptor elements of the ADH-releasing system. When the volume and osmotic stimuli were combined, the effect on ADH release was approximately additive. Thus, plasma ADH concentration remained unchanged when a 1.2% reduction of plasma osmolality was combined with a hemorrhage of about 10% of blood volume. From these studies, they concluded that with small changes in blood volume and plasma osmolality neither receptor element appears to dominate the other in the control of ADH release. Similar conclusions were reached by Moses and Miller (1971), who studied the osmotic threshold for ADH release in human subjects whose plasma osmolality was elevated by either hypertonic saline infusion or water deprivation. They found that in hydrated subjects, the plasma osmolality at which the water diuresis was inhibited was higher when the plasma osmolality was increased by hypertonic saline infusion (which also increases the extracellular fluid volume) than when it was increased by water deprivation (which also decreases the extracellular fluid volume).

In summary, available evidence indicates that both volume and osmotic elements of the ADH-releasing system act in concert to maintain the volume and osmolality of the extracellular fluid via the action of ADH on renal excretion of water. Moreover, within the normal physiological limits of changes in blood volume and osmolality, the effect of the two elements on ADH release is additive and neither element dominates the other in the control of ADH release.

D. ROLE OF RENIN-ANGIOTENSIN SYSTEM IN ADH RELEASE

In 1949, Gaunt and associates reported that patients with adrenal insufficiency have an impaired ability to excrete a water load. Since then, there has been growing evidence that the renin-angiotensin system plays an important role in the regulation of water balance through its effect on ADH release.

It is now well established (Hodge et al., 1966) that a reduction in blood volume by hemorrhage in the dog stimulates renin release and hence elevates the plasma concentration of angiotensin ($[Ang]_p$). Furthermore, similar alterations in blood volume have also been shown to stimulate ADH release and to increase its plasma level (Henry et al., 1968). In man, variations in the redistribution of blood volume induced by postural changes have been shown to produce directional changes in both renin release (Brown et al., 1966) and plasma level of ADH (Segar and Moore, 1968). Recently, Share and Travis (1971) reported that plasma level of ADH increased in adrenal insufficient dogs who had undergone bilateral adrenalectomy. Acute injection of glucocorticoids resulted in a decrease in ADH release. These authors attributed the rise in $[ADH]_p$ to a reduction in blood volume and blood pressure during the period of adrenal insufficiency. However, it is not known whether these responses of ADH secretion rate to adrenal function were due to an increase in the rate of release of ADH or a decrease in the rate of its removal.

Collectively, these studies indicate the possible existence of a functional interaction between the renin-angiotensin system and the control of ADH release. However, the nature of the interaction and a causal relationship, if any, remained to be determined.

Recently, Bonjour and Malvin (1970) studied this problem and have provided direct evidence for the control of ADH release by the renin-angiotensin system. They found that intravenous infusion of a small, non-pressor dose of angiotensin in conscious dog significantly increased $[ADH]_p$. Similar results were obtained by infusion of renin, suggesting that both exogenously administered and endogenously formed angiotensin were equally effective in stimulating ADH release. From these results, they concluded that there exists an intimate, causal relationship between the renin-angiotensin system and the control of ADH release. In a subsequent study from the same laboratory (Mouw et al., 1971), an attempt was made to define the locus of the receptor for angiotensin stimulation of ADH release. Intracarotid infusion of angiotensin in anesthetized dog was found to be a more potent stimulus of ADH release than its intravenous infusion. From this finding, they suggested that angiotensin can enter the brain tissue and that the angiotensin receptor must be located in the central nervous system. This concept was further supported by the observation that infusion of small amount of angiotensin II directly into the ventriculocisternal system stimulated ADH release. Since the paraventricular nucleus of the hypothalamus--a nucleus associated with ADH release--lies near the ventricular space, they hypothesized that this nucleus is the site of the angiotensin receptor. At present, confirmation of this hypothesis lacks direct neurophysiological evidence.

A recent study by Tagawa and associates (1971) suggests a negative feedback relationship between the renin-angiotensin and plasma concentration. They found that an increase in $[ADH]_p$ ranging from 0.4 to 4.4 µU/ml inhibited renin secretion in unanesthetized, sodium-deprived dogs. That this response may be of physiological importance was demonstrated by the fact that a 1.2 µU/ml increase in

[ADH]$_p$ resulted in a 30% reduction of renin release.

These studies suggest that there exists a negative feedback between the renin-angiotensin system and the ADH release, with the locus of interaction being in or near the hypothalamus. Thus, as depicted in Figure 12-3, an increase in [Ang]$_p$ stimulates ADH release, which in turn enhances the renal reabsorption of water, thereby closing the feedback loop. Although the studies cited above advance the thesis that the renin-angiotensin system plays an important role in water balance and hence osmoregulation, its singular and relative importance in the circumstances which stimulate the volume and osmotic elements of the ADH-releasing system have been questioned in a recent review of the subject (Share and Claybaugh, 1972). They suggest that the interrelationships between ADH, renin, and angiotensin may serve to minimize fluctuations in their plasma concentrations under resting conditions. Variations in the blood volume or plasma osmolality would then elicit appropriate responses from the volume receptors and osmoreceptors, thereby overriding this negative feedback relationship and bringing about appropriate changes in the secretion of ADH and renin.

In a recent study, Shade and Share (1975) have provided further evidence for the above point of view. Reporting their inability to repeat the results obtained by Bonjour and Malvin (1970) and Mouw and co-workers (1971), they suggest that angiotensin II may potentiate the effect of a known stimulus for ADH release, rather than directly stimulating its release. Thus, they found that intravenous infusion of small amounts of angiotensin II potentiated the release of ADH in bilaterally nephrectomized dogs subjected to nonhypotensive hemorrhage. However, this potentiating effect in response to the volume stimulus was found to be much smaller compared to that reported by Shimizu and associates (1973) for an osmotic stimulus. These latter investigators found that simultaneous intravenous infusion of angiotensin II and hypertonic solution caused a more significant increase in ADH release than infusion of hypertonic saline alone.

From these and other studies, Shade and Share (1975) conclude that "volume and osmotic control of ADH are to some degree independent and ... angiotensin does not affect the final common pathway for ADH release. Thus, angiotensin may potentiate osmotically stimulated ADH release, but has little or no effect on ADH release resulting from decreases in blood volume."

In conclusion, although the role of the renin-angiotensin system on ADH release and its possible role in water and electrolyte balance represents an attractive idea, the available evidence is conflicting. The unequivocal existence of such a relationship remains to be demonstrated.

REGULATION OF BLOOD VOLUME:
CONTROL OF SODIUM EXCRETION

As described in Chapter 2, potassium is the major cation of the intracellular fluid compartment, whereas sodium is the major cation of the extracellular fluid compartment. Accordingly, the availability of these ions, as determined by the dynamic balance between their rates of influx into and efflux out of the body, will largely determine the volume of water in these compartments.

Since the exchangeable sodium, which constitutes the major fraction of the total body sodium, is primarily confined in the extracellular compartment, its regulation will ultimately determine the volume and hydrostatic pressure of the extracellular fluid compartment and its extra- and intravascular components. Hence, in the final analysis, the regulation of blood volume and its associated hydrostatic pressure depends primarily on the careful adjustment of the dynamic balance between the rates of influx and efflux of sodium into and out of the body and secondarily on those of potassium. As mentioned previously, of these fluxes, only the rate of renal efflux is subject to internal regulation. Thus, in the absence of vomiting, diarrhea, or excessive sweating, the kidney can precisely adjust the excretion rates of sodium and potassium to match the wide variations in their intake, thereby stabilizing the volume and composition of the internal environment within normal limits.

The smooth operation of the mechanisms involved in the renal excretion of sodium and potassium depends on their continuous adjustment by *two* extrarenal mechanisms which respond to small changes in volume, hydrostatic pressure, and composition of the circulating blood. The *first* is a *humoral* mechanism consisting of the *renin-angiotensin-aldosterone system*, which plays the major role in the simultaneous regulation of all of the above three blood variables. The *second* is a *neural* mechanism, consisting of the *right atrial stretch-sensitive volume receptors*, which plays a minor but important role in regulating the above variables by reflexly modifying renin secretion by the kidney. It should be noted that the common pathway for the effects of both mechanisms is the fine adjustment of the rates of synthesis and release of aldosterone into the blood and its cellular action on the distal and collecting tubular epithelia of the nephron. It therefore follows that the renal regulation of blood volume ultimately depends on the careful adjustment of the renal excretion of sodium, which in turn depends on the factors which modify the rates of synthesis and release of aldosterone.

Let us now consider the stimulus-response characteristics of these two extrarenal mechanisms, component by component, as well as their relative contributions to the renal excretion of sodium and hence the regulation of blood volume.

I. THE RENIN-ANGIOTENSIN-ALDOSTERONE SYSTEM

A. HISTORICAL PERSPECTIVE

Our present knowledge of the role of the renin-angiotensin-aldosterone system in the renal regulation of blood volume is derived largely from those studies that were designed to delineate the causes of hypertension in general and of renal hypertension in particular.

Thus, to better understand the recent developments and their relevance to the regulation of blood volume (to be discussed later in this section), a brief survey of these early milestone studies is in order. For a more extensive treatment the interested reader is referred to an excellent recent review by Laragh and Sealey (1973).

Although in 1827 Richard Bright was first to recognize that hypertension may be a renal disease, the first "milestone" in the modern history of renal hypertension occurred 70 years later. In 1898 Tigerstedt and Bergman discovered that injection of a crude saline extract of rabbit kidney into anesthetized rabbits caused an increase in blood pressure. They attributed the hypertensive effect to a substance which they named *renin*. That the kidney is indeed involved in hypertension was subsequently reaffirmed by studies of Volhard and Fahr (1914), who defined an association between renal necrotizing arteriolitis and malignant hypertension.

The second milestone occurred in 1938, when Goldblatt demonstrated that *constriction of the renal artery* in dogs and rabbits caused a chronic, sustained elevation of blood pressure. The third milestone occurred in 1939 when both Page and Braun-Menéndez and colleagues independently discovered that renin is an enzyme that causes release of a pressor substance called *angiotensin* from its circulating plasma substrate, *α-2-globulin*. Subsequent studies by Goormaghtigh (1944) showed that renin secretion in both human and animal renal hypertension is associated with changes in the granularity of the *granular cells* of the juxtaglomerular apparatus (see Fig. 5-8). This directly implicated the kidney in the development of hypertension. As mentioned in Chapter 5, the granular cells are the sites of synthesis, storage, and release of renin.

The next milestone came between 1956 and 1957, when Skeggs and his associates (1956) and Elliot and Peart (1957) independently determined the amino acid sequence of angiotensin, which was later synthesized by Bumpus and his group (1957). Then, in 1960, Laragh and his associates showed that infusion of angiotensin II in man stimulates *aldosterone* release from the adrenal cortex. Thus, the link between renin, angiotensin, and aldosterone and their possible roles in the regulation of blood volume, composition, and hydrostatic pressure became firmly established.

Let us now consider some of the important physiological characteristics of the components of the renin-angiotensin-aldosterone system as revealed by subsequent studies.

B. COMPONENTS OF THE SYSTEM

1. RENIN. Renin is a proteolytic enzyme with a molecular weight of about 40,000. It is produced primarily by the granular cells of the juxtaglomerular apparatus of the kidney in response to a variety of stimuli (see page 420, *Control of Renin Release*). In addition, renin is also produced by two extrarenal organs, namely, the submaxillary gland and the uterus, with the pregnant uterus exhibiting a greater renin-like activity than the nonpregnant uterus. However, the available evidence indicates that these

extrarenal sources of renin contribute very little to the circulating plasma levels of renin.

Despite its molecular size, renin is found in urine, suggesting that it is partially filtered at the glomerulus. However, since its urinary excretion is normally less than 1% of the amount filtered, it is almost completely reabsorbed by the renal tubules (Brown et al., 1964).

Plasma renin activity (PRA) may be quantitated either by radioimmunoassay of generated angiotensin I or bioassay of generated angiotensin II. The latter is usually expressed in *Goldblatt units*. A Goldblatt unit is defined as that amount of renin which when injected into a conscious, trained dog raises the blood pressure by 30 mm Hg (Goldblatt et al., 1943). Using either method, Sealey and associates (1972) found a consistent dynamic relationship between the daily rate of renal sodium excretion ($\dot{E}_{Na}$) and midday PRA measured in 52 normal ambulatory subjects. In these subjects, PRA ranged from 0.5 to 2.8 ng/ml/hr when $\dot{E}_{Na}$ was above 150 mEq/day, from 1.4 to 6.3 ng/ml/hr when $\dot{E}_{Na}$ was between 50 and 150 mEq/day, and up to 21 ng/ml/hr when $\dot{E}_{Na}$ was below 50 mEq/day.

Several studies, reviewed by Lee (1969), have shown that the circulatory half-life of renin ranges from 10 to 20 minutes in rat, with somewhat higher values in dogs (45 to 79 minutes) and man (42 to 120 minutes). The variations in the circulatory half-life indicate the rapidity with which renin is secreted in response to various stimuli, such as hemorrhage, exercise, and changes in posture.

Normally, the plasma renin level is determined by a dynamic balance between the rate of its production and the rate of its destruction or removal from the circulation. Direct measurements of arteriovenous differences for renin across several vascular beds in dogs after elevation of arterial plasma renin (induced by stimulation of endogenous renin secretion by acute salt depletion) or infusion of exogenous renin have clearly shown that the liver is the major site of renin inactivation (Heacox et al., 1967). In these and subsequent studies (Schneider et al., 1970) the metabolic clearance of renin approached its hepatic clearance, suggesting that the rate of renin inactivation is a direct function of the hepatic blood flow. Thus, changes in plasma renin level in disease, such as congestive heart failure or liver cirrhosis, may reflect a reduction in normal hepatic renin inactivation.

Renin as such has no physiological effect other than causing liberation of angiotensin I from its plasma substrate. Intravenous infusion of renin causes an increase in blood pressure after a latent period of 15 to 20 seconds. The elevation of blood pressure is gradual and may last for 30 minutes or longer, depending on the amount of renin injected. In contrast, intravenous infusion of angiotensin II causes an immediate rise in blood pressure which is short-lived (Lee, 1969). The differences in the pressor action of renin and angiotensin II are attributed to the enzymatic properties of renin and the kinetics of endogenous liberation of angiotensin I from plasma renin substrate and its subsequent conversion to angiotensin II.

It is well known that repeated injection of renin over a short period of time results in progressively less elevation of blood pressure, a phenomenon called *renin tachyphylaxis*. Although the underlying mechanisms are not presently known, *angiotensin tachyphylaxis* and saturation of the vascular receptor sites, as well as prostaglandin release, have been implicated as contributing factors in renin tachyphylaxis.

Several studies (Lee, 1969) have demonstrated that endogenous renin secretion is highly correlated with the degree of granulation of the granular cells of the juxtaglomerular apparatus. Thus, hypergranulation is linked to hypersecretion of renin, whereas hypogranulation or degranulation is linked to hyposecretion. Experimentally, several conditions are known to produce hypergranulation of granular cells, and thus hypersecretion of renin. They include renal ischemia, prolonged anoxia, sodium deficiency, hyponatremia, experimental ascites, pregnancy, and adrenal insufficiency. In contrast, hypogranulation or degranulation, and hence hyposecretion of renin, occurs after sodium loading, increased arterial blood pressure, and expansion of body fluids by overtransfusion.

2. RENIN SUBSTRATE. Since the classic studies of Page (1939) and Braun-Menéndez and associates (1939), who identified α-2-globulin fraction of plasma as the renin substrate, a number of recent studies have attempted to identify the structure of the renin substrate molecule and the nature of the renin-renin substrate reaction. From degradation studies of horse renin substrate, Skeggs and co-workers (1964) identified the renin substrate as a 14-amino acid residue polypeptide (Fig. 12-5). Incubation of this tetradecapeptide with renin yielded angiotensin I, whose amino acid sequence was identical to the first 10 amino acids from the N-terminal group of the renin substrate. Furthermore, they showed that renin acts on the leucyl-leucyl bond of the tetradecapeptide renin substrate to yield angiotensin I (a decapeptide) and a tetrapeptide residue.

In a recent study, Sealey and associates (1972) reported a value of 1500 ng/ml for the concentration of renin substrate in human plasma, an amount capable of yielding 6 mg of angiotensin upon complete conversion by renin. Their findings clearly indicate that the concentration of renin substrate is normally far in excess of that needed to maintain the normal plasma level of angiotensin II. Furthermore, it shows that the large concentration of renin substrate excludes it from exerting a rate-limiting effect in the kinetics of the renin-renin substrate reactions.

Although their results are not unequivocal, most of the available studies implicate the liver as the main organ that manufactures the renin substrate. However, at present little is known about the mechanisms which maintain the plasma concentration of renin substrate at normal level. A recent review of the available evidence (Laragh and Sealey, 1973) suggests that a number of organ systems participate in the regulation of the plasma concentration of renin substrate. Of these, the kidney appears to be the most important. Thus, it has been found that bilateral nephrectomy in all species produces a rapid increase in the plasma concentration of the renin substrate. That this rise in substrate concentration may be a direct consequence of a reduction of renin synthesis following nephrectomy is not supported by recent experiments. For instance, it has been found that in salt-loaded or deoxycorticosterone-treated animals which exhibit a low plasma renin level, there is no accompanying rise in the plasma renin substrate concentration.

At present, little is known about the mechanisms responsible for the elevation of the plasma renin substrate concentration following nephrectomy. The most likely explanation offered to date is that of Laragh and Sealey (1973), who suggest that the kidney tissue may metabolize or utilize renin substrate, a factor accounting for the rise in its plasma concentration after nephrectomy. The precise nature of such a renal metabolism or utilization of renin substrate, however, remains to be determined.

In contrast to nephrectomy, the plasma concentration of the renin substrate is sharply reduced after adrenalectomy or hypophysectomy. In both cases, the reduction in the substrate concentration is attributed to a marked increase in plasma renin level consequent to excessive loss of sodium during adrenal insufficiency. Renin substrate concentration is also lowered in patients with cirrhosis of the liver. Since in these patients plasma renin is usually elevated due to a reduction in hepatic renin inactivation, it is not known whether the decrease in renin substrate level reflects a reduction in the capacity of the liver to synthesize the substrate or if it results from some other pathophysiological factors.

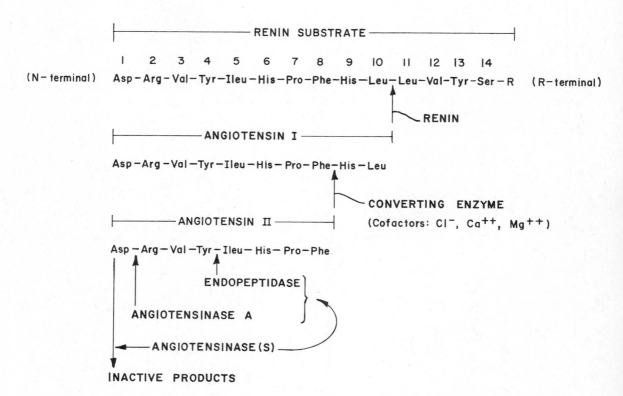

Figure 12-5. Steps involved in the formation and degradation of angiotensin II.

3. ANGIOTENSINS AND CONVERTING ENZYMES. As mentioned above and depicted in Figure 12-5, renin, by acting on its plasma substrate, splits off four amino acids from the R-terminal group, yielding a physiologically inactive decapeptide called *angiotensin I*. Upon passage through the lung, the peptidase enzymes found chiefly in this tissue split off the terminal histidyl-leucine amino acids from angiotensin I, yielding a potent octapeptide pressor substance called *angiotensin II*. Similar conversion can also take place by the action of peptidases found in the kidney tissue and blood. Collectively, these peptidases are called the *angiotensin converting enzymes*.

The structure of the amino acid sequence of horse angiotensin I was the first to be elucidated (Fig. 12-5). Subsequently, the amino acid compositions of angiotensin I isolated from bovine, hog, and human blood were determined. Of these, the amino acid sequence of human, hog, and horse angiotensin I were found to be identical. However, bovine angiotensin differed from these in that valine replaced isoleucine in the number five position (Laragh and Sealey, 1973).

Several studies reviewed by Lee (1969) have shown that the biological activity of angiotensin II is highly dependent on the structural integrity of the C-terminal amino acid phenylalanine (Phe). Its modification or replacement results in the virtual loss of potency of angiotensin II. In contrast, the structural integrity of the N-terminal amino acid aspargine (Asp) does not appear to be as crucial to angiotensin activity, although its modification or replacement does somewhat reduce its potency. Such information has led to the synthesis of a variety of angiotensin II analogues for both research and clinical applications.

A number of studies have shown that the lung is the major organ which contains the angiotensin converting enzymes. Ng and Vane (1968) were the first to show that angiotensin I is rapidly converted into angiotensin II in a single passage through the lungs. These *in vivo* studies have further been confirmed by *in vitro* studies of Huggins and Thampi (1968), who obtained angiotensin II upon incubating angiotensin I with lung tissues. Subsequent studies in intact anesthetized dogs by Oparil and her associates (1970) revealed that in addition to the lungs, renal tissue and blood can also convert tritium-labelled angiotensin I into angiotensin II. Furthermore, they found that both the lungs and kidneys can convert angiotensin I into angiotensin II much more rapidly than does the plasma. They found no evidence for hepatic conversion of angiotensin I into angiotensin II.

Recent kinetic studies (Huggins et al., 1970) have reaffirmed the relative difference in potency and speed of reaction between the lung and plasma angiotensin converting enzymes. Both enzymes had a broad, flattened pH curve, with a pH optimum of 7.25. However, there was a marked difference between the speed of conversion and the apparent K_m. Lung tissues required only 8 minutes of incubation to convert angiotensin I into angiotensin II, whereas plasma enzyme required 45 minutes of incubation. Furthermore, the apparent K_m for plasma enzyme was 4.8×10^{-5} M, whereas that for the lung enzyme was 5.2×10^{-6} M. Also, both enzymes required chloride ion as cofactor.

As shown in Figure 12-5, in addition to the monovalent ion

chloride, the converting enzyme requires the divalent cations calcium and magnesium for its activation. The enzyme is readily inhibited by chelating agents such as ethylenediamine tetraacetate (EDTA), suggesting that it is a metalloenzyme.

Plasma concentration of angiotensin II ($[Ang]_p$) in either arterial or venous blood varies considerably depending on the techniques used to measure it and on the state of sodium balance. Gocke and associates (1969) have recently developed a sensitive and specific radioimmunoassay method capable of measuring angiotensin II level directly from 0.1 ml of human plasma. Using this method, they found that $[Ang]_p$ was directly related to the plasma renin activity and inversely related to the state of sodium balance. Depending on the degree of sodium depletion, values for $[Ang]_p$ ranged from 42 to 139 $\mu\mu g/ml$ in 29 normal human subjects studied. In these subjects, the greater the daily sodium excretion rate, and hence the greater the degree of sodium depletion, the smaller were the values for $[Ang]_p$. These results provide direct confirmation of the interrelationship of renin, angiotensin, and sodium balance.

Angiotensin II has a very short circulating half-life--about 1 to 3 minutes in superinfusion and about 15 to 20 seconds in normal infusion. This suggests a mechanism for its rapid removal either by binding to receptor tissues or by degradation into inactive products by plasma angiotensinases, or both. A number of experiments have shown that nearly 70% of the infused angiotensin II is removed in one passage through the liver (Biron et al., 1968). Similarly, it has been found that angiotensin II is removed at the same rate by the kidney, but it is undestroyed as it passes through the lungs (Ng and Vane, 1968). Studies with intact-cell and broken-cell preparations have revealed selective uptakes of angiotensin I and II by other organs (Goodfriend and Lin, 1970). Both kidney and uterus showed a greater capacity to bind angiotensin II than angiotensin I, whereas adrenal cortex showed a greater capacity to bind angiotensin I than angiotensin II.

As shown in Figure 12-5, two major *angiotensinases*, capable of inactivating the circulating angiotensin II, have been identified in the plasma. Khairallah and associates (1963) have identified an *angiotensinase A*, also called *aminopeptidase*, which has a pH optimum of 7.5. It requires calcium for its activation and is inhibited by chelating agents, such as EDTA. Pickens and his group (1965) have isolated a second plasma angiotensinase, which they called *endopeptidase*. It has a pH optimum of 5.5 and is inhibited by diisopropylfluorophosphate (DFP).

Angiotensin II has three well-known physiological effects: (1) It causes vasoconstriction of the arterioles. As a vasoconstrictor, it is about 10 times more potent than norepinephrine on a weight basis, and about 50 times more potent on a molar basis. (2) It exerts a direct effect on the kidney; low doses cause sodium retention, whereas high doses cause natriuresis. The mechanisms mediating the renal response are not well understood. (3) It acts on the adrenal cortex, causing a prompt increase in aldosterone secretion, and it stimulates the release of epinephrine and norepinephrine from the adrenal medulla.

The vasoconstrictor effect of angiotensin II is believed to be

mediated via one or a combination of four pathways: (a) Direct
action on the arteriolar smooth muscle cells; (b) activation of the
sympathetic branch of the autonomic nervous system; (c) activation
of the central nervous system; and (d) stimulation of catecholamine
release from the adrenal medulla. At present, it is not known how
much of the initial or delayed cardiovascular effect of angiotensin
II is due to its *direct* action on the vascular smooth muscle
receptors and how much is due to its *indirect* activation of adrenal
medulla and the autonomic and central nervous systems.

Pressor responsiveness to angiotensin appears to be modified in
a variety of conditions in which there are associated changes in body
fluid volume (Laragh and Sealey, 1973). It is reduced in situations
in which there is volume depletion, such as hemorrhage, sodium
depletion, normal pregnancy, and pathological states of cirrhosis,
nephrosis, and congestive heart failure. The last three conditions
are characterized by transudation of fluid out of the circulation,
thereby reducing the effective volume of the circulating blood. In
contrast, the pressor responsiveness is increased in situations where
there is volume expansion, such as when sodium is given in excess or
when sodium intake is combined with administration of aldosterone.

Angiotensin II exerts a dual effect on the kidney: It causes
parallel dose-dependent changes in both renal hemodynamics and sodium
and water excretion. Thus, intravenous infusion of small amount of
angiotensin II (0.5 ng/kg/min) causes a significant decrease in RPF
and urine volume in man without any associated changes in the systemic
arterial blood pressure (DeBono et al., 1963). Furthermore,
intrarenal injection of small amount of angiotensin that does not
elevate the systemic arterial blood pressure causes renal
vasoconstriction (McGiff and Itskovitz, 1964).

Angiotensin II has been shown to be a potent stimulator of
aldosterone release from the adrenal cortex in man (Laragh et al.,
1960; Ames et al., 1965), sheep (Blair-West et al., 1962), and dog
(Carpenter et al., 1961). However, its stimulating effect on the
rat adrenal gland remains controversial.

The stimulatory effect of angiotensin II on sheep and dog
adrenal glands was demonstrated by direct perfusion studies. This
effect was found to be dependent on the electrolyte composition of
the perfusate. Thus, raising the sodium concentration in the
perfusate depressed the response to angiotensin, whereas raising
the potassium concentration or decreasing the sodium concentration
potentiated its stimulatory effect.

Like renin, repeated injection of large doses of angiotensin II
results in progressively less elevation of blood pressure. This
angiotensin tachyphylaxis has been attributed to a large extent to
the saturation of the vascular receptor sites by the presence of
excess hormone as well as to the release of prostaglandins.

Results of several experiments in both animal and man have
shown that although infusion of large doses of angiotensin causes
tachyphylaxis, continuous infusion of small doses results in
progressive elevation of blood pressure. This is attributed to
(a) angiotensin stimulation of aldosterone secretion, leading to
eventual salt and water retention, (b) increased sympathetic

activity, or (c) angiotensin-induced vascular damage. The mechanism mediating the latter effect remains obscure.

4. ALDOSTERONE. In Chapter 11, while describing the possible mechanisms of renal action of aldosterone, we stated that this hormone is synthesized exclusively in the zona glomerulosa of the adrenal cortex. Furthermore, as was depicted in Figure 11-15, we indicated that the biosynthesis of aldosterone is influenced primarily by changes in sodium balance whose effects were mediated via induced changes in the plasma levels of angiotensin II and potassium, with ACTH exerting only a supportive role in the steroidogenesis. In this section, we shall briefly discuss the major points of evidence that have established the role of angiotensin II as a *trophic hormone* for the stimulation of aldosterone release from the adrenal cortex. For a comprehensive analysis of the earlier as well as the recent literature on the subject, the interested reader is referred to excellent reviews by Tobian (1960), Davis (1962), Page and McCubbin (1968), and Laragh and Sealey (1973).

Beginning in the late 1950's, several studies led to the formulation of a negative feedback hypothesis for the control of renin release and its effects on aldosterone secretion. In 1958, Gross (1971) found an *inverse* relationship between sodium balance and renin content in the rat kidney. This information, coupled with the knowledge that sodium metabolism is primarily a renal function and that it is influenced by aldosterone, led to the concept that aldosterone secretion is somehow influenced by renin release. Furthermore, since changes in sodium balance were known to be associated with changes in the extracellular fluid and plasma volumes, it was deduced further that both aldosterone secretion and renin release were inversely related to the changes in the blood volume. Thus, the concept of aldosterone as a *volume control regulator* was born.

In support of this concept, Tobian (1960) found that the renin content of the granular cells of the juxtaglomerular apparatus was correlated with the degree of granulation of these cells, which, in turn, was a function of the degree of the renal arterial perfusion pressure. Thus, a reduction in the perfusion pressure induced by partial occlusion of the renal artery caused hypergranulation, and therefore increased renin release, whereas an increase in the renal perfusion pressure induced by elevation of systemic arterial pressure resulted in degranulation, and hence reduced renin release. Since the renal arterial perfusion pressure is ultimately a function of the blood volume, which in turn depends on the renal sodium metabolism and sodium balance, it follows that the renin release and consequently aldosterone secretion are inversely related to the renal arterial perfusion pressure, or some function thereof, induced by changes in the blood volume.

The direct role of angiotensin as the trophic hormone stimulating aldosterone secretion was subsequently defined by a number of investigators. Using the classic endocrine ablation techniques, in a series of experiments Davis and associates (1962) found that acute blood loss, which normally stimulated aldosterone secretion in hypophysectomized dogs, failed to evoke the same response in nephrectomized-hypophysectomized animals. However, injection of saline extracts of both kidneys of each animal resulted in a striking increase in aldosterone secretion. This suggested that the kidney is the source of the aldosterone stimulating agent.

That the stimulating agent is indeed angiotensin II was confirmed by Davis and his group in dogs and by Laragh and associates (1960) and Genest and co-workers (1961) in man. They found that intravenous infusion of synthetic angiotensin II in both dogs and man caused a prompt increase in aldosterone secretion as well as urinary excretion. Furthermore, in the dog experiments, both renin and angiotensin II stimulated steroidogenesis.

Subsequent studies by Ames and his associates (1965) extended these earlier observations by studying the effect of prolonged infusion of angiotensin II on sodium balance, aldosterone secretion and arterial blood pressure in normal subjects and in cirrhotic patients with ascites. They found that, in contrast to studies in dogs (Davis, 1962), infusion of angiotensin in doses required for stimulation of aldosterone secretion always produced a small but a definite elevation of the arterial blood pressure. This suggested that the trophic action of angiotensin appeared to be associated with its pressor effect. However, since infusion of pressor-equivalent amount of norepinephrine had no trophic effect on aldosterone secretion, they concluded that the pressor agents in general do not stimulate aldosterone secretion. They further observed that both the pressor and the trophic effect of exogenous angiotensin were related to the state of sodium balance. Thus, in normal subjects, prolonged infusion of angiotensin resulted in sustained sodium chloride retention. However, sodium depletion reduced the pressor responsiveness of angiotensin and enhanced the effectiveness of antipressor drugs. This suggested that the state of sodium balance is an important determinant of the vascular responsiveness to angiotensin. In contrast, in cirrhotic patients with ascites, prolonged infusion of angiotensin produced natriuresis, with diuresis of edema fluid. Furthermore, these patients exhibited pressor unresponsiveness and tachyphylaxis to angiotensin.

From these studies, Ames and co-workers (1965) have proposed the now well-accepted negative feedback concept of the renin-angiotensin-aldosterone system, whose function is to prevent sodium depletion and hypotension. Accordingly, loss of body sodium or a reduction in arterial blood pressure would eventually lead to a reduction of the renal perfusion pressure, thereby stimulating renin release and angiotensin II production. The latter causes sodium chloride retention both directly, by acting on the kidney, and indirectly, by increasing aldosterone production. The resulting sodium chloride retention causes expansion of the blood volume and elevation of the arterial blood pressure. The net effect of this would be the restoration of the renal perfusion pressure toward normal and the return of the renin-angiotensin-aldosterone system back to the normal operating point.

Although potassium has been shown to serve as a strong stimulus for aldosterone secretion, potassium homeostasis appears not to be the sole mechanism. Thus, potassium metabolism has been found to be normal in patients with hyperaldosteronism (e.g., congestive heart failure, cirrhosis, and nephrosis), who also have renal sodium chloride retention and edema (Laragh and Sealey, 1973).

Studies with radioactive labelled aldosterone have shown that the hormone is distributed in both the intracellular and the extracellular fluid compartments (Tait et al., 1961). These same studies have further shown that the circulatory half-life of aldosterone is about 30 minutes under normal conditions. However, it is found to be increased in patients with hepatic cirrhosis, a factor that may in part explain the formation of ascites and edema fluids in these patients (Coppage et al., 1962).

As stated in Chapter 11, the liver is the main site of inactivation of aldosterone. Furthermore, the metabolic clearance of aldosterone approaches its hepatic clearance, and it is influenced by postural changes. It is reduced in the upright position to about one half of that found in the supine position.

Aldosterone secretion rate has been found to range from 20 to 200 µg/day in human subjects with normal sodium intake (Laragh et al., 1966; Ledingham et al., 1967). These studies have further shown that aldosterone secretion fell to between 15 and 80 µg/day when subjects were placed on a high sodium diet, but increased to as much as 1000 µg/day after a period of sodium deprivation. Thus, it appears that the aldosterone secretion rate and hence its plasma concentration are highly sensitive to the state of sodium balance, a property resembling those described for both renin and angiotensin II.

C. CONTROL OF RENIN RELEASE

From the evidence presented in the preceding section, we learned that (1) renin is synthesized and stored in and released from the granular cells of the juxtaglomerular (JG) apparatus (Fig. 5-8); (2) there is a continuous release of renin from the kidney, which somehow is balanced by a continuous hepatic synthesis of the renin substrate; (3) the rate of formation of angiotensin follows a first-order kinetics, that is, its synthesis is proportional to the concentrations of renin and its plasma substrate; (4) the circulatory half-life of renin is considerably longer than that of angiotensin, so that neither the quantity of renin nor that of its plasma substrate are the limiting factors in the synthesis of angiotensin; and (5) depending on the state of body sodium and potassium balance, the synthesis of angiotensin and its short circulatory half-life will ultimately determine the rates of synthesis and release of aldosterone.

Since the discovery in 1960 of the role of the renin-angiotensin system in the control of aldosterone secretion, there has been a growing interest in delineating the nature of the mechanisms which control renin release. Elucidation of these mechanisms is important in understanding the pathophysiology of disturbances in water and electrolyte balance and the etiology of edema formation in such diseases as congestive heart failure, liver cirrhosis, and nephrosis, as well as the etiology of initiation and maintenance of benign and malignant hypertension.

Numerous studies in both man and animals (see reviews by Vander, 1967; Lee, 1969; Davis, 1973; Laragh and Sealey, 1973) have clearly established that at least three groups of mechanisms are involved in the control of renin release. As depicted in Figure 12-6, these include (1) an intrinsic mechanism with two intrarenal receptors, (2) the renal sympathetic nerves, and (3) a number of humoral agents. The two intrarenal receptors are (a) a vascular receptor, located in the media of the wall of the afferent arteriole, sensitive to changes in stretch or wall tension, and (b) a tubular receptor, located in the macula densa region, sensitive to changes in sodium concentration or load. Available evidence suggests a primary role for the intrarenal vascular receptors in the control of renin release. The renal sympathetic nerves, although not essential to the control of renin release, exert a modulating effect via β-adrenergic receptors on the magnitude of renin release in response to a given stimulus. The major humoral agents that control renin release include catecholamines (epinephrine and norepinephrine), ADH, and angiotensin II, as well as changes in body sodium and potassium balance. Thus, it is clear that renin release is controlled by a multiplicity of factors involving the interplay of all three of these mechanisms.

In this section, we shall consider in some detail each of these mechanisms and the major experimental evidence supporting them, as well as their strengths and weaknesses.

1. THE INTRINSIC MECHANISMS CONTROLLING RENIN RELEASE

A. THE INTRARENAL VASCULAR RECEPTOR THEORY. With the milestone discovery of Goldblatt (1938) that partial constriction of the renal artery produces a chronic, sustained elevation of the arterial blood pressure came the suggestion that this hypertension resulted from an excessive increase in renin release induced by *renal ischemia* (reduced blood flow) consequent to renal artery constriction. Subsequent studies (Peart, 1975), however, have revealed that the renal ischemia per se is not essential for renin release, since significant changes in renin secretion do occur during the autoregulation of renal blood flow, where changes in flow are minimized in the face of marked changes in the renal perfusion pressure. This has raised the question that perhaps a reduction in the *renal perfusion pressure*, or some function thereof, rather than renal ischemia, was the stimulus for renin release and the subsequent development of hypertension following renal artery stenosis.

The original idea that a reduction in the renal perfusion pressure stimulates some intrarenal baroreceptors to release renin was proposed independently by Goormaghtigh (1945) and Braun-Menéndez and co-workers (1946). Direct experimental evidence, however, in support of this theory came some 14 years later. In 1959, Tobian and his associates observed that the degree of granularity of the granular cells, which closely correlates with renin release, was *inversely* related to the degree of renal perfusion pressure, and hence the degree of stretch in the wall of the afferent arteriole. On the basis of these findings, Tobian and his group formulated the currently accepted *intrarenal vascular receptor theory* of renin release.

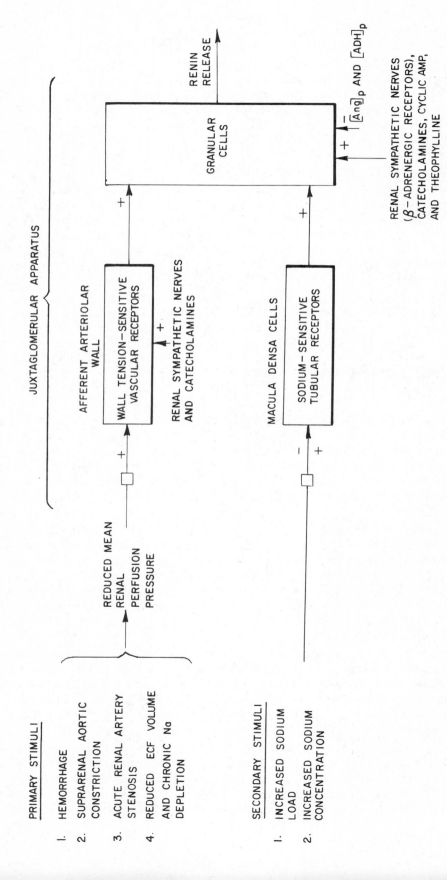

Figure 12-6. A functional block diagram showing the multiple factors involved in the control of renin release from the granular cells of the juxtaglomerular apparatus.

According to this theory, the granular cells of the juxtaglomerular apparatus, located in the media of the afferent arteriole (Fig. 5-8), are sensitive to changes in stretch in the wall of this vessel. Thus, as shown in Figure 12-6, any factor that decreases the renal perfusion pressure, such as hemorrhage, will tend to reduce the stretch in the wall of the afferent arteriole, which will tend to *increase* stimulation (stimulation is indicated by a plus sign) of the vascular receptors which monitor (designated by small box on the arrow) changes in the wall tension. This will in turn increase stimulation of the granular cells, thereby *increasing* renin release. In contrast, any factor that tends to increase the stretch in the wall of the afferent arteriole, such as an increase in the renal perfusion pressure, will tend to *reduce* stimulation of the vascular receptors. This will in turn reduce stimulation of the granular cells, thereby *decreasing* renin release. *In short, the release of renin from the granular cells is inversely related to the degree of stretch in the wall of the afferent arteriole containing these cells.*

Although the underlying mechanisms which somehow translate changes in the wall stretch into renin secretion remain unknown, a considerable body of experimental evidence has been marshalled for the support of the baroreceptor theory of renin release. The following represents highlights of some of the more important of these studies, which are summarized in part in Figure 12-6.

As stated above, the intrarenal baroreceptor theory rests on the premise that renin release is inversely related to changes in the *renal perfusion pressure.* Since the latter is normally a direct function of the systemic arterial blood pressure, it follows that renin release should also be inversely related to changes in the *systemic arterial blood pressure.* Thus, one would expect that acute *hemorrhage* sufficient to reduce the systemic blood pressure should increase renin release, whereas an increase in the systemic blood pressure, as by an expansion of the *extracellular fluid (ECF) volume,* should decrease renin release.

In support of the above concept, numerous studies in rats, rabbits, and dogs (Lee, 1969) have shown that both hypotensive and nonhypotensive acute hemorrhage causes an increase in renin release. These findings, coupled with the fact that acute hemorrhage also causes a reflex stimulation of the sympathetic nervous system, suggest that at least two mechanisms may mediate renin release in response to hemorrhage. The degree of participation of these two mechanisms is dependent upon the severity of hemorrhage and on the associated hypotension. Thus, in the case of mild, nonhypotensive hemorrhage, the increase in renin release is entirely due to activation of the renal sympathetics, whereas in the case of severe, hypotensive hemorrhage, both hypotension and renal sympathetic stimulation summate to produce a further increment in renin release.

Studies in the rabbit (McKenzie et al., 1966) have been particularly revealing in elucidating the site as well as the time course of renin release during acute hemorrhage. They found that within seconds after the onset of the hemorrhage, there was a large increase in plasma renin activity, which reached a value five times the control level 40 minutes later. This response was abolished 48 hours after bilateral nephrectomy, suggesting that the kidney may be the source of the released renin. The rapidity of this response led these investigators to suggest that renin release may have been due either to a direct stimulation of an intrarenal baroreceptor mechanism or to an indirect activation of the sympathetic nervous system, or both.

That *hypotension*, and not the hemorrhage per se, is the stimulus for renin release is supported by two different experiments. First, it has been found that an indirect reduction in the systemic arterial blood pressure produced by intravenous infusion of vasodilator drugs, such as histamine, sodium nitroprusside, and tetraethylammonium, causes an increase in renin release (Lee, 1969). The effect of the last drug, which is a sympathetic ganglion blocker, also implicates the role of the sympathetic nervous system in renin release; but more about this will be presented later. Second, it has been found that a small, direct reduction in the renal perfusion pressure, produced by graded suprarenal aortic constriction, causes an increase in renin release (Skinner et al., 1963). In this study, renin release was found to be highly sensitive to changes in the mean blood pressure and not the pulse pressure. Thus, there was no change in renin release when the pulse pressure was reduced, but renin release was increased when the mean renal perfusion pressure was reduced by as little as 10 mm Hg. Moreover, when the pulse pressure was abolished by a combination of suprarenal aortic constriction and vagotomy, renin release was not affected as long as the mean blood pressure remained constant. These latter results provide compelling evidence that a decrease in *mean renal perfusion pressure* rather than in the pulse pressure is the primary stimulus for renin release. This is consistent with Tobian's stretch-sensitive baroreceptor hypothesis, since the juxtaglomerular granular cells, which are located in the media of the afferent arterioles, undergo the same changes in stretch that affect the walls of these vessels.

The above evidence strongly supports the concept that changes in the mean renal perfusion pressure, induced by either acute hemorrhage, vasodilator drug infusion, suprarenal aortic constriction, renal artery stenosis, or chronic sodium depletion, constitute the primary stimulus for renin release via the intrarenal vascular receptor mechanism (Fig. 12-6). However, because of the nature of the experimental maneuvers used, these studies do not exclude the role of the sodium-sensitive macula densa receptors in renin release. Thus, it is not clear whether the increase in renin release occurs as a consequence of a reduction in the renal perfusion pressure or of a reduction in GFR (and hence reduced tubular sodium load to the macula densa cells). Or, alternatively, is the increase in renin release a consequence of a decreased stretch of the afferent arteriolar wall, or is it due to a change in some tubular function, such as a reduction in the sodium load delivered to the distal tubule in the vicinity of the macula densa cells? To answer these questions and to dissociate the effect of the reduced renal perfusion pressure from that of the reduced sodium load at the macula densa, Blaine and his associates (1970) developed a nonfiltering kidney model in the dog by constricting the left renal artery for two hours and ligating and cutting the left ureter. After the two hours of renal ischemia, the renal artery constriction was released and the animal was maintained on peritoneal dialysis for three days. On the fourth day, the right kidney was removed, and the response of the nonfiltering kidney to acute hemorrhage and aortic constriction was tested. This procedure resulted in cessation of the glomerular filtration rate and caused excessive tubular damage, thereby eliminating sodium delivery to the macula densa region. Hence, the model made it possible to study the response characteristics of the isolated intrarenal vascular receptors in the absence of functioning macula densa receptors. Blaine and associates found an increase in renin secretion (as determined from the measurements of the arterial-venous renin concentration) from the nonfiltering kidney in response to both an acute hemorrhage, of about 20 ml/kg of body weight, and suprarenal aortic constriction, which reduced renal perfusion pressure to 40 to 80 mm Hg.

Although these findings strongly support the role of the intrarenal vascular receptors in renin release, they do not exclude the possibility that increased renin secretion, particularly in acute hemorrhage, may have been mediated by either stimulation of the renal sympathetics (Vander, 1965) or increased catecholamine release from the adrenal medulla (Watts and Westfall, 1964). To eliminate these possibilities, Blaine and co-workers (1971) studied the response of the denervated, nonfiltering kidney in dogs which were bilaterally adrenalectomized. They observed a striking increase in renin secretion in this preparation in response to the same degree of acute hemorrhage and graded suprarenal aortic constriction. These findings provide unequivocal evidence in support of the baroreceptor theory and indicate further that the renin release was prompted only by activation of the intrarenal vascular receptors in the absence of any changes in the glomerular filtration rate, sodium delivery to the macula densa region, activation of the renal sympathetics, or catecholamine release. Moreover, these evidences strongly suggest that the intrarenal baroreceptor mechanism appears to be the primary receptor mechanism for the control of renin release and that it can override any signal from the macula densa receptors.

In a subsequent study from the same laboratory (Witty et al., 1971) an attempt was made to localize the site of the intrarenal vascular receptors and to elucidate the nature of the signal perceived by these receptors. As mentioned in Chapter 5, it is well known that intrarenal injection of papaverine (a smooth muscle relaxant) blocks renal autoregulation, which is an afferent arteriolar function (Fig. 5-6). Thus, these investigators reasoned that papaverine-induced dilation of the afferent arteriole should minimize the capacity of these vessels to constrict and hence to undergo a decrease in stretch following an acute hemorrhage. To test this hypothesis, papaverine was infused into the renal artery of denervated, nonfiltering kidney of dogs subjected to acute hemorrhage. They found that infusion of 4 mg/min of papaverine, sufficient to produce a maximal rise in renal blood flow, completely blocked renin secretion in response to acute hemorrhage. The increase in renal blood flow occurred with little change in renal perfusion pressure, reflecting a reduction in the renal vascular resistance. Since papaverine is known to dilate the renal afferent arterioles, then these results are consistent with the baroreceptor theory of renin release and suggest further that the afferent arteriole is the locus of the receptors involved.

The evidence cited above raises an important question. What is the specific signal perceived by these intravascular receptors? As mentioned earlier, Tobian (1960) suggested that the receptors are sensitive to the stretch transmitted through the wall of the afferent arterioles. Thus, in many situations, such as acute hemorrhage or sodium depletion, the increase in renin release is usually a consequence of a decrease in the stretch in the afferent arteriolar wall, a phenomenon which is also associated with an increase in the renal vascular resistance. However, there are exceptions to this *inverse* relationship between the diameter of the afferent arteriole and renin release. The most notable example is a decrease, not an increase, in renal vascular resistance, associated with an increase in renin release seen during the renal autoregulation of blood flow. Such findings, first reported by Skinner and his associates (1964) in normal dogs subjected to graded suprarenal aortic or renal artery constriction, were subsequently confirmed by Ayers and his group (1969) in conscious dogs with renal hypertension. The latter group found that partial constriction of the renal artery initially produced vasodilation, which was accompanied by a rise in plasma renin level. This was then followed by a gradual vasoconstriction, which returned the plasma renin to normal level during the chronic phase of the benign hypertension. Additionally, they found that intravenous infusion of the same dosages of the vasodilator drugs dopamine, isoproterenol, nitroprusside, and acetylcholine caused a marked increase in renin release in hypertensive dogs, but only slightly so in normal dogs.

More recently, Eide and co-workers (1973) reinvestigated the relationship between the diameter of the renal afferent arteriole and renin release. They measured renin secretion in response to stepwise reduction of the renal perfusion pressure in anesthetized dogs below the range of the autoregulation of the renal blood flow (Fig. 5-6). They found that renin release increased and reached its highest value when the renal perfusion pressure fell below the autoregulation range of 66 mm Hg. The renin release remained constant at this high level even when the perfusion pressure was further lowered below 66 mm Hg. This response was not significantly altered when sodium excretion was increased by intravenous infusion of the osmotic diuretic mannitol. This maneuver has been shown to blunt the increase in renin release following suprarenal aortic constriction, presumably by excluding the influence of the macula densa receptors on renin release (Vander and Miller, 1964).

Despite considerable evidence in support of the intrarenal baroreceptor theory of renin release, the exact nature of the signal perceived by these receptors remains unknown. As depicted in Figure 12-6, the intrarenal vascular receptors probably respond to changes in the wall tension in the afferent arteriole, and the magnitude of the receptor response (expressed as renin release) is influenced by several factors (Davis, 1973). These include (1) changes in the transmural pressure across the afferent arteriolar wall in the vicinity of the JG cells, (2) changes in the renal sympathetic activity which controls the tone of the afferent arteriolar wall,

(3) the intrinsic myogenic factors, as exemplified by the phenomenon
of autoregulation of the renal blood flow, and (4) changes in the
elasticity of the afferent arteriole. Accordingly, changes in any of
these variables could alter the state of tension in the afferent
arteriolar wall, thereby causing appropriate alterations in the rate
of renin release from the granular cells. The quantitative
relationship between these variables and their effects on the rate
of renin release, however, remains to be determined.

B. THE MACULA DENSA RECEPTOR THEORY. As mentioned in Chapter 5,
Goormaghtigh (1945) was the first to propose that the macula densa
cells are somehow involved in a negative feedback control of the
glomerular filtration rate. Nearly two decades elapsed, however,
before this concept received its first experimental support. In 1964,
Vander and Miller found that administration of osmotic diuretics,
chlorothiazide, or acetazolamide to dogs prior to suprarenal aortic
constriction minimized or completely prevented the usual increase in
renin release. Furthermore, infusion of these diuretics during the
aortic constriction returned the elevated plasma renin level toward
control values. They suggested that osmotic diuretics increased the
sodium load at the macula densa, thereby blocking the increase in
renin release. Accordingly, and as depicted in Figure 12-6, they
proposed the *macula densa sodium load theory* of renin release, which
states that *an increase in the sodium load at the level of the macula
densa by some unknown mechanism inhibits (designated by a negative
sign) the Na-sensitive tubular receptors, thereby decreasing renin
release from the JG granular cells*. It remained, however, for
subsequent studies to provide some clues as to the possible mechanism
by which the macula densa communicates changes in sodium load to the
renin-secreting granular cells.

It should be recalled (Chapters 8 and 11) that sodium load at
the level of the macula densa ultimately depends on changes in the
glomerular filtration rate and in the rates of sodium reabsorption
in the proximal tubule and the loop of Henle. Accordingly, this
theory is plausible if (1) changes in the sodium load reaching the
macula densa vary directly with changes in the filtered load of
sodium, and (2) sodium chloride reabsorption in the ascending limb
of the loop of Henle is unaffected by the diuretic-induced changes
in the tubular flow rate. The fact that sodium chloride reabsorption
in the ascending limb is markedly flow dependent (Fig. 8-16), coupled
with the evidence that these two diuretics inhibit sodium reabsorption
in both the proximal and distal tubules, does not lend credence to the
validity of these assumptions. Moreover, their findings and the
sodium load theory are inconsistent with a number of other studies
(Lee, 1969), which have shown that administration of natriuretic
agents in both man and dog cause an *increase* and not a decrease in
the plasma renin level. This occurs despite the fact that urinary
sodium loss (natriuresis) persists and that the sodium load at the
level of the macula densa presumably remains high.

To resolve this apparent discrepancy, Vander and Luciano (1967)
subsequently studied the effects of chlormerodin, a mercurial diuretic,
and acute sodium depletion on renin release in dogs. They found
that this mercurial diuretic exerted a dual effect on renin release:

(1) It inhibited the usual increase in renin release following a reduction in the renal perfusion pressure, and (2) it stimulated renin release secondary to the diuretic-induced salt and volume depletion, despite continuous natriuresis. From these results, they suggested that the mechanisms controlling renin release during the reduction of the renal perfusion pressure and during the acute salt depletion (induced by osmotic diuresis) must therefore be different. Thus, during chronic sodium depletion, the fluid loss and the resulting hypotension serve as potent stimuli for renin release and apparently override the inhibitory effect of the high distal tubular sodium load at the level of the macula densa on renin release. In this context, it should be pointed out that chronic sodium depletion in both man and dog, induced either by reduced dietary sodium intake or by administration of natriuretic agents, causes an increase and not a decrease in plasma renin level, accompanied by parallel changes in the JG cell granulation (Tobian, 1960).

In short, although renin release may be influenced by changes in the sodium load at the level of the macula densa, the nature of the signal perceived by the macula densa receptors and the mechanism mediating renin release, remain controversial.

Another theory which has received a wider acceptance is that proposed by Thurau and his associates (1967). As mentioned in Chapter 5, they found that retrograde perfusion of the rat distal tubule at the macula densa region (normally exposed to hypotonic solution) with isotonic saline resulted in a decrease in the proximal tubular diameter in the same nephron. This was interpreted to reflect a reduction in the GFR of that nephron and hence the tubular load. Similar results were obtained when the distal tubule was perfused with sodium bromide, but perfusion with choline chloride or isotonic mannitol had little effect. Assuming that the perfused solution reached the macula densa region, they suggested that these cells are sensitive to changes in sodium concentration of the tubular fluid and not to its osmolality. Thus, as depicted in Figure 12-6, they proposed the *macula densa intraluminal sodium concentration theory*, which states that *an increase in sodium concentration of the tubular fluid bathing the macula densa cells somehow stimulates (designated by a positive sign) the Na-sensitive tubular receptors, thereby increasing renin release from the JG granular cells*. The resulting intrarenal formation of angiotensin II causes constriction of the afferent arteriole for that nephron, thereby reducing P_g and hence GFR. This, in turn, will adjust by negative feedback the sodium concentration and load reaching the macula densa region, thereby closing the feedback loop. This function of the macula densa as the afferent limb of an intrarenal feedback mechanism regulating single nephron GFR has received considerable attention and experimental support from several types of studies.

In 1968, Meyer and his associates found that infusion of furosemide in rabbits caused an increase in plasma renin activity when systemic volume depletion was prevented by reinfuison of ureteral urine into the femoral vein. It should be recalled (Chapter 11) that furosemide inhibits sodium chloride reabsorption in the ascending limb of the loop of Henle, thereby increasing its concentration in the early distal tubular fluid near the macula densa region. These findings have also been confirmed by Cooke and co-workers (1970), who used ethacrynic acid instead of furosemide. In contrast, chlorothiazide, which inhibits sodium chloride reabsorption in the distal tubule beyond the loop of Henle, failed to increase renin release under similar conditions. From these findings, both groups of investigators concluded that an increased tubular sodium concentration near the macula densa caused by furosemide and ethacrynic acid stimulated renin release.

In 1970, Schnermann and co-workers provided direct quantitative evidence that single nephron glomerular filtration rate in the superficial nephrons is *inversely* related to the amount of sodium delivered to the distal tubule at the level of the macula densa. Specifically, they found that during sodium chloride perfusion of single loops of Henle, by micropuncture, both the sodium concentration and load in the early distal tubule increased with increasing flow rate, while at the same time the GFR of the same nephron decreased. However, perfusion with mannitol or sodium sulfate abolished this inverse relationship. The absence of an effect when sulfate ions were substituted for chloride ions was explained in two ways: (a) The presence of sulfate ions in the luminal fluid is known to reduce transmembrane flux of sodium (see Chapter 8). Furthermore, this indicates that to be effective, sodium ions must permeate the macula densa cells, raising the intracellular sodium concentration, and thereby stimulating renin release. (b) It is possible that both sodium and chloride ions are essential for activating the renin-secreting granular cells via the macula densa cells. This latter requirement is consistent with a recent finding that retrograde perfusion of the distal tubule with chloride-free solution did not increase renin activity in isolated juxtaglomerular apparatus (Thurau et al., 1972).

Further evidence in support of the intraluminal sodium concentration theory and its role in the tubuloglomerular feedback control of GFR is provided by Thurau and his group (1972), who showed a direct link between renin activity in JG apparatus and intraluminal sodium concentration at the level of macula densa. They found that retrograde perfusion of the distal tubule in the vicinity of the macula densa with isotonic saline produced a threefold increase in renin activity of the JG apparatus 20 minutes after the onset of perfusion. Perfusion of the macula densa region with iso-osmotic mannitol, choline chloride, lithium chloride, sodium bromide, or sodium ferrocyanide had no effect. The rapidity of this response suggested that release of *preformed* renin rather than its *de novo* synthesis was responsible for the effect. In addition, Granger and co-workers (1972) found that the juxtaglomerular apparatus, isolated from the rat kidney, contains the converting enzymes necessary for the conversion of angiotensin I into angiotensin II. Taken together, these data provide strong evidence in support of the intraluminal sodium concentration theory and its role in the tubuloglomerular feedback control of GFR. The essence of this theory may now be summarized as follows.

A rise in the sodium chloride concentration in the fluid issuing from the ascending limb of the loop of Henle increases

the amount of sodium chloride delivered to the early distal tubule
and the macula densa region. This would enhance sodium uptake by the
macula densa cells, raising the intracellular concentration of sodium
chloride. This, in turn, stimulates, by as yet unknown mechanisms,
the granular cells to release preformed renin into the adjacent
afferent arteriolar blood. The renin thus secreted will combine with
its plasma substrate angiotensinogen to form angiotensin I, which is
readily converted into the potent vasopressor substance angiotensin
II. This local increase in the angiotensin II level causes
constriction of the afferent arteriole, thereby reducing the
glomerular hydrostatic pressure and hence GFR. The reduction in
GFR will decrease the filtered load of sodium chloride and therefore
the amount of sodium chloride reaching the macula densa region,
thereby reducing the feedback signal and closing the loop. In this
manner, changes in the glomerular filtration rate, manifested by
changes in the amount of sodium chloride filtered and reaching the
macula densa and monitored by these cells, are kept within normal
limits.

This proposed tubuloglomerular feedback mechanism for control
of GFR, coupled with the finding of an inverse relationship between
juxtaglomerular granulation and the length of the loop of Henle,
suggests that the macula densa receptors may be involved in another
important renal function. They monitor the hypotonicity of the fluid
issuing from the ascending limb of the loop of Henle, thereby
maintaining the medullary transverse gradient so necessary for the
development of the longitudinal gradient by the countercurrent
mechanism. This function of the macula densa will be described
later in this chapter under the heading of the *intrarenal regulation*
of volume and osmolality of body fluids.

Despite these evidences, a recent microperfusion study of the
loop of Henle and macula densa in rats (Morgan, 1971) has disputed
the theory of tubuloglomerular feedback control of single nephron GFR.
Morgan found that single nephron glomerular filtration rate was
remarkably independent of flow and tubular composition at the macula
densa. He concluded that although changes in sodium concentration at
the macula densa may stimulate renin-secreting granular cells, its
effects are not at the level of the single nephron. Instead, the
renin so released may permeate into the surrounding interstitium,
where it combines with its substrate to form angiotensin I and
angiotensin II. The latter will cause constriction of the afferent
arterioles in that region. Accordingly, changes in the sodium
concentration at the level of the macula densa bring about a local
negative feedback control of GFR in a few surrounding nephrons.

The intraluminal concentration theory of renin release has been
further contested by Vander and Carlson (1969). Extending their
earlier studies, they found that infusion of 0.5, 2.5, or 10 mg/kg
of furosemide produced an increase in renal venous renin activity,
even when systemic volume depletion was prevented by isotonic saline
replacement. In contrast, infusion of 0.1 mg/kg furosemide
stimulated renin release when volume depletion was allowed to
occur. From these studies, they suggested that high doses of
furosemide stimulate renin release by directly inhibiting sodium

uptake by the macula densa cells, hence reducing the intracellular concentration of this ion. The latter effect would somehow inhibit renin release from the renin-secreting granular cells. They claimed that their findings are consistent with the sodium load theory but not with the intraluminal sodium concentration theory. However, this claim is not warranted in view of the fact that the assumption that furosemide somehow inhibits sodium uptake by the macula densa cells lacks direct experimental proof at present.

Nash and his associates (1968) have suggested that renal renin release is regulated primarily by the sodium sensitive macula densa tubular receptors, rather than the wall tension-sensitive vascular receptors. This conclusion was based on the finding that when dogs were volume-expanded to a similar extent by hypotonic or hypertonic saline solutions, renin release increased only in hyponatremic (low plasma sodium concentration) animals. This indicated that hyponatremia or reduced sodium supply to the tubular macula densa receptors was the mechanism mediating the increase in renin secretion.

Recently, based on electron microscopic examination of the juxtaglomerular apparatus, Barajas (1971) reported that the macula densa is more frequently associated with the efferent arteriole and mesangial cells than with the afferent arteriole. On the basis of a three-dimensional structural analysis of the juxtaglomerular apparatus, he has proposed that the degree of contact between the macula densa and the afferent arterioles (containing the renin-secreting granular cells) determines the release of renin. Thus, a reduction in sodium load and hence tubular volume leads to *decreased contact* and consequently *increased renin release*. Conversely, an increase in sodium load and therefore in tubular volume increases contact, which decreases renin release.

Although the results of various studies cited above implicate macula densa cells as sodium-sensitive receptors, the exact signal perceived by these receptors remains controversial at present. It is likely that the stimulating signal could be either a change in the luminal pressure or flow, or a change in sodium concentration or load, or a combination of these. The unequivocal proof, however, must await future critical experiments, in which simultaneous measurement of changes in these variables, as well as the factors mediating sodium uptake by the macula densa cells and their effects on renin release, are made.

2. THE ROLE OF RENAL SYMPATHETIC NERVES IN RENIN RELEASE

There is growing evidence that the sympathetic nervous system plays an important role in the control of renin release. Taquini and co-workers (1964) found that denervation of one kidney in rats decreased renin content in that kidney as compared to the intact kidney. In the same year, Tobian found that cutting the renal nerves reduced the granularity of the juxtaglomerular cells and hence their response to various stimuli. He suggested that renal sympathetics may be important in maintaining a basal level of renin production by the granular cells. Later, Hodge and associates (1966) found that application of anesthetic agents to the renal nerves eliminated renin release in response to mild but not to severe hemorrhage, thus implicating a direct effect of these nerves on renin release. Recently, infusion of catecholamines in both man (Gordon et al., 1967) and dogs (Johnson et al., 1971) has also been shown to stimulate renin release.

The above findings are further corroborated by several histological studies. Barajas and Latta (1967), using electron microscopy and histological techniques, have shown that the juxtaglomerular apparatus receives a rich supply of nonmyelinated fibers believed to be sympathetics. More recently, using similar techniques, Müller and Barajas (1972) found that both adrenergic and cholinergic nerve endings are in contact with the basement membranes of both the proximal and distal tubules. However, the most direct evidence implicating the role of renal sympathetics in renin release is the finding that in anesthetized dogs direct electrical stimulation of renal nerves caused an increase in renal venous renin activity (Vander, 1965). That the increase in renin release following renal nerve stimulation is indeed due to activation of the renal sympathetics has subsequently been confirmed by a variety of animal experiments (Loeffler et al., 1972; Coote et al., 1972).

A recent study in man (Gordon et al., 1967) has shown that both assumption of an upright posture and exercise increase renal sympathetic activity and produce renal arteriolar constriction, both maneuvers causing an increase in renin release. In addition, animal studies have clearly shown that activation of renal sympathetics exerts a modulating effect on the magnitude of renin release in response to a variety of stimuli. Thus, the increase in renin secretion following acute hemorrhage (Bunag et al., 1966) and during mild sodium depletion (Mogil et al., 1969) appears to be mediated in part by an increase in the renal sympathetic nerve activity.

The possible mechanisms mediating the effect of catecholamines and sympathetic stimulation on renin release have been investigated by a number of recent studies. Winer and associates (1969) have reported an increase in plasma renin activity in man after administration of ethacrynic acid and theophylline, and upon assumption of upright posture. The effect was blocked by propranolol (a β-adrenergic blocking drug) and phentolamine (an α-adrenergic blocker). Subsequently, Winer and co-workers (1971) investigated the mechanism of action of sympathomimetic amines in dogs. They found that epinephrine, isoproterenol, and cyclic AMP all increased renin secretion. These renin-stimulating effects were blocked by propranolol and phentolamine. From these studies, they suggested that intracellular accumulation of cyclic AMP mediates renin secretion via both the α- and β-receptors and that the α- and β-blockers act at a step distal to cyclic AMP production.

In contrast, recent studies of Assaykeen and his associates (1970) and Passo and co-workers (1971) favor the concept that the renin-stimulating effect of both renal sympathetic stimulation and catecholamines is mediated via β-adrenergic receptors. However, the specific mechanism mediating the effects remains to be elucidated.

In summary, available evidence supports the concept that at least five different mechanisms may mediate the effects of renal sympathetics and catecholamines on renin release: (1) Both the renal sympathetics and catecholamines produce constriction of the renal arterioles, thereby causing renin release via stimulation of the vascular receptors. (2) As mentioned in Chapter 5, glomerular filtration rate is in part determined by the hydrostatic blood pressure in the afferent arteriole, whose constriction will reduce GFR. A decrease in GFR produces a decrease in the filtered load of sodium chloride, which has the potential of changing the amount of sodium chloride reaching the macula densa receptors. This, in turn, would alter the rate of renin release by the macula densa mechanism. (3) As depicted in Figure 12-6, both renal sympathetics and catecholamines directly act on the afferent arteriolar vascular receptors and the granular cells, thereby modulating the rate of renin release from the granular cells. (4) Stimulation by both catecholamines and sympathetics causes a redistribution of the renal blood flow, so that the blood is shifted from the renin-rich cortical and outer cortical areas to the relatively renin-poor inner cortical and medullary regions. (5) As depicted in Figure 12-6, the effect of renal sympathetics and catecholamines on renin release is believed to be mediated via β-adrenergic receptors. This finding, coupled with the evidence that catecholamines and cyclic AMP can directly stimulate renin release (Michelakis et al., 1969) suggests a possible link between β-adrenergic stimulation and intracellular cyclic AMP accumulation. Thus, it is conceivable that activation of β-adrenergic receptors leads to stimulation of intracellular accumulation of cyclic AMP by inhibition of phosphodiesterase. Inhibition of this enzyme by theophylline also potentiates cyclic AMP stimulation of renin release.

3. CONTROL OF RENIN RELEASE BY SOME SELECTIVE HUMORAL AGENTS

As depicted in Figure 12-6, in addition to catecholamines, a number of other humoral agents, including some plasma electrolytes, influence the rate of renin release from the JG granular cells. In Chapter 11, in describing the factors influencing the biosynthetic pathway for aldosterone, we stated that changes in plasma concentrations of sodium and potassium influence aldosterone secretion, and hence indirectly affect renin release (Fig. 11-15).

Recent studies have demonstrated an inverse relationship between plasma sodium concentration and renin secretion in dogs (Nash et al., 1968). They found that an increase in sodium concentration in the renal artery suppressed renin release, while a decrease stimulated renin secretion. Similar results have been reported for humans by Brown and his associates (1965), who found an inverse relationship between plasma sodium concentration and plasma renin activity in 253 hypertensive patients. Newsome and Bartter (1968) and Gordon and Pawsey (1971) recently have shown that changes in the extracellular fluid (ECF) volume produced the opposite effect on this inverse relationship. Thus, an expansion of ECF suppressed plasma renin activity, even though plasma sodium concentration was low, whereas contraction of ECF produced the opposite effect. This supports the concept that the effect of changes in ECF volume on renin release may be mediated via the vascular receptor mechanism (Fig. 12-6).

In contrast, results of several studies suggest that the effect of alterations in plasma sodium concentration on renin secretion may be mediated via the sodium-sensitive macula densa receptors. Thus, Nash and co-workers (1968) found that stimulation of renin release by hyponatremic volume expansion, ureteral occlusion, or suprarenal aortic constriction was partially blocked by intrarenal infusion of hypertonic saline. Since in these experiments there were no detectable hemodynamic changes, they suggested that the macula densa receptor mediated the response. Essentially similar results were obtained by Shade and his associates (1972), who found that intrarenal infusion of hypertonic saline decreases renin release in dogs with thoracic caval constriction (a procedure causing sodium retention) and one filtering kidney. In contrast, intrarenal infusion of hypertonic saline had no effect on renin secretion in dogs with thoracic caval constriction and one nonfiltering kidney. This latter finding strongly supports the concept that the tubular macula densa receptor may be the mechanism mediating the response to changes in plasma sodium concentration.

The effect of potassium metabolism on renin secretion has also been investigated by a number of studies. Brunner and associates (1970) found that a high potassium intake resulted in a decrease in plasma renin activity in both normal and hypertensive subjects, whereas a low potassium intake produced the opposite effect. Moreover, they found that hyperkalemia, which inhibits renin secretion, stimulated aldosterone secretion, whereas hypokalemia produced the opposite effect. This relationship between chronic potassium loading and plasma renin activity has also been demonstrated in rats (Sealey et al., 1970) and dogs (Abbrecht and Vander, 1970).

The possible mechanism whereby changes in the plasma potassium concentration influence renin secretion has been studied by a number of investigators. Vander (1970) found that intrarenal infusion of potassium chloride into normal and salt-depleted dogs resulted in a decrease in renal vein renin activity. He suggested that the injected potassium inhibited sodium reabsorption in the proximal tubule, thereby increasing the sodium load reaching the macula densa region. That the tubular macula densa receptor may indeed play a role in potassium-induced changes in renin release was demonstrated by a recent study (Shade et al., 1972). These investigators observed that intrarenal infusion of potassium chloride in dogs with thoracic caval constriction and one filtering kidney produced a striking decrease in renin release. In contrast, intrarenal infusion of potassium chloride into dogs with thoracic caval constriction but with one nonfiltering kidney had no effect. Analogous to findings for sodium, these data strongly support the concept of the tubular macula densa mechanism as the mediator of the potassium effect.

However, recent micropuncture studies in dogs (Schneider et al., 1972), in which sufficient potassium chloride was given to depress renin release, showed that there was no increase in sodium delivery from the proximal tubules. These results do not support Vander's suggestion that potassium inhibits sodium reabsorption in the proximal tubule. They are, however, consistent with the concept that potassium inhibition of renin release may be mediated by a tubular mechanism, presumably the macula densa receptors. The specific nature of the mechanism remains to be determined.

Finally, as depicted in Figure 12-6, ADH and angiotensin II directly inhibit (designated by a negative sign) renin release from the granular cells. This concept is supported by a number of studies in mammalian species, including man. Thus, Shade and his co-workers (1973) demonstrated that intravenous infusion of ADH and angiotensin II inhibit renin release in sodium-depleted dogs with one nonfiltering kidney. These results suggest that both peptides act directly on the juxtaglomerular cells to inhibit renin release. Furthermore, they suggested that inhibition of renin release by angiotensin II involves a negative feedback loop, whereby the product of renin reaction with its substrate (angiotensin II) inhibits enzyme (renin) release.

SUMMARY

The evidence presented in the preceding sections indicates that renin release is normally controlled by the interplay of intrinsic and extrinsic mechanisms. Of the intrinsic mechanisms, the intrarenal wall tension-sensitive vascular receptors, located in the afferent arterioles, play a prominent role in control of renin secretion. As depicted in Figure 12-6, the primary input to these receptors is a reduction in the mean renal perfusion pressure, induced by four classes of systemic perturbations. Moreover, the sensitivity of the vascular receptor to a given stimulus is modulated by the degree of activation of renal sympathetics as well as the circulating blood levels of catecholamines.

The sodium-sensitive tubular receptors, located in the macula densa region, serve as a secondary mechanism for control of renin release. Although sodium concentration and sodium load in the tubular fluid at the level of the macula densa have been suggested as possible stimuli, the nature of the signal perceived by these receptors remains controversial. Nevertheless, the role of the macula densa receptors in an intrarenal negative feedback mechanism for the control of GFR in a single nephron or a few nephrons appears to be well documented.

The major extrinsic factor influencing renin release is the renal sympathetic nerves. Although the activity of renal sympathetics appears not to be essential for renin release, available evidence indicates that these nerves exert a modulating influence on renin secretion. As depicted in Figure 12-6, the renal sympathetics exert their effects on both the vascular receptors and the renin-secreting granular cells. These effects are believed to be mediated via the β-adrenergic receptors. In this way, renal sympathetics exert a dual effect: (1) They control the degree of arteriolar constriction and hence the renal perfusion pressure or the input to the vascular receptors. (2) They control the degree of constriction of both the afferent and efferent arterioles, which influences GFR, which in part determines the amount of sodium chloride reaching the tubular macula densa receptors. Both of these mechanisms influence renin release. Likewise, the catecholamines influence renin release by their effect on the renal arterioles and the juxtaglomerular cells.

Finally, a number of humoral agents, notably sodium and potassium ions, ADH, and angiotensin II, all influence renin secretion. The available evidence indicates that the effect of sodium and potassium ions is mediated via the tubular macula densa receptors, whereas both ADH and angiotensin II appear to act directly on the renin-secreting granular cells via a negative feedback mechanism.

II. RIGHT ATRIAL STRETCH-SENSITIVE RECEPTORS

As mentioned earlier, a second mechanism which influences urinary sodium excretion, and hence controls the blood volume, involves a reflex adjustment of renin release by the kidney. However, despite the evidence presented below in support of the existence of such a reflex, its role in the regulation of salt and water balance remains unresolved.

In 1957, Coleridge and co-workers successfully isolated nerve fibers from the right atrium, whose frequency of discharge could be reduced or abolished by constriction of the superior or inferior vena cava. Subsequently, Anderson and his associates (1959) demonstrated that stretching the right atrium with sutures produced a decrease in the plasma concentration of aldosterone. These findings, coupled with the observation that constriction of the inferior vena cava caused an increase in plasma aldosterone concentration (Davis et al., 1960), suggested that this response may be mediated by a reflex mechanism, whose afferent limb is the stretch-sensitive volume receptors located in the right atrium. Subsequently, Gupta and his group (1966) demonstrated that graded reductions in the blood volume were correlated with a decrease in the frequency of discharge recorded from the right atrial nerve fibers, thereby supporting this concept of the right atrial reflex.

Further evidence for this concept has recently been provided by Brennan and associates (1971). They showed that an increase in the right atrial pressure, produced by balloon inflation, resulted in a decrease in the plasma renin activity, presumably by a reflex suppression of renin secretion by the kidney. This finding provided a possible mechanism for the previously observed changes in the plasma aldosterone concentration. More recently, Stitzer and Malvin (1975) studied the effect of alterations in the right atrial pressure on renal sodium excretion. They found that inflation of a balloon in the right atrium in dogs resulted in salt and water retention not attributable to any renal or systemic hemodynamic changes. They found no significant difference between the responses of the intact or denervated kidney to the right atrial balloon distention. From these results, they suggested that a binary mechanism may mediate the renal response to right atrial balloon inflation. One mechanism involves a reflex reduction in the renal excretion of salt and water, induced by a fall in the mean arterial blood pressure consequent to right atrial balloon inflation. Another mechanism involves a reflex stimulation of renin release and aldosterone production, which leads to renal salt and water retention. From the similarity of the responses of the intact and denervated kidney, they further suggested that both mechanisms are hormonally mediated. However, the nature of the hormone involved remains unresolved at present.

In summary, available evidence supports the concept of a right atrial receptor reflex system for the control of urinary salt and water excretion. However, the identification of the neural pathway involved, the hormonal mechanism mediating the effect, and its significance in the body fluid regulation remain to be determined.

III. CONTROL OF SODIUM EXCRETION: A SYNTHESIS

The evidence presented in the preceding sections indicates that two general types of stimuli cause renin release: The *first* involves changes in the arterial blood pressure and the extracellular fluid (ECF) volume; the latter is induced by changes in the total body sodium. Thus, a decrease in either the blood pressure or ECF volume stimulates renin release, whereas an increase would suppress renin release. The *second* involves changes in potassium metabolism; potassium depletion stimulates renin release, whereas potassium excess depresses renin release. In addition, the magnitude of renin release in response to these stimuli is modified by the degree of activation of renal sympathetics and the circulating blood levels of catecholamines. Moreover, changes in the various stimuli to which renin secretion responds are, in turn, initiated by changes in the plasma levels of angiotensin II, which produces two systemic effects: (1) It alters the vascular resistance, thereby modifying the arterial blood pressure, and (2) depending on its plasma concentration, it influences aldosterone secretion, thereby controlling sodium and potassium balance and hence ECF volume.

It is therefore clear that the effectiveness of angiotensin-mediated regulation of both the arterial blood pressure and the ECF volume will ultimately depend on the rate of renin release into the circulation and the factors affecting its blood levels. These, in turn, will determine the rate of production of angiotensin II and hence its effects on the blood vessels, adrenal cortex, and ultimately the kidney.

As depicted in Figure 12-7, once renin is released into the plasma compartment, the rate of formation of angiotensin II, and hence its plasma concentration ($[Ang]_p$), depend on several factors. Angiotensin synthesis and therefore $[Ang]_p$ are enhanced in the presence of increased plasma levels of renin substrate concentration and increased pulmonary conversion rate, both designated by plus signs. However, $[Ang]_p$ is reduced by an increase in plasma volume, hepatic blood flow, and plasma levels of angiotensinase, all designated by negative signs.

Available evidence indicates that depending on its plasma concentration, angiotensin II may exert three effects (Bravo et al., 1975): At very low plasma concentration it acts only locally in the renal vasculature to cause constriction of the renal afferent arteriole, thereby reducing the GFR (designated by a negative sign) in one or a few adjacent nephrons. At somewhat higher concentrations, it acts on the smooth muscle cells lining the arterioles throughout the cardiovascular system, causing vasoconstriction and hence elevation of the systemic arterial blood pressure. At still higher

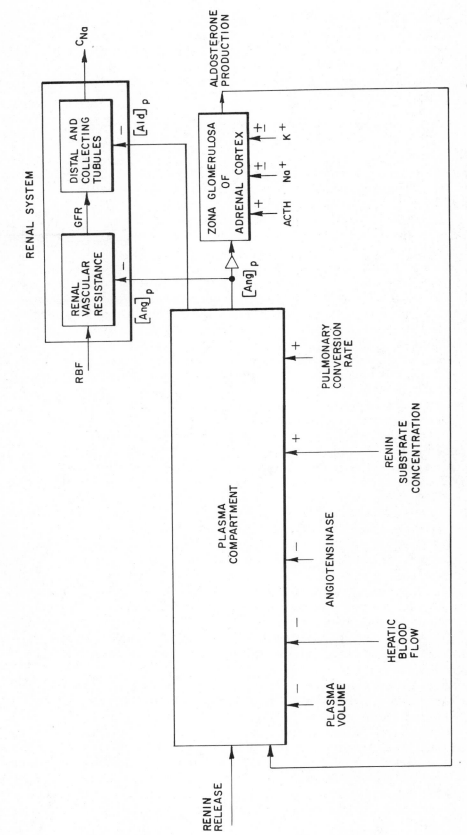

Figure 12-7. A functional diagram of the extrarenal regulation of aldosterone release and renal excretion of sodium.

concentrations, exceeding a threshold level (designated by a small triangle on the arrow), it stimulates the zona glomerulosa of the adrenal cortex to secrete aldosterone. The existence of a threshold concentration for aldosterone secretion is further supported by the findings of Ames and co-workers (1965) that in patients in a state of positive sodium-balance, infusion of a small amount of angiotensin II, insufficient to stimulate aldosterone production, was sufficient to maintain a hypertensive state.

The effectiveness of the trophic action of angiotensin II is enhanced by ACTH, as well as through sodium and potassium metabolism. Thus, as discussed previously (Fig. 11-15), aldosterone production is enhanced by potassium loading or sodium depletion, but is reduced by sodium loading or potassium depletion. These effects are indicated in Figure 12-7 by plus and minus signs next to the appropriate arrows impinging on the box labelled "zona glomerulosa of adrenal cortex." The aldosterone thus secreted enters the bloodstream, where for a given plasma volume it yields the circulating level of aldosterone ($[Ald]_p$). The latter, by the mechanism described in Chapter 11, acts on the epithelial cells of the distal and collecting tubules of the renal system to enhance isotonic sodium chloride reabsorption, and hence reduce (designated by a negative sign) renal clearance of sodium (C_{Na}).

In summary, the plasma renin level depends to a large extent on sodium and potassium metabolism and on the state of body sodium and potassium balance. These, in turn, determine the extracellular fluid (ECF) volume, plasma volume, arterial blood pressure, and renal perfusion pressure. Thus, for example, chronic low sodium intake leads to a reduction of the extracellular fluid volume and therefore of renal perfusion pressure as well. This leads to a reduction of the blood pressure in the afferent arteriole, which stimulates renin release by the intrarenal baroreceptor mechanism. The resulting increase in the plasma renin will eventually stimulate aldosterone secretion from the adrenal cortex. The elevation of the plasma aldosterone concentration will increase sodium and water reabsorption from the distal and collecting tubules as a compensatory mechanism, restoring the ECF volume to normal. The reduction of ECF volume will also reduce the hepatic blood flow, a factor which reduces the hepatic clearance of both renin and aldosterone. This would lead to a further increase in plasma concentration of aldosterone and hence to a further compensatory increase in renal reabsorption of sodium and water to restore ECF volume to normal.

RENAL-BODY FLUID REGULATING SYSTEMS: A SYNTHESIS

Having thus described the functional characteristics of the various components of the renal-body fluid regulating systems, we are now ready to combine and synthesize them into a unifying functional diagram. As discussed previously and illustrated in Figure 12-8, the renal regulation of volume and osmolality of the body fluids is ultimately achieved by the interplay of three major systems: (1) The renal system with its ultrafilter and tubular

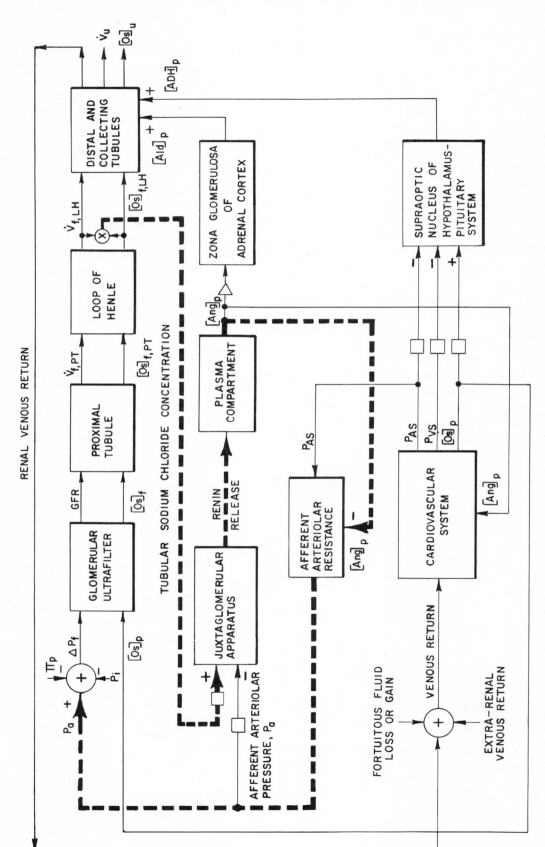

Figure 12-8. A functional diagram of the renal–body fluid regulating systems.

components, shown in the upper portion of the figure. (2) The juxtaglomerular apparatus-adrenal cortex system, shown in the middle of the figure, which controls the plasma volume and arterial blood pressure via the renin-angiotensin-aldosterone mechanism. And (3) the osmoreceptors-hypothalamus-pituitary system, shown in the lower part of the figure, which controls the plasma osmolality via the ADH mechanism.

As mentioned previously, the release of renin from the juxtaglomerular granular cells is controlled by two separate stimuli: One acting through the vascular receptors and the other through the tubular macula densa receptors. The vascular receptors respond to changes in the volume and hydrostatic pressure of the circulating blood, whereas the macula densa receptors are involved in an intrarenal negative feedback regulation of GFR. Accordingly, we may classify the various factors that influence renal regulation of volume and osmolality of body fluids under two general headings: *First* is the *intrarenal mechanism*, which operates via the sodium-sensitive macula densa receptors and the renin-secreting granular cells. This is depicted by the heavy broken pathways in the functional diagram. *Second* is the *extrarenal mechanisms*, consisting of the renin-angiotensin-aldosterone and ADH secreting systems. These are depicted by the other pathways in the functional diagram. Let us now consider the operation of each mechanism and its relative contribution to the renal regulation of volume and osmolality of body fluids, using the functional diagram in Figure 12-8 as our guide.

INTRARENAL MECHANISM

As depicted in this diagram, the intrarenal mechanism which regulates the volume and osmolality of excreted urine, and hence indirectly those of body fluids, involves monitoring the sodium chloride concentration or load in the tubular fluid emerging from the ascending limb of the loop of Henle as it passes by the *macula densa* receptor cells. This process is depicted by a small box on the heavy broken arrow which impinges on the large box labelled "juxtaglomerular apparatus." The latter includes both the sodium-sensitive tubular macula densa receptors and the afferent arteriolar wall tension-sensitive vascular receptors. Thus, an increase in the sodium chloride concentration in the tubular fluid stimulates (designated by a plus sign) the macula densa receptor component of the JG apparatus. This, in turn, will stimulate the *granular cells* to release renin, by an unknown intermediate step, possibly via secondary stimulation of the interstitial *mesangial cells*. The renin thus released into the plasma compartment combines with its plasma substrate angiotensinogen (found chiefly in the fraction of plasma containing α-2-globulin) to form the inactive decapeptide angiotensin I. This substance is then converted into the active, octapeptide vasopressor angiotensin II, by the action of plasma converting enzyme present locally in the renal tissue. This local synthesis of angiotensin II raises its plasma concentration ($[Ang]_p$) in the afferent arterioles supplying the same as well as a few adjacent nephrons, thereby constricting these vessels. For a given systemic arterial blood pressure (P_{AS}), the resulting increase in the afferent arteriolar resistance reduces the afferent arteriolar pressure (P_a), lowering the effective filtration pressure (ΔP_f) and hence GFR. This effect is depicted by a negative sign on the arrow labelled "$[Ang]_p$" which impinges on the box labelled "afferent arteriolar resistance." The resulting momentary decrease in GFR slows the filtrate flow along the various nephron segments, and in particular along the ascending limb of the loop of Henle. The increased tubular transit time increases the sodium chloride diffusion gradient at the luminal cell membrane, a factor tending to enhance the net transtubular sodium chloride transport from the fluid in the ascending limb, thereby lowering its concentration in the fluid emerging from this segment. The reduced concentration of sodium chloride in the tubular fluid bathing the macula densa cells will tend to reduce the stimulation of these cells and their associated receptors, leading to reduced stimulation of the renin-secreting granular cells and subsequent reduction in angiotensin II synthesis. In this manner, small transient changes in the sodium chloride concentration in the fluid emerging from the ascending limb of the loop of Henle, detected via the macula densa receptors-renin secreting granular cells system, by means of a negative feedback mechanism brings about a careful adjustment of the GFR in one or a few adjacent nephrons.

The importance of this mechanism in maintaining the constancy of the volume and osmolality of body fluids deserves special comment. As mentioned in Chapter 11, the fluid emerging from the ascending limb of the loop of Henle and entering the early distal tubule is normally hypotonic. Small changes in the tonicity of this fluid will have a profound effect on the magnitude of the *transverse gradient* developed between the fluids in the ascending and descending limbs at the corticomedullary level, a factor which ultimately determines the magnitude of the generated longitudinal gradient within the medullary interstitium, and hence the volume and osmolality of the excreted urine. Thus, operating at the level of single or few nephrons, the macula densa receptors, by monitoring the changes in the osmolality (due primarily to sodium chloride concentration) of the fluid emerging from the ascending limb, and via stimulation of the granular cells, can cause sufficient release of renin to adjust the GFR of individual nephrons. In this manner, the macula densa cells adjust filtrate flow through the loop of Henle, a factor which determines the activity of the chloride pump in the ascending limb of the loop of Henle, and therefore the osmolality of the tubular fluid leaving that segment of the nephron. The consequence of this *intrarenal* regulation of the glomerulotubular function in individual nephrons is the fine adjustment of the all-important *transverse gradient* between the fluids in the ascending and descending limbs. The magnitude of this gradient, as mentioned in Chapter 11, for a given loop length and GFR, is the primary determinant of the final steady state longitudinal gradient in the medullary interstitium, and hence the final volume and osmolality of the excreted urine.

In summary, the function of the *intrarenal mechanism*, as shown in Figure 12-8, is to adjust the glomerulotubular functions in individual nephrons. Since the overall kidney function represents the algebraic sum of the glomerulotubular functions of all the active nephrons, this intrarenal mechanism tends to coordinate and integrate the activity of the individual nephrons, and consequently the overall kidney function in response to body requirements.

The operation of the intrarenal mechanism just described is mediated by small, transient changes in local renal concentration of angiotensin II ($[Ang]_p$), a fact supported by a number of studies cited earlier. This is depicted in the functional diagram by the first *branching point* (or tie point) on the arrow labelled "$[Ang]_p$," which connects the box labelled "plasma compartment" to that labelled "zona glomerulosa of adrenal cortex." Needless to say, the elevation of $[Ang]_p$ brought about by extrarenal mechanisms will *override* the intrarenal effect and, depending on the magnitude of $[Ang]_p$, will act on the cardiovascular system to cause systemic vasoconstriction and hypertension, stimulation of aldosterone secretion, or both. The extrarenal mechanism mediating these effects are described next.

EXTRARENAL MECHANISMS

As depicted in Figure 12-8, the extrarenal regulation of the final volume and osmolality of urine, and hence indirectly that of body fluids, involves careful adjustment of the rates of synthesis and release of *ADH* and *aldosterone* and their respective plasma concentrations. As discussed previously, the plasma concentration of the antidiuretic hormone ($[ADH]_p$) is controlled by the integrated effects of both *volume* stimuli (mediated via the systemic arterial and venous stretch-sensitive volume receptors) and *osmotic* stimuli (mediated via the hypothalamic and hepatic osmoreceptors) on the supraoptic nucleus of the hypothalamus-pituitary system. The volume and osmotic stimuli may be activated separately or together by fortuitous loss or gain of fluids having different proportions of water and electrolytes. Hence, these perturbations or forcings may be isotonic, hypotonic, or hypertonic. Furthermore, since the fortuitous fluid influx or efflux represents fluid entry or loss from the blood, they tend to affect the function of the cardiovascular system and its regulated variables, including the systemic arterial (P_{AS}) and venous (P_{VS}) pressures and plasma osmolality ($[Os]_p$). Induced changes in these cardiovascular variables are monitored by the appropriate components of the volume and osmotic receptors, which send afferent neural signals to the hypothalamic centers. The dynamic integration of these signals will eventually lead to appropriate directional changes in the rates of synthesis and release of ADH and its plasma concentration. The latter, acting on the epithelial cells of the distal and collecting tubules, will induce appropriate directional changes in the osmotic reabsorption of water and its renal clearance (C_{H_2O}). The net effect is the negative feedback regulation of the volume and osmolality of the circulating blood.

As depicted in Figure 12-8, the other extrarenal mechanism influencing the renal regulation of volume and osmolality of body fluid is mediated via aldosterone-controlled isotonic sodium reabsorption in the distal and collecting tubules. As mentioned earlier, plasma concentration of aldosterone ($[Ald]_p$) is regulated primarily by plasma levels of angiotensin II and the state of sodium and potassium balance. Alterations in the latter two have profound effects on the volume and hydrostatic pressure of the circulating blood, which in turn influence the plasma levels of angiotensin II. Therefore, to facilitate presentation, we shall represent the effects of these three variables by a single process, namely, the renin-angiotensin-aldosterone mechanism.

As shown, any factor that tends to increase the afferent arteriolar pressure (P_a) will inhibit (designated by a negative sign) renin release from the juxtaglomerular apparatus and will reduce the synthesis of angiotensin II and hence its plasma concentration ($[Ang]_p$). Conversely, a decrease in P_a, induced by hemorrhage, sodium depletion, or renal artery stenosis, will stimulate the afferent arteriolar vascular receptors, which in turn stimulate granular cells to release renin. Once released into the blood, the renin will initiate the synthesis of angiotensin I and II.

The extrarenal conversion of angiotensin I by the lung converting enzyme, as the renal venous blood passes through the pulmonary tissues, produces the amount of angiotensin II required for its systemic effects. This extrarenal conversion of angiotensin I serves as a further check on the circulating plasma levels of angiotensin II and hence on its extrarenal effects. As depicted in Figure 12-7, besides pulmonary conversion rate, $[Ang]_p$ is further enhanced by the plasma concentration of renin substrate (angiotensinogen). However, $[Ang]_p$ is adversely affected by an increase in plasma volume, hepatic blood flow, and plasma angiotensinases.

Depending on its plasma concentration ($[Ang]_p$), angiotensin II will have one or both systemic effects. At relatively high concentration, it will act on the cardiovascular system, causing general systemic (including renal) vasoconstriction and systemic hypertension. This is depicted by the second branching point on the arrow connecting the box labelled "plasma compartment" to the box labelled "zona glomerulosa of adrenal cortex." At still higher concentrations, exceeding a *threshold* (depicted by a triangle on the arrow labelled "$[Ang]_p$"), it stimulates the zona glomerulosa of the adrenal cortex to increase synthesis and release of aldosterone, raising its plasma concentration ($[Ald]_p$). The increase in $[Ald]_p$ will enhance isotonic sodium reabsorption from the distal and collecting tubules, thereby reducing the renal excretion of sodium and its clearance (C_{Na}), yielding a relatively hypertonic urine. The net result would be an increase in the plasma volume, renal perfusion pressure, and afferent arteriolar pressure, with ultimate reduction of the juxtaglomerular cell stimulation. Thus, the juxtaglomerular vascular receptors, acting as "volume" receptors, constitute an important element in a negative feedback system which helps to restore the blood volume to normal.

In summary, as depicted in Figure 12-8, the final adjustment of urinary volume and osmolality, and hence that of body fluids, depends on the dynamic interplay of *three* regulatory processes: (1) The hemodynamic factors which modify the input to the renal regulator;

(2) the factors which influence the intrarenal regulation of the glomerulotubular function, as well as urinary concentration and dilution mechanisms; and (3) the neuroendocrine systems which through volume, pressure, and osmotic stimuli modify the plasma concentrations of ADH and aldosterone, thereby influencing the final volume and osmolality of the excreted urine.

Available evidence indicates that the first two mechanisms are involved in the minute-to-minute adjustment of the renal output and hence, indirectly, the volume and osmolality of body fluids. The neuroendocrine extrarenal mechanisms, on the other hand, are involved in the long-term adjustment of the extracellular fluid volume and osmolality, in response to wide variations in fluid influx or efflux under normal or abnormal conditions. Therefore, a thorough understanding of renal function under normal and disease conditions can only be achieved through an integrated analysis of the dynamic interactions of these three regulatory processes.

PROBLEMS

12-1. What are the stimuli and primary mechanisms for renin release (*a*) during nonhypotensive hemorrhage and (*b*) during hypotensive hemorrhage?

12-2. What extrarenal mechanisms are concerned in the regulation of (*a*) plasma osmolality, and (*b*) plasma volume? Of these, which ones are most important in the normal regulation of plasma volume and osmolality?

12-3. What are the factors that regulate the blood levels of angiotensin II?

12-4. Define tachyphylaxis and explain the possible factors responsible for angiotensin II tachyphylaxis.

12-5. Describe briefly the factors controlling the formation of angiotensin II and its fate in the circulation.

12-6. What are the renal and systemic effects of angiotensin II? Are these effects concentration dependent?

12-7. What is the most important factor determining the pressor responsiveness of angiotensin II?

12-8. Describe briefly the renin-angiotensin-aldosterone system in the control of blood volume. What is believed to be the main function of this system under normal conditions?

12-9. Describe (a) the baroreceptor theory of renin release and (b) the macula densa theory of renin release. Cite briefly the strengths and weaknesses for each.

12-10. Describe briefly the theory of tubuloglomerular feedback control of GFR and its physiological significance.

12-11. What is the role of sympathetics in the control of renin release?

12-12. Name some of the humoral agents and their effects on renin release.

12-13. In each of the following circumstances, indicate the expected directional deviation from normal (+ for increase, - for decrease, and 0 for no change) in the rate of renin release.
   A. After intravenous infusion of two liters of isotonic saline. _____
   B. Six hours after donating two pints of blood. _____
   C. Acute constriction of the renal artery. _____
   D. Chronic sodium deprivation from the diet. _____
   E. Assumption of upright posture. _____
   F. After intravenous infusion of a large dose of carbonic anhydrase inhibitor, acetazolamide. _____
   G. Chronic primary hyperaldosteronism. _____
   H. In congestive heart failure. _____

12-14. Of the two intrinsic intrarenal mechanisms for renin release, which is the primary mediator for the expected change in renin release in each of the circumstances in Problem 12-13?

12-15. Indicate by a checkmark whether the urine osmolality (and hence the urine concentration) increases or decreases in response to a sustained action of each of the following forcings:

Forcings	*Urine Osmolality (concentration)*	
	Increase	*Decrease*
A. An increase in GFR.	_____	_____
B. A decrease in medullary blood flow.	_____	_____
C. An increase in plasma ADH concentration.	_____	_____
D. A decrease in plasma aldosterone concentration.	_____	_____
E. Assumption of upright posture.	_____	_____
F. In congestive heart failure.	_____	_____
G. In severe sweating.	_____	_____

12-16.   Indicate by a checkmark in which of the following conditions
the ADH release is the highest:
A.   Sitting position. _____
B.   Recumbent position. _____
C.   Upright position. _____

12-17.   When a person stands up, there is increased venous pressure
in the lower extremities. The plasma protein concentration
rises and the volume of the legs increases, indicating a loss
of water from the vascular compartment into the interstitial
compartment. When the subject reclines, this fluid is
returned to the vascular compartment. Describe what probably
has happened in terms of capillary pressures.

12-18.   In an unanesthetized dog, the arterial pressure may be raised
reflexly to about 200 mm Hg for an hour by occluding both
common carotid arteries. Despite the rise in arterial
pressure and thus capillary hydrostatic pressure, there is
no change in plasma volume. Why?

12-19.   Muscular exercise has been shown to produce a marked change
in water and electrolyte distribution. For example, in
vigorous exercise, there is an increase in extracellular
fluid in the active tissue, which is reflected as an increase
in plasma protein concentration and in the percentage of red
cells. A normal student running for 90 seconds at top speed
may lose as much as 500 ml fluid from the plasma during this
run, but it will take 30 to 60 minutes for recovery. Explain,
in terms of capillary function, why this time difference may
occur.

12-20.   A hospital ship is wrecked. In the excitement of getting
ready to board the life raft, Mr. Jones, who has diabetes
insipidus, received an extra injection of ADH (too much),
while Mr. Smith, another patient with the same type of
diabetes, failed to receive the required amount. Among
the patients evacuated were a psychotic currently suffering
from water intoxication, a cardiac patient on a low salt
diet, and a burn patient who has lost a lot of plasma.
These five patients, along with their nurse, are set adrift
with food but without drinking water. Describe the changes
in water distribution (extracellular and intracellular) which
would probably occur in each *before* drinking sea water. *After*
three days, assuming all are still alive, they begin to drink
sea water. How would this alter the water distribution in
each of the six?

12-21.   The following table gives findings in five patients as
deviations from normal. From the list of distrubances
given below, select the one which *best* describes the
findings and then designate your choice by placing the
appropriate *letter* in the column under diagnosis.

Patients	Total Blood Volume	Inulin Clearance	Plasma Renin Level	Plasma ADH Level	Sodium Clearance	Diagnosis
1	−	−	+	+	+	_____
2	+	+	−	+	+	_____
3	−	−	+	+	−	_____
4	+	+	−	−	+	_____
5	+	−	+	−	−	_____

Disturbances:

A. Infusion of two liters of 3 gm% saline solution.
B. Congestive heart failure.
C. Two days following hemorrhage (about 20% of blood volume lost).
D. Excessive water ingestion.
E. Severe sweating.

12-22. The table given below gives the laboratory findings in four patients suspected of having renal disease. For comparison, the normal values for the same test are listed at the top of the table. (Assume permeability ratio for glucose is unity.)

Patients	Renal Function Tests		
	Inulin Clearance (ml/min)	Plasma Glucose Concentration (mg%)	Maximum Glucose Absorption Rate, $\dot{T}m_G$ (mg/min)
Normal	125	80	350
1. _____	75	80	60
2. _____	125	300	350
3. _____	125	80	90
4. _____	50	80	350

Match each patient's findings with the *most likely disease* from the list given below, by placing the corresponding *letter* designating the disease in the space provided under "Patients" in the above table.

A. *Glomerulonephritis* is a disease characterized by a marked reduction in GFR, but no change in $\dot{T}m$ for glucose.
B. *Renal glycosuria* is a disease characterized by a marked reduction in $\dot{T}m$ for glucose but with normal GFR.
C. *Diabetes mellitus* is a disease characterized by an elevated plasma glucose concentration with normal GFR and $\dot{T}m$ for glucose.
D. *Acute tubular necrosis* is a disease characterized by a decrease in GFR and extensive damage to tubules, leading to a *marked* reduction in $\dot{T}m$ for glucose.

12-23. Using the data in the table on the previous page, answer the following questions:

    A. The urine of which patient(s) gives a *positive test* for glucose? Enter patient(s)'s number(s) in the space provided _____.

    B. If you had to diagnose the renal function in these patients by clearance of para-aminohippurate (C_{PAH}), indicate your expected findings for each patient in the following table as deviations from normal (+ for increase, − for decrease, 0 for no change) for C_{PAH} and transport maximum for PAH ($\dot{Tm}_{PAH}$).

Patients	C_{PAH}	$\dot{Tm}_{PAH}$
1		
2		
3		
4		

    C. In which of these patients, if any, do you expect endogenous creatinine clearance (C_{Cr}) to be *least* and *most* reduced?
       (a) C_{Cr} is least reduced in _____.
       (b) C_{Cr} is most reduced in _____.

12-24. In each of the following circumstances, if you expect urine flow to increase, mark (+), if you expect it to decrease, mark (−), and if you expect no change to occur, mark (0).
    1. A rise in blood pressure at the glomerulus due to systemic hypertension. _____
    2. A marked decrease in the plasma protein concentration. _____
    3. An intravenous infusion of a large volume of an iso-oncotic solution (such as 6% dextran in normal saline). _____
    4. An intravenous injection of a large dose of ethacrynic acid. _____
    5. Consumption of three ounces of Old Kentuchy Bourbon. _____
    6. During a two-hour anesthesia for removal of an ovarian cyst. _____
    7. In congestive heart failure. _____
    8. An intravenous injection of isotonic saline sufficient to increase the renal medullary blood flow. _____
    9. A decrease in the active chloride transport in the thick ascending limb of the loop of Henle. _____
   10. In severe diarrhea. _____

12-25. For each of the five forcings listed in the table on Page 450 indicate deviation from normal (+ for increase; − for decrease; and 0 for no change), for the items listed in the table.

Forcings	Responses											
	V_E	V_C	$\overline{P}_{AS}$	$\overline{P}_{VS}$	GFR	$[Na]_p$	π_p	$[ADH]_p$	$[Ald]_p$	$\dot{V}_u$	C_{Na}	C_{H_2O}
1. Isotonic influx (e.g., edema)												
2. Hypotonic influx (e.g., water loading)												
3. Hypertonic influx												
4. Isotonic efflux (e.g., burns, hemorrhage)												
5. Hypotonic efflux (e.g., sweating)												

V_E = Extracellular fluid volume
V_C = Intracellular fluid volume
$\overline{P}_{AS}$ = Mean systemic arterial pressure
$\overline{P}_{VS}$ = Mean systemic venous pressure
GFR = Glomerular filtration rate
$[Na]_p$ = Plasma sodium concentration
π_p = Plasma protein oncotic pressure
$[ADH]_p$ = Plasma concentration of antidiuretic hormone
$[Ald]_p$ = Plasma concentration of aldosterone
$\dot{V}_u$ = Urine flow rate
C_{Na} = Sodium clearance
C_{H_2O} = Solute-free water clearance

REFERENCES

1. Abbrecht, P. H., and Vander, A. J.: Effects of chronic potassium deficiency on plasma renin activity. *J. Clin. Invest.* 49:1510-1516, 1970.

2. Ames, R. P., Borkowski, A. J., Sicinski, A. M., and Laragh, J. H.: Prolonged infusions of angiotensin II and norepinephrine and blood pressure, electrolyte balance, and aldosterone and cortisol secretion in normal man and in cirrhosis with ascites. *J. Clin. Invest.* 44:1171-1186, 1965.

3. Anderson, B.: Thirst and brain control of water balance. *Am. Scientist* 59:408-415, 1971.

4. Anderson, C. H., McCally, M., and Farrell, G. L.: The effects of atrial stretch on aldosterone secretion. *Endocrinology* 64:202-207, 1959.

5. Andrews, W. H. H., and Orbach, J.: Sodium receptors activating some nerves of perfused rabbit livers. *Am. J. Physiol.* 227:1273-1275, 1974.

6. Arndt, J. O., Reineck, H., and Gauer, O. H.: Ausscheidungsfunktion und Hämodynamik der Nieren bei Dehnung des linken Vorhofes am narkotisierten Hund. *Arch. Ges. Physiol.* 277:1-15, 1963.

7. Assaykeen, T. A., Clayton, P. L., Goldfien, A., and Ganong, W. F.: Effect of alpha- and beta-adrenergic blocking agents on the renin response to hypoglycemia and epinephrine in dogs. *Endocrinology* 87:1318-1322, 1970.

8. Ayers, C. R., Harris, R. H., Jr., and Lefer, L. G.: Control of renin release in experimental hypertension. *Circ. Res. 24 (Suppl. I)*:103-112, 1969.

9. Baisset, A., and Montastruc, P.: Polyurie par distension auriculaire chez le chien; role de l'hormone antidiuretique. *J. Physiol. Paris* 49:33-36, 1957.

10. Barajas, L., and Latta, H.: Structure of the juxtaglomerular apparatus. *Circ. Res. (Suppl. II) 20 and 21*:15-28, 1967.

11. Barajas, L.: Renin secretion: an anatomical basis for tubular control. *Science 172*:485-487, 1971.

12. Biron, P., Meyer, P., and Panisset, J. C.: Removal of angiotensins from the systemic circulation. *Can. J. Physiol. Pharmacol.* 46:175-178, 1968.

13. Blaine, E. H., Davis, J. O., and Witty, R. T.: Renin release after hemorrhage and after suprarenal aortic constriction in dogs without sodium delivery to the macula densa. *Circ. Res.* *27*:1081-1089, 1970.

14. Blaine, E. H., Davis, J. O., and Prewitt, R. L.: Evidence for a renal vascular receptor in control of renin secretion. *Am. J. Physiol.* *220*:1593-1597, 1971.

15. Blair-West, J. R., Coghlan, J. P., Denton, D. A., Goding, J. R., Munro, J. A., Peterson, P. E., and Wintour, M.: Hormonal stimulation of adrenal cortical secretion. *J. Clin. Invest.* *41*:1606-1627, 1962.

16. Bonjour, J. P., and Malvin, R. L.: Stimulation of ADH release by the renin-angiotensin system. *Am. J. Physiol.* *218*:1555-1559, 1970.

17. Braun-Menéndez, E., Fasciolo, J. C., Leloir, L. F., and Muñoz, J. M.: La substancia hipertensora de la sangre del riñon isquemiado. *Rev. Soc. Arg. Biol.* *15*:420-430, 1939.

18. Braun-Menéndez, E., Fasciolo, J. C., Leloir, L. F., Muñoz, J. M., and Taquini, A. C.: *Renal Hypertension* (translated by L. Dexter). Charles C Thomas, Springfield, Ill., 1946.

19. Bravo, E. L., Khosla, M. C., and Bumpus, F. M.: Vascular and adrenocortical responses to a specific antagonist of angiotensin II. *Am. J. Physiol.* *228*:110-114, 1975.

20. Brennan, L. A., Jr., Malvin, R. L., Jochim, K. E., and Roberts, D. E.: Influence of right and left atrial receptors on plasma concentrations of ADH and renin. *Am. J. Physiol.* *221*:273-278, 1971.

21. Bright, R.: Reports of medical cases selected with a view of illustrating the symptoms and cure of disease and by reference to morbid anatomy. Vol. 1. Longmans, Rees, and Company, London, 1827. Reprinted in Guy's Hospital Reports, *1*:338-400, 1836.

22. Brown, J. J., Davies, D. L., Lever, A. F., Lloyd, A. M., Robertson, J. I. S., and Tree, M.: A reninlike enzyme in normal human urine. *Lancet 2*:709-711, 1964.

23. Brown, J. J., Davies, D. L., Lever, A. F., and Robertson, J. I. S.: Plasma renin concentration in human hypertension. I. Relationship between renin, sodium, and potassium. *Brit. Med. J. 17*:144-148, 1965.

24. Brown, J. J., Davies, D. L., Lever, A. F., McPherson, D., and Robertson, J. I. S.: Plasma renin concentration in relation to changes in posture. *Clin. Sci. 30*:278-284, 1966.

25. Brunner, H. R., Baer, L., Sealey, J. E., Ledingham, J. G. G., and Laragh, J. H.: Influence of potassium administration and of potassium deprivation on plasma renin in normal and hypertensive subjects. *J. Clin. Invest. 49*:2128-2138, 1970.

26. Bumpus, F. M., Schwarz, H., and Page, I. H.: Synthesis and pharmacology of the octapeptide angiotonin. *Science 125*:886-887, 1957.

27. Bunag, R. D., Page, I. H., and McCubbin, J. W.: Neural stimulation of release of renin. *Circ. Res. 19*:851-858, 1966.

28. Carpenter, C. C. J., Davis, J. O., and Ayers, C. R.: Relation of renin, angiotensin II and experimental renal hypertension to aldosterone secretion. *J. Clin. Invest. 40*:2026-2042, 1961.

29. Coleridge, J. C., Hemingway, A., Holmes, R., and Linden, R. J.: The location of atrial receptors in the dog: a physiological and histological study. *J. Physiol., London 136*:174-196, 1957.

30. Cooke, C. R., Brown, T. C., Zacherle, B. J., and Walker, W. G.: Effect of altered sodium concentration in the distal nephron segments on renin release. *J. Clin. Invest. 49*:1630-1638, 1970.

31. Coote, J. H., Johns, E. J., Macleod, V. H., and Singer, B.: Effect of renal nerve stimulation, renal blood flow and adrenergic blockade on plasma renin activity in the cat. *J. Physiol. 226*:15-36, 1972.

32. Coppage, W. S., Jr., Island, D. P., Cooner, A. E., and Liddle, G. W.: The metabolism of aldosterone in normal subjects and in patients with hepatic cirrhosis. *J. Clin. Invest. 41*:1672-1680, 1962.

33. Davis, J. O.: The control of aldosterone secretion. *Physiologist 5*:65-86, 1962.

34. Davis, J. O.: The control of renin release. *Am. J. Med. 55*:333-350, 1973.

35. Davis, J. O., Carpenter, C. C. J., Ayers, C., and Bahn, R.: Relation of anterior pituitary function to aldosterone and corticosterone secretion in conscious dogs. *Am. J. Physiol. 199*:212-216, 1960.

36. Davis, J. O., Hartroft, P. M., Titus, E. O., Carpenter, C. C. J., Ayers, C. R., and Spiegel, H. E.: The role of the renin-angiotensin system in the control of aldosterone secretion. *J. Clin. Invest.* *41*:378-379, 1962.

37. DeBono, E., Lee, G. de J., Mottram, F. R., Pickering, G. W., Brown, J. J., Keen, H., Peart, W. S., and Sanderson, P. H.: The action of angiotensin in man. *Clin. Sci.* *25*:123-157, 1963.

38. Durham, R. M., and Novin, D.: Slow potential changes due to osmotic stimuli in supraoptic nucleus of the rabbit. *Am. J. Physiol.* *219*:293-298, 1970.

39. Eide, I., Løyning, E., and Kiil, F.: Evidence for hemodynamic autoregulation of renin release. *Circ. Res.* *32*:237-245, 1973.

40. Elliott, D. F., and Peart, W. S.: Amino acid sequence in a hypertensin. *Biochem. J.* *65*:246-254, 1957.

41. Gauer, O. H., and Henry, J. P.: Circulatory basis of fluid volume control. *Physiol. Rev.* *43*:423-481, 1963.

42. Gauer, O. H., Henry, J. P., and Behn, C.: The regulation of extracellular fluid volume. *Ann. Rev. Physiol.* *32*:547-595, 1970.

43. Gaunt, R., Birnie, J. H., and Eversole, W. J.: Adrenal cortex and water metabolism. *Physiol. Rev.* *29*:281-310, 1949.

44. Genest, J., Biron, P., Koiw, E., Nowaczynski, W., Chrétien, M., and Boucher, R.: Adrenocortical hormones in human hypertension and their relation to angiotensin. *Circ. Res.* *9*:775-791, 1961.

45. Gocke, D. J., Gerter, J., Sherwood, L. M., and Laragh, J. H.: Physiological and pathological variations of plasma angiotensin II in man. Correlation with renin activity and sodium balance. *Circ. Res. 24 (Suppl. I)*:131-146, 1969.

46. Goldblatt, H.: Studies in experimental hypertension: production of the malignant phase of hypertension. *J. Exp. Med.* *67*:809-826, 1938.

47. Goldblatt, H., Katz, Y. J., Lewis, H. A., and Richardson, E.: Studies on experimental hypertension. XX. The bioassay of renin. *J. Exp. Med.* *77*:309-314, 1943.

48. Goodfriend, T. L., and Lin, S.-Y.: Receptors for angiotensin I and II. *Circ. Res. 27 (Suppl. I)*:163-174, 1970.

49. Goormaghtigh, N.: *La fonction endocrine des artèrioles renales.* Librarie Fonteyn, Louvain, 1944.

50. Goormaghtigh, N.: Facts in favor of an endocrine function of renal arterioles. *J. Pathol. Bacteriol.* *57*:392-393, 1945.

51. Gordon, R. D., Kuchel, O., Liddle, G. W., and Island, D. P.: Role of the sympathetic nervous system in regulating renin and aldosterone production in man. *J. Clin. Invest.* *46*:599-605, 1967.

52. Gordon, R. D., and Pawsey, C. G. K.: Relative effects of serum sodium concentration and the state of body fluid balance on renin secretion. *J. Clin. Endocrin.* *32*:117-119, 1971.

53. Granger, P., Dalheim, H., and Thurau, K.: Enzyme activities of the single juxtaglomerular apparatus in the rat kidney. *Kidney International* *1*:78-88, 1972.

54. Gross, F.: The renin-angiotensin system and hypertension. *Ann. Internal Med.* *75*:777-787, 1971.

55. Gupta, P. D., Henry, J. P., Sinclair, R., and Von Baumgarten, R.: Responses of atrial and aortic baroreceptors to nonhypotensive hemorrhage and to transfusion. *Am. J. Physiol.* *211*:1429-1437, 1966.

56. Haberich, F. J.: Osmoregulation in the portal circulation. *Fed. Proc.* *27*:1137-1141, 1968.

57. Heacox, R., Harvey, A. M., and Vander, A. J.: Hepatic inactivation of renin. *Circ. Res.* *21*:149-152, 1967.

58. Henry, J. P., Gauer, O. H., and Reeves, J. L.: Evidence of the atrial location of receptors influencing urine flow. *Circ. Res.* *4*:85-90, 1956.

59. Henry, J. P., and Pearce, J. W.: The possible role of cardiac atrial stretch receptors in the induction of changes in urine flow. *J. Physiol., London* *131*:572-585, 1956.

60. Henry, J. P., Gupta, P. D., Heehan, J. P., Sinclair, R., and Share, L.: The role of afferents from the low-pressure system in the release of antidiuretic hormone during non-hypotensive hemorrhage. *Can. J. Physiol. Pharmacol.* *46*:287-295, 1968.

61. Heymans, C., and Neil, E.: *Reflexogenic Areas of the Cardiovascular System.* Little, Brown and Co., Boston, 1958.

62. Hodge, R. L., Lowe, R. D., and Vane, J. R.: The effects of alteration of blood volume on the concentration of circulating angiotensin in anesthetized dogs. *J. Physiol., London* *185*:613-626, 1966.

63. Huggins, C. G., and Thampi, N. S.: A simple method for the determination of angiotensin I converting enzyme. *Life Sci.* 7:633-639, 1968.

64. Huggins, C. G., Corcoran, R. J., Gordon, J. S., Henry, H. W., and John, J. P.: Kinetics of the plasma and lung angiotensin I converting enzymes. *Circ. Res.* 27 *(Suppl. I)*:93-108, 1970.

65. Jewell, P. A.: The occurrence of vasiculated neurons in the hypothalamus of the dog. *J. Physiol., London 121*:167-181, 1963.

66. Jewell, P. A., and Verney, E. B.: An experimental attempt to determine the site of the neurohypophyseal osmoreceptors in the dog. *Trans. Roy. Soc. London 240*:197-324, 1957.

67. Johnson, J. A., Moore, W. W., and Segar, W. E.: Small changes in left atrial pressure and plasma antidiuretic hormone titers in dogs. *Am. J. Physiol.* 217:210-214, 1969.

68. Johnson, J. A., Zehr, J. E., and Moore, W. W.: Effects of separate and concurrent osmotic and volume stimuli on plasma ADH in sheep. *Am. J. Physiol.* 218:1273-1280, 1970.

69. Johnson, J. A., Davis, J. O., and Witty, R. J.: Effects of catecholamines and renal nerve stimulation on renin secretion in the non-filtering kidney. *Circ. Res.* 29:646-653, 1971.

70. Karim, E., Kidd, C., Malpus, C. W., and Penna, P. E.: Effects of stimulation of the left atrial receptors on sympathetic efferent nerve fibres. *J. Physiol., London 213*:38P-39P, 1971.

71. Khairallah, P. A., Bumpus, F. M., Page, I. H., and Smeby, R. R.: Angiotensinase with a high degree of specificity in plasma and red cells. *Science 140*:672-674, 1963.

72. Korner, P. I.: Integrative neural cardiovascular control. *Physiol. Rev. 51*:312-367, 1971.

73. Koushanpour, E., and McGee, J. P.: Effect of mean pressure on carotid sinus baroreceptor response to pulsatile pressure. *Am. J. Physiol. 216*:559-603, 1969.

74. Laragh, J. H., Angers, M., Kelly, W. G., and Lieberman, S.: Hypotensive agents and pressor substances. The effect of epinephrine, norepinephrine, angiotensin II and others on the secretory rate of aldosterone in man. *J.A.M.A. 174*:234-240, 1960.

75. Laragh, J. H., Sealey, J. E., and Sommers, S. C.: Patterns of adrenal secretion and urinary excretion of aldosterone and plasma renin activity in normal and hypertensive subjects. *Circ. Res. 18 (Suppl. I)*:158-174, 1966.

76. Laragh, J. H., and Sealey, J. E.: The renin-angiotensin-aldosterone hormonal system and regulation of sodium, potassium, and blood pressure homeostasis. In: *Handbook of Physiology*. Sec. 8, *Renal Physiology*, edited by J. Orloff and R. W. Berliner. Washington, D.C., American Physiological Society, 1973, pp. 831-908.

77. Ledingham, J. G. G., Bull, M. B., and Laragh, J. H.: The meaning of aldosteronism in hypertensive disease. *Circ. Res. 21 (Suppl. II)*:177-186, 1967.

78. Lee, M. R.: *Renin and Hypertension; A Modern Synthesis*. Lloyd-Luke, Ltd., London, 1969.

79. Loeffler, J. R., Stockigt, J. R., and Ganong, W. F.: Effect of alpha and beta-adrenergic blocking agents on the increase in renin secretion produced by stimulation of the renal nerves. *Neuroendocrinology 10*:129-138, 1972.

80. Lydtin, H., and Hamilton, W. F.: Effect of acute changes in left atrial pressure on urine flow in unanesthetized dogs. *Am. J. Physiol. 207*:530-536, 1964.

81. McGiff, J. C., and Itskovitz, H. D.: Loss of renal vasoconstrictor activity of angiotensin II during renal ischemia. *J. Clin. Invest. 43*:2359-2367, 1964.

82. McKenzie, J. K., Lee, M. R., and Cook, W. F.: Effect of hemorrhage on arterial plasma renin activity in the rabbit. *Circ. Res. 19*:269-273, 1966.

83. Meyer, P., Menard, J., Papanicolaou, N., Alexandre, J. M., Devaux, C., and Milliez, P.: Mechanism of renin release following furosemide diuresis in rabbit. *Am. J. Physiol. 215*:908-915, 1968.

84. Michelakis, A. M., Caudle, J., and Liddle, G. W.: In vitro stimulation of renin production by epinephrine, norepinephrine, and cyclic AMP. *Proc. Soc. Exp. Biol. Med. 130*:748-753, 1969.

85. Mogil, R. A., Itskovitz, H. D., Russell, J. H., and Murphy, J. J.: Renal innervation and renin activity in salt metabolism and hypertension. *Am. J. Physiol. 216*:693-696, 1969.

86. Moore, W. W.: Antidiuretic hormone levels in normal subjects. *Fed. Proc. 30*:1387-1394, 1971.

87. Morgan, T.: A microperfusion study of influence of macula densa on glomerular filtration rate. *Am. J. Physiol. 220*:186-190, 1971.

88. Moses, A. M., and Miller, M.: Osmotic threshold for vasopressin release as determined by saline infusion and by dehydration. *Neuroendocrinology* 7:219-226, 1971.

89. Mouw, D., Bonjour, J. P., Malvin, R. L., and Vander, A. J.: Central action of angiotensin in stimulating ADH release. *Am. J. Physiol. 220*:239-242, 1971.

90. Müller, J., and Barajas, L.: Electron microscopic and histochemical evidence for a tubular innervation in the renal cortex of the monkey. *J. Ultrastr. Res. 41*:533-549, 1972.

91. Nash, F. D., Rostorfer, H. H., Bailie, M. D., Wathen, R. L., and Schneider, E. G.: Renin release: relation to renal sodium load and dissociation from hemodynamic changes. *Circ. Res. 22*:473-487, 1968.

92. Newsome, H. H., and Bartter, F. C.: Plasma renin activity in relation to serum sodium concentration and body fluid balance. *J. Clin. Endocrin. 28*:1704-1711, 1968.

93. Ng, K. K. F., and Vane, J. R.: Fate of angiotensin I in the circulation. *Nature 218*:144-150, 1968.

94. Niijima, A.: Afferent discharges from osmoreceptors in the liver of the guinea pig. *Science 166*:1519-1520, 1969.

95. Oparil, S., Sanders, C. A., and Haber, E.: In vivo and in vitro conversion of angiotensin I to angiotensin II in dog blood. *Circ. Res. 26*:591-599, 1970.

96. Page, I. H.: On the nature of the pressor action of renin. *J. Exp. Med. 70*:521-542, 1939.

97. Page, I. H., and McCubbin, J. W. (eds.): *Renal Hypertension.* Year Book Publishers, Inc., Chicago, 1968.

98. Passo, S. S., Assaykeen, T. A., Otsuka, K., Wise, B. L., Goldfien, A., and Ganong, W. F.: Effect of stimulation of the medulla oblongata on renin secretion in dogs. *Neuroendocrinology* 7:1-10, 1971.

99. Passo, S. S., Thornborough, J. R., and Rothballer, A. B.: Hepatic receptors in control of sodium excretion in anesthetized cats. *Am. J. Physiol. 224*:373-375, 1973.

100. Peart, W. S.: Renin-angiotensin system. *New Eng. J. Med. 292*:302-306, 1975.

101. Perlmutt, J. H.: Reflex antidiuresis after occlusion of common carotid arteries in hydrated dogs. *Am. J. Physiol.* *204*:197-201, 1963.

102. Pickens, P. T., Bumpus, F. M., Lloyd, A. M., Smeby, R. R., and Page, I. H.: Measurement of renin activity in human plasma. *Circ. Res. 17*:438-448, 1965.

103. Schneider, E. G., Davis, J. O., Baumber, J. S., and Johnson, J. A.: The hepatic metabolism of renin and aldosterone. *Circ. Res. 27 (Suppl. I)*:175-183, 1970.

104. Schneider, E. G., Lynch, R. E., Willis, L. R., and Knox, F. G.: The effect of potassium infusion on proximal sodium reabsorption and renin release in the dog. *Kidney International 2*:197-202, 1972.

105. Schnermann, J., Wright, F. S., Davis, J. M., v. Stackelberg, W., and Grill, G.: Regulation of superficial nephron filtration rate by tubuloglomerular feedback. *Arch. Ges. Physiol. 318*:147-175, 1970.

106. Sealey, J. E., Gerten-Banes, J., and Laragh, J. H.: The renin system: variations in man measured by radioimmunoassay or bioassay. *Kidney International 1*:240-253, 1972.

107. Sealey, J. E., Clark, I., Bull, M. B., and Laragh, J. H.: Potassium balance and the control of renin secretion. *J. Clin. Invest. 49*:2119-2127, 1970.

108. Segar, W. F., and Moore, W. W.: The regulation of antidiuretic hormone release in man. I. Effect of changes in position and ambient temperature on blood ADH levels. *J. Clin. Invest. 47*:2143-2151, 1968.

109. Shade, R. E., Davis, J. O., Johnson, J. A., and Witty, R. T.: Effects of renal arterial infusion of sodium and potassium on renin secretion in the dog. *Circ. Res. 31*:719-727, 1972.

110. Shade, R. E., Davis, J. O., Johnson, J. A., Gotshall, R. W., and Spielman, W. S.: Mechanism of action of angiotensin II and antidiuretic hormone on renin secretion. *Am. J. Physiol. 224*:926-929, 1973.

111. Shade, R. E., and Share, L.: Vasopressin release during nonhypotensive hemorrhage and angiotensin II infusion. *Am. J. Physiol. 228*:149-154, 1975.

112. Share, L.: Effects of carotid occlusion and left atrial distention on plasma vasopressin titer. *Am. J. Physiol. 208*:219-223, 1965.

113. Share, L.: Role of peripheral receptors in the increased release of vasopressin in response to hemorrhage. *Endocrinology 81*:1140-1146, 1967.

114. Share, L., and Levy, M. N.: Cardiovascular receptors and blood titer of antidiuretic hormone. *Am. J. Physiol. 203*:425-428, 1962.

115. Share, L., and Levy, M. N.: Carotid sinus pulse, a determinant of plasma antidiuretic hormone concentration. *Am. J. Physiol. 211*:721-724, 1966.

116. Share, L., and Travis, R. H.: Interrelations between the adrenal cortex and the posterior pituitary. *Fed. Proc. 30*:1378-1382, 1971.

117. Share, L., and Claybaugh, J. R.: Regulation of body fluids. *Ann. Rev. Physiol. 34*:235-260, 1972.

118. Shimizu, K., Share, L., and Claybaugh, J. R.: Potentiation of angiotensin II of the vasopressin response to increasing plasma osmolality. *Endocrinology 93*:42-50, 1973.

119. Shu'ayb, W. A., Moran, W. H., and Zimmerman, B.: Studies of the mechanism of antidiuretic hormone secretion and post-commissurotomy dilutional syndrome. *Ann. Surg. 162*:690-701, 1965.

120. Skeggs, L. T., Jr., Lentz, K. E., Kahn, J. R., Shumway, N. P., and Woods, K. R.: Amino acid sequence of hypertensin II. *J. Exp. Med. 104*:193-197, 1956.

121. Skeggs, L. T., Lentz, K. E., Hochstrasser, H., and Kahn, J. R.: The chemistry of renin substrate. *Can. Med. Assoc. J. 90*:185-189, 1964.

122. Skinner, S. L., McCubbin, J. W., and Page, I. H.: Renal baroreceptor control of acute renin release in normotensive, nephrogenic, and neurogenic hypertensive dogs. *Circ. Res. 15*:522-531, 1963.

123. Skinner, S. L., McCubbin, J. W., and Page, I. H.: Control of renin secretion. *Circ. Res. 15*:64-76, 1964.

124. Stitzer, S. O., and Malvin, R. L.: Right atrium and renal sodium excretion. *Am. J. Physiol. 228*:184-190, 1975.

125. Stricker, E. M.: Osmoregulation and volume regulation in rats: inhibition of hypovolemic thirst by water. *Am. J. Physiol. 217*:98-105, 1969.

126. Tagawa, H., Vander, A. J., Bonjour, J. P., and Malvin, R. L.: Inhibition of renin secretion by vasopressin in unanesthetized sodium-deprived dogs. *Am. J. Physiol. 220*:949-951, 1971.

127. Tait, J. F., Tait, S. A. S., Little, B., and Laumas, K. R.: The disappearance of 7-H^3-d-aldosterone in the plasma of normal subjects. *J. Clin. Invest. 40*:72-80, 1961.

128. Taquini, A. C., Blaquier, P., and Taquini, A. C., Jr.: On the production and role of renin. *Can. Med. Assoc. J. 90*:210-213, 1964.

129. Thurau, K., Schnermann, J., Nagel, W., Horster, M., and Wohl, M.: Composition of tubular fluid in the macula densa segment as a factor regulating the function of the juxtaglomerular apparatus. *Circ. Res. 21 (Suppl. II)*:79-89, 1967.

130. Thurau, K., Dahlheim, H., Grüner, A., Mason, J., and Granger, P.: Activation of renin in the single juxtaglomerular apparatus by sodium chloride in the tubular fluid at the macula densa. *Circ. Res. 31 (Suppl. II)*:182-186, 1972.

131. Tigerstedt, R., and Bergman, P. G.: Niere und Krieslauf. *Skand. Arch. Physiol. 8*:223-271, 1898.

132. Tobian, L., Tomboullan, A., and Janecek, J.: Effect of high perfusion pressures on the granulations of juxtaglomerular cells in an isolated kidney. *J. Clin. Invest. 38*:605-610, 1959.

133. Tobian, L.: Interrelationship of electrolytes, juxtaglomerular cells and hypertension. *Physiol. Rev. 40*:280-312, 1960.

134. Tobian, L.: Sodium, renal arterial distention and the juxtaglomerular apparatus. *Can. Med. Assoc. J. 90*:160-162, 1964.

135. Vander, A. J.: Effect of catecholamines and the renal nerves on renin secretion in anesthetized dogs. *Am. J. Physiol. 209*:659-662, 1965.

136. Vander, A. J.: Control of renin release. *Physiol. Rev. 47*:359-382, 1967.

137. Vander, A. J.: Direct effects of potassium on renin secretion and renal function. *Am. J. Physiol. 219*:455-459, 1970.

138. Vander, A. J., and Miller, R.: Control of renin secretion in the anesthetized dog. *Am. J. Physiol. 207*:537-546, 1964.

139. Vander, A. J., and Luciano, J. R.: Effects of mercurial diuresis and acute sodium depletion on renin release in dog. *Am. J. Physiol. 212*:651-656, 1967.

140. Vander, A. J., and Carlson, J.: Mechanism of the effects of furosemide on renin secretion in anesthetized dogs. *Circ. Res.* 25:145-152, 1969.

141. Verney, E. B.: The antidiuretic hormone and the factors which determine its release. *Proc. Roy. Soc., London, Ser. B.* 135:25-106, 1947.

142. Volhard, F., and Fahr, T.: *Die Brightsche Nierenkranheit: Klinik, Pathologie und Atlas.* Springer, Berlin, 1914.

143. Watts, D. T., and Westfall, V.: Studies on peripheral blood catecholamine levels during hemorrhagic shock in dogs. *Proc. Soc. Exp. Biol. Med.* 115:601-604, 1964.

144. Winer, N., Chokshi, D. S., Yoon, M. S., and Freedman, A. D.: Adrenergic receptor mediation of renin secretion. *J. Clin. Endocrin.* 29:1168-1175, 1969.

145. Winer, N., Chokshi, D. S., and Walkenhorst, W. G.: Effects of cyclic AMP, sympathomimetic amines and adrenergic receptor antagonists on renin secretion. *Circ. Res.* 29:239-248, 1971.

146. Witty, R. T., Davis, J. O., Johnson, J. A., and Prewitt, R. L.: Effects of papaverine and hemorrhage on renin secretion in the nonfiltering kidney. *Am. J. Physiol.* 221:1666-1671, 1971.

147. Zehr, J. E., Johnson, J. A., and Moore, W. W.: Left atrial pressure, plasma osmolality and ADH levels in the unanesthetized ewe. *Am. J. Physiol.* 217:1672-1680, 1969.

Chapter 13

PATHOPHYSIOLOGY OF RENAL FUNCTION IN DISEASE

This chapter is an attempt to provide the physiological bases for the etiology, clinical manifestations, and rationale for the therapeutic management of some of the most frequently encountered primary and secondary renal diseases that compromise normal renal function, based on the knowledge and the concepts developed in the preceding chapters. Because this is a textbook of physiology, the discussion of these diseases must by necessity be brief. For a more detailed treatment of the clinical aspects of these diseases, the interested reader may wish to consult the references cited at the end of this chapter and other excellent textbooks on renal diseases.

Classification of Renal Diseases

Disturbances in the normal renal function may result from either a primary renal disease or a nonrenal systemic disease which secondarily compromises the normal renal function. Of course, this does not preclude the possibility that a patient may have both renal and nonrenal systemic diseases, or a combination of diseases. For the purpose of this presentation, the major renal and nonrenal systemic diseases affecting renal function may be classified into three general categories (Table 13-1): *First*, those diseases that affect primarily the *renal parenchyma*. For convenience, they may be subdivided, in accordance with the two components of the nephron, into those affecting the *glomeruli*, such as *glomerulonephritis* and *nephrotic syndrome*, and those affecting the *tubules*, such as *toxic nephropathy, transfusion reactions, nephrogenic diabetes insipidus,* and *renal tubular acidosis*. The *second* category includes those diseases that affect primarily the *urinary tract*, such as *obstructive uropathy* and *pyelonephritis*. And *third*, there are those nonrenal systemic diseases which secondarily affect renal function, such as *renovascular*

TABLE 13-1

A Simplified Classification of the Major
Renal and Systemic Diseases Affecting Renal Function

I.   Primary Renal Parenchymal Diseases
     A.   Glomerular Diseases
          1.   Glomerulonephritis
               a.   Acute
               b.   Chronic
          2.   Nephrotic Syndrome
     B.   Tubular Diseases
          1.   Acquired Tubular Diseases
               a.   Toxic nephropathy
               b.   Renal ischemia
               c.   Transfusion reactions
          2.   Inherited Tubular Disorders
               a.   Nephrogenic diabetes insipidus
               b.   Renal tubular acidosis
               c.   Specific tubular disorders

 II.   Diseases of the Urinary Tract
       A.   Obstructive Uropathy
       B.   Pyelonephritis

III.   Systemic Diseases and Renal Function
       A.   Renovascular Hypertension
       B.   Congestive Heart Failure
       C.   Liver Cirrhosis

 IV.   Renal Failure
       A.   Acute
       B.   Chronic

---

hypertension, congestive heart failure, and *liver cirrhosis.* Since
all three classes of diseases mentioned, in one form or another,
produce a variable reduction in renal mass and hence in renal
function, they could also lead to various degrees of *renal failure.*
Therefore, to underscore this potentiality, renal failure is placed
at the end of Table 13-1, and will be discussed in some detail
following the sections on diseases in this chapter. To facilitate
presentation, for each disease we shall briefly describe its etiology,
the major pathological and clinical findings, as well as the known
physiological bases for these findings. Also, when appropriate, the
rationale for the management and therapy will be given. Finally, we
will conclude this chapter with a brief discussion of the
physiological basis of azotemia and clinical tests for evaluating
renal function.

I. Primary Renal Parenchymal Diseases

As shown in Table 13-1, the major diseases that affect renal parenchyma may be classified as those that impair either glomerular or tubular functions. Although, in some circumstances, a particular disease may spread from the glomerular to the tubular component of the nephron or vice versa, for convenience of presentation, we shall describe the etiology and clinical manifestations of each separately.

A. GLOMERULAR DISEASES

As shown in Table 13-1, there are two general types of renal diseases that impair glomerular function. They are (1) *glomerulonephritis* and (2) *nephrotic syndrome*.

1. GLOMERULONEPHRITIS

As the name implies, *glomerulonephritis* refers to an inflammatory disease that affects primarily the glomeruli. If the inflammation is widespread, the disease is called *diffuse glomerulonephritis*. The most common cause of diffuse glomerulonephritis is *streptococcal infection*. On the other hand, if the inflammation is localized, so that only some of the glomeruli are involved, the disease is called *focal glomerulonephritis*. The most common cause of focal glomerulonephritis is *bacterial endocarditis*.

Like most other renal diseases, clinical manifestations of the glomerulonephritis depend on the severity of the disease and on whether the disease is in the *acute* or *chronic* stage. Although the prognosis is good, 1 to 3% of the patients die during the acute phase as a result of *hypertensive encephalopathy*, and fewer than 1% develop chronic glomerulonephritis.

A. ACUTE GLOMERULONEPHRITIS. This disease, also called *hemorrhagic Bright's disease* or *post-infectious hemorrhagic nephritis*, is an inflammatory disease that generally occurs in children. It follows some 4 to 12 days after onset of infection with a nephritogenic strain (of which types 12 and 47 account for about 95% of all cases) of group A β-hemolytic streptococcus. Males are affected twice as often as females.

Pathogenesis of Acute Glomerulonephritis. Although the precise *etiology* remains to be elucidated, recent studies (Dixon, 1968; Wilson and Dixon, 1973; Zabriskie et al., 1973) suggest that glomerulonephritis is the result of immunologically induced morphological changes in the glomerular capillaries, mediated by two different mechanisms. One mechanism involves formation of antibodies which react with the *glomerular basement membrane* (GBM) antigens. The other mechanism involves formation of antibodies which react with *nonglomerular antigens*. In both cases, the antigen-antibody complexes formed act as *nephritogenic* "toxic compounds" which are deposited in the glomerular capillary lumen. Although clinical manifestations of

the glomerulonephritis caused by either mechanism are indistinguish-
able, the two mechanisms produce distinct morphological changes in the
glomerular capillaries. The anti-GBM antibody induces antigen-
antibody complexes which are deposited in a uniform and regular
pattern on the inner aspect of the glomerular basement membrane.
In severe cases, the antigen-antibody reaction may cause separation
of the endothelial cells from the thickened GBM. On the other hand,
the antigen-antibody complexes induced from the nonglomerular
antibodies are deposited as discrete, irregular, and lumpy granules
on the outer aspect of the glomerular basement membrane beneath the
epithelial cells. Available morphological and immunological evidence
strongly supports the view that the pathogenesis of *poststreptococcal
glomerulonephritis* is mediated by the deposition of nonglomerular
antigen-antibody complexes which induce characteristic pathologic
proliferative changes in the glomeruli. Thus, infection, serving
as the antigen, stimulates antibody formation. In the circulation,
the antigen-antibody reaction leads to the formation of nephritogenic
"toxic compounds," which secondarily stimulate *complement* (a lytic
substance that combines with the antigen-antibody complex and produces
lysis) activation. This in turn causes the release of *mediators*, such
as *anaphylatoxin* and *histamine*, which lead to the deposition of the
antigen-antibody complexes in the wall of the glomerular capillary as
the focus of the inflammatory process. The inflammatory process,
which affects both kidneys, though it is initially confined to the
glomeruli, may spread to the tubules as the disease progresses to the
chronic stage.

Histopathological and physiological studies (Metcoff, 1967) have
revealed that the inflammatory process results in extensive damage to
the glomerular capillary, markedly reducing its lumen and filtering
surface, increasing its permeability to large molecules (e.g.,
proteins), and causing a generalized increase in the permeability
of capillaries throughout the body.

As shown in Figure 5-2, the *endothelial cells* lining the
glomerular capillary lumen are separated from the *capsular* (Bowman's)
epithelial cells by the thick *basement membrane*. The *mesangial cells*
(not shown in the figure) lie in the interstitial space, which is
located between the capillary endothelial cells and the basement
membrane. Microscopic examination of the renal tissues obtained from
renal biopsy and from postmortem specimens has shown that the
inflammatory process leads to excessive proliferation of all three
glomerular cell types, especially the mesangial cells. Depending on
the severity of the disease, the mesangial cells proliferate and lay
down thin layers of matrix, thereby increasing the size of the
mesangial space at the expense of the glomerular capillary lumen.
Additionally, the epithelial cells may swell and exhibit focal
proliferation, commonly referred to as the *cellular crescents*. There
is also swelling of the glomerular capillary tuft, due to proliferation
of the capillary endothelium. Also present are considerable number of
polymorphonuclear leukocytes in the capillary lumen. The net effect
is a marked reduction in the capillary lumen and in the surface
available for filtration, which together are responsible for the

reduced glomerular filtration rate. These morphological changes
are reversible, especially in children, since they heal and recover
completely.

Physiological Bases of Clinical Symptoms. The sequence of
pathological changes in the structure of the glomerular capillaries
mentioned above induces marked alterations in the glomerular function.
Clinically, the most common symptoms are proteinuria, hematuria,
leukocyturia, and elevated blood urea nitrogen (BUN) or azotemia,
accompanied by variable degrees of oliguria (diminished urine output),
edema, and hypertension. The physiological explanations for these
blood and urinary abnormalities are as follows.

As mentioned in Chapter 5 and depicted in Figure 5-1, the
glomerular filtration rate depends on (1) the effective filtration
pressure (ΔP_f), (2) the permeability of the glomerular ultrafilter
(K_g), and (3) the glomerular capillary surface area available for
filtration. As mentioned above, the inflammation-induced
proliferation of the glomerular cells, along with intercapillary
accumulation of polymorphonuclear leukocytes, diminishes the
capillary lumen and surface area for filtration, thereby reducing
the glomerular filtration rate. The reduction in GFR decreases the
filtered load of all the solutes normally filtered, thus resulting
in azotemia and elevated BUN levels.

Another inflammation-induced change in the glomerular function
is the increase in the capillary permeability. This allows substances
with large molecular weight, particularly proteins, to pass into the
glomerular filtrate. Despite the reduction in GFR, this increase in
the protein permeability increases the filtered load of the proteins
to such an extent that filtered load exceeds tubular reabsorption.
The net effect is the excretion of protein in the urine, and hence
the observed moderated *proteinuria* (more than 1 to 2 g/day).

A corollary event associated with these inflammatory reactions
is the rupture of the glomerular capillary membrane. This allows the
red and white blood cells to pass into the glomerular filtrate. Their
subsequent excretion in the urine is the cause of observed
leukocyturia and *hematuria* (due to release of hemoglobin from red
cells). The latter is responsible for the darkish color of the
excreted urine. In addition to proteinuria and hematuria, numerous
granular and hyaline casts are found in the urine. All of these
urinary changes presumably represent the leakage of materials through
the imperfect glomeruli, and their subsequent concentration as they
pass through the tubules.

Clearance studies (Earle et al., 1944) have shown that the early
phase of the disease is characterized by a marked reduction in GFR
with a lesser decrease in renal plasma flow (RPF). Furthermore,
measurement of RPF by PAH clearance (Bradley et al., 1950) has
revealed a distinct increase in renal blood flow above normal
(hyperemia), a finding consistent with the inflammatory cause of
the glomerulonephritis. In addition, the observed reduction in Tm
for both PAH and Diodrast (Earle et al., 1944; Bradley et al., 1950)
suggests presence of moderate tubular damage. However, the extent
and consequence of the tubular damage are not as serious compared to
the induced glomerular damage.

The reduced GFR results in excessive renal reabsorption of salt and water, and hence edema formation, accompanied by oliguria. The onset of edema formation stems from a variety of physiological changes occurring at the *renal* and *systemic* circulation levels.

At the renal level, as described in Chapter 8, the reduced GFR will increase the tubular transit time for the glomerular filtrate, a factor which enhances the renal tubular reabsorption of salt and water and diminishes urine output *(oliguria)*. This will cause a transient rise in the *volume* and a transient fall in the plasma protein concentration (due to dilution), and hence a reduced plasma *protein oncotic pressure* of the blood returning to the heart.

At the systemic level, the transient rise in the blood volume (and hence in the venous return) leads to a transient increase in the systemic arterial blood pressure, and consequently in the hydrostatic pressure at the systemic capillaries (P_C). The increase in P_C, coupled with the decrease in the protein oncotic pressure in the systemic circulation and in the capillaries (π_C) as well, by the mechanisms described in Chapter 3 (Fig. 3-3), leads to outward filtration of fluid from the capillary into the interstitial space, and therefore the development of systemic edema. The development of edema is further exacerbated by the proteinuria and the continuous exudation of the plasma proteins into the interstitial space, caused by a marked increase in the capillary permeability to proteins consequent to a generalized *vasculitis*. The latter may in part be a consequence of deranged sodium metabolism manifested by the systemic edema, a condition also characteristics of the malignant phase of hypertension (Gavras et al., 1975).

The continuous outward filtration of fluid and proteins into the interstitial space not only precipitates the development of edema, but also leads to a *decrease* in the "effective" circulating blood volume. The latter causes a reduction in the cardiac output, and hence of the renal blood flow. The resulting decrease in the renal perfusion pressure will stimulate the baroreceptor component of the juxtaglomerular apparatus (Fig. 12-6), leading to the release of renin and subsequent formation of angiotensin II and stimulation of aldosterone secretion *(secondary aldosteronism)*. The consequent increase in the blood levels of aldosterone will enhance isotonic sodium reabsorption from the distal and collecting tubules. This, by the mechanism just described, will eventually lead to further outward filtration of fluid and proteins into the extravascular spaces, and hence to further edema. This vicious cycle continues until a new equilibrium for the distribution of fluid between the intra- and extravascular compartments is reached.

In addition to the development of edema, patients with acute glomerulonephritis frequently have an elevated arterial blood pressure *(hypertension)*. Since clearance measurements in these patients (Bradley et al., 1950) have shown that renal plasma flow decreases somewhat less than the GFR, the development of the arterial hypertension must be due to factors other than the reduced renal blood flow and the renin-angiotensin system. It has been suggested that reduced clearance of some "pressor" agents, as a result of the reduced GFR, might be a contributing factor for the development of hypertension.

The hypertension of variable degree found in the majority of patients with acute glomerulonephritis suggests possible vascular spasm, either from direct vascular changes or from the renal pressor substances (renin-angiotensin system) released by the diseased kidneys. In about 5% of cases the hypertension can be so severe as to cause *hypertensive encephalopathy* and death.

Clinical Management of Acute Glomerulonephritis. Treatment of the acute glomerulonephritis is directed toward the control of the pathophysiological complications of the disease. This includes management of hypertension and edema by control of the diet and administration of drugs. Hypertension can be controlled by restricting dietary salt intake, and, if severe, by judicious administration of antihypertensive drugs and diuretics. The success of antihypertensive therapy depends on a controlled reduction of the arterial blood pressure without impairing the renal blood flow, or reducing the effective filtration pressure at the glomerulus. A reduction in one or both will exacerbate the development of hypertension and systemic edema. An adjunct to the antihypertensive therapy is control of the diet. Restriction of dietary salt intake helps to reduce the filtered load of sodium and water, thereby reducing their tubular reabsorption. This would decrease salt and water retention and the accompanying edema and hypertension. Restriction of protein intake may have therapeutic value only in those patients with high levels of BUN and recognized clinical symptoms caused by it.

B. CHRONIC GLOMERULONEPHRITIS. This is a disease of multiple etiology. Clinically, it is characterized by renal *insufficiency*, whose symptoms include massive proteinuria, hematuria, hypoproteinemia, hypercholesterolemia, edema, and hypertension. About 85 to 90% of the cases have insidious onset with no apparent previous renal history. About 10% of the cases probably result from a late manifestations of acute poststreptococcal glomerulonephritis.

In severe conditions in which renal insufficiency is advanced and GFR is markedly reduced, the clinical findings include variable edema, sustained diastolic hypertension, increasing azotemia, anemia, and metabolic acidosis. The last three symptoms are characteristic of *frank uremia* and are due to reduced number of functioning nephrons and a reduced tubular function, as well as excessive loss of hemoglobin in the urine.

Treatment consists of preventing complications and relief of symptoms of renal failure. The latter will be discussed later. The therapy includes administration of antihypertensive drugs and diuretics for hypertension and edema along with steroid therapy to reduce the urinary loss of proteins.

2. NEPHROTIC SYNDROME

PATHOGENESIS AND PHYSIOLOGICAL BASES OF THE DISEASE. Unlike the *childhood nephrosis* (previously called lipoid nephrosis), which is a distinct disease and for which the prognosis is good, the *nephrotic syndrome* in the adult is a serious disease of multiple etiologies with poor prognosis. It occurs as an associated phenomenon in a variety of disease states, including *primary renal disease* (e.g., glomerulo-nephritis); *metabolic disease* (e.g., diabetes mellitus); *circulatory disorders* (e.g., right heart failure and renal vein thrombosis); *nephrotoxins* (e.g., mercury and lead poisoning); *allergic reactions*, including snake and insect bites; *infections*, including malaria, syphilis, and tuberculosis; and *pregnancy*. In all these conditions, the underlying cause of the renal malfunction is a marked increase in the permeability of the glomerular capillaries to plasma proteins, with possible accompanying defects in tubular reabsorption of proteins. This glomerulotubular defect is responsible for the four major clinical characteristics of this disease: (1) massive proteinuria, (2) hypoalbuminemia, (3) hyperlipemia, and (4) edema. Because of the multiple etiology and the above clinical findings, Kark and associates (1958) have defined the *nephrotic syndrome* as a disease manifested by the metabolic, nutritional, and clinical consequences of the continued massive proteinuria. Furthermore, to be diagnosed as nephrotic syndrome, the proteinuria must exceed 3.5 g/24 hours/1.73 m^2 surface area in the absence of reduced GFR (Berman and Schreiner, 1958).

In severe nephrotic syndrome, proteinuria (primarily of albumin) may be as high as 30 to 40 g per day. Although the resulting hypoalbuminemia stimulates the liver to increase albumin synthesis, the rate of hepatic synthesis cannot keep pace with the rate of urinary loss of protein. As a result, there would be a marked decrease in plasma protein concentration and hence of the protein oncotic pressure, which may fall from a normal value of 28 mm Hg to as low as 6 to 8 mm Hg.

The reduced plasma protein oncotic pressure throughout the systemic circulation alters the balance of capillary Starling forces in favor of outward filtration. This would lead to a net shift of fluid (primarily salt and water) from the vascular compartment into the interstitial compartment, and hence to the formation of edema. In severe cases, the marked increase in the interstitial volume reduces the "effective" circulatory blood volume, which leads to a reduction of the cardiac output and the renal perfusion pressure. The reduction in the renal perfusion pressure, by the mechanism described in Chapter 12, stimulates the baroreceptor component of the JG apparatus to increase renin release and the subsequent production of angiotensin II. At moderate concentrations, angiotensin II causes vaso-constriction of the blood vessels, leading to hypertension, and at high concentrations stimulates the zona glomerulosa of the adrenal cortex to increase synthesis and release of aldosterone (secondary aldosteronism). The increase in the blood levels of aldosterone causes an increase in the reabsorption of sodium and water, as isotonic solution, from the distal and collecting tubules. The resulting increase in the plasma volume causes a further transient increase in the capillary hydrostatic pressure, which further exacerbates the edema formation. Thus, *as long as the proteinuria exists, the reabsorbed salt and water do not remain in the vascular system but diffuse into the interstitial space. Hence, edema formation and secondary aldosteronism continue, and a vicious cycle is established.* Eventually, the increase in the interstitial volume leads to increased tissue hydrostatic pressure, favoring the return of fluid into the blood, thereby compensating for the reduced plasma protein oncotic pressure. The net result is the establishment of a new equilibrium state.

CLINICAL MANAGEMENT. Treatment consists of correcting the hypoproteinemia by increasing plasma protein concentration and suppressing proteinuria. Plasma protein concentration can be increased by administration of salt-poor albumin solution. Proteinuria can be reduced by administration of ACTH and corticosterone to repair the damaged glomerular capillary membrane, and by administration of immunosuppressive drugs to inhibit the antigen-antibody reactions responsible for the altered glomerular capillary membrane (Michael et al., 1973). In addition, the edema can be alleviated by administration of appropriate diuretics, such as furosemide, ethacrynic acid, and thiazides.

TOXEMIA OF PREGNANCY. Of the various conditions that lead to manifestation of nephrotic syndrome, *toxemia of pregnancy* serves as a useful example. Clinically, toxemia of pregnancy is classified into (1) an early stage, called *pre-eclampsia*, characterized by edema, albuminuria, and hypertension, and (2) a late stage, called *eclampsia*, which is characterized by convulsions (Norden and Kass, 1968).

The chief pathological change is the reduction in the size of the glomerular capillary lumen as a result of swelling of the endothelial and epithelial cells of the glomerulus. Consequently, there is a reduction of intrarenal blood flow, which is one of the causes of accompanying hypertension. The glomerular basement membrane appears essentially normal in these patients when toxemia of pregnancy is uncomplicated by other renal diseases.

There is also albuminuria, suggesting an increase in permeability of the glomerular capillary membrane to protein. The resulting proteinuria, which may occur before or after the development of hypertension, is in part responsible for edema and excessive weight gain in these patients.

The treatment of toxemia of pregnancy consists of controlling the diet, administration of diuretics, sedation, and rest. This treatment controls 80 to 90% of the cases. In rare cases, antihypertensive drug therapy may be necessary. If these treatments cannot control the hypertension and albuminuria, termination of the pregnancy should be considered in order to prevent eclampsia with convulsive seizures.

B. TUBULAR DISEASES

As shown in Table 13-1, tubular diseases may be classified according to whether they are *acquired* or *inherited*. In the case of an acquired tubular disease, such as *toxic nephropathy* and *transfusion reaction*, there is extensive destruction of the tubular epithelial cells leading to *tubular necrosis*. In the case of an inherited tubular disorder, the involved tubular segment is unable to carry out its normal function. Examples include *nephrogenic diabetes insipidus*, a disease characterized by ADH-unresponsiveness of the epithelial cells of the distal and collecting tubules, and *renal tubular acidosis*, a disease characterized by inability of the proximal tubule to reabsorb bicarbonate and/or the distal tubule to secrete hydrogen ions.

1. ACQUIRED TUBULAR DISEASES

Acquired tubular diseases causing tubular necrosis may result from at least three conditions: (a) nephrotoxic agents producing toxic nephropathy, (b) severe renal ischemia, and (c) transfusion reactions. Regardless of the causative agents, tubular necrosis results in acute renal failure, severe oliguria, and rapidly developing uremia.

A. TOXIC NEPHROPATHY. Toxic nephropathy can be induced by a variety of agents (Schreiner, 1975). The list includes *heavy metals* and their compounds (e.g., mercury and lead), *analgesic agents*, especially those containing phenacetin, and *carbon tetrachloride*, a volatile liquid. Unlike the other nephrotoxic agents, carbon tetrachloride can rapidly enter the body via the lungs and skin. Because carbon tetrachloride is heavier than air, it is very difficult to ventilate. Moreover, its nephrotoxic effect is potentiated by intake of alcoholic beverages.

Since these nephrotoxic agents are usually blood-borne, they cause *diffuse* tubular damage. The damaged tubular epithelial cells slough away from the basement membrane into the tubular lumen, thereby plugging the lumen and reducing tubular flow. If the basement membrane is not damaged, the tubular epithelial cells are usually repaired within 2 to 3 weeks.

B. RENAL ISCHEMIA. A severe reduction in renal blood flow, such as may occur in severe circulatory shock due to hemorrhage or heart failure, can cause tubular necrosis. However, because the resulting renal ischemia may differ both in nature and in distribution, the tubular necrosis is *patchy* rather than diffuse. The pathological findings are similar to those seen with toxic nephropathy. Again tubular epithelial cells are repaired within 2 to 3 weeks if basement membrane is intact.

C.   TRANSFUSION REACTIONS.   Transfusion of mismatched blood results in the hemolysis of the red blood cells and the release of hemoglobin.   Since the molecular size of hemoglobin is somewhat less than the pores of the glomerular capillary membrane (Table 5-1), hemoglobin passes through the ultrafilter membranes and enters the glomerular filtrate.   If a large volume of blood is transfused, the filtered load of hemoglobin would far exceed the amount of hemoglobin that can be reabsorbed by the proximal tubules.   The unreabsorbed hemoglobin will remain in the tubules, causing tubular blockage, reduced flow, tubular necrosis, and eventually acute renal failure.

Another condition in which tubular epithelia are destroyed is the so-called *crush syndrome*.   This condition results when a person has both circulatory shock and severely crushed muscles as a result of trauma.   The circulatory shock causes renal ischemia with variable tubular damage, as explained above.   The severely crushed muscles release large amounts of myoglobin into the circulation.   Myoglobin, like hemoglobin, is filtered at the glomerulus.   However, when its filtered load exceeds its reabsorption in the proximal tubule, the unreabsorbed myoglobin remains in the tubule, causing tubular blockage.   This would diminish tubular flow, cause tubular necrosis, and eventually lead to acute renal failure.

It is clear that the underlying cause of the acute renal failure is the tubular necrosis resulting from various tubular disorders already mentioned.   Physiologically, depending on whether the lesion is diffuse or patchy, tubular necrosis produces variable reduction in the tubular mass and hence glomerulotubular imbalance.   The extent of the induced glomerulotubular imbalance will determine the degree of oliguria and the resulting acute renal failure.   A detailed discussion of the clinical manifestations of renal failure and their physiological basis, as well as the rationale of treatment, is given later in this chapter.

2.   *INHERITED TUBULAR DISORDERS*

As discussed in Chapters 8 and 9, tubular processing of the various components of the filtrate involves one or a combination of several types of transport processes.   Of these the carrier-mediated transport is by far the most important.   The efficiency of such a transport mechanism depends on the nature and specificity of the carrier system, which are genetically determined.   Therefore, the absence of the appropriate genes leads to a defect in the tubular transport, which is manifested as a disease process.   For convenience of presentation, we shall consider three types of inherited tubular disorders: (a) nephrogenic diabetes insipidus, (b) renal tubular acidosis, and (c) some specific tubular disorders.

A.   NEPHROGENIC DIABETES INSIPIDUS.   As mentioned in Chapter 11, this is a disease characterized by polyuria and the loss of ability of the kidney to concentrate urine when fluid intake is restricted. Except for this defect, the kidney function is normal in all other aspects. The inability of the kidney to concentrate urine is attributed to unresponsiveness of the epithelial cells of the distal and collecting tubules to either endogenous or exogenous ADH. Histological studies, however, have failed to reveal obvious lesions in these tubules. Although the exact mechanism underlying the pathogenesis of this disease remains unknown, available evidence from studies with isolated renal tissue suggests that the defect may be due to a decrease in ADH-stimulated cyclic AMP formation within the distal and collecting tubular cells (see Fig. 11-14, page 355). Since these patients continually lose water, the condition leads to severe dehydration and hyperosmolality of the extracellular fluids. The problem can be prevented by replacing the excreted water.

B. RENAL TUBULAR ACIDOSIS. This condition is characterized by primary hyperchloremic metabolic acidosis and secondary disturbances in body potassium and calcium metabolism resulting from inability of the kidney to reabsorb bicarbonate in the proximal tubule and to secrete hydrogen ions in the distal tubule. Since, as mentioned in Chapter 10, hydrogen secretion is coupled with sodium reabsorption at the luminal membrane of the renal tubules, the failure of the hydrogen secreting mechanism leads to a marked reduction in hydrogen-sodium exchange. Since this exchange mechanism serves to generate bicarbonate ions within the renal cell, which promotes reabsorption of sodium and bicarbonate, failure of this exchange mechanism results in marked depletion of the body bicarbonate pool. The condition, however, can be corrected by adequate replacement therapy of alkali and potassium.

Depending on the site of defect, two forms of renal tubular acidosis have been recognized (Morris, 1969). Although the validity of such a distinction is open to question, it serves as a convenient basis for describing the biochemical variations seen in patients with renal tubular acidosis.

Proximal Renal Tubular Acidosis. This condition results from a defect in the proximal tubular reabsorption of bicarbonate ion. Reduced proximal reabsorption of bicarbonate increases its delivery to the distally located nephron segments, thereby exceeding the bicarbonate reabsorptive capacity of these tubular segments. The result is an increase in the urinary loss of bicarbonate along with potassium. Furthermore, presence of excess bicarbonate in the distal tubule effectively competes with the acidification of urine in the distal tubules by ammonia production and titratable acid excretion. As a consequence of these changes, plasma bicarbonate concentration will be lowered, whereas chloride concentration will be elevated (hyperchloremia). As described in Chapter 10, this leads to the development of extracellular metabolic acidosis and excretion of alkaline urine.

Distal Renal Tubular Acidosis. This is due to a defect in the distal tubule leading to the impaired ability of this tubular segment to secrete hydrogen ions against an unfavorable concentration gradient, and hence to impaired ability to acidify urine. As a result, the urinary phosphate remains in the dibasic form (Na_2HPO_4) rather than being converted into its monobasic form (NaH_2PO_4). Furthermore, there is a reduced production of ammonia and trapping of it in the tubules (due to reduced H^+ in the tubular lumen). This results in excretion of bicarbonate along with potassium, yielding an alkaline urine and making the blood hyperchloremic, as well as causing extracellular metabolic acidosis.

In both proximal and distal renal tubular acidosis, the induced metabolic acidosis may lead to the development of *nephrocalcinosis* (excess calcium phosphate deposition in the renal tubules) and *rickets* (bone deformation caused by Vitamin D deficiency). Treatment includes administration of sodium citrate or other sodium salts along with sufficient potassium to replace urinary loss. Alkali therapy should correct the nephrocalcinosis, whereas large doses of Vitamin D are required to correct the rickets. Prognosis of nephrocalcinosis depends on the degree of renal damage prior to the start of the treatment and the degree of reversibility of the renal damage with alkali therapy.

C. SPECIFIC TUBULAR DISORDERS. There are a number of other inborn defects of tubular transport that cause abnormal urinary excretion of some of the important constituents of the glomerular filtrate (Mudge, 1958). The following is a brief account of three of these.

Renal Glycosuria. This is a condition in which excessive quantity of glucose is excreted into the urine as a result of a deficiency in or complete absence of glucose reabsorption in the proximal tubule. Since blood glucose level is usually within the normal range, glycosuria in this renal tubular disease must not be confused with glycosuria in diabetes mellitus. In the latter condition, due to absence or deficient amount of pancreatic insulin, the plasma glucose concentration and hence its filtered load are exceedingly high, whereas the tubular transport maximum for glucose is normal.

Renal Hypophosphatemia. This hereditary disease is transmitted as a sex-linked dominant and is characterized by inadequate tubular reabsorption of phosphate ions (marked reduction in $\dot{T}m$ for phosphate) even when phosphate concentration of the extracellular fluid is very low. Although hypophosphatemia poses no immediate danger to cellular function, if it persists, it would lead to reduced bone calcification, causing the development of rickets or *osteomalacia* (bone softening due to Vitamin D deficiency), depending on the age of the patient. In contrast to the usual type of rickets, which responds to Vitamin D therapy, the renal hypophosphatemic rickets does not respond to Vitamin D administration.

Aminoaciduria. This condition, which is a genetic disease, results from a deficiency in the reabsorption of one or more amino acids (Frimpter et al., 1962). The most notable examples include glycinuria and cystinuria. The latter condition is characterized by an increase urinary excretion of cystine, lysine, arginine, and ornithine. Another example is the *Fanconi syndrome*. This is a disease most commonly characterized by renal glycosuria, renal hypophosphatemia, and renal aminoaciduria.

II. Diseases of the Urinary Tract

Besides the primary parenchymal diseases mentioned above, renal dysfunction may also result from the retrograde effects of disorders that chiefly affect the *urinary tract* (urethra, bladder, ureters, renal pelvis and calyces). The resulting pathophysiological changes in renal function may best be illustrated by two classes of urinary tract disorders: (a) *obstructive uropathy* and (b) *pyelonephritis*.

A. OBSTRUCTIVE UROPATHY

Obstructive uropathy refers to the pathological changes resulting from the mechanical obstruction of urine flow by deposition of renal stones along the urinary tract (Strauss and Welt, 1971). If the stone is not removed the condition will lead to *obstructive nephropathy*. Furthermore, the problem becomes very serious if it is accompanied by infection. Unless obstruction is distal to the bladder, the obstructive uropathy leads to the distention of the tubular structures with urine proximal to the obstruction, a condition called *hydronephrosis*.

The major cause of the obstructive uropathy is the formation of renal *calculi* (mineral salt stones), which are subsequently deposited in the renal calyces and the renal pelvis, whence they enter the ureters, bladder, and urethra. Depending on their size and location, the renal calculi may obstruct urine flow, which eventually could lead to obstructive nephropathy.

Urinary tract calculi is one of the oldest renal diseases known. It may affect persons of all ages, including children. The prime age group for urinary calculi is between 20 and 55 years of age. Most calculi are formed within the kidney. They consist of a framework of organic matrix with variable mixtures of calcium phosphate or magnesium ammonium phosphate. Occasionally, urinary stones contain uric acid.

The etiology of the urinary calculi is variable. Calculi are found in patients with gout, hyperparathyroidism, and excessive intake of calcium (e.g., milk) and Vitamin D. Formation of urinary calculi is also favored by urinary tract infection. Conversely, calculi formation may cause urinary obstruction and urinary stasis, which predispose the kidney to urinary tract infection.

Regardless of the etiology of renal calculi, the best treatment is achieved by adequate fluid intake so as to maximize urine output and minimize the likelihood of precipitation of urinary salts. In specific metabolic diseases, appropriate adjunct drug therapy is also recommended. In the event that the stone is too large to pass through spontaneously or to be reduced in size, as revealed by radiographic examination, surgical removal is required.

B. PYELONEPHRITIS

Pyelonephritis is an infectious disease affecting both the interstitial renal tissue and the renal pelvis. It is caused by several pathogenic bacteria, including *Escherichia coli* and staphylococci. The retrograde secondary spread of the inflammation to the renal tubules and eventually to the blood vessels and glomeruli results in the associated clinical manifestations of renal malfunction. These commonly include a reduction in renal medullary function associated with obstructive lesions of the lower urinary tract (Jackson et al., 1962).

Pyuria (pus in urine) and *leukocyte casts* in urine are strong indications of pyelonephritis. Depending on the extent of infection and the involvement of the renal parenchyma, renal function may be considerably reduced. Of these, the most important is the inability of the kidney to concentrate urine (Quinn and Kass, 1960). In fact, measurement of osmolar clearance (C_{Osm}) and solute-free water clearance (C_{H_2O}) after fluid restriction in such patients provides a sensitive diagnostic test of the degree of diminished ability of the kidney to concentrate urine (Brod, 1956). As discussed in Chapter 11, the ability of the kidney to concentrate urine is the function of the loop of Henle and the collecting tubules. Therefore, the diminished urine concentration may be interpreted as evidence of the localization of the lesion in the distally located nephron segments, including the loop of Henle and the collecting tubules. However, such tests are not specific.

Accompanying these destructive tubular lesions are significant reductions in renal function manifested by progressive depression of renal blood flow (RBF) and glomerular filtration rate (GFR). However, since the disease mostly affects the tubules, measurement of PAH clearance has shown that RBF decreases more than GFR, yielding an increase in filtration fraction (Bradley et al., 1950).

As mentioned above, obstructive uropathy predisposes the patient to the development of pyelonephritis. Although the mechanism of the relationship between obstruction and infection is not known, it is related to development of infection consequent to urinary tract obstruction. Such an obstruction causes stagnation of urine, making it an excellent medium for bacterial growth. Thus, any condition that reduces urine flow increases the tendency for development of pyelonephritis. An example of the relationship between obstruction and infection is *nephrocalcinosis*, a condition resulting from calcium phosphate precipitation within the renal tubules and obstructing the flow of urine. The incidence of pyelonephritis in patients with nephrocalcinosis is close to 100%.

Among young people, the incidence of pyelonephritis is more frequent in children and females. Infants, during the diaper period, are more susceptible to pyelonephritis. Beyond one year of age, females are likely to have renal infections nine times more frequently than males (Riley, 1968). In the older age group, the incidence of pyelonephritis becomes comparable in both males and females, due to the prevalence of *prostatic hypertrophy* in males.

There is also a high incidence of pyelonephritis during the second and third trimesters of pregnancy (Norden and Kass, 1968). This is attributed to the physiologic hydronephrosis (distention of renal pelvis with urine) which is present throughout this period of pregnancy.

In short, there are several predisposing factors for the development of pyelonephritis. They include anomalies of the kidney and ureter, presence of renal calculi, obstruction of urine flow at any level along the urinary tract, pregnancy, and insertion of instruments into the bladder, including catheterization.

Approximately 90% of patients with acute pyelonephritis will recover from the initial episode with careful antibiotic therapy and show no detectable residual renal damage. The remaining 10% do not recover completely and develop chronic pyelonephritis, the clinical manifestations of which include hypertension, azotemia, and some proteinuria. The latter is due to the impaired tubular reabsorption of the normally small amount of filtered proteins. However, if proteinuria exceeds 3.5 g/day, it indicates nephrotic syndrome rather than chronic pyelonephritis. Hypertension is presumably due to stimulation of renin-angiotensin system consequent to severe sclerosis and narrowing of the interlobar, arcuate, and interlobular arteries caused by secondary spread of inflammation to the renal parenchyma. The treatment consists of controlling the disease process by judicious and long-term use of antibiotics.

III. Systemic Diseases and Renal Function

Of the various known systemic diseases that result from or produce secondary changes in renal function, we have selected three (Table 13-1) for consideration in this section. These are *renovascular hypertension, congestive heart failure,* and *liver cirrhosis.* Our choice was based largely on the fact that although there are considerable differences in the etiology of each disease, in the *chronic state*, a common denominator (namely, a derangement in the renin-angiotensin-aldosterone system) underlies the induced pathophysiological alterations in renal function and their clinical manifestations.

Hypertension and Its Classification

Before describing the etiology of renovascular hypertension and the physiological basis for its treatment, it is necessary to define the clinical meaning of hypertension and its varied classifications.

Hypertension generally refers to the elevation of both the *systolic* and the *diastolic* components of the blood pressure. Clinically, a patient may be classified as hypertensive when both the systolic and diastolic blood pressures are consistently higher than 140 and 90 mm Hg, respectively (compared to 120 and 80 mm Hg for normal). Of course, either systolic or diastolic blood pressure

alone could be elevated, in which case the hypertension is referred
to as either systolic or diastolic hypertension. Of these, the
diastolic hypertension is considered to be more serious than the
systolic hypertension.

In most hypertensive patients with normal renal function, cardiac
output is found to be either normal or decreased. However, cardiac
output is increased in patients with hypertension of renal origin,
such as *renovascular hypertension* (Frohlich et al., 1969). This
suggests that in the absence of renal disease, the primary hemodynamic
change in hypertension is an increase in the peripheral resistance
(Fries, 1960), which is responsible for the increase in the diastolic
pressure. The induced rise in the systolic pressure is considered to
be secondary to the elevation of the diastolic blood pressure.

Hypertension is generally classified according to whether its
primary etiology is known or not. If the primary etiology is known,
it is called *secondary hypertension* and it usually bears the name of
the diseased organ and/or causative factors. Examples include
hypertension due to primary renal parenchymal disease, such as
glomerulonephritis or *pyelonephritis, renovascular hypertension,
primary aldosteronism,* and *pheochromocytoma*. Pathogenesis of
hypertension in *glomerulonephritis* and *pyelonephritis* have already
been discussed. Pathogenesis of *renovascular hypertension* will be
discussed later in this section. *Primary aldosteronism* (Conn's
syndrome) is caused by an aldosterone-secreting adrenocortical
adenoma, a tumor in the zona glomerulosa of the adrenal cortex.
The consequent continued aldosterone-stimulated renal reabsorption
of salt and water leads to hypertension, accompanied by hypokalemia,
alkalosis, and low plasma renin activity (Cain et al., 1972).
Pheochromocytoma refers to a disease in which there is a
catecholamine-secreting (epinephrine and norepinephrine) tumor
in the adrenal medulla. The excessive secretion of catecholamines
leads to vasoconstriction, increased peripheral resistance, and
hence hypertension. In cases where the specific primary etiology
is not known, the elevated blood pressure is called *primary* or
essential hypertension, or more specifically hypertension of unknown
origin. Whether the etiology of hypertension is known or not,
clinically hypertension may be considered as *benign* if it develops
slowly over many years and if it can be treated and controlled. On
the other hand, if hypertension develops rapidly and over a short
period of time, it is called *malignant*, and in these cases the
treatment is usually unsuccessful.

Of the patients who die from essential malignant hypertension,
nearly 65% succumb to complications from associated cardiovascular
diseases, such as congestive heart failure and coronary thrombosis
(heart attack), 25% die from either the hemorrhagic or thrombotic types
of cerebral vascular accident (stroke), and the remaining 10% die
from chronic renal disease (Page and Sidd, 1972). The high incidence
of hypertensive patients who die from cardiovascular complications
suggests that the heart and its vasculature are more sensitive to the
damaging effects of the high blood pressure than are the vasculatures
of the brain and the kidney.

A recent comprehensive review of the possible factors contributing to the etiology of essential hypertension (Page and Sidd, 1972) suggests that "...genetic factors, modified by environmental influences, combine to determine the emergence of hypertension in early middle age." Of the various environmental influences that have been studied, it has been found that dietary sodium intake, a culturally related factor, is very important. Thus, excess dietary sodium intake early in life and genetic predisposition appear to be among the leading underlying factors in the development of essential hypertension in early middle age.

Besides the etiology, the clinical course in patients with malignant essential hypertension is quite different from that in other patients who have hypertension of known etiology and similar levels of high blood pressure. If untreated, nearly all patients with malignant hypertension will die within two years, and two thirds within 9 months after the presumable onset of the condition. Treatment involves the control of high blood pressure with appropriate antihypertensive drugs in order to prevent cerebrovascular accidents, acute congestive heart failure, and renal failure. Although the available evidence for the beneficial effects of antihypertensive therapy is inconclusive, the consensus is that such a therapy would not only promote healing of damaged renal tissues and restoration of renal function but would also in part correct the underlying cause and hence aid in the management of hypertension. Furthermore, anti-hypertensive drug therapy reduces the risk of cerebrovascular accidents of both hemorrhagic and thrombotic types and of cardio-vascular complications. Needless to say, the earlier the anti-hypertensive drug therapy is instituted the greater is its potential for beneficial results. Patients with superimposed renal failure who do not respond to antihypertensive drug therapy should be evaluated for possible bilateral nephrectomy and renal transplant.

A. RENOVASCULAR HYPERTENSION

Renovascular hypertension results from a reduction in the intrarenal blood flow consequent to a reduction in the renal perfusion pressure. Depending on the underlying pathological changes that affect the renal blood vessels, two types of renovascular hypertension have been recognized: (1) *intrarenovascular hypertension*, caused by a progressive sclerotic stenosis of the intrarenal blood vessels, and (2) *extrarenovascular hypertension*, caused by stenosis of the main renal artery and/or its branches. In both cases, the underlying mechanism that initiates the hypertension is believed to be a reduction in the afferent arteriolar pressure, which, by the mechanism described in Chapter 12, leads to excessive stimulation of the renin-angiotensin system and the development of hypertension. However, the role of the renin-angiotensin system and other neural and humoral factors in the maintenance of hypertension is less certain and is presently the subject of intensive investigation.

1. *INTRARENOVASCULAR HYPERTENSION*

Progressive pathological changes in the wall of the intrarenal vasculature results in *nephrosclerosis*, which may lead to a marked reduction in the intrarenal blood flow and the development of hypertension. Since the primary etiology of these vascular changes is at present ill defined, the resulting hypertension may be classified as *essential hypertension*. Pathologically, depending on the extent of the vascular lesion, two forms of nephrosclerosis have been recognized: benign and malignant. In *benign nephrosclerosis*, the primary pathological findings consist of proliferation of the intima of the small arteries and arterioles accompanied by subintimal deposition of fatty and hyaline materials and hypertrophy of media (Anderson and Scotti, 1972). The induced vascular sclerosis and hyalinization leads to structural narrowing of the lumen of the affected blood vessels. This reduces the intrarenal blood flow, which may lead to patchy degeneration of glomeruli and tubular atrophy. In contrast, *malignant nephrosclerosis* is characterized by hyperplastic arteriosclerosis with necrosis in the walls of the small arteries and arterioles (Anderson and Scotti, 1972).

Physiologically, the progressive sclerotic stenosis of the intrarenal arteries and arterioles gradually decreases their lumens and therefore increases the intrarenal vascular resistance. This would reduce the intrarenal perfusion pressure and hence the intrarenal blood flow distal to the sites of sclerotic lesions. The resulting reduction in the intrarenal perfusion pressure at the level of the afferent arterioles, by the mechanism described in Chapter 12 (Fig. 12-6), stimulates the baroreceptor component of the juxtaglomerular apparatus to release renin. Depending on the degree of reduction of the afferent arteriolar pressure, the increase in renin release leads to a proportional increase in the synthesis of angiotensin II and its plasma concentration. Depending on its circulating levels (Fig. 12-8), angiotensin II could cause both vasoconstriction of the systemic blood vessels, including those of the kidney, and stimulation of the zona glomerulosa of the adrenal cortex to secrete aldosterone. Both of these effects would lead to the elevation of the diastolic blood pressure, which induces a secondary rise in the systolic blood pressure, and hence the development of hypertension. Although considerable experimental evidence supports the above sequence of events as the possible mechanism initiating the hypertension, the nature of the underlying mechanisms that maintain the hypertension is at present controversial and remains to be elucidated. A possible mechanism (Laragh, 1973; Kurtzman et al., 1974) might be that as the disease progresses, the peripheral vascular bed becomes more sensitive to angiotensin II, so that a smaller amount of angiotensin II is required to maintain the high blood pressure. The degree of vascular sensitivity to angiotensin II appears to be set by aldosterone-induced sodium retention and extracellular volume expansion. Thus, sodium depletion reduces the vascular sensitivity to angiotensin II, whereas sodium retention increases the vascular sensitivity to angiotensin II. The physiological significance of the renin-angiotensin-aldosterone system and its role in the clinical diagnosis and treatment of hypertension of renal and nonrenal origin will be described in the next section.

2. EXTRARENOVASCULAR HYPERTENSION

The possibility that the stenosis of the main renal artery could produce hypertension came under consideration when Goldblatt and his associates (1934) showed that partial occlusion of one renal artery in the dog with contralateral nephrectomy resulted in the development of sustained chronic arterial hypertension. In the ensuing years (see Page and McCubbin, 1968, for review) numerous studies have confirmed the production of experimental extrarenovascular hypertension by this method--known as the *one-kidney Goldblatt model*--in other species, including rat, rabbit, and sheep. In addition, these studies have shown that renovascular hypertension could also be produced by several variations of the original method. Notable among these are (1) the *two-kidney Goldblatt model*, which consists of partial occlusion of one renal artery, with the contralateral kidney left untouched, (2) partial occlusion of both renal arteries, (3) subtotal removal of the renal mass of the sole remaining kidney in the one-kidney Goldblatt model, and (4) bilateral nephrectomy. The hypertension resulting from the latter procedure is known as the *renoprival hypertension*.

MECHANISM OF GOLDBLATT HYPERTENSION. In 1950, the clinical recognition that hypertension may be caused secondarily to either unilateral or bilateral renal artery stenosis in man generated considerable interest in delineating the underlying mechanisms of the development and maintenance of hypertension in both the one-kidney and two-kidney Goldblatt models. As early as 1946, following the discovery of the renin-angiotensin system, Braun-Menéndez and his associates postulated that the increase in renin secretion subsequent to the renal artery stenosis might be responsible for the development and maintenance of hypertension in the one-kidney Goldblatt model. Experimental proof for this hypothesis, however, had to await the development of more reliable assays for the measurement of plasma levels of both renin and angiotensin. Despite the discovery and application of these new assay techniques, the numerous studies carried out between the years 1946 to 1968 have yielded conflicting evidence on the role of the renin-angiotensin system in the development and maintenance of both types of Goldblatt renal hypertension (see Page and McCubbin, 1968, for review). Considered briefly, these studies have revealed that although constriction of the renal artery caused an increase in renin release, the blood patterns of the renin-angiotensin system in the two types of Goldblatt hypertension were quite different both during the transient and during the established phase of hypertension. Thus, in the one-kidney Goldblatt model, there was an initial transient rise in the renal venous blood, which reached a maximum after a few days and returned to normal thereafter. In contrast, in the two-kidney Goldblatt model, there was an increase in the renin level in the renal venous blood from the occluded ischemic kidney, which reached a maximum after a few weeks. However, the renin level in the renal venous blood from the untouched contralateral kidney remained normal or was slightly decreased. Taken together, in the two-kidney model, the systemic plasma renin level was found to be elevated during both the initial transient and established phases of hypertension. In short, these studies implied that in the one-kidney model, only the initial phase of hypertension was pressor-mediated, whereas in the two-kidney model both the initial and established phases were pressor-dependent. However, the probable mechanisms mediating this difference in plasma renin profile during the transient and established phases of hypertension in the two Goldblatt models remained largely unexplained until the late 1960's, when a number of studies implicated an interaction between sodium metabolism and plasma renin level in hypertension.

In 1965, Gross and his associates found that removal of the occluded ischemic kidney in the two-kidney Goldblatt model during the established phase of hypertension lowered the plasma renin level, but did not cure the hypertension and in fact worsened it. They reasoned that this was somehow related to the manner by which the two kidneys (ischemic and normal) handled sodium transport. In the same year, Brown and his colleagues reported a highly significant inverse relationship between plasma renin levels and plasma sodium concentration in 253 hypertensive patients studied. The lowest plasma renin levels were found in patients with hypernatremia (high plasma sodium level), whereas the highest plasma renin levels were found in patients with hyponatremia. Moreover, this inverse relationship was found to be remarkably independent of the etiology of hypertension, the height of the blood pressure, complications, or treatment. In a subsequent study, Conway (1968) reported a significant sodium retention in dogs with one-kidney Goldblatt hypertension, thereby confirming the above inverse relationship between body sodium and plasma renin levels.

PRESSOR- AND VOLUME-MEDIATED COMPONENTS OF HYPERTENSION. These and similar studies led to the formulation of the following probable mechanism through which the renin-angiotensin system and sodium metabolism mediate the transient and established phases of hypertension in the one-kidney Goldblatt model. Partial occlusion of the renal artery reduces the renal arterial pressure, which results in renal ischemia. The reduced renal arterial pressure lowers the pressure at the afferent arteriole, which stimulates the baroreceptor component of the juxtaglomerular apparatus to release renin (Fig. 12-6). The resulting elevated plasma renin level causes a proportional increase in the synthesis of angiotensin II, which produces peripheral vasoconstriction and leads to the development of hypertension. Moreover, continued production of renin raises the plasma angiotensin II to the level which stimulates the zona glomerulosa of the adrenal cortex to secrete aldosterone. The resulting increase in the plasma level of aldosterone enhances reabsorption of salt and water from the distal and collecting tubules, thereby expanding the plasma volume and further elevating the blood pressure. The resulting hypertension produced by angiotensin II-induced vasoconstriction and aldosterone-induced sodium retention will increase renal perfusion pressure, which decreases stimulation of renin production. The renin production is further reduced by additional sodium retention owing to reduced GFR (by the mechanism described in Chapter 8) consequent to partial renal artery occlusion. As the hypertension enters the established phase, the continued sodium retention progressively increases the pressor responsiveness to angiotensin II (Ames et al., 1965), a factor which further returns the plasma renin-angiotensin II levels to normal, where it is sufficient to cause vasoconstriction and maintain hypertension in the presence of sodium retention. Thus, in the one-kidney Goldblatt model, the initial phase of hypertension is *pressor-mediated*, whereas the established phase of hypertension is related to sodium retention and hence is *volume-mediated*.

The relative roles of sodium metabolism and the renin-angiotensin system in the development and maintenance of hypertension in both the one-kidney and two-kidney Goldblatt models have been further elucidated by a number of recent studies in which antirenin antibodies or specific angiotensin antagonists were used to lower the blood pressure. Thus, Brunner and his associates (1971) found that treatment of the two-kidney Goldblatt hypertensive rats with antirenin antibodies or specific angiotensin antagonists resulted in a reduction of the blood pressure. However, such a treatment had no effect when the normal contralateral kidney had been removed. When such a one-kidney animal was then sodium-depleted, it responded to anti-hypertensive treatment. These results clearly indicate that in both Goldblatt models, the expression of the pressor effects of the renin-angiotensin system were somehow related to the state of body sodium balance. Thus, when there was salt retention, as in the one-kidney model (due to reduced sodium excretion by the sole remaining kidney), the antihypertensive treatment was ineffective, confirming that hypertension was volume-mediated. In contrast, when there was salt depletion, as in the two-kidney model (due to increased sodium excretion by the contralateral kidney), the antihypertensive treatment was effective, confirming that hypertension was pressor-mediated.

The interrelationship between sodium metabolism and the renin-angiotensin system in the development and maintenance of renal hypertension has now been clearly established by studies in both experimental animals and man (Brunner et al., 1972; Brunner et al., 1974; Kurtzman et al., 1974). To summarize, these studies have demonstrated the existence of an inverse relationship between plasma renin activity (PRA) and body sodium balance. Thus, sodium depletion, which reduces the extracellular fluid (ECF) volume and hence the renal perfusion pressure, is found to stimulate renin secretion, whereas sodium loading, which expands ECF volume, suppresses renin secretion. Moreover, it has been shown that the apparent affinity of the vascular receptors for angiotensin II is increased during sodium loading, whereas it is decreased during sodium depletion. In short, angiotensin II pressor responsiveness correlates directly with body sodium balance and inversely with plasma renin level. Thus, as Brunner and his associates (1972) suggest, the kidney plays a central role in the regulation of blood pressure by virtue of the fact that it can control simultaneously both production of angiotensin II via renin release and the pressor responsiveness of the vascular receptors to the liberated angiotensin II via induced changes in aldosterone secretion and hence sodium metabolism. The mechanism of these sodium-induced changes in the vascular affinity to angiotensin II, however, remains to be elucidated. Brunner and his group (1972) have proposed that salt loading leads to an increase in sodium uptake by the arterial walls, and therefore raises sodium concentration within the wall. The resulting accumulation of salt and water causes swelling of the wall, which increases the exposure of the vascular receptor sites and hence their accessibility to angiotensin II, thereby promoting their interaction and consequently favoring vasoconstriction and hypertension. However, in a more recent study, Thurston and Laragh (1975) found that a decrease in the pressor responsiveness of angiotensin II during salt depletion was the result of a prior occupancy of the vascular receptor sites by endogenous angiotensin II. Therefore, they have suggested that "a change in the number or the affinity of receptors consequent to changes in sodium balance need not be postulated to explain the phenomenon."

Regardless of the underlying mechanism, the proposed effect of sodium metabolism on pressor responsiveness of angiotensin II may also explain the differences in the renin profile in the two types of Goldblatt hypertension. Thus, in the one-kidney Goldblatt model, excessive stimulation of renin-angiotensin system initiates the development of hypertension. However, the accompanying sodium retention, due to decreased salt excretion by the ischemic kidney, not only suppresses the renin-angiotensin system, reverting it toward normal, but also enhances the vascular affinity for angiotensin II sufficient to maintain the hypertension. *In short, in the one-kidney Goldblatt model, the development of hypertension is pressor-mediated, whereas its maintenance is volume-mediated.* In contrast, in the two-kidney Goldblatt model, salt depletion caused by increased sodium excretion by the normal contralateral kidney not only stimulates the renin-angiotensin system, but also reduces vascular affinity for angiotensin II. *In short, in the two-kidney Goldblatt model, both the development and maintenance phases of hypertension are renin-angiotensin dependent.*

In summary, these studies clearly indicate that hypertension is not due solely to the stimulation of the renin-angiotensin system but it also results from the indirect mediation of other factors. Chief among them are the body sodium balance and the ECF volume. Although the renin-angiotensin system plays an important role in the initiation of the hypertension, its subsequent vasoconstriction effect (vascular sensitivity) is adversely affected by the renal handling of sodium, the resulting state of sodium balance and the ECF volume. The extent of the involvement of the latter effects determines the magnitude as well as the nature of the established phase of the renovascular hypertension.

ANTIHYPERTENSIVE ROLE OF THE KIDNEY

A considerable body of evidence has shown that in addition to producing *prohypertensive* substances, such as renin and angiotensin, the kidney is also capable of secreting *antihypertensive* agents. This may explain why removal of the contralateral normal kidney in the two-kidney Goldblatt model in the dog enhances the hypertension, and why bilateral nephrectomy in man leads to renoprival hypertension.

The best evidence in support of the antihypertensive function of the kidney is the recent finding of Muirhead and his associates (1970) that implantation of renal medullary fragments under the skin of hypertensive rats and rabbits lowered their blood pressures. This observation was subsequently confirmed by Tobian and Azar (1971), who showed further that removal of such implants resulted in the return of the blood pressure to the previous hypertensive levels. Moreover, microscopic examination of these fragments revealed a great abundance of large stellate interstitial cells containing numerous cytoplasmic vacuoles, large Golgi complexes, and lipid granules. When grown in tissue culture, these cells released prostaglandin E_2 (PGE_2), a substance normally found in large amounts in the inner renal medulla. In addition, it has been shown that PGE_2 and PGA_2, another prostaglandin which is a possible product of PGE_2, have the property of lowering the blood pressure (Kadowitz, 1972). Of the two prostaglandins, PGE_2 is 95% destroyed as it passes through the lung, and therefore it is an unlikely candidate for the role of a peripheral hormone. On the other hand, PGA_2 is less completely degraded by the lung, so that it could serve as a peripheral antihypertensive hormone (Tobian, 1974).

Recent studies have suggested a possible role for another humoral system, namely, the *kallikrein-kinin system* in the pathogenesis of hypertension. *Kallikrein* is a renal enzyme that cleaves kallidin (lysyl-bradykinin), a potent vasodilator kinin, from the kininogen substrates. In a series of studies in rat and man Margolius and associates (1974a, 1974b) reported that urinary excretion of kallikrein is increased in normal rats and humans fed a low-sodium diet or after administration of sodium-retaining steroids, *fludrocortisone*. Moreover, they found that patients with essential hypertension excrete less kallikrein in urine, and when placed on a low-sodium diet, the increase in excretion is much less than that in normotensive patients. In contrast, patients with primary aldosteronism excrete large amounts of kallikrein, which is unresponsive to altered dietary sodium intake. Despite this evidence, at present the roles of the prostaglandins and kallikrein-kinin humoral systems in the pathogenesis and maintenance of renovascular hypertension remain to be elucidated.

CLINICAL EVALUATION OF RENOVASCULAR AND ESSENTIAL HYPERTENSION

Available evidence suggests that in the chronic state, the sustained elevation of blood pressure in patients with renovascular hypertension may represent an imbalance between the pressor-mediated and the volume-mediated mechanisms. Whether either one of these two mechanisms or some combination thereof is responsible for the chronic hypertension can best be deduced from determination of the plasma renin levels. Such a determination of plasma renin profile not only serves to diagnose the underlying cause but also can be used as a guide to the selection of the appropriate course of therapy. Thus, in patients with high plasma renin levels (as in the two-kidney Goldblatt model) maintenance of hypertension is most likely pressor-mediated. These patients respond to antihypertensive therapy, such as treatment with propranolol hydrochloride (Inderal), a β-adrenergic blocking agent that lowers the blood pressure and also reduces renin secretion. On the other hand, in patients with low plasma renin levels (as in the one-kidney Goldblatt model), maintenance of the hypertension is most likely volume-mediated. These patients respond to appropriate diuretic therapy, such as administration of ethacrynic acid, furosemide, spironolactone, triamterene, or amiloride. In cases in which plasma renin level is normal, the mechanism maintaining hypertension is most likely due to an inappropriate interaction between the pressor- and volume-mediated mechanisms. In such cases, treatment should consist of a judicious and appropriate mixture of both antihypertensive and diuretic drug therapies. That this same imbalance between the pressor-dependent and volume-dependent mechanisms may be responsible for the pathogenesis and maintenance of chronic essential hypertension has been proposed recently by Laragh (1973). He has classified hypertensive patients into high, normal, and low renin groups and has suggested that the morbidity is correlated with their plasma renin levels. On the basis of this classification, Laragh has suggested that the development and maintenance of essential hypertension may be characterized as either purely pressor-mediated or purely volume-mediated or as a combination of these. A purely pressor-mediated hypertension may arise from a primary renal disease, such as unilateral or bilateral renal artery stenosis or nephrosclerosis, which are all characterized by an excessive stimulation of the renin-angiotensin-aldosterone system. A purely volume-mediated hypertension may arise from oversecretion of aldosterone, as in primary aldosteronism (Conn's syndrome). The increased blood level of aldosterone enhances renal reabsorption of salt and water, leading to the expansion of the extracellular fluid volume, increased renal perfusion pressure, and hence suppressed renin release. Of course, hypertension could arise from an inappropriate interaction between the pressor- and volume-mediated mechanisms, leading to renin-angiotensin-aldosterone blood levels different from those mentioned above. Of the two extreme mechanisms mediating essential hypertension, the volume-mediated hypertension is considered to be less serious, since it results in less severe vascular damage than does the pressor-mediated hypertension. In both types, the maintenance of hypertension is thought to be due to a greater increase in the vascular volume relative to the vascular capacity, with the expansion of the vascular volume resulting largely from excessive renal retention of salt and water. As outlined previously, determination of plasma renin levels should be used as a guide to the diagnosis of the probable factors contributing to the hypertension and the selection of the appropriate antihypertensive or diuretic therapies or both.

In cases in which plasma renin level is normal, possible presence of unilateral or bilateral renal artery stenosis as a cause of hypertension may be confirmed by *intravenous pyelography* (IVP). This test involves intravenous injection of sodium iodohippurate-I^{131}, a contrast material, and then visualizing its subsequent disappearance from renal circulation by x-ray. Since the renal clearance of the sodium iodohippurate is similar to that of the para-aminohippurate (PAH)--that is, it is cleared by filtration and tubular secretion--its excretion is affected by renal artery stenosis. Careful evaluation of the results could reveal the presence, location, and type of renovascular lesion. If IVP test reveals the presence of a lesion, it should be further confirmed by simultaneous measurement of renin levels in the renal veins from both kidneys. This procedure is called the *split-function test* (Howard and Connor, 1964).

If the results of these tests prove to be positive, then surgical removal of the renal artery obstruction should help to reduce the elevated blood pressure. However, if renal artery stenosis is accompanied by intrarenal damage (nephrosclerosis), such corrective surgery will not provide long-term cure. Presence of intrarenal parenchymal damage may be assessed by *renal biopsy*.

Another type of hypertension whose clinical manifestation is mediated in part by an alteration in electrolyte balance and the renin-angiotensin-aldosterone system is the *primary aldosteronism* of Conn's syndrome. Since in these patients plasma renin activity is low, estimation of PRA may provide a valuable diagnostic tool for separating these patients from other hypertensive patients. Thus, failure of PRA to rise during volume depletion maneuvers, such as hemorrhage, sodium depletion, administration of diuretics, and postural changes, provides a major criterion for primary aldosteronism. However, because reduced PRA occurs in 25% of patients with essential hypertension as well as in patients with aldosteronism secondary to bilateral adrenal hyperplasia and other mineralocorticoid excess syndromes, Cain and associates (1972) suggest that PRA test should be combined with measurement of aldosterone secretion. Since aldosterone secretion may be normal in patients on a restricted sodium diet, they suggest that nonsuppressibility of aldosterone secretion must be demonstrated. This is accomplished by volume expansion maneuvers, such as mineralocorticoid administration, oral sodium loading, and intravenous infusion of saline or other plasma expanders. Furthermore, when performing *aldosterone suppression tests*, potassium balance must be carefully maintained in such patients. In view of the pronounced effect of potassium on aldosterone secretion rate (Fig. 11-15), failure to achieve potassium balance may lead to false results.

As yet, it is not possible to differentiate patients with primary aldosteronism from those with bilateral adrenal hyperplasia by the PRA and aldosterone suppression tests. It is generally agreed, however, that patients with bilateral adrenal hyperplasia have a less severe hypokalemia, lower aldosterone secretion, and higher levels of PRA than do patients with primary aldosteronism (Cain et al., 1972).

B. CONGESTIVE HEART FAILURE

Before describing the changes in renal function resulting from congestive heart failure, we need to define the meaning of heart failure, its underlying physiological mechanisms, and its clinical manifestations.

The term *"heart failure"* simply means the failure of the heart to pump an adequate amount of blood to the tissues. When heart failure is accompanied by an abnormal increase in blood volume and interstitial fluid volume (edema), the condition is known as *congestive heart failure*. The term "congestive" implies sequestration or congestion of edema fluid, usually in the pulmonary tissues.

The heart failure may be *unilateral*, involving either the left or the right ventricle, or *bilateral*, involving both ventricles. Of these, the failure of the left ventricle is more common, and it may eventually lead to the failure of the right ventricle and therefore to bilateral heart failure.

Regardless of the type, heart failure is caused by a decreased contractility of the myocardium, resulting in a reduction of the cardiac output. The decrease in myocardial contractility may follow a direct damage to the myocardium or it may be an indirect effect of a secondary disease. The most common direct cause of heart failure is a reduction in the coronary blood flow. This may result from an atherosclerotic coronary heart disease, which may lead to narrowing of the coronary artery or coronary thrombosis, precipitating an acute heart attack. Direct myocardial damage and heart failure may also result from any type of valvular lesions, such as mitral valve stenosis. Heart failure may also be caused indirectly by diseases that secondarily affect myocardial function. Examples include pericaridal hemorrhage (cardiac tamponade), pulmonary venous obstruction (pulmonary embolism), or reduced venous return, as in shock.

Depending on whether the heart failure is unilateral or bilateral, the resulting clinical manifestations may be ascribed to one or a combination of *three* underlying physiological abnormalities (Guyton et al., 1973): (1) A reduction in the cardiac output, causing a decrease in the blood flow to the systemic tissues, including the kidneys; (2) an increase in the left atrial pressure, consequent to left ventricular failure, causing the blood to be backed up in the pulmonary tissues, resulting in pulmonary venous congestion (pulmonary edema); and (3) an increase in the right atrial pressure, consequent to right ventricular failure, causing the blood to be backed up in the systemic tissues, resulting in systemic venous congestion (systemic edema).

Cardiac failure associated with reduced cardiac output is called "low output heart failure." This is in contrast to "high output heart failure," in which the cardiac output is increased, as in hyperthyroidism.

LEFT VENTRICULAR FAILURE. Whether one or more of these factors are operating depends largely on the underlying nature of the heart failure. Thus, in acute left ventricular failure, there is a marked reduction in the cardiac output, which may lead to some pulmonary edema. In contrast, in chronic left ventricular failure, because of the operation of the compensatory mechanisms described on page 491, the cardiac output returns to normal but the left atrial pressure remains elevated and the pulmonary edema persists. In severe cases, pulmonary venous congestion may lead to pulmonary hypertension and eventual failure of the right ventricle. Moreover, pulmonary congestion interferes with normal breathing, causing *dyspnea* (rapid, shallow or "labored" breathing), and impeding pulmonary gas exchange, resulting in cyanosis. The latter results from (1) an increase in resistance to air flow, and (2) a reduction in the alveolar air consequent to flooding of the alveolar space with edema fluid (Rushmer, 1976).

RIGHT VENTRICULAR FAILURE. Unlike the left ventricle, the right ventricle is adapted to handle large transient changes in the blood volume. Therefore, it rarely fails as a result of a pure volume load (Rushmer, 1976). The principal cause of right ventricular failure is a pressure load which may result from several conditions, including (1) left ventricular failure and pulmonary hypertension, (2) primary lung disease, and (3) pulmonary valvular stenosis. Thus, in chronic right ventricular failure, cardiac output remains normal while the elevated right atrial pressure causes the blood to be sequestered in the systemic circulation. As a result, there will be demonstrable subcutaneous edema, especially in the dependent extremities (the so-called "pitting edema"), hydrothorax (edema fluid in pleural cavity), ascites (edema fluid in abdominal cavity), generalized venous congestion, and cyanosis.

In serious bilateral failure, all of these physiological abnormalities may of course be present. In short, one may classify heart failure as (1) cardiac failure with low cardiac output, (2) cardiac failure with pulmonary congestion, and (3) cardiac failure with systemic congestion.

COMPENSATORY MECHANISMS IN HEART FAILURE. Following an acute, moderate heart attack, a number of cardiovascular changes occur that tend to compensate for the decreased myocardial contractility and the resulting reduced cardiac output. These compensatory changes usually occur in sequential phases, as follows (Guyton, 1976): (1) In the acute phase, the reduced cardiac output causes a secondary decrease in the systemic arterial blood pressure. The latter reduces the inhibitory afferents from the carotid sinus and aortic arch baroreceptors to the vasomotor center, thereby causing an instantaneous increase in the sympathetic efferents to the heart and blood vessels. The result is an increase in heart rate (tachycardia) and peripheral vasoconstriction, both of which tend to elevate the blood pressure and restore the cardiac output to normal. In congestive heart failure with chronic elevation of systemic venous pressure, the vagal afferents arising from the left atrial stretch receptors tend to diminish (saturate), thereby reducing the inhibition of the sympathetic outflow (see Fig. 12-3, page 399). This may in part explain the increased sympathetic activity which may cause the hypertension in congestive heart failure. (2) In the chronic phase, the continued reduction in the cardiac output is compensated by (a) recovery of damaged myocardium along with cardiac hypertrophy, and (b) renal retention of salt and water. The continuous operation of these two mechanisms leads to the state of *"compensated heart failure."*

RENAL FUNCTION IN CONGESTIVE HEART FAILURE

Renal compensation of chronic heart failure consists of simultaneous operations of both hemodynamic and humoral mechanisms. Let us see how.

Normally 20 to 25% of the cardiac output flows through the kidneys. In congestive heart failure, because of the reduction of cardiac output, the renal blood flow (RBF) may be reduced to less than 10% of the cardiac output. The reduction in the renal blood flow activates two compensatory mechanisms, both intrarenal, to restore the renal blood flow. One mechanism involves activation of the renal autoregulation described in Chapter 5, and the other involves the stimulation of the renin-angiotensin system described in Chapter 12. Both of these mechanisms constitute the hemodynamic component of the renal compensatory mechanisms. Briefly, the reduced RBF is partially compensated for by the intrarenal autoregulatory mechanism, which causes an increase in the vascular resistance across the glomerular capillary bed. This will tend to maintain the glomerular filtration rate (GFR) near normal, even though RBF is decreased. The increase in the vascular resistance may in part be mediated by an increase in angiotensin II synthesis consequent to reduced RBF caused by low cardiac output. The decreased RBF and normal GFR implies an increase in filtration fraction (FF), a factor which increases protein concentration in the postglomerular peritubular capillary blood. Consequently, there will be a rise in the protein oncotic pressure relative to the hydrostatic pressure. This will tend to upset the balance of the capillary Starling forces (Fig. 12-2) in favor of enhanced fluid reabsorption, a factor contributing to the formation of edema. Another contributory factor is the enhanced urea reabsorption, thereby elevating its blood level *(azotemia)*. Since the underlying cause of azotemia is extrarenal (reduced cardiac output), this is called *"extrarenal azotemia."* (See also discussion under *Physiological Basis of Azotemia* on page 503.

Another factor which may contribute to the enhanced renal reabsorption of salt and water in congestive heart failure is the redistribution of the renal blood flow (Barger, 1966). This has been confirmed recently by Sparks and associates (1972) who, using Krypton-85 washout method (see Chapter 6), along with anatomical localization by silicone rubber injection, found a decrease in the outer cortical blood flow and an increase in inner cortical and outer medullary blood flow in dogs with chronic congestive heart failure. Similar results were obtained during sympathetic nerve stimulation, hemorrhagic hypotension, and norepinephrine infusion. These investigators suggested that the intrarenal redistribution of the renal blood flow and decreased cortical blood flow, which reduces GFR in the cortical nephrons by the mechanism described in Chapter 8, leads to enhanced renal reabsorption of sodium and water and hence to enhanced sodium retention and edema in congestive heart failure.

In addition to the hemodynamic mechanism just described, the reduced RBF stimulates a humoral mechanism, namely, the renin-angiotensin-aldosterone system. As described in Chapter 12, a decrease in the renal perfusion pressure stimulates the baroreceptor component of the juxtaglomerular apparatus to secrete renin (Fig. 12-6). This increases the synthesis of angiotensin II, which at relatively high plasma concentration stimulates the zona glomerulosa of the adrenal cortex to secrete aldosterone. The latter, acting on the epithelia of the distal and collecting tubules, enhances the renal reabsorption of salt and water and hence the development of edema. Another factor that contributes to the elevation of plasma aldosterone level is its reduced hepatic clearance. As depicted in Figure 12-7, hepatic blood flow is an important determinant of the plasma levels of both angiotensin II and aldosterone. This fact, coupled with the finding that hepatic blood flow is reduced in congestive heart failure (Davis, 1965), tends to underscore the significance of reduced hepatic clearance of aldosterone in the pathogenesis of sodium retention in congestive heart failure. This role of aldosterone in the pathogenesis of edema in patients with congestive heart failure has received considerable attention. As described previously in Chapter 11, normally 95% of the aldosterone in the plasma is cleared in one circulation through the liver. In congestive heart failure, there is a reduction in both renal blood flow and splanchnic (visceral, including liver) blood flow, both of which tend to reduce the metabolic clearance of aldosterone (Davis, 1965). This factor, coupled with the increased production of aldosterone consequent to reduced renal blood flow, leads to marked elevation of the plasma aldosterone level and hence to enhanced renal retention of salt and water. As mentioned above, the reduced RBF is largely due to a decreased cortical blood flow, a factor tending to enhance sodium retention.

This concept has been confirmed recently by Ayers and his associates (1972), who investigated the relative importance of aldosterone secretion, via stimulation of the renin-angiotensin system, and metabolic clearance of aldosterone in patients with congestive heart failure at rest and during exercise. They found that plasma renin activity (PRA) and aldosterone secretion rate were normal, but metabolic clearance of aldosterone was decreased in these patients at rest. However, during exercise, PRA increased while metabolic clearance of aldosterone decreased. Moreover, creatinine clearance decreased, but urinary excretion of catecholamines increased. The latter was taken as evidence of increased sympathetic nerve activity. From these studies, Ayers and his colleagues (1972) concluded that the sympathetic nervous system-induced alteration in the renal hemodynamics, coupled with reduced metabolic clearance of aldosterone, was primarily responsible for sodium retention in patients with congestive heart failure.

CLINICAL MANAGEMENT OF CONGESTIVE HEART FAILURE

Treatment of the congestive heart failure is usually twofold: (1) strengthening the myocardium, and (2) improving the renal excretion of salt and water. Myocardium is strengthened by administration of digitalis or other similar cardiotonic drugs. These drugs are believed to improve myocardial contractility by enhancing the entry of calcium into the muscle fibers, thereby facilitating the formation of actomyosin complex and muscle contraction. Renal excretion of salt and water can be increased by administration of appropriate diuretic agents, such as the aldosterone antagonist spironolactone. Since these patients show adverse reactions to the slightest degree of exertion, strict bed rest is necessary. In addition, to reduce the formation of edema, salt intake should be restricted or completely excluded from the diet.

C. LIVER CIRRHOSIS

Liver cirrhosis is a disease characterized by progressive degeneration of the hepatic cells leading to fibrosis or scarring of the liver. There are several types of cirrhosis, differing in etiology and pathophysiological manifestations. However, for convenience, they may be classified into three general categories (Anderson and Scotti, 1972): *portal cirrhosis* (e.g., alcoholic cirrhosis), *postnecrotic cirrhosis* (e.g., toxic cirrhosis), and *biliary cirrhosis* (e.g., biliary duct obstruction).

In the present context, regardless of the specific etiology, in the chronic state the major clinical manifestations include (1) hypoalbuminemia, (2) portal hypertension, (3) ascites and impairment of renal function or renal failure (Papper, 1963; Sodeman and Sodeman, 1974). Let us briefly examine the physiological bases for these findings.

It is well known that destruction of hepatic parenchymal cells leads to diminished hepatic function, including reduced synthesis of albumin. This accounts for the decreased blood level of albumin and therefore *hypoalbuminemia*. When the concentration of plasma albumin falls considerably below 3 gm%, a generalized edema usually ensues. Of course, hypoalbuminemia may result from other factors besides liver disease. Examples include (1) excessive urinary loss of albumin, as in nephrotic syndrome, (2) loss of albumin from the G.I. tract or from the burned skin, (3) dilution or maldistribution of plasma albumin, as in excessive fluid infusion, and (4) accelerated degradation of albumin.

The sequence of events that lead to a *generalized edema* following hypoalbuminemia in cirrhosis may be summarized as follows. The reduction in the hepatic synthesis of albumin lowers the protein oncotic pressure. This alters the Starling forces across the systemic capillary bed, resulting in the shift of fluid from the intravascular compartment into the interstitial space, thereby resulting in systemic edema. The localized sequestration of this edema fluid in the peritoneal cavity is known as *ascites*. A contributing factor to the formation of ascites is the rise in the portal venous pressure, which may result from either *intrahepatic* or *extrahepatic* mechanical obstruction to the venous outflow from the liver. Thus, progressive fibrosis of the liver causes intrahepatic compression of the hepatic vasculature, thereby increasing the resistance to the hepatic blood flow, which leads to the development of *portal hypertension*. Frequently, localization of edema fluid in the peritoneal cavity precedes the formation of a generalized edema as a result of extrahepatic mechanical obstruction of the venous outflow from the liver. For example, enlargement of the liver, which may accompany cirrhosis, could compress the inferior vena cava just above the entry of the hepatic vein. The consequent engorgement of the liver with blood leads to development of portal hypertension, and hence to formation of ascitic edema. Other examples in which extrahepatic venous obstruction leads to portal hypertension and formation of ascites include right ventricular heart failure, constrictive pericarditis, and pulmonary thrombosis.

Despite accumulation of fluid in the body, cirrhotic patients with ascites are unable to excrete sodium and water. Urinary sodium concentration in these patients is frequently very low, less than 10 mEq/L. This is due to the impaired renal function and renal failure, a factor contributing to sodium and water retention and consequently to edema. Another striking feature of these patients is their inability to excrete a water load, suggesting enhanced renal reabsorption of solute-free water, a factor responsible for

the abnormal *hyponatremia*. Although the primary mechanism leading
to impaired renal function and renal failure is not known, available
evidence strongly implicates a reduction in the renal circulation as
the major cause. This may account for the elevated blood urea
nitrogen (BUN) and plasma creatinine levels in these patients.

It is well known that cirrhotic patients with ascites have an
increased total blood volume (McCloy et al., 1967). However, because
of hypoalbuminemia the distribution of plasma fluid between the intra-
and extravascular compartments is significantly altered, leading to a
reduction in the "effective" circulating blood volume (Papper and
Vaamonde, 1968). The result is a reduction in the renal blood flow
and glomerular filtration rate (Schroeder et al., 1970) and hence
impairment of renal function.

As described in Chapter 12 (Fig. 12-6), a decrease in the renal
perfusion pressure consequent to a reduction in the renal blood flow
stimulates the baroreceptor component of the juxtaglomerular apparatus
to increase renin release. This increases the synthesis of angiotensin
II, raising its plasma concentration. Depending on its plasma concentration, angiotensin II causes vasoconstriction of the peripheral
vascular beds, including those of the kidney, and stimulation of the
zona glomerulosa of the adrenal cortex to secrete aldosterone
(secondary aldosteronism). Since cirrhotic patients with ascites are
known to develop increased tachyphylaxis to angiotensin (Laragh et al.,
1964), the level of endogenous angiotensin produced may be insufficient
to cause hypertension but it is ample to cause renal vasoconstriction
and stimulation of aldosterone secretion. This explains the high
plasma renin level usually found in cirrhotic patients with ascites
(Brown et al., 1964; Schroeder et al., 1970). Another factor which
helps to further increase plasma concentration of aldosterone is the
decreased metabolic clearance of all hormones by the liver and kidney,
owing to a decrease in hepatic and renal blood flow as a result of
reduction in the "effective" circulating blood volume. The most
familiar example is the estrogenic effect in the male cirrhotic
patient. The high plasma concentration of estrogen increases the
permeability of the hepatic capillaries, thereby promoting peritoneal
effusion and formation of ascitic edema fluid. The inadequate hepatic
inactivation of aldosterone further increases its plasma level. The
elevation of plasma aldosterone concentration caused by stimulation of
synthesis and decreased degradation enhances the renal reabsorption of
sodium and water from the distal and collecting tubules, thereby
causing expansion of plasma volume. However, because of hypoalbuminemia, this leads to further exudation of fluid from the
intravascular compartment into the interstitial compartment, hence
causing more edema formation. This situation is further exacerbated
by the decrease in GFR, which enhances sodium reabsorption from the
proximal tubule (see Chapter 8) and the distal tubules (Chaimovitz
et al., 1972). Another factor contributing to water retention is
enhanced renal reabsorption of solute-free water, presumably as a
consequence of an increase in plasma ADH level. The latter is
probably due to a combination of factors, including reduced metabolic
clearance of the hormone by the liver and the kidney.

The net result of hypoalbuminemia and the hormonal effects just described is the whole-body retention of sodium and water, leading to a generalized edema formation. As long as the hypoalbuminemia persists, the increase in plasma volume, consequent to enhanced renal retention of sodium and water, leads to further formation of edema. Eventually, the transcapillary distribution of body fluid stabilizes at a new steady-state level.

Cirrhotic patients usually die *in* renal failure rather than *of* renal failure. The pathogenesis of renal failure in these patients is not known. However, as outlined above, a reduced effective renal perfusion pressure secondary to renal vasoconstriction has been implicated.

Clinical management of cirrhotic patients with ascites consist of improving the hepatic function, including enhancement of albumin synthesis, reduction of portal hypertension, and control of systemic edema and ascites. The administration of salt-poor albumin not only improves hypoalbuminemia, but also increases renal circulation. This will improve renal function, promote natriuresis, and reduce total body sodium and the systemic edema. In some severe cases the use of selective diuretic agents, such as spironolactone, may be beneficial in controlling the edema.

IV. Renal Failure

As described in the preceding sections, the primary and secondary diseases that affect renal function could potentially produce variable degrees of renal damage, resulting in temporary or permanent impairment of renal function. In circumstances in which renal function is so reduced that formation of urine or its elimination from the body is drastically diminished, a state of *renal failure* will supervene. Thus, renal failure represents the terminal stage in the clinical course of the various renal and nonrenal diseases (Table 13-1) that affect renal function. It constitutes a life-threatening illness, with poor prognosis, and is characterized by multiple clinical manifestations in addition to those of the primary or secondary renal disease. Therefore, a detailed consideration of renal failure and its clinical manifestations had to be deferred until the student has acquired a basic knowledge of the pathophysiology of the various primary and secondary diseases that affect renal function. Since the clinical course and management of renal failure depends on the severity of the underlying disease, we will discuss the pathophysiology of renal function in renal failure during the *acute* and *chronic* phases.

A. ACUTE RENAL FAILURE

The hallmark of acute renal failure is a reduction in urine flow to such an extent that it is insufficient to meet the metabolic demands of the body. Such a reduction in urine output is called *oliguria*. The onset of acute renal failure is the result of a sudden reduction in the function of all nephrons, a condition which is potentially totally reversible. Besides the small volume, the urine is characterized by a low specific gravity of about 1.010 (compared to 1.025 for normal), a pH near 7.0, and a high amount of sodium and chloride ions. In short, the urine resembles a poorly modified proximal tubular fluid (see Chapter 8), as a consequence of the reduced number of functioning nephrons and the reduced function of the distal tubular systems--loop of Henle and distal and collecting tubules. Because of the reduced renal function and oliguria, there will also be a marked reduction in urinary excretion of the end-products of the nitrogenous metabolism, notably urea and creatinine. This may lead to *azotemia* and development of uremia (Merrill and Hampers, 1970a, 1970b). (See also discussion under *Physiological Basis of Azotemia* on page 503.) In some cases and for unexplained reasons, there may be a complete failure of the kidneys to form urine, leading to cessation of urine output or *anuria*.

Acute renal failure may be caused by *prerenal, renal,* and *postrenal* factors (Bernstein, 1965). *Prerenal* factors include hypotension, heart failure, shock, hemorrhage, dehydration (vomiting, diarrhea, etc.), burns, or trauma. *Renal* factors include glomerulo-nephritis, pyelonephritis, toxic nephropathy, mismatched blood transfusion, and crush syndrome. *Postrenal* factors include obstruction to outflow of urine distal to the kidney, as in obstructive uropathy. Since the pathophysiology of renal function in these diseases has already been discussed in this chapter, no further details will be given here. It should be noted, however, that the resulting acute renal failure will continue for as long as the underlying disease persists.

Regardless of the initial cause, the underlying factor leading to the development of the acute renal failure is a marked reduction in the renal blood flow, particularly in the cortex of the kidney (see Chapter 6). The resulting renal ischemia causes tubular necrosis, which is in part responsible for oliguria and azotemia, and reduced afferent arteriolar pressure, which stimulates the renin-angiotensin system. The net result is the formation of peripheral edema and hypertension.

Although acute renal failure is a serious, life-threatening illness, the patient may recover completely without any residual functional or anatomical sequelae. Nevertheless, the mortality rate is about 50%. In patients who survive, the onset of recovery is signaled by diuresis, return of the concentrating ability of the kidney, and the return of plasma urea and creatinine levels to normal. Although the initial phase of recovery may begin about 10 days after the onset of the original insult, full recovery may take as long as 3 to 4 months. Because treatment is very difficult and prognosis very uncertain, it behooves the physician to recognize the early signs of the onset of acute renal failure and to take appropriate preventive measures. Treatment usually consists of adjustment of fluid intake (in the absence of dehydration), a restricted protein diet with adequate nonprotein calories, control of hyperkalemia by cation exchange small-mesh resin, control of acidosis by administration of appropriate alkali and dialysis if necessary, and isolation of the

patient to prevent pulmonary, urinary tract, and soft tissue
infections, which are the main causes of death in acute renal
failure. For a more extensive treatment of the subject and the
clinical management of acute renal failure, the interested reader
is referred to the monographs by Bernstein (1965) and Dean (1966).

B. CHRONIC RENAL FAILURE

Chronic renal failure results from progressive *reduction in
the total number of the functioning nephrons* as sequelae to other
renal diseases. The patient with chronic renal failure usually
excretes a large volume of urine *(polyuria)*, which remains high
until before death. Additionally, the excreted urine has a specific
gravity of about 1.010, a pH close to 7.0, and high amounts of sodium
and chloride, despite low salt intake. In all respects the composition
and volume of urine excreted in chronic renal failure resembles the
response of the normal kidney to severe osmotic diuresis (see Chapters
8 and 11), and except for its large volume, it also resembles the
urine excreted in acute renal failure.

The major causes of chronic renal failure are: primary glomerular
diseases (e.g., *glomerulonephritis*), primary tubular diseases (e.g.,
toxic nephropathy), renovascular diseases (e.g., *nephrosclerosis*),
obstructive diseases of the urinary tract (e.g., *obstructive uropathy*),
metabolic diseases (e.g., *gout* and *primary hyperparathyroidism*), and
congenital anomalies of the kidney (e.g., *polycystic kidneys*). Of
these, the most common cause of chronic renal failure in man is the
diffuse, bilateral, progressive types of glomerulonephritis as well as
other types of renal inflammatory diseases.

Clinically, chronic renal failure results in several characteristic
changes in renal functions, which may secondarily affect other organ
systems of the body. The following is a brief summary of some of these
disturbances.

1. URINE VOLUME AND CONCENTRATION

Animal and clinical studies (Gottschalk, 1971) have clearly shown
that the common denominator of the chronic renal failure is the
progressive reduction in the total number of the functioning nephrons,
with the remaining nephrons exhibiting both structural hypertrophy and
functional hyperactivity. As a result, assuming that dietary intake
of water and electrolytes and other nutrients is unaltered, fewer
nephrons must excrete the same osmotically active solute load as the
intact normal kidneys. This can only be accomplished by an increase
in the filtered load of these solutes in these nephrons far in excess
of their reabsorptive capacities, leading to the excretion of more
solutes in urine, accompanied by more water. The result is the
paradoxical finding of an increase in urine output *(polyuria)* of up
to three times normal, and excretion of a *dilute* urine (specific
gravity 1.010), both of which are the early signs of chronic renal
failure.

The excretion of dilute urine reflects the loss of the ability of the kidneys to concentrate urine, a direct consequence of polyuria. The increase in urine output causes an increase in the tubular flow rate in all segments of the nephron, especially the loop of Henle--the site of the countercurrent multiplication mechanism for concentrating urine. The increase in the tubular flow rate in the loop of Henle, by the mechanism described in Chapter 11, leads to a decrease in the magnitude of the corticomedullary transverse gradient, thereby reducing the medullary longitudinal gradient, and hence the osmolality of the excreted urine. As a result, as progressively more and more nephrons are destroyed, the osmolality of the excreted urine decreases, eventually approaching the osmolality of the glomerular ultrafiltrate, a condition known as *isosthenuria*.

2. ACID-BASE DISTURBANCES

Continued loss of renal function in chronic renal failure progressively diminishes the capacity of the kidneys to excrete metabolic acid, thus precipitating the development of metabolic acidosis. The major defects are the reduced tubular synthesis of ammonia, and the gradual fall in the availability of the urinary buffers, principally the phosphate buffers. However, bicarbonate reabsorption and hydrogen ion secretion mechanisms appear to be well preserved. As the disease progresses, the reduction in GFR lowers the filtered load of phosphate and thus raises its plasma concentration. The latter induces a rise in plasma calcium concentration, which stimulates release of parathyroid hormone (PTH). This hormone, as described in Chapter 9, reduces tubular reabsorption of phosphate. The reduced tubular synthesis of ammonia, together with the reduced tubular reabsorption of phosphate, accounts for the greater excretion of the metabolic acid in the form of titratable acid rather than ammonium salt in the early stages of chronic renal failure. However, as the disease advances, the marked reduction in the total number of the functioning nephrons reduces the availability of urinary phosphate buffers, resulting in the development of secondary *tubular acidosis*.

The retained acid, that is hydrogen ions, must be buffered by both the intra- and extracellular buffers, including the bone buffers. The involvement of the latter causes the liberation of calcium and phosphate from the bones, resulting in diminished mineral content of the bone and development of *rickets* (see discussion under *Calcium and Phosphate Metabolism* on page 500).

The metabolic acidosis is partially compensated for by the respiratory pH regulator (Chapter 10). The fall in blood pH stimulates the respiratory center to increase the depth of breathing *(hyperpnea)*, resulting in *Kussmaul breathing* pattern (Sodeman and Sodeman, 1974), a characteristic finding in patients with advanced renal failure and uremic syndrome. In such patients, blood pH, pCO_2 and $[HCO_3]_p$ are all characteristically low, while blood concentration of phosphate is high. Urine pH is quite low and urine contains few ammonium ions (Bernstein, 1965).

3. SODIUM AND POTASSIUM METABOLISM

The reduced GFR, due to the decrease in the total number of functioning nephrons, results in a decrease in the absolute filtered load of sodium in the remaining nephrons. Although the reduced GFR causes a maximal increase in sodium reabsorption (see Chapter 8), because sodium is not reabsorbed by a Tm-limited process, there will be an *obligatory* loss of sodium in urine. Since these patients may also have nausea and vomiting along with reduced dietary sodium intake, they are highly prone to sodium depletion.

The dietary restriction of sodium along with the obligatory loss of sodium in urine leads to progressive, cumulative reduction in the extracellular fluid (ECF) volume, which further reduces GFR. Consequently, the clinical symptoms and abnormalities of blood and urine are intensified. The situation may be reversed by proper administration of salt and water to these patients. Correction of dehydration by water intake alone leads to the development of a condition of *dilutional hyponatremia*.

Another factor influencing sodium metabolism in chronic renal failure is the *secondary aldosteronism*, caused by reduction of ECF volume and blood volume secondary to sodium depletion, the mechanism of which was described in Chapter 12.

As discussed in Chapters 8, 9, and 10, the kidney is the chief organ for disposing of excess potassium from the body. Normally, the filtered potassium is completely reabsorbed in the proximal tubule, so that any potassium excreted in the urine must come from secretion of potassium by the distal and collecting tubules.

In advanced stages of chronic renal failure, there is an increase in plasma potassium concentration as a result of several factors. These include (1) reduced GFR, (2) release of cellular potassium from continuous destruction of nephrons, (3) diminished ability of the kidney to excrete acid, and hence metabolic acidosis, and (4) administration of diuretics, such as spironolactone and triamterene. The danger of elevation of plasma concentration of potassium is that when hyperkalemia approaches 12 to 15 mEq/L (it is normally 4 to 5 mEq/L) it causes the heart to stop in diastole. The emergency treatment for the control of hyperkalemic manifestations consists of intravenous administration of calcium in the form of calcium gluconate.

4. CALCIUM AND PHOSPHATE METABOLISM

Plasma concentration of ionized calcium ($[Ca^{++}]_p$) is normally determined by three factors: (1) The degree of protein binding, (2) the plasma phosphate concentration ($[HPO_4^=]_p$), and (3) the blood pH. The protein binding of calcium is fixed and remains relatively invariant under a variety of conditions. The plasma phosphate and ionized calcium are in equilibrium with the solid phase of calcium-phosphate, found principally in the bone, so that their solubility product ($[Ca^{++}]_p$ x $[HPO_4^=]_p$) remains constant. As a result, their plasma concentrations are reciprocally related. Thus, an increase in the plasma concentration of phosphate results in a decrease in the plasma concentration of ionized calcium, and vice versa. Because of this reciprocal relationship, the plasma concentration of phosphate becomes a virtual determinant of the parathyroid hormone(PTH) secretion. Thus, just as a fall in plasma concentration of ionized calcium stimulates PTH secretion, a rise in plasma phosphate concentration stimulates PTH secretion.

As described briefly in Chapter 10, PTH has several functions: It increases calcium absorption from the G.I. tract and mobilizes calcium from the bone, both affects requiring Vitamin D. In addition, PTH increases renal reabsorption of calcium, thereby decreasing its urinary excretion. It is not known whether this effect is Vitamin D-dependent. Furthermore, PTH reduces the Tm for renal reabsorption of phosphate, thereby reducing its tubular reabsorption and increasing its urinary excretion. This action is also Vitamin D-dependent.

Patients with chronic renal failure do exhibit some degree of hyperparathyroidism and Vitamin D insufficiency. Hyperparathyroidism causes elevation of plasma calcium and reduction of plasma phosphate concentrations. This will tend to increase calcium-phosphorus product in the blood, which may lead to deposition of calcium salts in the kidney, a condition known as *nephrocalcinosis*. Furthermore, despite PTH stimulation of tubular reabsorption of calcium, its filtered load is even more increased, owing to marked elevation of plasma calcium levels. The result is an increase in urinary excretion of calcium, resulting in *hypocalcemic state*.

The cause of Vitamin D insufficiency in chronic renal failure is not well known. It has been attributed to nutritional deficiency or increased resistance to the action of Vitamin D. Nutritional deficiency is probably due to inadequate food intake. This becomes an especially serious problem in childern and in patients with intestinal malabsorption. Resistance to Vitamin D action may in part be due to the inability of the kidney to convert Vitamin D into its active form. This occurs in tubular acidosis and in patients with *familial syndrome of hypophosphatemic rickets.*

Regardless of the causative factors, Vitamin D insufficiency produces hypocalcemia, probably by reducing intestinal absorption of calcium. The accompanying hypophosphatemia is due to hyperparathyroidism secondary to hypocalcemia. In advanced stages of renal failure, when GFR becomes extremely low, there will be overt hypocalcemia and hyperphosphatemia despite hyperparathyroidism.

Another feature of renal insufficiency is *osteomalacia*, a condition characterized by softening of the bone resulting from absorption of bone constituents. The cause of bone absorption is twofold. First, chronic acidosis in renal failure enhances solubility of the bone salts and increases their absorption. Second, the elevated plasma phosphate concentration leads to an increased secretion of parathyroid hormone, which stimulates the osteoclast cells to absorb bone.

Treatment includes reducing the blood levels of phosphate by decreasing its intestinal absorption. In patients with accompanying bone disease, subtotal parathyroidectomy may prove beneficial. Patients with *osteomalacia* usually benefit from treatment with Vitamin D. However, this should be done carefully and in conjunction with bone biopsy.

5. ANEMIA

Another clinical manifestation of chronic renal failure is *anemia*. The probable cause of anemia is the following: The kidneys normally produce *erythropoietin*, a polypeptide which stimulates bone marrow to produce red blood cells. The reduced renal mass in chronic renal insufficiency, therefore, results in a marked reduction in the production of erythropoietin, and hence in the number of circulating red blood cells, with consequent anemia. In the absence of a hemolytic component, anemia may be treated by transfusion of red cells.

6. UREA AND CREATININE METABOLISM

As described in Chapter 6, both urea and creatinine are filtered at the glomerulus. Nearly half of the filtered urea is subsequently reabsorbed in the proximal tubule, the reabsorption being highly flow-dependent. In contrast, creatinine is secreted in the proximal tubule, and its secretion is not flow-dependent. Normally, urea excretion amounts to 500 mOsm/day, in contrast to 30 mOsm/day for creatinine. Thus, urea excretion accounts largely for the osmotic diuresis and polyuria in chronic renal failure.

The flow dependency of urea is in part responsible for some of the discrepancies seen between blood urea and creatinine levels in certain clinical situations. The following is a brief explanation of these differences.

The dynamics of renal function when GFR is reduced by prerenal factors, such as shock, are different from that caused by renal factors in which there is a reduction of renal mass, such as glomerulonephritis. In renal failure caused by prerenal factors, GFR per nephron is lower than normal. In contrast, in renal failure caused by renal factors, GFR per functioning nephron is much higher than normal. Thus, although the creatinine clearance may be the same in both types of renal failure, the urea clearance will be much lower in the prerenal-induced and much higher in the renal-induced renal failure. Therefore, when the urea-to-creatinine concentration ratio ($[U/Cr]_p$) in the blood exceeds its normal range of 10 to 15, a prerenal cause, including spontaneous hemorrhage, for the elevated blood urea nitrogen *(azotemia)* should be considered. Other causes may include trauma, tissue catabolism, corticosteroid administration, increased dietary protein intake, as well as obstructive uropathy of recent onset.

As mentioned earlier, *azotemia* is a condition in which there is a high concentration of *nonprotein nitrogen* compounds, especially *urea,* in the blood, due to reduced renal excretion. The accumulation of these substances (normally excreted) in the extracellular fluid compartment leads to a condition known as *uremia* (Merrill and Hampers, 1970a, 1970b). Uremic patients often lapse into coma as a result of metabolic acidosis. Their respiration becomes deep and rapid to compensate for this acidosis. However, because respiratory compensation is incomplete (see Chapter 10), death ensues when the blood pH falls to about 7.0.

Because of the clinical importance of azotemia in differential diagnosis of the possible factors causing renal failure, it is discussed in more detail in the following section.

Physiological Basis of Azotemia

Azotemia means simply an abnormal elevation of plasma concentrations of nonprotein nitrogenous (NPN) end-products of protein and purine metabolism. The blood NPN substances include urea, ammonia, uric acid, creatinine, creatine, and amino acids. Of these, because blood urea nitrogen (BUN) is by far the largest fraction (BUN is roughly half the NPN), and because variations in the non-urea NPN are relatively small, changes in NPN follow closely those of BUN. Hence, variations in BUN in disease have received considerable clinical attention.

Blood urea nitrogen level, normally 10 to 20 mg%, is determined by the relative rates of urea synthesis and urinary excretion, which are both influenced by a wide variety of renal and metabolic diseases. Thus, abnormal changes in BUN reflect abnormal alterations either in the rates of urea synthesis or in its renal excretion, or in both. The rate of urea synthesis is influenced by several factors, including protein intake, protein metabolism and its hormonal modification, and protein catabolism. The rate of renal excretion of urea is influenced by alterations in renal function, principally the glomerular filtration rate and the tubular transport. Table 13-2 presents a summary of some of the factors affecting blood urea nitrogen concentration. The physiological mechanisms underlying their effects and the manner in which they influence the development of clinical azotemia are described below.

FACTORS TENDING TO INCREASE BUN

1. PROTEIN CATABOLISM. Protein catabolism is by far the most important factor affecting BUN. The blood urea level increases with high and decreases with low protein catabolism. Two factors that influence protein catabolism are the caloric intake and protein ingestion. They determine the metabolic pathway pursued by the

TABLE 13-2

Factors Affecting Blood Urea Nitrogen
Concentration (BUN)

Factors Tending to Increase BUN

1. *Protein Catabolism:*
   increased nitrogen release.

2. *Thyroid Hormone, Corticotrophin,
   and Glucocorticoids:*
   these stimulate increased tissue
   breakdown and nitrogen excretion.

3. *Stress (Surgery, Infection, Burns,
   Severe Toxicity:*
   causes increased tissue breakdown
   and nitrogen excretion.

4. *Congestive Heart Failure:*
   causes decreased glomerular
   filtration rate.

5. *Acute and Chronic Renal Failure:*
   these result in failure of nitrogen
   excretion because of severe oliguria
   and reduced nephron function and
   mass.

6. *Contraction of Total Body Water:*
   causes a relative increase in
   urea nitrogen concentration.

Factors Tending to Decrease BUN

1. *Insulin and Growth Hormone:*
   these stimulate increased
   synthesis of protein and
   of adipose tissue and
   decreased nitrogen
   excretion.

2. *Pregnancy:*
   increased tissue formation,
   decreased protein breakdown,
   hemodilution, and increased
   GFR.

3. *Hepatic Disease:*
   reduced urea synthesis.

4. *Skin:*
   loss of urea in sweat.

5. *Expansion of Total Body Water:*
   causes a relative decrease
   in urea nitrogen concentration.

amino acids derived from protein digestion. During inadequate protein intake, a large fraction of the diet is used for energy production rather than tissue anabolism. Whenever carbohydrate metabolism is impaired (as in fasting or in uncontrolled diabetes mellitus), protein and fat metabolism is markedly increased. Thus, variations in the dietary intake of protein and its catabolism profoundly influence the metabolic production of urea, and therefore its blood levels.

2. THYROID HORMONE, CORTICOTROPHIN, AND GLUCOCORTICOIDS. These hormones tend to increase BUN by stimulating protein metabolism. Thyroid hormone, in stimulating overall body metabolism, enhances protein catabolism and urea formation. Adrenal cortical hormones produce contrasting effects. The glucocorticoids are catabolic, causing increased tissue breakdown and urinary excretion of nitrogen, phosphorus and potassium. The adrenocorticotrophic hormone (ACTH), in stimulating the adrenal cortex, has both catabolic and anabolic effects. Presumably, the catabolic effect is mediated via the glucocorticoids and the anabolic effect is mediated via the androgens.

3. STRESS (SURGERY, INFECTION, BURNS, SEVERE TOXICITY). Clinically, the most frequently seen cause of increased protein breakdown and increased urinary nitrogen excretion is tissue destruction in any of its varied forms. Examples of causative agents include surgery, burns, or severe toxicity. The metabolic degradation of proteins released from the tissues leads to increased urea formation and hence an increase in its blood levels.

4. CONGESTIVE HEART FAILURE. As discussed earlier in this chapter, in congestive heart failure the resulting decrease in the cardiac output reduces the renal blood flow, which in turn lowers the glomerular filtration rate (GFR). The decrease in GFR not only lowers the filtered load of urea, but also increases urea reabsorption from the proximal tubules, thereby decreasing urea clearance and increasing BUN.

As mentioned in Chapter 6, the kidney is the primary organ which eliminates metabolically formed urea. The mechanism of renal excretion of urea consists of glomerular filtration followed by partial reabsorption in the proximal tubule. Moreover, the fraction of filtered urea reabsorbed depends on the tubular flow rate. Thus, urea clearance rises at high urine flows, and falls in oliguria. Consequently, BUN is lowered by the markedly increased urine flow in diabetes insipidus, and is elevated by the reduced urine flow in dehydration or after ADH administration.

5. ACUTE AND CHRONIC RENAL FAILURE. As discussed in the section on *Renal Failure*, there is an increase in BUN in both acute and chronic renal failure. The probable mechanisms accounting for the elevated BUN level in both conditions have already been described.

6. CONTRACTION OF TOTAL BODY WATER. Another factor which increases BUN is a reduction in the total body water, such as may occur in severe dehydration (vomiting, diarrhea, etc.). This leads to contraction of the intravascular volume, hemoconcentration, and hence an increase in BUN.

FACTORS TENDING TO DECREASE BUN

1. INSULIN AND GROWTH HORMONE. In contrast to thyroid and adrenal cortical hormones, insulin and growth hormone are anabolic. They promote protein deposition and nitrogen retention. In previously untreated diabetes mellitus, administration of insulin, together with adequate carbohydrate to permit normal carbohydrate metabolism, obviates the need for energy derived from amino and fatty acids, and allows increased synthesis of fat and protein. Thus, less appears as urea. Growth hormone, like insulin, is anabolic. It stimulates protein deposition and nitrogen retention, thereby reducing urinary nitrogen excretion. Testosterone, the male sex hormone, and other androgens produce a similar effect.

2. PREGNANCY. During the latter half of pregnancy, much of the maternal protein intake is used for tissue synthesis in mother and fetus. This process reduces urea formation, and hence decreases BUN. Simultaneously, the increased GFR, secondary to the increased plasma volume, results in increased urea clearance and reduced BUN.

3. HEPATIC DISEASES. Urea is formed exclusively in the liver. In severe hepatic disease, such as liver cirrhosis, there is a marked reduction in protein metabolism and hence metabolic formation of urea. This results in a redcution of the nonprotein nitrogenous substances in the blood, and hence in a decrease in BUN.

4. SKIN. As mentioned in Chapter 3, cutaneous loss of urea in sweat represents a secondary but important route of urea excretion from the body. Thus, sweating of any degree tends to reduce BUN.

5. EXPANSION OF TOTAL BODY WATER. Finally, any factor that increases the total body water, such as intravenous fluid infusion, leads to an expansion of the intravascular volume, hemodilution, and hence a decrease in BUN.

UREMIA AND UREMIC SYNDROMES

Clinically, *uremia*, which results from renal failure, manifests itself as a constellation of symptoms reflecting a general disturbance in the internal environment of the body. Although the reduction in renal function is the underlying cause, uremia is a generalized disease that affects every major organ of the body. The following is a brief description of some of the major symptoms of uremia.

1. NEUROLOGICAL MANIFESTATIONS. Uremia causes mental depression and drowsiness, which may lead to coma in the last stages of the disease. Uremic patients may exhibit acute psychotic episodes and convulsive seizures. In addition, they may show a variety of defects in a sensory and motor function, which are collectively called *peripheral neuropathies*.

2. CARDIOVASCULAR MANIFESTATIONS. Hypertension is a common finding in uremia, which if uncontrolled could lead to congestive heart failure accompanied by pulmonary and systemic edema.

3. GASTROINTESTINAL MANIFESTATIONS. Loss of appetite, nausea, and vomiting are some of the early signs of uremia. Diarrhea may become a problem in the late stage of the disease. These manifestations are accompanied in many patients by gastrointestinal bleeding. These disturbances in the G.I. system could result in serious dehydration of the body and acid-base abnormalities.

4. SKIN MANIFESTATIONS. Generalized itching is a common complaint of uremic patients. There is a tendency for darkening of the skin as a result of deposition of urinary pigments. Presence of urea crystals on the surface of the skin is not uncommon, giving rise to the descriptive term "uremic frost."

CLINICAL MANAGEMENT OF UREMIA

Because urea itself is nontoxic, clinical management of uremia must be directed at identifying the underlying cause rather than reducing the blood levels of urea *per se*. Thus, the major aim of the treatment should be twofold: (1) to determine the pathogenesis of uremia, and (2) to remedy the functional deficits that the disease has imposed on the patient.

The first step in delineating the pathogenesis of uremia should be a careful review of the past clinical history of the patient in search of the possible factors that might have precipitated the illness. In the absence of finding a clear-cut etiology, several tests may be performed, which could provide a clue to the underlying causes of uremia. Of the various tests (Ravel, 1973), the most commonly used are the determination of BUN and endogenous creatinine clearance. For reasons explained earlier in this chapter and in Chapter 6, these tests, coupled with complete urinalysis and renal biopsy, could provide valuable clues in the differential diagnosis of uremia and its underlying causes. Needless to say, recognition of the pathogenesis of uremia greatly facilitates its clinical management.

When elevation of BUN or uremia is due to such nonrenal factors as dehydration, circulatory insufficiency, or fluid losses, appropriate replacement therapy is indicated. A rise in BUN resulting from rapid protein breakdown, such as during cortisone therapy, is usually of short duration and spontaneously reversible; hydration will accelerate the return to normal. In gastrointestinal bleeding, elevated BUN is also transient. A high BUN due to renal or genitourinary tract disease (e.g., *obstructive uropathy*) poses a more difficult diagnostic problem. As a rule, a detectable rise in BUN in these cases does not occur until about 50% of renal function is lost.

The choice of treatment largely depends on the etiology of uremia (Bernstein, 1965; Dean, 1966). Thus, in both acute and chronic renal failure, provision of diet rich in nonprotein calories spares protein catabolism and hence prevents azotemia. In chronic renal failure, continuous loss of salt and water in urine due to polyuria must be replaced to prevent dehydration, reduction of the extracellular volume, reduced renal circulation, and hence deterioration of uremia. Metabolic acidosis resulting from deficient ammonia formation and acid excretion may be treated with appropriate alkaline therapy, such as sodium bicarbonate. Calcium may be administered to enhance renal excretion of phosphate and to prevent the possibility of osseous changes. In this way, by artificial means the delicate homeostatic balance of the volume and composition of the body fluids is maintained despite deficiency in or deterioration of renal function. If these fail, of course, the use of peritoneal dialysis and hemodialysis may become necessary to maintain the patient and prolong life. In some cases, renal transplant may represent the ultimate therapy.

Clinical Tests for Evaluating Renal Function

With a few exceptions, the various types of renal function tests described below can only provide a "gross" measure of the overall performance of the kidney. However, despite this limitation, if results are interpreted in the light of the physiological principles described in the preceding chapters, these tests can provide considerable useful diagnostic information about impairment of renal function and its possible location, as well as the prognosis during the recovery.

From clinical standpoint, the various types of renal function tests that are routinely performed may be classified into three categories (Table 13-3): (1) general, (2) specific, and (3) exotic.

The *general tests* usually includes routine *urinalysis* and SMA-12 *blood analysis* performed on every patient upon admission to the hospital. The SMA-12 stands for Sequential Multiple Analyzer which determines the blood levels of 12 biochemicals from a single blood sample. The graphic display of the results, which includes normal range of values, permits *pattern recognition* of the 12 blood biochemicals. The analysis of urine and blood biochemicals provides

TABLE 13-3

Summary of the Major Types of Renal Function Tests

I. *General Tests*

    A. Urinalysis
        1. Appearance
        2. Specific gravity or osmolality
        3. pH
        4. Glucose
        5. Proteins
        6. Microscopic examination of urine sediment

    B. Blood Analysis
       Measurement of plasma solutes, such as the SMA-12, which is
       the biochemical profile of 12 blood substances.

II. *Specific Tests*

    A. Tests to Measure Glomerular Function
        1. Endogenous urea clearance
        2. Endogenous creatinine clearance

    B. Tests to Measure Tubular Function
        1. Phenolsulfonphthalein (PSP) excretion
        2. Concentration tests
            a. Urine specific gravity test
            b. Osmolar clearance
            c. Intravenous pyelography (IVP)

    C. Tests to Localize Defective Tubular Function
        1. Measurement of $\dot{T}m$ for glucose and PAH to assess
           proximal tubular function.
        2. Measurement of solute-free water clearance (C_{H_2O}) to
           assess distal tubular function.

III. *Exotic Tests*

    Measurement of plasma renin levels, split-function tests,
    aldosterone suppression tests, renal biopsy, etc.

---

a "gross" input-output profiling of the kidneys and their overall performance. These tests also serve as the initial general screening tests for patients suspected of having renal disease, and the results can serve as a guide for more specific tests.

The *specific tests* consist of those laboratory tests designed to reveal presence of parenchymal renal disease and to "grossly" differentiate the involvement of glomerular or tubular components of the nephron. These tests may be subdivided into (1) tests to measure glomerular function, (2) tests to measure tubular function, and (3) tests to localize defective tubular function.

The *exotic tests* refer to those clinical tests which are not routinely performed but may be required for more specific differential diagnosis of renal disease. Examples include determination of plasma renin levels, split-function tests, aldosterone suppression tests, renal biopsy, and so forth.

The following is a brief description of the physiological principles underlying these tests, their clinical use and potential diagnostic values, as well as their advantages and shortcomings.

I. GENERAL TESTS

A. URINALYSIS

Routine urinalysis provides much useful information about the presence of both structural and functional abnormalities of the kidney and the urinary tract. The following is a brief description of some of these tests and their clinical significance. For a detailed treatment, the reader is referred to the excellent monograph by Kark and associates (1966).

1. APPEARANCE. The appearance of a urine specimen is determined by three qualities: color, odor, and turbidity.

The *color* of the urine is affected by many factors, including concentration, presence of blood and blood pigment, etc. The yellow or amber color of the normal urine is due to the presence of a yellow pigment, called *urochrome*. The intensity of the color is increased when the urine is concentrated; it is decreased when the urine is dilute. Presence of red blood cells in the urine *(hematuria)* will impart a hazy, ground glass appearance to the urine. Products of red cell destruction (primarily hemoglobin and hemosiderin) may give the urine a reddish-brown color.

The characteristic *odor* of the normal urine is due to the presence of volatile acids. The voided urine upon standing develops an ammoniacal odor which is caused by decomposition of the urine specimen. The urine odor is affected by a variety of diseases. Examples include patients with diabetes mellitus, who usually have

urine with a fruity odor (due to the presence of acetone),
and patients with urinary tract infection, who usually have a
foul-smelling urine. However, because urinary odor is nonspecific,
it is of no special diagnostic significance.

A freshly voided normal urine is usually transparent. If the
urine is alkaline, the presence of phosphates and carbonates will
impart a cloudy or *turbid* appearance to the urine. This turbidity
disappears when the urine is acidified. Patients with urinary tract
infections usually have cloudy urine, mainly due to the presence of
alkali in the urine.

2. SPECIFIC GRAVITY. As described in Chapter 3, specific
gravity of urine is defined as the ratio of the weight of the urine
to that of distilled water under standard conditions. Hence, specific
gravity reflects the weight of the solutes in the urine and is not a
measure of the number of particles of solute present in the urine.
The latter is obtained by measuring the freezing point depression of
the urine specimen by an osmometer, and expressing the result as
osmolality. Osmolality of normal urine ranges from 500 to 850
mOsm/kg water, and may vary between 50 to 1400 mOsm/kg water,
depending on the state of body fluid and electrolyte balance.

Since measurement of urine osmolality requires a specialized
instrument, it is not a routine clinical test. On the other hand,
the ease of measurement of urine specific gravity (measured by
urinometer or refractometer) and the fact that it approximates
urine osmolality (Fig. 3-1) has made it a widely used clinical
tool. Since specific gravity of urine indicates the quantity of
water relative to the solute reabsorbed from the glomerular filtrate
as it travels through the various tubular segments, it has been used
as a means of testing the concentrating and diluting ability of the
kidney. This test will be described later.

Specific gravity of normal urine may range from 1.005 to 1.030.
The highest value is usually obtained in the first morning specimen.
The specific gravity of urine is affected by a variety of diseases.
For example, it is reduced in patients with diabetes insipidus,
glomerulonephritis, and pyelonephritis. It is increased in patients
with diabetes mellitus, adrenal insufficiency, hepatic disease and
congestive heart failure.

3. URINE pH. As described in Chapter 10, the pH of the urine
is a measure of the ability of the kidney to respond to disturbances
in acid-base balance. Normally, a freshly voided urine is acid and has
a pH of about 6.0. It becomes alkaline upon standing as a result of
loss of CO_2 and bacterial conversion of urea into ammonia.

Patients on high protein diets excrete highly acid urine. The
same is true of patients with uncontrolled diabetes mellitus and
acidosis. Normally, urine becomes alkaline after a meal, because
blood becomes alkaline as a result of HCl secretion into the gastric
juice. This is called *alkaline tide*. Individuals on vegetarian diets

and patients with renal tubular acidosis excrete alkaline urine.

4. GLUCOSE. As described in Chapter 9, normally clearance of glucose is zero, indicating that normal urine is glucose-free. However, when filtered load of glucose exceeds the reabsorptive capacity of the tubules, glucose will appear in urine (*glucosuria* or *glycosuria*).

Clinically, detection of glucose in urine suggests two possible abnormalities, one of renal origin *(renal glucosuria)* and the other of nonrenal origin *(diabetes mellitus)*. *Renal glucosuria* results from reduced tubular reabsorption of glucose in the presence of normal blood glucose levels. This is usually a benign condition which may occur after a heavy meal or with emotional stress. *Diabetes mellitus*, on the other hand, is a pathological state resulting from excessive elevation of blood glucose levels, and hence of its filtered load, consequent to diminished pancreatic insulin secretion.

5. PROTEINS. Normally a small amount of protein (40 to 80 mg) may be excreted in urine per day. The urinary proteins include primarily albumin and globulins. When protein excretion exceeds the normal range, clinical *proteinuria* may be present. Depending on the etiology of the pathologic disease, several types of proteinuria have been recognized:

Marked proteinuria refers to excretion of more than 4.0 gm of protein per day. This is a common finding in several types of diseases especially in patients with nephrotic syndrome.

Moderate proteinuria refers to excretion of proteins less than 4.0 gm/day. This is a common finding in several disorders, including chronic glomerulonephritis and toxic nephropathy.

Postural proteinuria refers to the excretion of protein when the patient is standing. It usually disappears when the individual lies down. It occurs in small percentage of healthy people with no evidence of renal pathology.

Functional proteinuria refers to the excretion of protein in association with fever, exposure to cold, severe exercise, and emotional stress. The underlying physiological mechanism causing proteinuria is renal vasoconstriction.

Bence Jones proteins refer to specific low molecular weight proteins excreted by more than half of the patients with *multiple myeloma*, a primary malignant tumor of bone marrow.

6. MICROSCOPIC EXAMINATION OF URINARY SEDIMENT. Examination of the urine sediment yields useful information about the presence of renal disease, the nature of this disease, and prognosis during recovery. There are many pitfalls in the procedure, however, and unless performed properly, erroneous conclusions may be drawn.

The urinary sediments of general interest are: red blood cells, white blood cells, epithelial cells, casts, crystals, and bacteria. Presence of one or more of these sediments in urine represents an abnormal condition resulting from renal and a variety of systemic diseases.

To examine the sediment, 10 to 15 ml of freshly voided urine is centrifuged at 1500 to 2000 rpm for 5 minutes. Most of the supernatant is discarded and the sediment is suspended in 1 ml of the supernatant fluid. Then, one drop of the sediment is placed on a glass slide and covered with a coverslip. The sediment is first examined under low power to localize the various types of sediment, which are then identified under high power.

Presence of more than one or two *red blood cells* (RBC) per high power field is an abnormal condition. It indicates renal disease, such as renal carcinoma, tuberculosis of the genitourinary tract, and prostatitis. The presence of large number of of *white blood cells* (WBC) usually indicates bacterial infection in the urinary tract.

The finding of *epithelial cells* in the urine indicates active tubular degeneration, as in patients with acute tubular necrosis.

Casts are pieces of gelled protein-like material which have been formed in the tubule and carried by the flowing urine. Red and white blood cell casts are usually found in the urine of patients with some level of renal inflammation, such as acute glomerulonephritis, pyelonephritis, and nephrotic syndrome.

Presence of urinary *crystals* depends largely on the pH of the urine. Some of the crystals in abnormal urine include cystine, leucine, tyrosine, and cholesterin.

Normal urine is free of *bacteria.* In the absence of contamination, presence of bacteria in the urine indicates urinary tract infection.

B. BLOOD ANALYSIS

Measurement of blood concentrations of those substances normally excreted in the urine can also provide a "gross" measure of renal function. Such a blood biochemical profile can be obtained by ordering a standard SMA-12 blood test. This type of test gives the blood concentrations of the following 12 substances (Preston and Troxel, 1971): Serum glutamic oxaloacetic transaminase (SGOT), lactic acid dehydrogenase (LDH), alkaline phosphatase, bilirubin, cholesterol, calcium, inorganic phosphorus, glucose, urea nitrogen, uric acid, total protein, and albumin. The following is a brief description of the clinical significance of each.

SGOT is an enzyme of the Krebs' cycle and its elevation may be indicative of several diseases, most frequently heart or liver disease. *LDH* is also an intracellular enzyme, and its elevation usually indicates cellular death. LDH is elevated in a number of diseases, including acute myocardial infarction, acute renal infarction, and hepatic disease. *Alkaline phosphatase* is an enzyme that splits phosphate from an ester substance. It is elevated in a variety of disorders, including primary malignant neoplasm, particularly those involving bones, obstructive liver disease, acute or chronic liver disease, and primary or secondary hyperparathyroidism. *Bilirubin* levels are usually increased in liver disease of either hepatic, obstructive, or hemolytic varieties. *Cholesterol* levels are elevated in a number of diseases, including cardiovascular disease, uncontrolled diabetes mellitus, obstructive jaundice, and pregnancy. *Calcium* levels are elevated in several diseases, including primary hyperparathyroidism, long-term use of diuretics, and acidosis. The plasma concentration of calcium is lowered in chronic renal failure and alkalosis. *Inorganic phosphorus* levels are inversely related to blood calcium levels. Thus, many of the factors that cause hypercalcemia also cause hypophosphatemia, and vice versa. *Glucose* levels are increased in several diseases, including diabetes mellitus, Cushing's disease, and pheochromocytoma. *Urea nitrogen* or BUN levels are influenced by several factors already described (see section on *Physiological Basis of Azotemia*). *Uric acid* levels are influenced by overproduction or inability of the kidney to excrete them, as was described in Chapter 9. Factors affecting *total proteins* and *albumin* levels have already been discussed (Chapters 3 and 9).

II. SPECIFIC TESTS

A. *TESTS TO MEASURE GLOMERULAR FUNCTION*

As described in Chapter 6, clinical evaluation of glomerular function is made by determination of either *endogenous urea* or *endogenous creatinine clearance*. For the reasons described in that chapter, endogenous creatinine clearance is the preferred test. Briefly, plasma creatinine levels virtually depend on the integrity of the nephron. In contrast, blood urea levels are affected by several factors, including the diet, hepatic function, gastro-intestinal bleeding, and protein catabolism. Moreover, unlike urea, which is reabsorbed, and the reabsorption of which is highly urine flow-dependent, creatinine is secreted, and its urinary excretion is independent of urine flow. Urea clearance is normally about 60% of inulin clearance. When urine flow is greater than 2 ml/min, its value ranges from 64 to 99 ml/min/1.73 m^2 body surface area. Normal values for creatinine clearance range from 80 to 110 ml/min/1.73m^2 body surface area.

Clinically, clearance of either urea or creatinine may be used to assess GFR and overall renal function in a variety of circumstances, such as to follow the course of acute glomerulonephritis and to differentiate acute glomerulonephritis from diffuse chronic renal structural damage (Ravel, 1973).

B. *TESTS TO MEASURE TUBULAR FUNCTION*

Clinically, two procedures may be used to assess the integrity of the tubular function: (1) the phenolsulfonphthalein (PSP) excretion test, and (2) the concentration tests.

1. PHENOLSULFONPHTHALEIN (PSP) EXCRETION. PSP is an alkaline dye which binds plasma proteins. Consequently, tubular secretion of PSP accounts for most of its urinary excretion. Less than 5% of the injected PSP is filtered at the glomerulus. Of the remaining 95%, over 85% is actively secreted by the proximal tubule, and the balance by the other distally located nephron segments. Accordingly, its urinary excretion depends on (1) the integrity of the tubular blood supply and the involved blood vessels, (2) the integrity of the tubular functions, (3) a patent and normal urinary tract, and (4) the presence or absence of competing drugs.

Clinically, the procedure for PSP excretion test is as follows. The patient is hydrated by drinking 2 to 3 glasses of water to insure an adequate urine flow. Then, 30 minutes later, exactly 6 mg of PSP contained in 1 ml is injected intravenously. Urine specimens are then collected at exactly 15 minutes, 1 hr and 2 hr. Because the collection of the 15 minute specimen is the most important in detecting early renal damage, the patient may start the test with full bladder to insure the ability to void at 15 minutes. The amount of PSP excreted in each voided urine specimen is then quantitated by standard colorimetric technique and the final results are expressed as percentage of the amount injected.

Normally about 25% or more of the injected dye is excreted in 15 minutes, 40% or more in 1 hr, and 60% or more in 2 hr. Since the amount of dye excreted in the 1 hr and 2 hr specimens represents an additive or cumulative effect, these specimens provide little diagnostic value for the detection of early or mild bilateral renal damage. For this reason, the collection of the 15 minute specimen is very important.

PSP excretion test is primarily a measure of tubular function. It is therefore of little practical value in the differential diagnosis of glomerular versus interstitial or tubular disease.

2. CONCENTRATION TESTS. As described in Chapter 11, the ability of the kidneys to concentrate urine depends on the integrity of the distally located nephron segments--the loop of Henle and the distal and collecting tubules. Clinically, this may be tested by three methods, depending on the particular patient: (a) the urine specific gravity test, (b) the osmolar clearance, and (c) the intravenous pyelography (IVP). Following is a brief description of each.

A. The Urine Specific Gravity Test. This procedure consists of restricting the patient's fluid intake for at least 16 to 18 hr, and measuring the specific gravity of the last voided urine. In normal individual, the specific gravity of such a urine should be about 1.025 or higher. A urine specific gravity less than 1.025 indicates decreased ability of the kidneys to concentrate urine, as in patients with pyelonephritis. This test should not be used in patients who are on diuretics or are having spontaneous diuresis. The concentration test is of little value and is dangerous to perform on patients with chronic renal failure who are polyuric and are already dehydrated.

B.   Osmolar Clearance.   A more precise test of the ability of the kidneys to concentrate urine is the measurement of urine osmolality or, more specifically, the osmolar clearance, which was fully described in Chapter 11.   The urine osmolality is low (urine is less concentrated) in patients with parenchymal renal disease, such as pyelonephritis and chronic renal failure.   In contrast, urine osmolality is high (urine is more concentrated) in patients with prerenal types of renal failure, such as hypotensive shock.

C.   Intravenous Pyelography (IVP).   As described earlier in this chapter, this test is used to visualize renal structure and to aid in diagnosing the presence of unilateral or bilateral renal artery stenosis.   Since the renal excretion of the injected contrast material (usually organic iodine compounds) is by a combination of glomerular filtration and tubular secretion, such a test also provides a means of assessing renal function and testing the ability of the kidney to concentrate urine.   Since a normal kidney can maximally excrete the contrast material, it concentrates it in the tubular system, the calyces, the pelvis, and the ureter, thereby providing a good visualization of these structures on the x-ray film.   Therefore, a poor visualization of these structures may be taken as evidence of depressed renal function and reduced ability of the kidneys to concentrate urine.

C.   TESTS TO LOCALIZE DEFECTIVE TUBULAR FUNCTION

From the physiological standpoint, it is possible to localize defective tubular function by virtue of the knowledge of selective tubular transport of various constituents of the filtrate along the nephron.   As described in Chapter 9, since glucose is reabsorbed only in the proximal tubule and PAH is secreted primarily in this nephron segment, measurement of $\dot{T}m$ for glucose and PAH could provide useful diagnostic information about the functional integrity of the proximal tubule.   Similarly, as described in Chapter 11, measurement of solute-free water clearance (C_{H_2O}) could reveal possible abnormalities in the tubular segments beyond the proximal tubule.   In addition, since manifestations of abnormal renal function in some diseases are the result of defective function of specific tubular segments, these manifestations can provide useful diagnostic information.   Thus, Fanconi syndrome, renal glucosuria, or Vitamin D-resistant rickets are all examples of disorders of proximal tubular function.   Another example is renal tubular acidosis which, as described earlier, may result from either a defect in bicarbonate reabsorption (proximal tubular acidosis) or a decreased ability to secrete hydrogen ions against an unfavorable concentration gradient (distal tubular acidosis).

III. EXOTIC TESTS

In addition to the above tests, the resolution of certain diseases may require the use of more specific and exotic tests. Examples include measurement of plasma renin levels in the diagnosis of hypertension, split-function tests in the diagnosis of unilateral or bilateral renal artery stenosis, aldosterone suppression test in the diagnosis of primary aldosteronism, and renal biopsy, which is used occasionally to diagnose renal parenchymal disease. The clinical applications of these tests have already been described in the earlier sections of this chapter.

We conclude this chapter with a clinical example of renal disease in the form of a case history.

CASE HISTORY

A 15 year old male student was admitted to the hospital with the chief complaint of headaches, puffiness around the eyes, and a decreasing urine output. The urine was wine colored in appearance. The onset of the present symptoms was rapid, starting on the day of admission. The patient had pharyngitis 10 days prior to the onset of the present symptoms, which had completely healed.

PHYSICAL EXAMINATION

The patient was a well developed, well nourished male who was becoming increasingly lethargic. There was a +1 pitting edema of both ankles and periorbital edema. Respirations were 22 per minute, pulse rate 88 per minute, temperature 99.0°F, and blood pressure 180/105 mm Hg. Patient's first urine specimen amounted to 5 cc of cloudy urine. Approximately one week from the date of admission, the patient suffered an attack ot vomiting, his respirations became labored, he suffered a convulsion, and then sank into a coma. The blood pressure reading was 185/120 mm Hg, and respirations were 26 per minute. Rales were heard over most of the chest.

LABORATORY FINDINGS

Date	Fluid Intake (ml/day)	Urine Output (ml/day)	BUN (mg%)	$[Na]_p$, mEq/L	$[K]_p$, mEq/L	CO_2 Content (mEq/L)	Plasma Creatinine (mg%)	Hematocrit (%)
1/5		20		Quantity not sufficient				
1/6	2500	120	40	128	5.0	13	6.0	38
1/7	1400	180	65	120	4.8	18	7.9	33
1/8	1500	200	95	121	5.2	10	8.4	26
1/9	1400	200	144	119	4.8	9	10.3	23
1/10	1500	300	115	127	5.2	11	8.7	25
1/11	1100	525	92	129	5.6	14	6.5	30
1/12	1700	675	65	130	5.0	18	3.6	38
1/13	1600	810	32	134	4.8	22	3.3	42
1/14	1800	985	15	136	4.3	24	2.5	45
1/15	1750	990	20	139	4.0	25	2.0	40

Blood cultures were negative for the first three days after admission. On January 10 the urine protein was 2.0 gm/24 hr. RBC casts were numerous, with scattered WBC's. Blood studies revealed a normochromic-normocytic anemia.

HOSPITAL COURSE

The patient's condition declined steadily from the day of admission until Janurary 11; thereafter the patient steadily improved until dismissal from the hospital 47 days after admission. The patient was placed on steroid therapy (Dexamethasone, 4 mg per day).

Tests for kidney function (PSP and IVP) were negative, whereas urea and creatinine clearances were below normal limits.

Renal biopsy was performed on January 11 and confirmed the working diagnosis.

QUESTIONS

1. What do you think probably precipitated this condition?
2. Where was the basic renal lesion?
3. What was the cause of the anemia?
4. What did the biopsy of the kidney probably reveal?

5. Why was the PSP test within normal limits and the clearance tests abnormal?
6. What are the effects of high potassium levels?
7. Why did the patient have hypertension, edema, and rales?
8. Why was steroid chosen, and why this particular one?
9. Why was the IVP done?

REFERENCES

1. Ames, R. P., Borkowski, A. J., Sicinski, A. M., and Laragh, J. H.: Prolonged infusion of angiotensin II and norepinephrine and blood pressure, electrolyte balance, and aldosterone and cortisol secretion in normal man and in cirrhosis with ascites. *J. Clin. Invest. 44*:1171-1186, 1965.

2. Anderson, W. A. D., and Scotti, T. M.: *Synopsis of Pathology.* C. V. Mosby Company, St. Louis, 1972.

3. Ayers, C. R., Bowden, R. E., and Schrank, J. P.: Mechanisms of sodium retention in congestive heart failure. In: *Advances in Experimental Medicine and Biology, Vol. 17. Control of Renin Secretion.* Edited by T. A. Assaykeen. Plenum Publishing Corp., New York, pp. 227-243, 1972.

4. Barger, A. C.: Renal hemodynamic factors in congestive heart failure. *Ann. N. Y. Acad. Sci. 139*:276-284, 1966.

5. Berman, L. B., and Schreiner, G. E.: Clinical and histologic spectrum of the nephrotic syndrome. *Am. J. Med. 24*:249-267, 1958.

6. Bernstein, L. M.: *Renal Function and Renal Failure.* The Williams and Wilkins Co., Baltimore, 1965.

7. Bradley, S. E., Bradley, G. P., Tyson, C. I., Curry, J. J., and Blake, W. D.: Renal function in renal diseases. *Am. J. Med. 9*:766-798, 1950.

8. Braun-Menéndez, E., Fasciolo, J. C., Leloir, L. F., Munoz, J. M., and Taquini, A. C.: *Renal Hypertension.* Charles C Thomas, Springfield, Ill., 1946.

9. Brod, J.: Chronic pyelonephritis. *Lancet 1*:973-981, 1956.

10. Brown, J. J., Davies, D. L., Lever, A. F., and Robertson, J. I. S.: Variations in plasma renin concentration in several physiological and pathological states. *Can. Med. Assoc. J. 90*:201-206, 1964.

11. Brown, J. J., Davies, D. L., Lever, A. F., and Robertson, J. I. S.: Plasma renin concentration in human hypertension. I. Relationship between renin, sodium, and potassium. *Brit. Med. J. 2*:144-148, 1965.

12. Brunner, H. R., Kirshman, D. J., Sealey, J. E., and Laragh, J. H.: Hypertension of renal origin: Evidence for two different mechanisms. *Science 174*:1344-1346, 1971.

13. Brunner, H. R., Chang, P., Wallach, R., Sealey, J. E., and Laragh, J. H.: Angiotensin II vascular receptors: Their avidity in relationship to sodium balance, the autonomic nervous system, and hypertension. *J. Clin. Invest. 51*:58-67, 1972.

14. Brunner, H. R., Gavras, H., Laragh, J. H., and Keenan, R.: Hypertension in man: Exposure of the renin and sodium components using angiotensin II blockade. *Circ. Res.* (Suppl. 1) *34,35*:35-46, 1974.

15. Cain, J. P., Tuck, M. L., Williams, G. H., Dluhy, R. G., and Rosenoff, S. H.: The regulation of aldosterone secretion in primary aldosteronism. *Am. J. Med. 53*:627-637, 1972.

16. Chaimovitz, C., Szylman, P., Alroy, G., and Better, O. S.: Mechanism of increased renal tubular sodium reabsorption in cirrhosis. *Am. J. Med. 52*:198-202, 1972.

17. Conway, J.: Changes in sodium balance and hemodynamics during development of experimental renal hypertension in dogs. *Circ. Res. 22*:763-767, 1968.

18. Davis, J. O.: The physiology of congestive heart failure. In: *Handbook of Physiology*, Section 2, *Circulation*. Edited by W. F. Hamilton and P. Dow. Washington, D. C., American Physiological Society, 1965, Volume 3, pp. 2071-2122.

19. Dean, N.: *Kidney and Electrolytes - Foundations of Clinical Diagnosis and Physiologic Therapy*. Prentice-Hall, Inc., Englewood Cliffs, N. J., 1966.

20. Dixon, F. J.: The pathogenesis of glomerulonephritis. *Am. J. Med. 44*:493-498, 1968.

21. Earle, D. P., Jr., Taggart, J. V., and Shannon, J. A.: Glomerulonephritis: A survey of the functional organization of the kidney in various stages of diffuse glomerulonephritis. *J. Clin. Invest.* *23*:119-137, 1944.

22. Fries, E. D.: Hemodynamics of hypertension. *Physiol. Rev.* *40*:27-54, 1960.

23. Frimpter, G. W., Horwith, M., Furth, E., Fellows, R. E., and Thompson, D. D.: Inulin and endogenous amino acid renal clearances in cystinuria: Evidence for tubular secretion. *J. Clin. Invest.* *41*:281-288, 1962.

24. Frohlich, E. D., Tarazi, R. C., and Dustan, H. P.: Re-examination of the hemodyanmics of hypertension. *Am. J. Med. Sci.* *257*:9-23, 1969.

25. Gavras, H., Brunner, H. R., Laragh, J. H., Vaughan, Jr., E. D., Koss, M., Cote, L. J., and Gavras, I.: Malignant hypertension resulting from deoxycorticosterone acetate and salt excess: Role of renin and sodium in vascular changes. *Circ. Res.* *36*:300-309, 1975.

26. Goldblatt, H., Lynch, J., Hanzal, R. F., and Summerville, W. W.: Studies on experimental hypertension. I. The production of persistent elevation of systolic blood pressure by means of renal ischemia. *J. Exper. Med.* *59*:347-379, 1934.

27. Gottschalk, C. W.: Function of the chronically diseased kidney: The adaptive nephron. *Circ. Res.* (Suppl. 2) *28*:1-13, 1971.

28. Gross, F., Brunner, H., and Ziegler, M.: Renin-angiotensin system, aldosterone and sodium balance. *Recent Progr. Hormone Res.* *21*:119-177, 1965.

29. Guyton, A. C.: *Textbook of Medical Physiology*, 5th ed. W. B. Saunders Co., Philadelphia, 1976.

30. Guyton, A. C., Jones, C. E., and Coleman, T. G.: *Circulatory Physiology: Cardiac Output and Its Regulation.* 2nd ed. W. B. Saunders Co., Philadelphia, 1973.

31. Howard, J. E., and Connor, T. B.: Use of differential renal function studies in the diagnosis of renovascular hypertension. *Am. J. Surg.* *107*:58-66, 1964.

32. Jackson, G. G., Arana-Sialer, J. A., Anderson, B. R., Grieble, H. G., and McCabe, W. R.: Profiles of pyelonephritis. *Arch. Internal Med.* *110*:663-675, 1962.

33. Kadowitz, P. J.: Effect of prostaglandins E_1, E_2, and A_2 on vascular resistance and response to noradrenaline, nerve stimulation, and angiotensin in the dog hindlimb. *Brit. J. Pharmacol.* *46*:395-400, 1972.

34. Kark, R. M., Pirani, C. L., Pollak, V. E., Muehrcke, R. C., and Blainey, J. D.: The nephrotic syndrome in adults: A common disorder with many causes. *Ann. Internal Med.* *49*:751-774, 1958.

35. Kark, R. M., Lawrence, J. R., Pollak, V. E., Pirani, C. L., Muehrcke, R. C., and Silva, H.: *A Primer of Urinalysis.* 2nd ed., Hoeber Medical Division, Harper and Row, Publishers, New York, 1966.

36. Kurtzman, N. A., Pillay, V. K. G., Rogers, P. W., and Nash, D., Jr.: Renal vascular hypertension and low plasma renin activity: Interrelationship of volume and renin in the pathogenesis of hypertension. *Arch. Internal Med.* *133*:195-199, 1974.

37. Laragh, J. H., Cannon, P. J.,and Ames, R. P.: Interaction between aldosterone secretion, sodium, and potassium balance, and angiotensin activity in man: Studies in hypertension and cirrhosis. *Can. Med. Assoc. J.* *90*:248-256, 1964.

38. Laragh, J. H.: Vasoconstriction - volume analysis for understanding and treating hypertension: The use of renin and aldosterone profiles. *Am. J. Med.* *55*:261-274, 1973.

39. Margolius, H. S., Horwitz, D., Geller, R. G., Alexander, R. W., Gill, J. R., Jr., Pisano, J. J., and Keiser, H. R.: Urinary kallikrein excretion in normal man: Relationships to sodium intake and sodium-retaining steroids. *Circ. Res.* *35*:812-819, 1974a.

40. Margolius, H. S., Horwitz, D., Pisano, J. J., and Keiser, J. R.: Urinary kallikrein excretion in hypertensive man: Relationships to sodium intake and sodium-retaining steroids. *Circ. Res.* *35*:820-825, 1974b.

41. McCloy, R. M., Baldus, W. P., Tauxe, W. N., and Summerskill, W. H. J.: Plasma volume and renal circulatory function in cirrhosis. *Ann. Internal Med.* *66*:307-311, 1967.

42. Merrill, J. P., and Hampers, C. L.: Uremia. I. *New Eng. J. Med.* *282*:953-961, 1970a.

43. Merrill, J. P., and Hampers, C. L.: Uremia. II. *New Eng. J. Med.* *282*:1014-1021, 1970b.

44. Metcoff, J. (ed.): *Acute Glomerulonephritis*. Little, Brown and Company, Boston, 1967.

45. Michael, A. F., McLean, R. H., Roy, L. P., Westberg, N. G., Hoyer, J. R., Fish, A. J., and Vernier, R. L.: Immunologic aspects of the nephrotic syndrome. *Kidney International 3*:105-115, 1973.

46. Morris, R. C., Jr.: Renal tubular acidosis. Mechanisms, classification, and implications. *New Eng. J. Med. 281*:1405-1413, 1969.

47. Mudge, G.: Clinical patterns of tubular dysfunction. *Am. J. Med. 24*:785-804, 1958.

48. Muirhead, E. E., Brown, G. B., Germain, G. S., and Leach, B. E.: The renal medulla as an antihypertensive organ. *J. Lab. Clin. Med. 76*:641-651, 1970.

49. Norden, C. W., and Kass, E. H.: Bacteriuria of pregnancy - a critical appraisal. *Ann. Rev. Med. 19*:431-470, 1968.

50. Page, I. H., and McCubbin, J. W. (eds.): *Renal Hypertension*. Year Book Medical Publishers, Inc., Chicago, 1968.

51. Page, L. B., and Sidd, J. J.: Medical management of primary hypertension. *New Eng. J. Med. 287*:960-967, 1972.

52. Papper, S.: The kidney in liver disease. In: *Diseases of the Kidney*. Edited by M. B. Strauss and L. G. Welt. Little, Brown and Co., Boston, 1963.

53. Papper, S., and Vaamonde, C. A.: Renal failure in cirrhosis - role of plasma volume. *Ann. Internal Med. 68*:958-959, 1968.

54. Preston, J. A., and Troxel, D. B.: *Biochemical Profiling in Diagnostic Medicine*. Technicon Instruments Corporation, Tarrytown, N. Y., 1971.

55. Quinn, E. L., and Kass, E. H. (eds.): *The Biology of Pyelonephritis*. Little, Brown and Co., Boston, 1960.

56. Ravel, R.: *Clinical Laboratory Medicine - Application of Laboratory Data*. 2nd ed. Year Book Medical Publishers, Inc., Chicago, 1973.

57. Riley, H. D., Jr.: Pyelonephritis. *Adv. Pediatr. 15*:191-269, 1968.

58. Rushmer, R. F.: *Cardiovascular Dynamics*. 4th ed. W. B. Saunders Co., Philadelphia, 1976.

59. Schreiner, G. E.: Toxic nephropathy. In: *Textbook of Medicine*. Edited by P. B. Beeson and W. McDermott. 14th ed. W. B. Saunders Comapny, Philadelphia, 1975.

60. Schroeder, E. T., Eich, R. H., Smulyan, H., Gould, A. B., and Gabuzda, G. J.: Plasma renin level in hepatic cirrhosis. *Am. J. Med. 49*:186-191, 1970.

61. Sodeman, W. A., Jr., and Sodeman, W. A. (eds.): *Pathologic Physiology - Mechanisms of Disease*. 5th ed. W. B. Saunders Co., Philadelphia, 1974.

62. Sparks, H. V., Kolpald, H. H., Carriere, J., Chimoskey, J. E., Kinoshita, M., and Barger, A. C.: Intrarenal distribution of blood flow with chronic congestive heart failure. *Am. J. Physiol. 223*:840-846, 1972.

63. Strauss, M. B., and Welt, L. G., (eds.): *Diseases of the Kidney*. 2nd ed. Little, Brown and Company, Boston, 1971.

64. Thurston, H., and Laragh, J. H.: Prior receptor occupancy as a determinant of the pressor activity of infused angiotensin II in the rat. *Circ. Res. 36*:113-117, 1975.

65. Tobian, L., Jr., and Azar, S.: Antihypertensive and other functions of the renal papilla. *Trans. Assoc. Am. Physicians 84*:281-288, 1971.

66. Tobian, L., Jr.: Hypertension and the kidney. *Arch. Internal Med. 133*:959-967, 1974.

67. Wilson, C. V., and Dixon, F. J.: Anti-glomerular basement membrane antibody-induced glomerulonephritis. *Kidney International 3*:74-89, 1973.

68. Zabriskie, J. B., Utermohlen, V., Read, S. E., and Fischetti, V. A.: Streptococcus-related glomerulonephritis. *Kidney International 3*:100-104, 1973.

INTRODUCTION TO QUANTITATIVE DESCRIPTION OF BIOLOGICAL CONTROL SYSTEMS

The most apparent and yet fundamental characteristic of living organisms is their capacity to self-maintain, self-regulate, and self-reproduce. The ability to do each of these separate but related functions depends on the smooth, coordinated functioning of the different organ systems and their components. Because of the inherent complexity of these diverse regulatory functions and the multiplicity of their responses to a variety of external and internal stimuli, living organisms may be classified as *biological control systems*.

The ultimate goal in studying the biological control systems, such as the various organ systems of the human body, is to understand the mechanism of these diverse regulatory processes in health and to identify the causes of their failure in disease.

Because of the complex nature of the regulatory processes that compose the physiological systems, the most logical investigative approach is to examine systematically each component and to describe quantitatively its behavior. This investigative process is called *system analysis*. Having thus characterized the operation of each component, it should then be possible to describe the behavior of the overall system by combining the responses of the individual components. This process is called *system synthesis*.

The purpose of this Appendix is to introduce some basic principles and techniques of *control system theory*, aiming to provide the framework for a quantitative analysis and synthesis of the renal-body fluid regulating system.

GENERAL DESCRIPTION OF A SYSTEM

A regulatory biological control system consists of a group of interconnecting and interacting components for which there will be an identifiable *output* (response or dependent variable) that is related to a known *input* (stimulus or independent variable). The response of such a system to a normal or an abnormal stimulus depends

on the *static* (time-invariant) and *dynamic* (time-dependent) properties
of the components of the system. Understanding the static and the
dynamic characteristics of such a response depends on a complete
knowledge of the system as revealed by a description of (1) the
input-output relationship of each of the components of the system,
and (2) the *arrangement* and the nature of the paths connecting these
components and the *rules* governing their relationships.

One way to begin such a system analysis and synthesis is to
assemble the current knowledge about the overall function of the
system and the arrangement of its components in the form of a *block*
or *flow diagram*. In such a representation, each block serves as a
simplified mathematical operator through which the input to the
block is transformed into the output. Moreover, the block diagram
representation is a powerful device for making the knowledge about the
system explicit and rigorous. Figure A-1A shows a schematic block
diagram representation of an isolated system. Note that two arrows
impinge on the end and the side of the block, representing two kinds

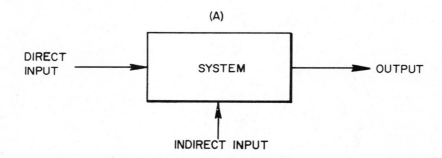

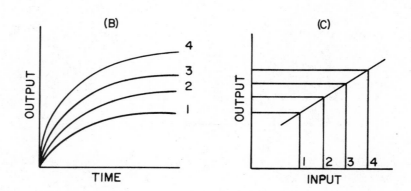

Figure A-1. (*A*) A schematic representation of an isolated system.
(*B*) Time course of the output of an hypothetical system to a series
of four step inputs of increasing magnitude. (*C*) Steady state
input-output relationship for this system.

of inputs, and one arrow leaves the block, as the output. As shown, the two inputs are called the *direct* and the *indirect*, respectively. Applying an input to a system is a way of *forcing* that system to respond. Hence, the terms input, stimulus, and forcing may be used synonymously.

The direct input is the primary forcing, while the indirect input is a function of system properties. For example, the electrical activity recorded from the carotid sinus baroreceptor nerve (the output) is a function of both the applied intrasinus pressure (the direct input) and the distensibility of the carotid sinus wall (the indirect input). Thus, when the effects of these two inputs are dissociated experimentally, it is found that for a given applied intrasinus pressure, the changes in the carotid sinus wall distensibility alter the amplitude and frequency of the action potentials recorded from the baroreceptor nerve.

INPUT-OUTPUT RELATIONSHIPS

The ultimate goal in the analysis of a complex biological system is to define, in mathematical terms, the input-output relationships of the overall system, as well as its components. Of particular interest is the time-behavior of the output as the input is varied. In general, the response of a system to a given input shows two distinct characteristics--an initial *transient* phase, followed by a *steady state* phase. During the transient phase the response is changing with time, even if the stimulus is not, while during the steady state the response remains time-invariant. The steady state response should not be confused with equilibrium, which characterizes the non-living systems. In biological systems equilibrium is achieved only at death.

Knowledge of how a system's response varies with time is provided by the time constant (τ), or constants, of each component of the system. Stated another way, the time constant is the time required for the system's response to reach its final steady state value. Therefore, calculation of the time constant from the transient response allows us to predict the steady state response of the system.

In general, the input-output relationship of a system may be described either mathematically in the form of an *equation* or visualized by a *graph*. Although the steady state response of a system, or its components, may adequately be described by an algebraic expression, description of the transient response requires a *differential* equation, in which the dependent variable varies with time.

The response characteristics of a system may be determined by applying one or more of several types of forcings (Fig. A-2). The most commonly used input is the *step forcing*, characterized by a sudden onset which is maintained until the steady state response is reached. The presence of transient response during step forcing is due to the dynamics of the system and not the changing input. For example, a sudden bilateral occlusion of the common carotid arteries

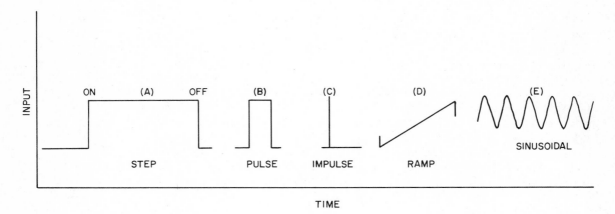

Figure A-2. Types of forcings used in analysis of physiological systems. (*A*) Step; (*B*) pulse; (*C*) impulse; (*D*) ramp; and (*E*) sinusoidal.

would result in a reflex rise of the systemic arterial blood pressure. The changes in the blood pressure, during the occlusion, usually show an initial transient phase of short duration followed by a steady state response lasting as long as the occlusion persists.

The magnitude of both the transient and the steady state response to the step input is a function of the intensity of the forcing. Therefore, applying a series of step inputs of increasing intensities would result in a family of response curves, each with its own transient and steady state characteristics. Figure A-1B shows the plot of the time-response of an hypothetical system to *four* step forcings of increasing magnitudes. The steady state or static input-output relationship may be obtained by plotting the final steady state value in each response curve against the magnitude of the step input. Such a plot is shown in Figure A-1C. Of course, this static input-output relationship may also be expressed algebraically by an equation, in this case by an equation for a straight line. The input-output relationship shown in Figure A-1C illustrates the response of a *linear system* in which the output is always a constant multiple of the input.

As depicted in Figure A-2, there are other types of forcings, with time-dependent patterns, which may be applied to determine the static as well as the dynamic response of a system. These include impulse, pulse, ramp, and sinusoidal forcings: The *impulse* is a forcing with essentially no duration at all. The *pulse* is similar in pattern to step forcing, except that it has a much shorter duration, hence the response has no chance to reach steady state. The intravenous injection of a drug or a dye solution resembles quali- tatively a pulse forcing. The *ramp* is a forcing characterized by a uniformly changing intensity. It is often used to determine the rate-sensitive properties of a system. The *sinusoidal* forcing is characterized by a cyclic variation of intensity (amplitude) with adjustable duration (period). The reciprocal of duration of each sinusoidal cycle is called the frequency, f (equal to $\omega/2\pi$), where ω is the angular frequency in radians. The amplitude of a sinusoidal forcing may be described in four ways: the *peak* value (A_p), the *peak-to-peak* value ($2A_p$), the *average* value (A_{av}), and the *rms* (or *root-mean-square*) value (A_{rms}). These values may be calculated from the following expressions:

$$A_p = \frac{1}{2} \text{ (peak-to-peak amplitude)} \qquad (A-1)$$

$$A_{av} = \frac{1}{\pi} \int_0^{\pi} A_p \sin \omega t = \frac{2A_p}{\pi} = 0.637 \, A_p \qquad (A-2)$$

$$A_{rms} = \sqrt{\frac{A_p^2}{2}} = \frac{A_p}{2} \sqrt{2} = 0.707 \, A_p \qquad (A-3)$$

The sinusoidal forcing is usually used to determine the dynamic response of a system.

OPEN-LOOP AND CLOSED-LOOP CONTROL SYSTEMS

There are two types of control systems: *open-loop* and *closed-loop*. In an open-loop system the input is not affected by the output, whereas in a closed-loop system a portion of the output signal is "fed back," thereby affecting the input. In general, every control system is a closed-loop system, but every closed-loop system is not necessarily a control system.

The first step in applying systems analysis to the study of a closed-loop control system is to open the feedback loop and then determine the open-loop input-output relationship. Once every component of the system is thus characterized, it should be possible to synthesize the whole system and to determine its overall closed-loop static and dynamic response characteristics.

A self-regulating, physiological control system may be considered to consist of three components: *controlling element*, *controlled element*, and *feedback element*. Figure A-3 illustrates schematically the arrangement of these elements with their associated inputs and outputs. Grossly, a control system may be divided into two subsystems: a *controlling system*, consisting of the controlling and the feedback elements, and a *controlled system*, consisting of the controlled element.

Operationally, the controlling element detects deviations of the stabilized variable or the output signal (S_o) monitored through the feedback element (S_f) from the input or the reference signal (S_i).

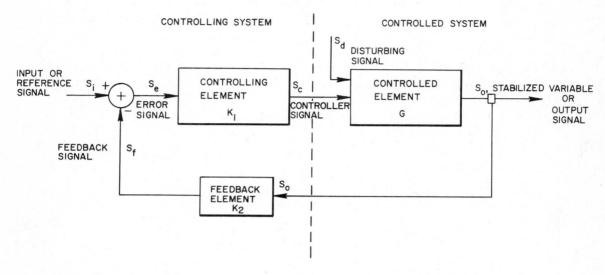

Figure A-3. A generalized closed-loop control system.

The error signal, S_e (equal to $S_i - S_f$), thus produced causes the controlling element to issue appropriate corrective orders as the *controller* signal (S_c), to the controlled element. If the deviations in the stabilized variable are caused by a disturbing signal, adjustments through the feedback and the controlling elements should minimize the error and restore the output to the desired level.

The small box on the arrow representing the output signal indicates that this signal is being monitored at that point by the feedback element. The letters K_1, K_2, and G inside the boxes represent mathematical operators and may be used to describe the input-output relationship of these elements. For example, $S_c = K_1 S_e$, $S_o = G S_c$, and $S_f = K_2 S_o$.

There are two types of closed-loop control systems: regulator and servomechanism. A *regulator* is a closed-loop control system, such as that shown in Figure A-3, which stabilizes the output signal in the presence of a disturbing signal, by manipulating the feedback element. Thus, if a step-like disturbing signal is imposed on the system, the regulator responds by manipulating the feedback and the controlling elements so as to stabilize the output signal at its pre-disturbed level. Such a response characteristic is shown in Figure A-4. Note that imposing a sudden (step) disturbing signal causes a transient change in output which levels off to a steady state value, somewhat higher than its pre-disturbed level (dashed lines). This steady state error in the output persists, due to the imperfect operation of the regulator.

A *servomechanism* is a closed-loop control system which makes the output signal follow a changing input as closely as possible. Figure A-5 (upper panel) shows schematically the arrangement of such a system. Note that there is no feedback element in such a

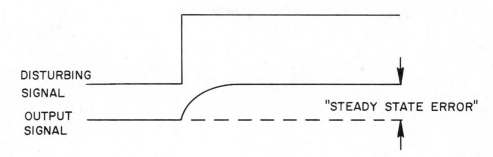

Figure A-4.   Response of a regulator to a step disturbing signal.

system; instead, a portion of the output is compared with the
controller signal and the difference forces the controlled element.
In this manner, a servomechanism control system can follow the
changes in the input, but with a steady state error due to imperfect
operation. The response of a servomechanism to a step change in the
input is shown in the lower panel of Figure A-5.

   Both the regulator and the servomechanism control systems
minimize the steady state errors. The regulator minimizes the
deviations of the output from a constant input, whereas the
servomechanism minimizes deviations from a variable input.

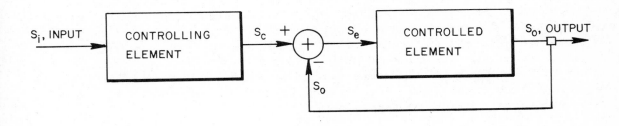

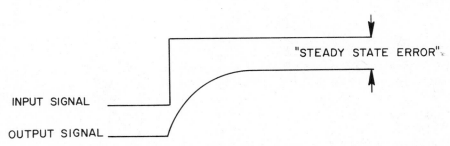

Figure A-5. *Upper panel:* A schematic diagram of a servomechanism
closed-loop control system. *Lower panel:* Response of a servomechanism
to a step input signal.

TYPES OF CONTROLLER SIGNALS

The effectiveness of a regulator as a control system depends on the *type* and the *sensitivity* of the controller signal (S_c) used to force the controlled element. There are three types of controller signals which may be found singly or arranged in combination in a control system. They are *proportional, rate-sensitive,* and *integral* controller signals.

PROPORTIONAL CONTROLLER

In a control system with a proportional controller, there is a constant and linear relationship between the magnitude of the controller signal and the error signal. Using the symbols defined in Figure A-3, this relationship may be expressed as

$$S_c = -K_p S_e \tag{A-4}$$

where K_p is the proportionality constant. Thus, deviations of the output signal from its stabilized level cause a continuous corrective response from the controlling element via the controller signal, the magnitude of which is linearly proportional to the magnitude of the error signal.

The steady state response of a control system with a proportional controller to a step disturbing signal will always show some error in the desired output. This *steady state error* is due to a *lag* in the response of the controlling element, which does not begin to respond until it detects an error that has already occurred. Then, it responds by sending a controller signal whose magnitude is proportional to the magnitude of the error signal, but of the opposite sign. Hence, the time course of the response of such a system shows transient oscilla- tions followed by a steady state error, as shown in Figure A-15. To eliminate these undesired oscillations in the system's response, a rate-sensitive controller may be added.

RATE-SENSITIVE CONTROLLER

In a control system with a rate-sensitive controller, the magnitude of the controller signal is proportional to the rate of change (time-derivative) of the error signal. This relationship may be expressed as

$$S_c = -K_r \frac{dS_e}{dt} \tag{A-5}$$

where K_r is the proportionality constant. Thus, the magnitude of the correction induced in the system's response is proportional to the rate of deviation of the output from the desired stabilized position, but with the opposite sign. The importance of a rate-sensitive controller in a control system is that it can stabilize the response during its dynamic rather than its steady state phase. Hence, it adds stability to the system's operation by minimizing or eliminating the rapid oscillations in the system's response to a sudden, undesired disturbance. This is illustrated in Figure A-16.

Despite the rapid rate of correction in the response of a system with a rate-sensitive controller, the steady state error persists. To eliminate this error an integral controller may be added.

INTEGRAL CONTROLLER

In a control system with an integral controller, the rate of the correction induced in the stabilized signal is proportional to the magnitude of the error signal. This may be expressed as

$$\frac{dS_c}{dt} = -K_I S_e \tag{A-6}$$

where K_I is the proportionality constant. Upon integrating this equation, we get

$$\int dS_c = -K_I S_e \int dt \tag{A-7}$$

$$S_c = -K_I S_e t + C_1 \tag{A-8}$$

where the symbol $\int$ indicates integration. The result of integration is given by Equation A-8, where C_1 is the constant of integration, and has a value of S_o, that is the value of S_c when t = 0. Substituting S_o for C_1 in Equation A-8, and rearranging terms, we get

$$S_c - S_o = -K_I S_e t \tag{A-9}$$

This equation states that the magnitude of the correction signal ($S_c - S_o$), produced by an integral controller, is proportional to the *summation* of the error signal over the interval of disturbance. Hence, the idea of the *integral* controller. Consequently, the correction process, although very slow, continues until the steady state error is abolished. This is illustrated in Figure A-17.

MATHEMATICAL DESCRIPTION OF RESPONSE CHARACTERISTICS OF A CONTROL SYSTEM

A better understanding of a physiological control system will ultimately be linked to a mathematical description of its static and dynamic response characteristics. In addition, such a quantitative analysis allows us to (1) predict the future behavior of the system; (2) formulate a possible isomorphic model of the system; (3) synthesize rigorously the available information about the system; and (4) design future experiments that might be of great value in developing a complete understanding of the behavior of the system.

Mathematical characterization of a system's response must include a description of both the steady state and the transient components. In general, although algebraic equations may be sufficient to characterize the static response, the transient or dynamic response can only be described by differential equations. In this section, without attempting to be complete, we shall discuss the basic steps involved in formulating the static as well as the dynamic input-output functions of a control system.

STATIC CHARACTERISTICS

Analysis of the static characteristics involves the input-output description of a system in a steady state condition. The simplest system for which this may be done is a single-component, open-loop system as shown in Figure A-1A. Physiologically, the carotid sinus baroreceptor, after its physical isolation from the circulation, may exemplify such an open-loop system. For this isolated system, we could identify the intrasinus pressure (P) as the direct input, the carotid sinus wall distensibility (D) as the indirect input, and the action potentials in the Hering nerve (N) as the only output.

The first step in characterizing the static input-output function is to determine the open-loop *gain*, that is, the ratio of the output signal to the input signal. This is also called the system's *transfer function*. In the carotid sinus example, it has been shown that in response to static pressures the baroreceptors operate as "linear" pulse frequency modulated transducers. However, as shown in Figure A-6, when the isolated carotid sinus is forced with a pulsatile pressure, the amplitude and frequency of action potentials recorded from the Hering nerve increase (receptor recruitment) during the rising phase of pressure and decrease during its falling phase. Since within the normal pressure range, the changes in the recorded action potentials vary linearly with the forcing pressure, we may express the open-loop transfer function by

$$\frac{N(t)}{P(t)} = K(t) \tag{A-10}$$

where $K(t)$ is the transfer function; it is the value by which the input must be multiplied to generate the output. Note that in Equation A-10 both intrasinus pressure and the nerve action potentials are written as a function of time. Hence, the transfer function is also time-dependent. However, if we determine the steady state response of the baroreceptors to a static (time-invariant) forcing, such as a step pressure increase or decrease, then a time-independent form of Equation A-10 yields the static transfer function:

$$\frac{N}{P} = K \tag{A-11}$$

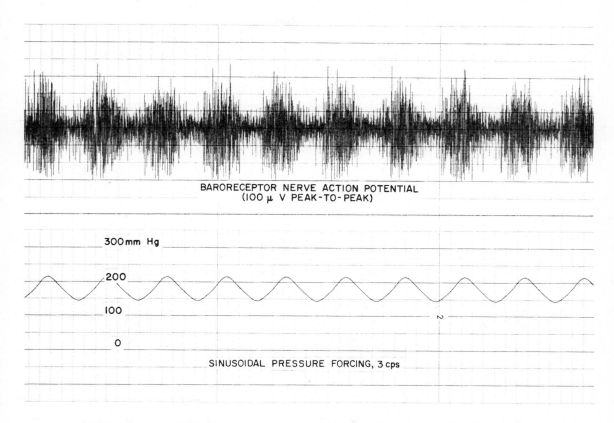

BARORECEPTOR NERVE ACTION POTENTIAL
(100 μ V PEAK-TO-PEAK)

300mm Hg

200

100

0

SINUSOIDAL PRESSURE FORCING, 3 cps

Figure A-6. Simultaneous records of the carotid sinus pressure and the action potentials in the Hering nerve.

If K is a direct proportion, the transfer function is linear and its value gives the "gain" of the system.

We can now extend the idea of open-loop transfer function to a closed-loop system. To illustrate the technique, we shall consider the carotid sinus baroreceptor as a component of a feedback system involved in the regulation of the systemic arterial pressure. The primary elements of this complex feedback system are shown in their simplest form in Figure A-7. Note that in this scheme, the controlling element consists of the carotid sinus baroreceptor and the vasomotor center lumped as one component, and the cardiovascular system, representing the controlled element, as the other component of the overall system. The input to the controlling element is the difference (ΔP) between the carotid sinus pressure (P_C) and systemic arterial pressure (P_{AS}). An increase in the controller signal, determined by the magnitude of ΔP, causes a net inhibition of the vasomotor center and hence a decrease in the sympathetic outflow (N_S) to the cardiovascular system. The result is to decrease P_{AS} and to minimize ΔP, thereby restoring the blood pressure at the carotid sinus to the normal level.

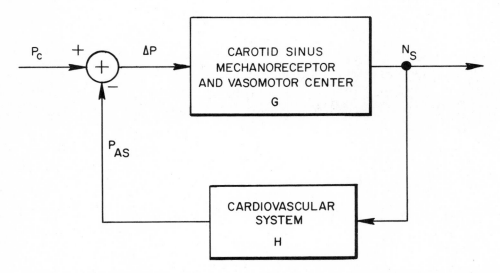

Figure A-7. A schematic diagram of the blood pressure control system.

The closed-loop gain of this system, defined as the ratio of the sympathetic outflow to the carotid sinus pressure (N_S/P_C) may be found as follows. First, we write a defining equation for the controller signal:

$$\Delta P = P_C - P_{AS} \qquad (A-12)$$

Next, we write two equations expressing ΔP and P_{AS} as a function of static gains of the controlling (G) and the controlled (H) elements, respectively:

$$\Delta P = \frac{N_S}{G} \qquad (A-13)$$

$$P_{AS} = H \cdot N_S \qquad (A-14)$$

Substituting Equations A-13 and A-14 into Equation A-12, and rearranging terms, we get

$$P_C = N_S \left(\frac{1 + GH}{G} \right) \qquad (A-15)$$

Rearranging Equation A-15 yields the closed-loop gain of the system:

$$\frac{N_S}{P_C} = \frac{G}{1 + GH} \qquad (A-16)$$

The product GH in Equation A-16 is a measure of the effectiveness of the regulatory control of the system. Hence, the larger the numerical value of GH, the closer the output (N_S) will follow changes in the input (P_C). Therefore, the value of GH determines the closeness with which a physiological variable is controlled at a desired level.

DYNAMIC CHARACTERISTICS

The time-dependent characteristics of an open-loop or a closed-loop control system can best be described if we resolve the dynamic transfer function, K(t), into its "gain" and "phase" components. As before, the gain is defined as the ratio of the amplitude of the output signal to that of the input signal. The phase is defined as the number of degrees (or the time unit per cycle of revolution) the output signal leads or lags the input.

There are several methods of characterizing the gain and phase components of the dynamic transfer function. In this section, we shall describe only two of these methods because their understanding and application requires minimal mathematical foundation. Both methods consist of determining the response of the system to a sinusoidal input at various frequencies. Since both the gain and the phase are time-dependent parameters, their numerical values vary as the frequency of the input sinusoids changes.

The first method for determining the dynamic transfer function and its components consists of plotting the output signal at a given frequency against the input signal. Since both the input and the output signals are functions of time, the resulting path traced out will not be a sinusoid but a loop. This is called a *dynamic* or a *Lissajous'* plot. The shape of the loop varies with the relative time phase of the input and the output signals and with their relative frequency. Returning to the carotid sinus example, if we apply sinusoidal pressure of a given mean and peak-to-peak amplitude, but different frequencies, to the isolated (open-loop) system, we find that the action potentials recorded from the Hering nerve lag behind the input as the frequency of the input sinusoidal pressure increases. Figure A-8 illustrates the resulting Lissajous' plots of the computed

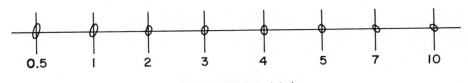

FREQUENCY (Hz)

Figure A-8. Lissajous' plots relating the averaged action potentials in the Hering nerve to pressure, as the frequency of the sinusoidal pressure input is varied from 0.5 to 10 cycles/sec.

electrical activity in the Hering nerve action potentials versus the intrasinus pressure, as the frequency of the sinusoidal pressure is varied between 0.5 and 10 cycles/sec.

To obtain the gain and phase values of the transfer function from these plots, we first draw a line bisecting each ellipsoid Lissajous' loop along its major axis (Fig. A-9). Next, we draw two lines parallel to the horizontal axis through the two points intersecting the ellipsoid with the bisecting line. The vertical distance B between these two horizontal lines is a measure of the gain of the transfer function. The ratio of vertical distance A to that of B is equal to the sine of the phase difference between the input and the output. Figure A-9 shows schematically the graphic determination of the gain and phase components of the dynamic transfer function from the Lissajous' plot of the input-output signals.

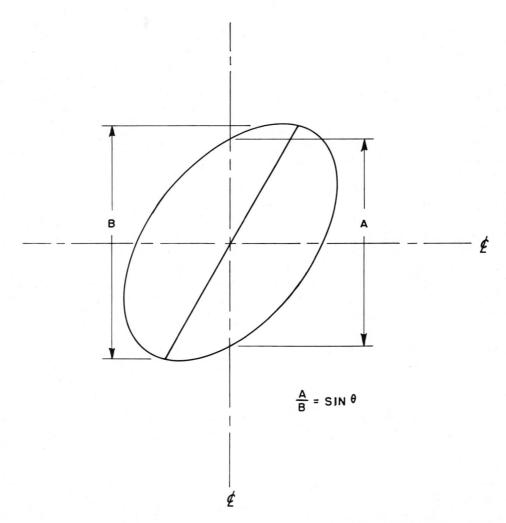

$$\frac{A}{B} = \text{SIN } \theta$$

Figure A-9. Graphic determination of the gain and phase components of a transfer function from a Lissajous' plot.

The second method for determining the dynamic transfer function involves the use of *Bode* analysis. Strictly speaking, this method is applicable only for a linear system. A *linear system*, as defined earlier, is one whose output is always a constant multiple of the input. Under certain conditions, the Bode method could be extended to determine the transfer function of a *non-linear system*, in which the output is not a constant multiple of the input.

In a linear system, Bode analysis consists of plotting both the gain and the phase shifts against the logarithm of frequency of the input sinusoids. The advantage of Bode plot analysis, compared to the Lissajous' plot, is that it provides a direct method of deriving the differential equation describing the behavior of the system. To illustrate the technique, let us consider a linear system whose input-output relationship is described by the following differential equation:

$$y = x + a \frac{dx}{dt} \tag{A-17}$$

where y is the output, x is the input, and a is a proportionality constant. Both the input and output signals are obviously functions of time. Equation A-17 states that the instantaneous value of the output is a function of the instantaneous value of the input, plus the rate of change of the input with respect to time. Suppose that we deliver a sinusoidal input of frequency $f = \omega/2\pi$ and peak amplitude A to this system. Then, according to Equation A-17, the input and output can be expressed by the following equations:

$$x(t) = A \sin \omega t \tag{A-18}$$

$$y(t) = A \sin \omega t + A\omega \cos \omega t \tag{A-19}$$

where ω is the angular frequency in radians, and ωt is the phase of the sinusoidal input. Equation A-19 was obtained by substituting $A \sin \omega t$ for x, and its derivative (rate of change with respect to time) for dx/dt in Equation A-17. Using trigonometric rules, Equation A-19 can be rewritten to show the sinusoidal form of the output, as follows:

$$y(t) = [A \sqrt{1 + (a\omega)^2}] \sin (\omega t + \tan^{-1} a\omega) \tag{A-20}$$

where the quantity in the bracket represents the amplitude of the output sinusoid, and $\tan^{-1}$ is the arctangent. The gain of the system at each input frequency, $G(\omega)$, defined as the ratio of the output amplitude to that of the input at that frequency, is given by the following equation:

$$G(\omega) = \frac{A \sqrt{1 + (a\omega)^2}}{A} = \sqrt{1 + (a\omega)^2} \tag{A-21}$$

and the phase shift at each input frequency, $\emptyset(\omega)$, between the output and the input is given by

$$\emptyset(\omega) = (\omega t + \tan^{-1}a\omega) - (\omega t) = \tan^{-1}a\omega \qquad \text{(A-22)}$$

The gain and phase may be obtained by still another method, the *Laplace transformation*. This procedure consists of transforming the differential Equation A-17 from the time domain to Laplace domain, that is, replacing (t) by (s). Applying this transformation, Equation A-17 becomes

$$y(s) = x(s) + asx(s) = (1 + as) \cdot x(s) \qquad \text{(A-23)}$$

where sx(s) is the Laplace transformation of dx/dt. Since Equation A-23 is the Laplace transformation of the system's differential equation, we can obtain the transfer function, in Laplace domain, as follows:

$$\frac{y(s)}{x(s)} = 1 + as \qquad \text{(A-24)}$$

In order to obtain the gain and phase components of this transfer function, as a function of the input frequency, we transform Equation A-24 back to the complex frequency domain by replacing (s) with (jω):

$$\frac{y(j\omega)}{x(j\omega)} = (1 + aj\omega) \qquad \text{(A-25)}$$

where $j = \sqrt{-1}$, $\omega = 2\pi f$, f is the real frequency in cycles per second, and $a = 1/\omega_c$ or the time constant (τ) of the system. ω_c is the so-called *corner* or break frequency; it is the frequency at which the gain and phase curves change slope. The gain of the system, $G(\omega)$, is the magnitude of this equation, given by

$$G(\omega) = \sqrt{1 + (a\omega)^2} \qquad \text{(A-26)}$$

and the phase shift, $\emptyset(\omega)$, is the phase angle of this equation, given by

$$\emptyset(\omega) = \tan^{-1}(a\omega) \qquad \text{(A-27)}$$

Note that Equations A-26 and A-27 are exactly the same as Equations A-21 and A-22.

The Bode analysis consists of plotting Equations A-26 and A-27 against the logarithm of the input frequency. By convention, the gain values in such a plot are expressed in decibels (db), and are defined by

$$G(db) = 20 \log G \qquad (A-28)$$

Converting the gain Equation A-26 to decibels yields:

$$G(db) = 20 \log \sqrt{1 + (a\omega)^2} = 10 \log [1 + (a\omega)^2] \qquad (A-29)$$

At low frequencies, where $(a\omega)$ is very much less than 1, Equation A-29 becomes

$$G(db) = 10 \log 1 = 0 \qquad (A-30)$$

At high frequencies, where $(a\omega)$ is very much greater than 1, Equation A-29 becomes

$$G(db) = 10 \log (a\omega)^2 = 20 \log (a) + 20 \log (\omega) \qquad (A-31)$$

Equation A-31, on a logarithmic frequency scale, plots as a straight line with a slope of 20 db per log unit, or 20 db per decade increase in frequency. At the corner frequency, where $a\omega = 1$, the gain obtained from Equation A-29 is

$$G(db) = 10 \log 2 = 3 \text{ db} \qquad (A-32)$$

To understand the significance of these equations, we have plotted the gain and phase curves for the system described by Equation A-17 in Figure A-10. A portion of the gain curve covering a decade increase in frequency (between frequencies 1 and 10 cycles/sec) is fitted to a straight line (dashed line) whose slope is 20 db per decade. Note that the phase shift approaches zero degrees as the input frequency decreases, and it approaches 90 degrees as the input frequency increases. At the corner frequency, where $a\omega = 1$ and the gain is 3 db, the phase shift is

$$\phi(\omega) = \tan^{-1} 1 = 45 \text{ degrees} \qquad (A-33)$$

From the Bode plot of the gain and phase shift curves several observations may be made. (1) The gain curve can be approximated by a number of straight lines whose slopes will be a multiple of 20 db/decade. (2) For each 20 db/decade slope there is a phase shift of 45 degrees at the corner frequency. (3) The sign of the phase

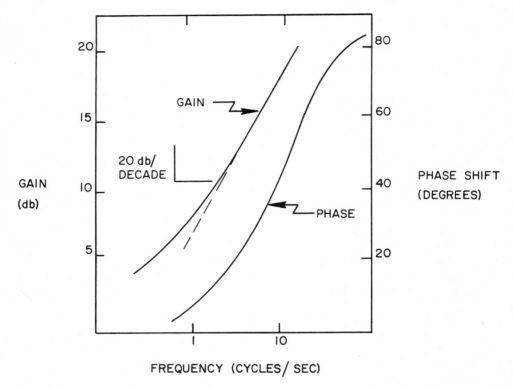

Figure A-10. Bode plot representation of Equation $y = x + a \dfrac{dx}{dt}$.

shift corresponds to the slope of the linearized gain curve. That is, if the slope is negative the phase shift will also be negative. (4) For a linear system, the gain and phase shifts are not independent. Thus, either gain or phase shift curve may be used to determine the shape of the other, as well as the transfer function.

As mentioned above, the advantage of the Bode analysis is that it allows us to determine the differential equation of the system. To illustrate, we use the gain and phase curves plotted in Figure A-10 as the starting point. In general, for each straight line with a multiple of 20 db/decade slope there is associated a specific time constant. In this example, since the gain curve is fitted to only one straight line, there is one time constant ($\tau = 1/\omega_c = 1/2\pi f$). Since the gain has a slope of 20 db/decade and the phase shift goes through 45 degrees at $f = 10$, $\tau = 0.016$ sec. Also, a 20 db/decade slope indicates that the gain at all frequencies must be multiplied by 20 db. From these two pieces of information we can now write the system's transfer function:

$$\frac{y(s)}{x(s)} = 10 \ (1 + 0.016 \ s) \qquad\qquad \text{(A-34)}$$

where the factor of 10 is the gain constant that gives 20 db gain at all frequencies without changing the phase shift. Transforming Equation A-34 into the time domain, we get

$$y = 10 \ (x + 0.016 \ \frac{dx}{dt} \ ) \qquad\qquad (A-35)$$

This equation, except for a scale factor, is identical to Equation A-17.

SOLUTION OF SYSTEM DIFFERENTIAL EQUATION

The problem thus far has been to derive the system differential equation from empirical input-output data. The next phase in the analysis is to solve the differential equation. The solution consists of finding a functional relationship between the dependent variable, or the output y, and the independent variable time, t. There are two ways that such a solution may be obtained: by *analytical procedure* or by a *computer*. Before considering either method, let us examine the general form of a differential equation commonly encountered in the analysis of physiological systems:

$$A \ \frac{d^2y}{dt^2} + B \ \frac{dy}{dt} + C \ y = X(t) \qquad\qquad (A-36)$$

This equation is called a *linear, ordinary, non-homogeneous, second order, first degree differential equation with constant coefficients.* Let us examine the meaning of each term separately. It is a *differential equation*, because it has derivatives; that is, the value of the dependent variable in the equation is a function of time. It is *linear*, because the dependent variable and its derivatives do not contain power or product terms. It is *ordinary*, because it has only one independent variable, namely, time. If more than one independent variable were involved, it would be called a *partial* equation with respect to a specific independent variable. It is *non-homogeneous*, because it has a non-zero term on the right-hand side. This implies that the differential equation describes the response of a system to a forcing whose form is specified by the term on the right-hand side. It is *second order*, because the highest derivative is the second derivative of the dependent variable. It is *first degree*, because the algebraic power of its highest derivative is unity. Finally, it has *constant coefficients*, because the coefficients A, B, C do not vary with time.

In general, the solution of a differential equation, y(t), is the sum of two components, $y_c(t)$ and $y_p(t)$:

$$y(t) = y_c(t) + y_p(t) \qquad\qquad (A-37)$$

where $y_c(t)$ is called the *complementary* solution or transient (force-free) response and $y_p(t)$ is called the *particular* integral or forced response.

The coefficients in Equation A-36, when rearranged, describe some important physical characteristics of the system. Before we proceed with the solution, let us rearrange the coefficients and rewrite Equation A-36 in the so-called standard form,

$$\frac{1}{\omega_n^2} \frac{d^2y}{dt^2} + \frac{2\zeta}{\omega_n} \frac{dy}{dt} + y = \frac{1}{c} x(t) \qquad \text{(A-38)}$$

where $\omega_n = \sqrt{C/A}$, which is the *undamped, natural frequency*, and $\zeta = B/2 \sqrt{AC}$, which is the *damping ratio*. For example, if there is *zero damping* (i.e., $B = 0 = \zeta$), then, if the system is forced with a step input, it will oscillate sinusoidally indefinitely at the natural frequency (ω_n), and an amplitude equal to the magnitude of the step forcing. Now, if we introduce damping, and force the system with the same step input, it will oscillate sinusoidally at a frequency less than the natural frequency and an amplitude which decays exponentially to zero.

Now, to obtain the force-free or the complementary solution, we replace $x(t)$ in Equation A-38 by zero:

$$\frac{1}{\omega_n^2} \frac{d^2y}{dt^2} + \frac{2\zeta}{\omega_n} \frac{dy}{dt} + y = 0 \qquad \text{(A-39)}$$

The solution of this equation consists of the sum of two exponential terms (because it is a second order equation):

$$y_c(t) = C_1 e^{\beta_1 t} + C_2 e^{\beta_2 t} \qquad \text{(A-40)}$$

where β_1 and β_2 are the reciprocals of the time constants and C_1 and C_2 are constants.

To obtain the forced response component of the solution, $y_p(t)$, we need to know the form of the input signal $x(t)$. For most cases, the input signal consists of one or more of the types listed in Table A-1. The final solution of the differential Equation A-38 is given by the following equation, after substituting an appropriate expression for $y_p(t)$ from Table A-1:

$$y(t) = C_1 e^{\beta_1 t} + C_2 e^{\beta_2 t} + y_p(t) \qquad \text{(A-41)}$$

For a more detailed treatment of Equation A-36 and its solution the reader is referred to the references at the end of this Appendix.

TABLE A-1

Form of Particular Integral, $y_p(t)$, for
Different Input Functions, $x(t)$

$x(t)$	Form of $y_p(t)$
Constant, k	K
Power, kt^n	$K_0 t^n + K_1 t^{n-1} + \ldots K_{n-1} t + K_0$
Real Exponential, $ke^{\alpha t}$	$Ke^{\alpha t}$
Sine, $k \sin \omega t$	$K_0 \cos \omega t + K_1 \sin \omega t$
Cosine, $k \cos \omega t$	$K_0 \cos \omega t + K_1 \sin \omega t$

[From Grodins, F. S. (1963).]

COMPUTER SOLUTION OF RESPONSE CHARACTERISTICS OF A CONTROL SYSTEM

The solution of a differential equation is not mathematically always as straightforward as that just described. Nevertheless, it is imperative to obtain some kind of a solution, even if incomplete, if we want to get an insight into the response characteristics of the system. To get around the mathematical difficulty of solving a differential equation, we can resort to electronic computers. There are two general types of computers: (1) an *analogue* computer which performs addition, subtraction, multiplication, and division on *continuous* physical quantities in the form of electric voltages; and (2) a *digital* computer which performs the same mathematical operations on *discrete* physical data.

Most instruments used in biomedical research display their output in analogue form. Very often a *transducer* of some sort is employed to convert the biomedical quantity being measured into electrical signals. Therefore, it is necessary to use an *analogue-to-digital* converter before we can perform useful mathematical and statistical calculations on a digital computer. The fundamental difference between the two types of computers is one of speed. The advantage of the analogue computer is that it allows the analysis and synthesis of a system with moderate speed and efficiency. However, there are certain types of problems which can be solved with greater speed and accuracy with a digital computer than with an analogue computer. Therefore, the type of computer used depends on the type of problem to be solved. In this section, we shall provide a brief introduction to the use of the analogue computer to simulate a control system. For the application of digital computers in the simulation and mathematical modeling of renal function the reader is referred to the work of Koushanpour, Tarica, and Stevens (1971).

Our immediate goal now is to study the response characteristics of a system, regardless of the method we choose to solve the system's differential equation. In short, we do not care how we obtain the solution, but we are interested in what it tells us about the transient and steady state response of the system. The use of the analogue computer not only allows us to solve a differential equation, it also enables us to observe the response of the system to any desired forcing without having to go through cumbersome mathematical manipulations required to solve one or more differential equations.

Let us now see how we can solve the differential Equation A-36 by an analogue computer. To simplify notation, it is customary to represent d/dt (the rate of change with respect to time or the *time-derivative*) of a variable by a *dot* placed above the letter designating it. Thus, we can represent dy/dt by $\dot{y}$ (pronounced y-dot) and d^2y/dt^2 by $\ddot{y}$ (pronounced y-double dots). Using this notation, we first consider the force-free form of Equation A-36, with x(t) = 0:

$$\ddot{y} = -\frac{B}{A}\dot{y} - \frac{C}{A} \tag{A-42}$$

Equation A-42 states that the second time-derivative of y is equal to the algebraic sum of y and its first time-derivative. The implication is that given $\ddot{y}$, we could obtain $\dot{y}$ and y by *inverse of differentiation*, which is *integration*. We can do this by an analogue computer using three of its basic electronic components: an *integrator*, a *summer*, and a *potentiometer*, which are shown symbolically in Figure A-11. The mathematical operation of each component is represented by the equation written below the symbol.

The first step in solving Equation A-42 is to represent it in terms of these analogue computer circuit components. This is shown in Figure A-12. Since the analogue computer operates on voltage, the solution, y(t), can be displayed on the face of a cathode ray oscilloscope. Therefore, it is possible to observe the behavior of $\ddot{y}$, $\dot{y}$, and y as functions of time in response to any desired forcing.

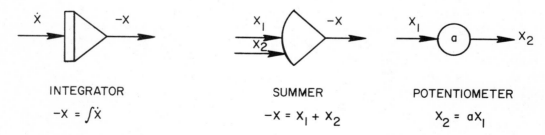

INTEGRATOR
$$-X = \int \dot{X}$$

SUMMER
$$-X = X_1 + X_2$$

POTENTIOMETER
$$X_2 = aX_1$$

Figure A-11. Basic operating components of an analogue computer. Note that both the integrator and the summer change the sign of the input signal.

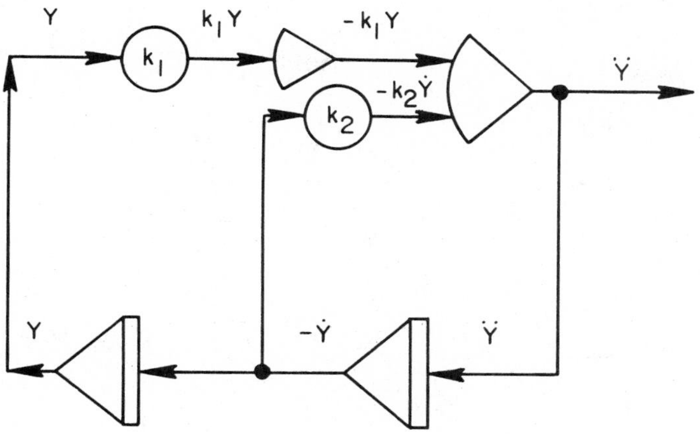

Figure A-12. Analogue computer representation of Equation A-42, where $k_1 = C/A$ and $k_2 = B/A$.

We shall now investigate, by means of an analogue computer, the static and dynamic response characteristics of the second order system represented by Equation A-38, to a step input. First, we look at the response of the open-loop system, then close the loop and insert various types of controller signals and observe the static and dynamic responses. Figure A-13 shows the analogue computer circuit and the different types of controller signals (S_c) used to simulate the response of the second order system represented by the equation

$$\ddot{y} + k_1\dot{y} + k_2 y = k_3 x(t) \tag{A-43}$$

For the purpose of simulation, in the analogue circuit diagram, we have assigned arbitrary values for the natural frequency and the damping ratio such that:

$$k_1 = 0.2\zeta\omega_n = 0.126 \text{ volt} \tag{A-44}$$

$$k_2 = 0.01\omega_n^2 = 0.0986 \text{ volt} \tag{A-45}$$

$$k_3 = 0.1\omega_n^2 = 0.986 \text{ volt} \tag{A-46}$$

These coefficient values are written below the potentiometers designated as k_1, k_2, k_3, on the right side of the circuit diagram. The numerical values 1 or 10 which appear at the input side of either an integrator or a summer are called the *gain factors*. They refer to the "gain" of the electronic amplifier which makes up the integrator or the summer.

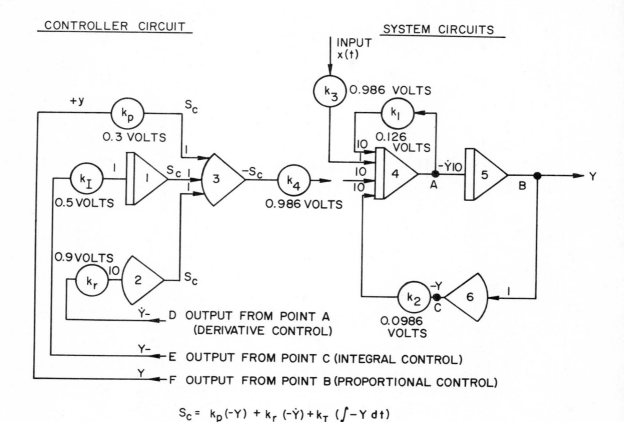

$$S_c = k_p(-Y) + k_r(-\dot{Y}) + k_I\left(\int -Y\,dt\right)$$

Figure A-13. Analogue computer circuit representing a second order control system with proportional, rate-sensitive, and integral controllers.

The left side of Figure A-13 shows the analogue computer circuits for the controller signals. The potentiometers labelled k_p, k_r, and k_I represent the proportionality coefficients for the proportional, rate-sensitive, and integral controller signals, respectively. The values of these coefficients are written below the appropriate potentiometers.

Figure A-14 shows the reponses of an open-loop system (the controller signal is disconnected) to a step input traced from photographs taken from the face of an oscilloscope. Both the input and output traces start at the same horizontal position. The output oscillates about the input and finally the two are superimposed during the steady state. Hence, in the absence of a controller signal, the output cannot be stabilized at the predisturbed position. When the loop is closed and a proportional controller is added to the controlling system, the steady state error is reduced, as seen in Figure A-15. However, the output still shows oscillation before reaching steady state.

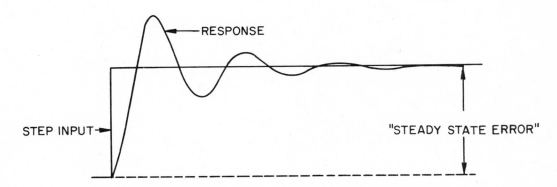

Figure A-14.   Response of an open-loop control system to a step input.

In terms of the analogue computer simulation, shown in Figure A-13, the closing of the loop and addition of a proportional controller is equivalent to connecting the output of the integrator (5) at B to the potentiometer k_p at F. The controller signal (S_C) is connected through potentiometer k_4 with a "gain" factor of 10 to the integrator (4). As mentioned previously in this Appendix, the response of a closed-loop control system, with a proportional controller, to a step input shows both transitory oscillations and steady state errors. The transient oscillations in response can be eliminated by adding a rate-sensitive controller to the controlling system. In Figure A-13, this is equivalent to connecting the output of integrator (4) at A to the potentiometer k_r at D. When this is done, the response of the system to a step input is that shown in Figure A-16. Note that the only difference in response between a closed-loop control system with

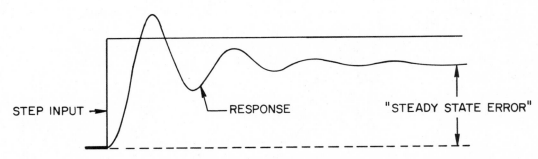

Figure A-15.   Response of a closed-loop control system with a proportional controller to a step input.

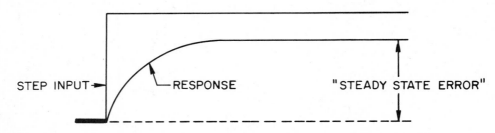

Figure A-16. Response of a closed-loop control system with proportional and rate-sensitive controllers to a step input.

a proportional controller and one with both proportional and rate-sensitive controllers is that the transient oscillations are absent, but the steady state error still persists.

The steady state error can be eliminated by adding an integral controller to the controlling system. In Figure A-13, this is equivalent to connecting the output of the summer (6) at C to the potentiometer k_I at E. When this is done, the response of the system to a step input shows no oscillation and no steady state error, as shown in Figure A-17.

For a more extensive treatment of the materials presented here, the reader may wish to consult the selected references cited at the end of this Appendix.

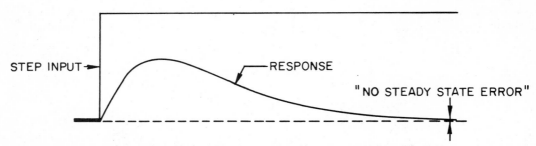

Figure A-17. Response of a closed-loop control system with proportional, rate-sensitive and integral controllers to a step input.

PROBLEMS

A-1. Discuss the similarities and differences between the flow and functional diagrams.

A-2. Define the various forcings commonly used to study the response characteristics of a biological system.

A-3. What is the difference between a transient and a steady-state response?

A-4. Define time constant and briefly describe its physiological significance.

A-5. What distinguishes steady-state from equilibrium?

A-6. What is the characteristic difference between a linear and a nonlinear system?

A-7. What is the difference between a control system and a closed-loop system?

A-8. What is the difference between a regulator and a servomechanism?

A-9. Define (a) controlling system, (b) controlled system, and (c) feedback.

A-10. What are the three types of controllers and their functions in a control system?

A-11. Define static gain of an open-loop system.

A-12. Define dynamic gain of an open-loop system and describe its components.

A-13. Describe three methods used to determine the dynamic transfer function of a linear system.

A-14. What are the main differences between an analogue and a digital computer?

REFERENCES

1. Cannon, R. H., Jr: *Dynamics of Physical Systems*. McGraw-Hill Book Co., Inc., New York, 1967.

2. Gray, J. S.: *Physiology Study Book*. Lecture notes in physiology, Department of Physiology, Northwestern University Medical School, Chicago, 1968.

3. Grodins, F. S.: *Control Theory and Biological Systems*. Columbia University Press, New York, 1963.

4. Johnson, C. L.: *Analog Computer Techniques*. McGraw-Hill Book Co., Inc., New York, 1963.

5. Koushanpour, E., and Kelso, D. M.: Partition of the carotid sinus baroceptor response in dogs between the mechanical properties of the wall and the receptor elements. *Circ. Res. 31*:831-845, 1972.

6. Koushanpour, E., and McGee, J. P.: Effect of mean pressure on carotid sinus baroceptor response to pulsatile pressure. *Am. J. Physiol. 216*:599-603, 1969.

7. Koushanpour, E., Tarica, R. R., and Stevens, W. F.: Mathematical simulation of normal nephron function in rat and man. *J. Theor. Biol. 31*:177-214, 1971.

8. Milhorn, H. T., Jr.: *The Application of Control Theory to Physiological Systems*. W. B. Saunders Co., Philadelphia, 1966.

9. Randall, J. E.: *Elements of Biophysics*. Year Book Medical Publishers, Inc., Chicago, 1962.

10. Riggs, D. S.: *The Mathematical Approach to Physiological Problems*. The Williams & Wilkins Co., Baltimore, 1963.

11. Trimmer, J. D.: *Response of Physical Systems*. John Wiley & Sons, Inc., New York, 1950.

Appendix B

MATHEMATICAL BASIS OF DILUTION PRINCIPLE

As described in Chapter 2, the volume of a body fluid compartment, in practice, may be determined from a graphic analysis of a plot of the logarithm of the plasma concentration of the test substance against time. Experimental collection of the necessary data and the successful analysis of such a time-plot requires satisfactory resolution of two time-dependent characteristics of the test substance: (1) its *mixing* in the plasma and (2) its *distribution* into other compartment(s).

The initial non-linearity seen in the semi-logarithmic plot of the plasma concentration against time (Fig. 2-1, page 13) strongly suggests that the mixing of the test substance is not at all instantaneous, but actually follows an exponential decay process. Likewise, the distribution of the test substance into other compartment(s) is not instantaneous, but proceeds exponentially. Furthermore, while the test substance is being mixed in the plasma, it may also be penetrating and distributing into other compartment(s). Therefore, the time-dependent decrease in the plasma concentration of the test substance is in part determined by the rates at which the substance mixes in the plasma and distributes into other compartment(s). Hence, the overall shape of the semi-logarithmic plot of the plasma concentration against time depends largely on these two rates and their interaction.

To get a better insight into the effect of these processes on the application of the dilution principle, let us examine the mathematical basis of the often used *single dose injection method* and the rationale for the graphical analysis of the resulting data.

Consider the hypothetical compartment illustrated in Figure B-1. As shown, $\dot{V}_i$ is the rate of volume flow into the compartment in ml/min, $[x]_i$ is the concentration of the injected test substance in the inflow stream in mg/ml, $[x]_o$ is the concentration of the test substance leaving the compartment in mg/ml, $[\dot{x}]_o$ is the rate of change of concentration of the test substance in the compartment V in mg/ml/min, and $\dot{V}_o$ is the rate of volume flow out of the compartment V in ml/min.

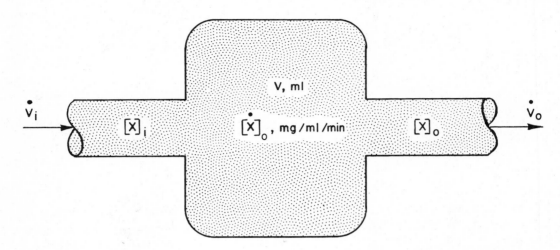

Figure B-1. An idealized representation of a body fluid compartment.

Applying the principle of conservation of mass to this system, we see that the rate of change of mass of the test substance injected into the compartment is equal to the rate of the test substance entering the compartment minus the rate leaving the compartment, provided that the test substance is neither formed nor metabolized by the body. In mathematical notation, we can write

$$V \cdot [\dot{x}]_o = \dot{V}_i \cdot [x]_i \cdot \delta(t) - \dot{V}_o \cdot [x]_o \qquad (B-1)$$

Rate of change = Rate of inflow − Rate of outflow
of mass (mg/min) of mass (mg/min) of mass (mg/min)

where $\delta(t)$ is the *Dirac delta function* and represents mathematically the fact that the test substance is administered as an impulse over a small time interval rather than continuously.

The first term on the right hand side of Equation B-1 is a measure of the amount of the administered test substance which when mixed completely in the volume V would yield the initial concentration, $[x(t = 0)]_o$. This would be the concentration if the test substance had been delivered and mixed instantaneously in the compartment. In practice, for the period after the test substance has been injected, $\delta(t) = 0$--and hence the term containing this function--disappears, and Equation B-1 becomes

$$V \cdot [\dot{x}]_o + \dot{V}_o \cdot [x]_o = 0 \qquad (B-2)$$

Dividing Equation B-2 through by $\dot{V}_O$ yields

$$\frac{V}{\dot{V}_O} \, [\dot{x}]_O + [x]_O = 0 \tag{B-3}$$

Equation B-3 is a first order linear differential equation with constant coefficients and with initial conditions as given in Figure B-1. The coefficient of the derivative term $(V/\dot{V}_O)$ is called the time constant (τ) or the *residence time*; it is the time during which the test substance remains in the compartment. In the steady state, when the rate of volume inflow is equal to the rate of volume outflow, $\dot{V}_i$ equals $\dot{V}_O$, and the above homogeneous differential equation would have the following force-free solution:

$$[x(t)]_O = [x(t = 0)]_O e^{-(\dot{V}_O/V)t} \tag{B-4}$$

The coefficient of t in the exponent of the exponential term is the reciprocal of the time constant $(\dot{V}_O/V = 1/\tau)$ and hence makes the exponent dimensionless. Substituting this relationship, Equation B-4 may be written in a more conventional form:

$$[x(t)]_O = [x(t = 0)]_O e^{-t/\tau} \tag{B-5}$$

Equation B-5 describes a process represented by an exponential decay. In studying the behavior of many biological systems, the physiologist is interested in the *half-time* $(t_{1/2})$ (also called *half-life*) which is the time required for half of the initially administered test substance to disappear from the compartment under study. To determine the half-time, Equation B-5 may be rearranged as follows:

$$[x(t_{1/2})]_O / [x(t = 0)]_O = 1/2 = e^{-t_{1/2}/\tau} \tag{B-6}$$

Taking the natural logarithm of both sides of Equation B-6 and rearranging terms, we get

$$t_{1/2} = 0.693\tau \tag{B-7}$$

The time constant (τ) which appeared in Equations B-5 to B-7 is the time required for the concentration of the administered test substance to decrease to $1/e = 1/2.718 = 0.367$ or 36.7 per cent of the initial value. The time constant is also called the *turnover time*, because it is the time required for the fluid flowing out at a rate of $\dot{V}_O$ to "turnover" and make one complete pass through the volume V.

To obtain the value of the time constant $(\tau = t_{1/e})$, t is set equal to τ in Equation B-5. This makes the exponent of the exponential term equal to -1, and the exponential term e^{-1} may be written as 1/e. Using these relationships Equation B-5 may be rewritten to yield

$$[x(\tau)]_o/[x(t = o)]_o = 1/e \tag{B-8}$$

It should be noted that Equation B-4 in logarithmic form is similar to an equation for a straight line:

$$\ln [x(t)]_o = \ln [x(t = 0)]_o - (\dot{V}_o/V)t \tag{B-9}$$

The semi-logarithmic plot of Equation B-9 is a straight line with a negative slope of magnitude $\dot{V}_o/V$ which is the reciprocal of the time constant, and the value of $\ln [x(t = 0)]_o$ as its ordinate intercept.

Equation B-9 is the basis for the semi-logarithmic plot of the plasma concentration of the test substance against time and the subsequent graphical analysis (linear extrapolation, etc.) of the results.

To get a better "feel" for the mathematical formulations just presented, try to answer the questions posed in the following problem.

PROBLEM

B-1. The data listed below were obtained from an 80 kg patient after he had received 4.5 g of inulin in a single dose.

Time (min)	Plasma Inulin Concentration (mg/ml)
10	440
20	320
40	200
60	150
90	110
120	80
150	60
175	48
210	35
240	25

Calculate (a) the time constant of the exponential decay curve, (b) the half-time for the disappearance of inulin, (c) volume of inulin space, and (d) the renal excretion rate of inulin.

ANSWERS TO PROBLEMS

CHAPTER 1

1-1. a. Osmolality = 308 mOsm/L; osmotic pressure = 5240 mm Hg
      b. Osmolality = 300 mOsm/L; osmotic pressure = 5100 mm Hg
1-2. (a) 55.5 g; (b) 54 g
1-3. a. 3000 mM/L; 3000 mEq/L; 3000 mOsm/L
      b. 3000 mM/L; 3000 mEq/L; 6000 mOsm/L
      c. 500 mM/L; 500 mEq/L; 500 mOsm/L
1-4. 96 mOsm/L
1-5. 490 mOsm/L

CHAPTER 2

2-1. (a) 55.3%; (b) 24.5%; (c) 22.05 kg; (d) 1.05
2-2. 20.8%
2-3. 41.4 mEq/kg body weight
2-4. (a) 20.6 liters; (b) 0.0425 mg%/min (log scale)
2-5. 25.4 liters
2-6. a. Should not be toxic.
      b. Should distribute uniformly within the compartment.
      c. Should not be metabolized.
      d. Should not alter the volume of the compartment.
2-7. (a) 14.4 kg; (b) 475 mOsm/L
2-8. (a) Sodium; (b) chloride; (c) potassium; (d) phosphate;
      (e) albumin; (f) large extracellular volume; (g) increase
      in the number of the cells; (h) increase in tissue with
      greater intracellular water; (i) increase in body fat

CHAPTER 3

3-1. (a) 2020 ml; (b) 1510 ml; (c) 865 ml

3-2. (a) 70 g in plasma; (b) 82 g in tissues

3-3. a. $[Os] = 331$ mOsm/L; $V_E = 19.7$ liters; $V_C = 22.6$ liters
      b. $[Os] = 300$ mOsm/L; $V_E = 19$ liters; $V_C = 25$ liters
      c. $[Os] = 298$ mOsm/L; $V_E = 21$ liters; $V_C = 25$ liters

3-4. a. $V_C = 29$ liters; $V_E = 13$ liters; $[Os]_p = 310$ mOsm/L;
          $[Na]_p = 155$ mEq/L
      b. $V_C = 26.8$ liters; $V_E = 21.2$ liters; $[Os]_p = 338$ mOsm/L;
          $[Na]_p = 169$ mEq/L
      c. $V_C = 31.3$ liters; $V_E = 15.7$ liters; $[Os]_p = 287.6$ mOsm/L;
          $[Na]_p = 143.8$ mEq/L

3-5. _Forcings_   _Condition or Disease_
      1. Isotonic Influx   Edema
      2. Hypotonic Efflux   Sweating
      3. Hypertonic Influx   Nephritis
      4. Isotonic Efflux   Hemorrhage
      5. Hypotonic Influx   Water Intoxication

CHAPTER 5

5-1. a. + ; b. - ; c. + ; d. - ; e. + ; f. + ; g. +

5-2. a. 133.3 mEq/L; b. 0.93 for sodium and 1.10 for chloride

5-3. $(P_C - \pi_C)$ is lower in the lung, accounting for the relative
      dryness of this organ.
      $(P_C - \pi_C)$ is higher in the kidney, accounting in part for the
      large quantity of fluid processed by this organ.

5-4. a. + ; + ; + ; -
      b. - ; - ; - ; 0
      c. + ; + ; + ; 0
      d. 0 ; 0 ; - ; 0
      e. 0 ; 0 ; + ; 0

CHAPTER 6

6-1. a. 80.0; b. 0.2; c. 5.0; d. 0.75

6-2. a. 10; 0.2
      b. 100; 0
      c. 4; 1.0
      d. 0; 4
      e. 20; 5

6-3. 0

6-4. Arterial plasma concentration

6-5. a. 728; 129
      b. 480; 126
      c. 229; 275
      d. 179; 224
      e. 47.8; 129
      f. 30.4; 140

6-6.   778 ml/min
6-7.   1730 ml/min
6-8.   43%
6-9.   16.5%
6-10. and 6-11.   a.   565; 4400; 0.165
                  b.   380; 2960; 0.162
                  c.   229; 1780; 0.155
                  d.   179; 1390; 0.162
                  e.   85; 660; 0.167
                  f.   50; 388; 0.180
6-12.   a.   1; b.   3; c.   3; d.   secretion
6-13.   Only filtered and having a permeability ratio of unity.
6-14.   Filtered, secreted, and having a high extraction ratio.
6-15.   Filtration and secretion.
6-16.   a.   Glomerular filtration.
        b.   Tubular reabsorption.
6-17.   a.   1.0; b.   0.57; c.   0.257; d.   0.186; e.   0
6-18.   a.   560; 280; 140
6-19.   (a) 9 mg%; 45 mg%; 0.36 per min; 0.57 per min
        (b) 0.063 min; 0.02 min
6-20.   a.   Secreted at a rate of 40 mg/min.   (Note negative sign in
             calculations.)
        b.   20 mg/min
6-21.   a.   130; 700; 0; 0; 130
        b.   650; 3500; 55; 0.08; 375
6-22.   a.   1, 3, 6; b.   2, 9; c.   1, 5, 8, 9; d.   1, 5, 8;
        e.   1, 5, 8, 9; f.   1, 10
6-23.   a.   14 mEq/L
        b.   13.5 mEq/L
        c.   300 mg/min
        d.   300 mg%
        e.   20%
6-24.   35.5 mOsm/L
6-25.   (a) 90 mg%; (b) 62%
6-26.   (a) 300 mg%; (b) none
6-27.   a.   none; b.   X; c.   Z; d.   Y

CHAPTER 7

7-1.   a.   For drug-receptor complex, K_m = 25.
       b.   For inhibitor-receptor complex, K_m = 47.5.
       c.   Since V_{max} = 51.5 for both, the inhibitor is a competitive
            one.
7-2.   a.   Ordinate intercept = $1/V_{max}$; a measure of the efficiency
            of the process.
       b.   Abscissa-intercept = $- 1/K_m$; a measure of the affinity of
            the enzyme and substrate.
7-3. $J_S = J_{CS} = - \dfrac{D}{\xi} [SC_1 - SC_2]$

7-4. When $S \gg K_{CS}$, then $J_S = - \dfrac{D}{\zeta} \cdot C_T \left[1 - \dfrac{S_2}{S_2 + K_C} \right]$

7-5. a. $\dfrac{[Z_1]}{[C_1]} = \dfrac{[Z_2]}{[C_2]}$, that is, symmetrical metabolic reactions on

both sides of the membrane.

b. $K_{CS} = K_{ZS}$, that is, the two carriers have equal affinities for the substrate on both sides of the membrane.

7-6. Let $S_1 = 0.2$ M and $K_C = S_2 = 0.02$ M

Fraction of maximum flux = $\left[\dfrac{S_1}{S_1 + K_C} - \dfrac{S_2}{S_2 + K_C} \right] = \dfrac{9}{11}$

CHAPTER 8

8-7. 15.96 mEq/min or 95% of the filtered sodium is reabsorbed.

8-8. 1. − ; 2. + ; 3. − ; 4. + ; 5. + ; 6. − ; 7. + ;
8. − ; 9. − ; 10. + ; 11. − ; 12. + ; 13. +

CHAPTER 9

9-1. 650; 375

9-2. 5.7; 36.3

9-3. a. 65; 65; 350; 0; 0
b. 130; 130; 700; 0; 0
c. 375; 375; 2020; 0; 0
d. 650; 375; 3500; 55; 0.0785
e. 910; 375; 4900; 76.5; 0.109
f. 1300; 375; 7000; 92.5; 0.132

9-6. 288

9-7. 375

9-8. a. 260; 520; 780; 1170
b. 260; 375; 375; 375
c. 0; 140; 400; 790
d. 0; 27; 51; 68

9-9. It varies monotonically toward an asymptote.

9-10. a. Since $\dfrac{U_G V}{GFR \cdot P_G} = 1$, $C_G = C_{In} = GFR = 130$

b. $\dfrac{130}{700} = 0.186$ (See Fig. 6-3)

9-11. a. 2.16; 11.84; 14; 700; 1
b. 6.48; 35.52; 42; 700; 1
c. 14.0; 77; 91; 700; 1
d. 21.6; 77.9; 140; 497.5; 0.71
e. 43.2; 77.3; 280; 300.0; 0.43
f. 64.8; 77.7; 420; 238.0; 0.34

9-13. 13
9-14. 77.5
9-15. a. 4; 8; 16; 32; 54; 76
       b. 22; 46; 77.5; 77.5; 77.5; 77.5
       c. 28; 54; 94; 109; 130; 151
       d. 18.2%; 17.4%; 20.6%; 41.3%; 70%; 98%
9-16. Varies linearly and proportionally when plasma concentration
       increases above 15 mg%.
9-17. a. Since $U_{PAH}\dot{V} = GFR \cdot P_{PAH} + \dot{Tm}_{PAH}$, then, if $\dot{Tm}_{PAH} \to 0$,
           $C_{PAH} = C_{In} = GFR$ (see Fig. 6-3)
       b. 0.186
9-20. a.
9-21. a.
9-22. 13

CHAPTER 10

10-1.   (a) 7.41 (b) 25.0 (c) 25.0
10-2.   (a) 7.32 (b) 27.5 (c) 25.0 (d) acidemia (e) acidosis
        (f) respiratory (g) uncompensated (h) displacement
10-3.   (a) 7.50 (b) 22.0 (c) 25.0 (d) alkalemia (e) alkalosis
        (f) respiratory (g) uncompensated (h) displacement
10-4.   (a) Oppositely (b) together (c) of course
10-5.   (a) 34.0 (b) 19.0 (c) metabolic (d) compensated for
        respiratory disturbance
10-6.   (a) Down the $pCO_2 = 40$ line, until $pCO_2 = 40$, $[HCO_3^-]_p = 18$,
            and pH < 7.32.
        (b) Low respiratory pathway until $pCO_2 = 34$, $[HCO_3^-]_p = 18$,
            and pH = 7.32.
        (c) No, because respiratory regulator responds rapidly.
        (d) Normal metabolic pathway.
10-7.   (a) Up the $pCO_2 = 40$ line, until $pCO_2 = 40$, $[HCO_3^-]_p = 34.0$,
            and pH > 7.50.
        (b) High gain respiratory pathway until $pCO_2 = 45.5$,
            $[HCO_3^-]_p = 35.0$, and pH = 7.50.
        (c) No, because respiratory regulator responds rapidly.
        (d) Normal metabolic pathway.
10-8.   (a) Normal respiratory pathway.
        (b) Uncompensated respiratory alkalosis.
10-9.   (a) Yes--pO_2 is still low; (b) yes; (c) renal; (d) slow;
        (e) yes--integral control; (f) $[HCO_3^-]_{40}$; (g) high gain
        metabolic pathway; (h) 7.41, 15, 24.5; (i) respiratory
        alkalosis, fully compensated; (j) more, because pH inhibition
        is removed; (k) better, because of still greater
        hyperventilation.
10-10. (a) Yes, pO_2 returns to normal; (b) still 19.0; (c) only
        moderate, because pH is now low; (d) low gain respiratory
        pathway; (e) 34, 7.32, 18.0; (f) metabolic acidosis, partially
        compensated (correcting the respiratory disturbance leaves the
        compensatory metabolic acidosis exposed).

10-11. (a) Will rise to normal, by renal action; (b) normal metabolic
        pathway; (c) 7.41, 25.0, 40; (d) slow; (e) yes, back to
        normal, having followed a four-sided loop.
10-12. You will have to check yourself this time.
10-13. (a) Fully compensated respiratory acidosis and alkalosis.
        (b) Respiratory alkalosis and metabolic acidosis.
        (c) Metabolic acidosis, or compensated respiratory alkalosis.
        (d) Metabolic acidosis or respiratory acidosis, but beware of
            dissociated disturbances.
        (e) No--it takes more than one.
10-14. Don't forget combinations, like simultaneous respiratory and
        metabolic acidosis.
10-15. (a) High gain metabolic pathway.
        (b) It will become abnormally high.
        (c) Hinders--in fact, frustrates--renal compensation.
10-16. (a) The low gain respiratory pathway.
        (b) It will become even lower.
        (c) Hinders--in fact, frustrates--respiratory compensation.
10-17. (1) a. 6; b. 2; c. 1; d. 5; e. 7; f. 3; g. 4; h. 8
        (2) 2, 3, 4, 5 and 1, 6, 7, 8
        (3) 1 and 5
        (4) 6, 7, 8 and 2, 3, 4
        (5) 1, 2, 8 and 4, 5, 6
        (6) 3, 4, 5 and 1, 7, 8
        (7) 1, 2, 8
        (8) 4, 5, 6
        (9) 3, 2, 1, N
        (10) 1, 7, 8
        (11) 3, 4, 5
        (12) 4

CHAPTER 12

12-13. (a) - ; (B) + ; (C) + ; (D) + ; (E) + ; (F) + ; (G) - ; (H) +
12-14. Vascular receptors for all except F, the response of which is
        mediated via the macula densa receptors.
12-15. (A) Decrease; (B) increase; (C) increase; (D) decrease;
        (E) increase; (F) increase; (G) increase
12-16. (C) Upright position
12-21. (1) E; (2) A; (3) C; (4) D; (5) B
12-22. (1) D; (2) C; (3) B; (4) A
12-23. (A) 2 and 3
        (B) Patient 1: -, -; patient 2: 0, 0; patient 3: -, -;
            patient 4: -, 0
        (C) a. Patient 2
            b. Patient 1
12-24. (1) + ; (2) + ; (3) + ; (4) + ; (5) + ; (6) - ; (7) - ;
        (8) + ; (9) + ; (10) -
12-25. (1) +, 0, +, +, +, 0, -, -, -, +, +, +
        (2) +, +, +, +, +, -, -, -, -, +, +, +
        (3) +, -, +, +, +, +, -, +, -, -, +, -

(4) -, 0, -, -, -, 0, 0, +, +, -, -, -
(5) -, -, -, -, -, +, +, +, +, -, -, -

CHAPTER 13

13-1. Probably streptococcus infection, which led to the development of acute glomerulonephritis.

13-2. The glomerulus.

13-3. Probably loss of blood cells from the ruptured and leaky glomerular capillaries.

13-4. Probably presence of inflamed glomeruli and little or no tubular damage.

13-5. Since PSP test measures primarily tubular function, it was normal because there was no tubular damage. In contrast, since creatinine clearance measures primarily GFR, it was below normal because of the altered glomerular function.

13-6. The most important effects are on the heart, as manifested by abnormal electrocardiogram patterns. A very high plasma potassium level causes the heart to stop in diastole.

13-7. The patient developed hypertension probably as a consequence of two mechanisms. First, the reduction in the intrarenal blood flow stimulated the renin-angiotensin system. Second, the reduced GFR led to increased salt and water retention, thereby expanding the intravascular volume and increasing the blood pressure. The edema resulted from the renin-angiotensin stimulation of aldosterone secretion, reduced plasma proteins due to proteinuria, and reduced GFR. Rales were probably due to pulmonary congestion, which is another manifestation of edema.

13-8. Steroid was given to repair the glomerular capillary membrane and to reduce proteinuria. This particular steroid was chosen because it has anti-inflammatory effect and has no effect on renal sodium reabsorption.

13-9. The IVP test was probably done to determine whether the hypertension was caused by prerenal or renal causes, and to evaluate the integrity of the renal tubular system, including the urinary tract distal to the kidney.

APPENDIX B

B-1. (a) $\tau = 1.6$ min
      (b) $t_{1/2} = 1.1$ min
      (c) Volume of inulin space = 16.0 liters
      (d) Excretion rate = 0.63 mg/ml/min

INDEX

Note: Numbers in *italics* refer to illustrations; (t) indicates tables.